NSCA's Essentials of Tactical Strength and Conditioning

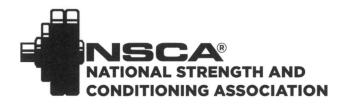

NSCA®
NATIONAL STRENGTH AND CONDITIONING ASSOCIATION

Brent A. Alvar, PhD, CSCS,*D, RSCC*D, FNSCA

Rocky Mountain University of Health Professions, Provo, UT

Katie Sell, PhD, CSCS,*D, TSAC-F

Hofstra University, Hempstead, NY

Patricia A. Deuster, PhD, MPH, CNS

Consortium for Health and Military Performance (CHAMP)

Uniformed Services University of the Health Sciences, Bethesda, MD

Editors

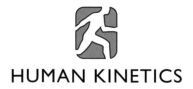

HUMAN KINETICS

Library of Congress Cataloging-in-Publication Data

Names: Alvar, Brent A., editor. | Sell, Katie, editor. | Deuster, Patricia
  A., editor. | National Strength & Conditioning Association (U.S.), issuing
  body.
Title: NSCA's essentials of tactical strength and conditioning / Brent A.
  Alvar, Katie Sell, Patricia A. Deuster, editors.
Other titles: National Strength and Conditioning Association's essentials of
  tactical strength and conditioning | Essentials of tactical strength and
  conditioning
Description: Champaign, IL : Human Kinetics, [2017] | Includes
  bibliographical references and index.
Identifiers: LCCN 2016035892| ISBN 9781450457309 (print) | ISBN 9781492546146
  (e-book)
Subjects: | MESH: Physical Fitness | Resistance Training--methods | Emergency
  Responders | Military Personnel
Classification: LCC RA781 | NLM QT 256 | DDC 613.7/1--dc23 LC record available at https://lccn.loc.gov/2016035892

ISBN: 978-1-4504-5730-9 (print)

The web addresses cited in this text were current as of September 2016, unless otherwise noted.

Acquisitions Editor: Roger W. Earle; **Senior Developmental Editor:** Christine M. Drews; **Managing Editor:** Karla Walsh; **Copyeditor:** Alisha Jeddeloh; **Indexer:** Susan Danzi Hernandez; **Permissions Manager:** Dalene Reeder; **Senior Graphic Designer:** Joe Buck; **Cover Designer:** Keith Blomberg; **Photographer (interior):** Neil Bernstein, unless otherwise noted; photographs © Human Kinetics, unless otherwise noted; figure 17.9 © David Royal/The Monterey County Herald via AP; figure 17.10 © Shari L. Morris/age fotostock; figure 17.12 © David I. Gross/ZUMA Press; figure 18.1 © Oleg Zabielin/Dreamstime.com; figures 22.3 and 22.4 © Frank Palkoska; **Photo Asset Manager:** Laura Fitch; **Visual Production Assistant:** Joyce Brumfield; **Photo Production Manager:** Jason Allen; **Art Manager:** Kelly Hendren; **Illustrations:** © Human Kinetics, unless otherwise noted; **Printer:** Walsworth

We thank the National Strength and Conditioning Association in Colorado Springs, Colorado, for assistance in providing the location for the photo shoot for this book.

Study questions written by Shelby Williamson.

Printed in the United States of America   10 9 8 7

The paper in this book was manufactured using responsible forestry methods.

Human Kinetics
1607 N. Market Street
Champaign, IL 61820
USA

United States and International
Website: **US.HumanKinetics.com**
Email: info@hkusa.com
Phone: 1-800-747-4457

Canada
Website: **Canada.HumanKinetics.com**
Email: info@hkcanada.com

E5975

Tell us what you think!
Human Kinetics would love to hear what we
can do to improve the customer experience.
Use this QR code to take our brief survey.

Contents

Chapter 5   Basic Nutrition for Tactical Populations 69

Steve Hertzler, PhD, RD, LD

Amanda Carlson-Phillips, MS, RD, CSSD

Chapter 6   Tactical Fueling 101

Maj. Nicholas D. Barringer, PhD, RD, CSCS,*D, CSSD

Maj. Aaron P. Crombie, PhD, RD

Chapter 7   Ergogenic Aids 113

Abbie E. Smith-Ryan, PhD, CSCS,*D, FNSCA, FISSN

Colin D. Wilborn, PhD, CSCS, ATC

Eric T. Trexler, MA, CSCS

Chapter 8   Testing and Evaluation of Tactical Populations 135

Maj. Bradley J. Warr, PhD, MPAS, CSCS

Patrick Gagnon, MS

Dennis E. Scofield, MEd, CSCS,*D

Suzanne Jaenen, MS

Chapter 9   Development of Resistance Training Programs 157

Nicholas A. Ratamess, PhD, CSCS,*D, FNSCA

Chapter 19 Physiological Issues Related to Military Personnel 505

William Kraemer, PhD, CSCS,*D, FNSCA
LTC David Feltwell, PT, OCS, TSAC-F
Tunde Szivak, PhD, CSCS

Chapter 20 Physical Training to Optimize Load Carriage 535

Paul C. Henning, PhD, CSCS
Barry A. Spiering, PhD, CSCS
Dennis E. Scofield, MEd, CSCS
Bradley C. Nindl, PhD

Chapter 21 Wellness Interventions in Tactical Populations 551

Robin Orr, PhD, MPhty, BFET, TSAC-F
John R. Bennett, MS, CSCS, EMT-P

Chapter 22 Organization and Administration Considerations. 563

John Hofman, Jr, MS, CSCS
Frank A. Palkoska, MS, CSCS

Preface

NSCA's Essentials of Tactical Strength and Conditioning is the most comprehensive evidence-based presentation on the scope of practice as well as the theoretical and applied approaches of strength and conditioning for exercise professionals working with tactical athletes—Special Weapons and Tactics (SWAT), Special Operations Forces, conventional military forces, law enforcement, and fire and rescue personnel. The Tactical Strength and Conditioning (TSAC) program offered by the National Strength and Conditioning Association (NSCA) continues to experience exponential growth since its inception in 2005. As such, there is a need for qualified individuals with high levels of professional competence to work with tactical athletes. The material presented in this book will serve as a primary resource for individuals intending to achieve the NSCA Tactical Strength and Conditioning Facilitator (TSAC-F) certification.

The TSAC concept was conceptualized, created, and initially developed by Mark Stephenson. The NSCA's TSAC program was developed during the tenure of Jay Hoffman's NSCA presidency, as well as during his time as a member of the NSCA board of directors, and he was a major developer of the TSAC concept for and on behalf of the NSCA. The NSCA's TSAC program continues to grow as a leader in tactical strength and conditioning.

The authors of this book include professionals who have served or are currently serving in law enforcement, firefighting, or military arenas; college and university professors; physical therapists; strength and conditioning coaches; athletic trainers; and nutritionists actively conducting research and engaging in practical application of evidence-based information. Consequently, the information presented in this book supports the need for subject matter expertise in the realm of strength and conditioning for those currently implementing physical conditioning programs for tactical athletes.

To work with tactical populations, a foundational understanding of exercise physiology and biomechanical movement patterns is necessary. Therefore, three early chapters overlap with those in other NSCA *Essentials* texts. Chapters 2, 3, and 4 discuss fundamental cardiopulmonary and skeletal muscle function and adaptation to exercise, biomechanics, and bioenergetics and metabolism. Each subsequent chapter builds on this foundation to help the reader toward understanding optimal development and implementation of population-specific training in tactical athletes.

A comprehensive training program for tactical athletes must account for their population-specific nutritional requirements (chapters 5, 6, and 7); physical fitness testing requirements (chapter 8); needs concerning exercise selection, technique, and program design (chapters 9, 10, 11, 12, 13, and 14); biomechanical, physiological, and metabolic needs (chapters 17, 18, 19, and 20); injury and illness risk (chapter 21); and the influence of numerous factors including governing organization over program implementation and administration (chapter 22). The material presented in this book will help TSAC Facilitators understand the importance of a needs analysis for each group of tactical athletes with whom they are currently working or may work in the future, all with the goal of ensuring that they can implement a program that will optimize performance and decrease the risk of injury and mortality. Examples of such evidence-based guidelines and programs are presented throughout chapters 9, 10, and 15; however, these programs will need to be adapted, depending on the tactical athletes for whom they are being applied. Each chapter also discusses the scope of practice for the TSAC Facilitator, including, for example, when to refer a tactical athlete to a nutritionist (chapters 5 and 6) or an allied healthcare professional to assist with rehabilitation (chapter 16).

Chapters begin with objectives and include key terms (boldfaced in text and listed at the end of the chapter), diagrams, detailed photographs, and key points to help guide the reader and emphasize important concepts. Sidebars, sample programs, and case studies are also included to assist with the application of theoretical concepts to professional practice.

To assist instructors using this text, a presentation package including almost 900 PowerPoint slides of text, photos, and artwork from the book has been created. These slides facilitate discussion and illustrate key concepts found in the book. They can be used directly in PowerPoint or can be printed to make transparencies or handouts. Presenters can easily add, modify, and rearrange the order of the slides as well as search for slides based on key words.

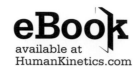

eBook available at HumanKinetics.com

The presentation package has an image bank that includes all of the illustrations, artwork, content photos, and tables from the text, sorted by chapter. The image bank provides flexibility for presenters creating their own resources, including customized presentations, handouts, and other resources.

The presentation package plus image bank is free to course adopters and is available online. Contact your Sales Manager for details about how to access HK*Propel*, our ancillary delivery and learning platform. For use outside of a college or university course, this presentation package plus image bank may be purchased separately at **US.HumanKinetics.com**.

Chapter 1

Tactical Strength and Conditioning: An Overview

Brent A. Alvar, PhD, CSCS,*D, RSCC*D, FNSCA

Katie Sell, PhD, CSCS,*D, TSAC-F

Patricia A. Deuster, PhD, MPH, CNS

After completing this chapter, you will be able to

- describe the NSCA Tactical Strength and Conditioning Facilitator (TSAC-F) program,
- describe what it means to be a tactical athlete,
- summarize and explain general concepts related to tactical strength and conditioning, and
- discuss the differences between a tactical athlete and a sport athlete.

Tactical strength and conditioning is an important emphasis for the National Strength and Conditioning Association (NSCA). The roots of conditioning athletes have a far-reaching history: It can be argued that the ancient Olympic Games were showcases of how warriors needed to train to high levels of fitness and athleticism for a tactical advantage. Today the focus of research and programming for tactical strength and conditioning is directed toward occupational and mission preparedness, including the ability to not only excel in job performance and capability but also minimize injuries and premature mortality. This chapter introduces the NSCA's Tactical Strength and Conditioning Facilitator (TSAC-F) program as well as key concepts that will be further discussed throughout the book.

NSCA TSAC PROGRAM

The Tactical Strength and Conditioning (TSAC) program began within the NSCA as an effort to educate professionals who want to train, direct, and prepare tactical athletes to meet the physical demands of their occupations. These athletes include personnel in special weapons and tactics (SWAT), special operations forces, conventional military forces, law enforcement, and fire and rescue response.

History of the NSCA TSAC Program

The **TSAC program** originated in 2005, and since then it has strived to meet goals through translating cutting-edge research, applying population-specific training methods and field experiences, and implementing evidence-based approaches to reduce injury risk, improve or maintain overall health, and increase specific areas of fitness (e.g., strength, agility, aerobic fitness) pertinent to the tactical athlete. In collaboration with leaders in the tactical communities, academic institutions, and multiple governmental and nongovernmental first responder positions, the NSCA developed the TSAC program to "provide the highest level of physical training possible to those who serve and protect our country, state, and local communities" (1).

The **TSAC Facilitator (TSAC-F) certification** was developed by the NSCA for people who have an interest in working with tactical athletes. The certification provides a standardized credential to people who have the knowledge, skills, and experiences to apply scientific principles for training various tactical athlete populations. The certification also helps establish a high level of professional competence for those who work with tactical athletes. Anyone certified by the NSCA for the training of tactical athletes will henceforth be referred to as a **Tactical Strength and Conditioning Facilitator (TSAC Facilitator)**.

The TSAC Facilitator is a specialized trainer who uses an evidence-based approach (evaluating current research and proven training methodologies) in conjunction with personal field experience to optimize occupational physical preparedness and reduce the risk of injury. All TSAC Facilitators are trained to develop strength and conditioning programs for tactical athletes based on the athlete's individual needs.

Historically, many tactical training protocols focused primarily on cardiorespiratory fitness without considering occupational mission or job performance. This book emphasizes the opportunity to integrate multiple aspects of strength and conditioning for tactical athletes. It provides guidance and the scientific underpinnings of the concepts behind evidence-based tactical strength and conditioning. Chapters 2, 3, 4, and 5 provide an overview of the physiological, anatomical, biomechanical, metabolic, and nutrition-related information upon which a TSAC Facilitator should be building population specific knowledge.

However, training tactical athletes also requires specialized knowledge, skills, and experiences. The certification process focuses on understanding the physiological, environmental, logistical, and cultural factors that influence training as well as successfully implementing and maintaining programming.

Scope of Practice of a TSAC Facilitator

TSAC Facilitators need to understand and work within their **scope of practice**. Acquiring this level of knowledge, skills, and experience, along with engaging in professional development and continuing education, should allow the TSAC Facilitator to work autonomously with a thorough understanding of when it is appropriate to reach out to other professionals. Further, TSAC Facilitators must be able to recognize when issues fall outside their area of expertise (e.g., nutritional counseling, injury treatment). TSAC Facilitators are part of a team of experts working to improve the health, performance, and longevity of tactical athletes.

In addition, TSAC Facilitators have a duty to provide appropriate supervision and instruction to meet a reasonable standard of care and to provide a safe environment for the tactical athletes under their supervision. Their duties also involve informing users of risks inherent in their activities and preventing unreasonable risk or harm resulting from negligent instruction or supervision (14).

Prerequisites of the TSAC-F Certification

To participate in the TSAC-F certification, applicants must be at least 18 years of age and have a high school diploma or equivalent. In addition, applicants must have CPR (cardiopulmonary resuscitation) and AED (automated external defibrillator) certification. Although no formal postsecondary course work is required, candidates are expected to understand the fundamentals of biomechanics, training adaptations, anatomy, exercise physiology, program design, and guidelines that pertain to the unique needs of law enforcement, fire and rescue, and military or special operations. No other NSCA certification is required as a prerequisite for the TSAC-F certification.

Goals of the TSAC Program

The NSCA TSAC-F certification was developed to establish a level of competence in fundamental knowledge, skills, and experiences. The intent is to ensure certified individuals can train tactical athletes to improve the fitness-related attributes of job performance, promote wellness (chapter 21), and decrease injury risk across the spectrum of military, fire and rescue, law enforcement, protective services, and other emergency personnel.

DUTIES OF A TACTICAL ATHLETE

Tactical athletes use their minds and bodies to serve and protect individuals, communities, states, countries, and themselves. They may be employees or volunteers for community, state, or national organizations (governmental or nongovernmental) whose missions are to protect against various threats. In addition, they may be the first to respond to and assist at emergencies, accidents, local and international natural disasters, and terrorist attacks. A tactical athlete must be ready to face any and all threats—physical, environmental, or psychological. Thus, a key requirement for a tactical athlete is physical fitness. Unless tactical athletes are in top physical condition, their ability to protect and serve others is limited.

Key Point

> The TSAC-F certification was developed by the NSCA to provide a standardized credential that ensures a high level of professional competence among individuals with the knowledge, skills, and experiences to apply scientific principles to training tactical athletes.

Tactical athletes share several attributes with recreational, collegiate, professional, and Olympic athletes (e.g., need for physical fitness, teamwork), but they also differ in many ways. Table 1.1 presents some of the differences between tactical athletes and other athletes. These differences will be discussed in more detail in subsequent chapters. Tactical athletes rarely have the resources commonly available to elite or professional sport athletes, and their mission is distinct—surviving and ensuring the survival of others is key, whereas sport athletes strive to win sporting events.

Exercise Testing and Prescription

The tactical athlete training program may incorporate periodic testing for muscular strength and endurance, power, speed, agility, anaerobic power, and cardiorespiratory components of fitness. Chapter 8 presents the principles of testing and evaluating tactical athletes to identify strengths and weaknesses. The test results must then be analyzed and appropriate exercises prescribed to promote the requisite improvements in the fitness and preparedness of tactical athletes. Chapters 9 and 10 discuss the principles of resistance training program design as well as how to sequence a resistance training program to optimize the resultant outcomes (periodization).

Table 1.1 Comparisons Between Tactical Athletes and Professional Sport Athletes

Attribute	Tactical athletes	Professional sport athletes
Outcome of event	Life or death	Win or lose
Commitment	Year-round training cycle	Seasonal training
Scope of training	Multiple skills	Sport specific
Motivation to participate	Volunteer or paid	Sponsored or paid
Work shifts and predictability of assignment	24/7 potential for being deployed; unpredictable assignments	Well-scheduled, well-orchestrated, predictable events
Attire	Personnel protective gear; must carry load	Uniform and protective sport gear
Performance arena	Any and all environmental conditions	Protected environment with varying environmental conditions
Dietary lifestyle	Eat on the fly; help yourself	Help from sports nutritionists and psychologists
Accommodations	Anywhere possible (tents, trucks, rough terrain)	Hotels when traveling
Coverage	Covert operations; some media coverage	Limelight and enthusiastic audience
Magnitude of impact	Local, state, national, or global impact	Self-promotion; local, national, or global enthusiasm or following
Job demands	Unexpected is the norm	Structured and controlled
Rewards for participation	Primarily private reflection and satisfaction; some administrative or public recognition	Public approval, appreciation, recognition
Cohesion	Unit at risk	Team effort
Leadership	Buddy-reliant, commander	Coach-, team-, and captain-directed goals

Key Point

> The TSAC Facilitator evaluates the physical demands of the operational tasks and then designs training programs to address the weaknesses in fitness attributes pertaining to specific occupational needs.

Occupational Specificity

Following testing, training prescriptions are based on an occupation-specific training paradigm—that is, **occupational specificity**. The TSAC Facilitator needs to consider the physical demands of the operational and occupational activities and design the training program accordingly. This requires an understanding of the principles and concepts that guide program development and **periodization** used for specific training time frames (chapters 9 and 10). However, it is not sufficient to use a generalized exercise prescription across tactical populations. Each individual's occupational demands should be assessed, and subsequent program specifications should be guided by the gaps or weaknesses in fitness attributes that pertain to the specific occupational needs. Therefore, the TSAC Facilitator must clearly understand the occupational tasks—what the key tasks are and what physical attributes are required to perform those tasks.

Using a sport analogy, the training program for a football player is specific to the skills and demands of the sport (American football); likewise, the training programs for baseball, tennis, and soccer need to address the specific demands of those sports. This holds true for tactical athletes as well: Law enforcement officers, infantry soldiers, and firefighters all need to train according to the physical demands of their occupational profiles, with their specific occupational tasks forming the foundation for program development (e.g., assessment choices, exercise selection). These considerations are further complicated when taking into account the differential needs of the athlete in terms of flexibility, mobility, speed, agility, aerobic endurance, strength, and power needs. These factors (discussed in chapters 12, 13, 14 and 15) are among the components that make up the job analysis.

JOB ANALYSIS OF A TACTICAL ATHLETE

As noted earlier, one key requirement of a TSAC Facilitator is **job analysis**, or analyzing the occupational tasks of interest. Directly observing tactical athletes performing their job tasks is essential for obtaining firsthand knowledge about the physical demands and skills of the occupation. These observations allow the TSAC Facilitator to quantify the physical demands and skills for future training and tracking progress. Specifically, the TSAC Facilitator must analyze movements, know what energy systems are required for the movements, and identify what potential injuries might arise from the biomechanical demands of the occupational tasks.

Movement Analysis

Fundamental movement competency is essential for occupational performance and mitigation of injury risk (3-5, 10, 11). When conducting a **movement analysis**, the TSAC Facilitator must consider the types of movements performed in the occupation of interest (chapters 17, 18, and 19). For example, a firefighter might have to breach and pull down a ceiling, a soldier will have to carry a heavy rucksack while wearing body armor, and a police officer might have to scale a wall. Those specific tasks would likely be paired with multiple other tasks before the mission is finished. A TSAC Facilitator must be aware of the major movements (symmetry and balance) and muscle contractions (concentric, eccentric, isometric, or combination) performed daily in the occupational tasks. In addition, the types of loads carried in the movements (e.g., tools, scuba gear, rucksack, body armor) should be considered. Consequently, a TSAC Facilitator must understand how the application and distribution of load influence functional capacity, movement patterns, and gait mechanics (chapter 20) as well as exercise technique (chapter 11).

Key Point

A TSAC Facilitator must be able to assess the major physical movements common to occupational tasks, evaluate the types of equipment and loads carried, and apply this knowledge to optimize functional capacity, movement patterns, and gait mechanics.

Energy System Usage

The scientific basis for energy pathways and basic metabolic pathways will be explored in chapter 2 and then applied in subsequent chapters, particularly chapter 14. This topic is critical because the speed, intensity, and duration of movements and occupational tasks drive **energy system** preferences, ensuing fatigue, and the need for rest and recovery. Understanding and training the energy systems used during occupational tasks is also important for preventing injuries, guiding nutritional practices, and optimizing recovery. See chapters 6 and 7 for nutritional recommendations for tactical populations and a discussion of common supplements.

Key Point

The TSAC Facilitator must be able to implement programs to improve cardiorespiratory fitness and minimize the risk of musculoskeletal injuries and illness in tactical athletes.

Injury and Illness Analysis

Injury prevention relies in part on assessing fundamental movements and identifying muscle strength asymmetries (left versus right). A TSAC Facilitator must be knowledgeable about the screening tools that help identify range of motion (ROM) or movement deficits that may compromise performance and lead to injury; **injury analysis** is part of the job task analysis. Muscle strength and anaerobic power also influence performance, and appropriate levels of muscular strength may be key to preventing musculoskeletal injuries (9, 12). TSAC Facilitators must also be aware of illness and injury concerns prevalent in specific tactical populations, as well as the etiology of such conditions and how it might affect training practices. For example, sudden cardiac death is the major killer of structural firefighters while in the line of duty (7). Based on this **illness analysis**, the TSAC Facilitator can implement programs to improve fitness and reduce cardiovascular risk in firefighters by emphasizing aerobic fitness (2, 8, 13, 15), as described in chapter 17. In addition, the TSAC Facilitator should be capable of working with other healthcare providers in the care and rehabilitation process if an injury should occur (chapter 16).

ASSESSMENT OF THE INDIVIDUAL

The TSAC Facilitator usually plays an integral role in the design, implementation, and evaluation of physical fitness testing for tactical athletes. Fitness testing batteries may be required as part of a department wellness program or administered independently as a way to evaluate progress through a physical conditioning program. The TSAC Facilitator must be aware of the recommendations and standards for fitness testing put forth by governing organizations that oversee physical training for tactical athletes (e.g., National Fire Protection Agency [NFPA], United States Department of Defense, Ontario Ministry of Community Safety and Correctional Services), including the standard procedures for use in specific disciplines (e.g., test selection, frequency of administration). In addition, the TSAC Facilitator may be asked to develop a department test battery based on the fitness needs of the tactical athletes and therefore must consider the physiological, metabolic, and biomechanical demands of the occupational tasks, as well as cultural and motivational factors. These will help guide test selection. More information can be found in chapters 8, 17, 18, and 19.

Training Status

One aim of fitness testing is to determine the fitness and health status of a tactical athlete. However, the choice of test may be influenced by the current training status of the individual and any additional physical training endeavors the individual or group may be required to perform in the days before and after testing. The TSAC Facilitator needs to understand and comply with prescreening procedures and be aware of any protocols necessary to clear tactical personnel for participating in physical testing or training practices. The choice of fitness test may need to be adjusted based on recommendations of other allied health care providers (e.g., physicians, physical therapists), particularly if a tactical athlete is being tested when returning to training following an injury or illness.

Key Point

The TSAC Facilitator must be able to prescreen tactical athletes to clear them for participation in physical testing and training for selection and to screen them for return to training following an injury or illness.

Individual Versus Group Testing and Evaluation

Test selection may be influenced by whether testing is occurring with an individual or a group of tactical athletes, the time frame available for testing, and the outcomes of the test itself. Additional logistical considerations include available equipment, training age of participants, location of available testing space, and number and intensity of tests to be administered.

Goal Development

The purpose of physical fitness testing should be clearly presented to the tactical athletes by the TSAC Facilitator. This rationale may address multiple areas in need of goal development, such as improvement or maintenance of physical fitness or various components of overall health. It is the TSAC Facilitator's job to implement tests that quantify current fitness and health status, and then use the test results to help the tactical athlete set realistic (and modifiable) goals for a given time frame. The TSAC Facilitator therefore needs to be aware of current fitness requirements of tactical populations, as well as specific illnesses or injuries to which specific tactical athletes are susceptible, in order to identify health-related goals attained through improved physical fitness.

Key Point

The TSAC Facilitator must be able to apply program design variables to the training of tactical athletes and know when to refer clients to other professionals.

PROGRAM DESIGN

Physical training or conditioning (including long-term periodization programs and acute training sessions) may need to be adjusted to accommodate the unpredictable occupational demands facing tactical athletes. For example, if a firefighter has returned from a long, arduous callout, then a high-intensity training session may not be appropriate during the same shift, given the elevated stress level already experienced and the possibility of another callout during the same shift. The training session planned for that day may need to be adjusted to decrease the risk of accumulated stress and fatigue that affect occupational performance and injury risk (6).

As noted in subsequent chapters, key issues for TSAC Facilitators relate to the scientific foundation of physical training and the application of that knowledge. A TSAC Facilitator should be able to take many of the principles and training guidelines used for athletic populations and apply them in a population-specific manner for various tactical athletes. In particular, a TSAC Facilitator must be able to determine how the following program design variables apply to tactical athletes (e.g., year-long periodization program, isolated six-week predeployment program):

- Specificity
- Progressive overload
- Variation
- Volume
- Frequency
- Duration
- Intensity

Guidelines for designing training programs for military, law enforcement, and fire and rescue (emergency services) personnel are described in chapters 17, 18, 19 and 20.

CONCLUSION

The professional need for TSAC Facilitators is clear. The NSCA has committed to being the leader in this ever-evolving arena. It is our hope that this book will be the touchstone for people seeking a reference for the knowledge they need to design and implement safe, effective training programs for tactical athletes. Whether TSAC Facilitators are working with military, fire and rescue, law enforcement, protective service, or other emergency personnel, the principles in this book can serve as a framework.

Key Terms

duration	progressive overload
energy system	scope of practice
frequency	specificity
illness analysis	tactical athlete
injury analysis	Tactical Strength and Conditioning Facilitator
intensity	(TSAC Facilitator)
job analysis	TSAC Facilitator (TSAC-F) certification
movement analysis	TSAC program
occupational specificity	variation
periodization	volume

Study Questions

1. The prerequisites to become a certified TSAC Facilitator include being 18 years or older, having a CPR/AED certification, and what other component?

   a. postsecondary education

   b. another NSCA certification

   c. high school diploma

   d. college coaching experience

2. Which of the following is a component of a tactical athlete's lifestyle that must be considered by a TSAC Facilitator when designing a program?

   a. seasonal training

   b. unpredictable schedule

   c. structured job demands

   d. protected environment

3. A TSAC Facilitator observes that a police officer may have to jump out of a car and hop a barricade to chase a suspect. Which of the following describes that type of analysis?
   a. holistic
   b. injury
   c. movement
   d. illness

4. The role of a TSAC Facilitator includes all of the following EXCEPT
   a. designing training programs
   b. preventing common injuries
   c. reinforcing physical preparedness
   d. providing nutrition counseling

Chapter 2

Cardiopulmonary and Endocrine Responses and Adaptations to Exercise

Denise Smith, PhD

After completing this chapter, you will be able to

- describe the structure and function of the cardiovascular and pulmonary systems,
- describe the cardiopulmonary responses to exercise,
- describe the endocrine responses to exercise, and
- discuss the chronic adaptations of the cardiopulmonary and endocrine systems to exercise and high-stress situations.

The respiratory system and the cardiovascular system work together to bring oxygen into the body and deliver it to active tissues, such as muscle, so that energy in the form of **adenosine triphosphate (ATP)** can be produced for cellular work (figure 2.1). The respiratory system includes the airways and lungs. The cardiovascular system includes the heart, blood vessels, and blood. Together, these systems are often referred to as the **cardiopulmonary system** because of their closely entwined functions.

CARDIOVASCULAR STRUCTURE AND FUNCTION

The heart is a hollow muscular pump located in the thoracic cavity. It is approximately the size of a clenched fist and weighs 250 to 350 g (<1 lb). The heart beats approximately 70 times per minute at rest, and its contractions provide the force to pump blood throughout the vascular system.

Key Point

The cardiovascular system pumps blood and provides the force to perfuse working tissues during physical activity.

Cardiac Structure

The muscular walls of the heart are called **myocardium** (*myo* = muscle; *cardium* = heart) and are composed primarily of cardiac muscle cells, or **myocytes**, that produce the force to eject blood from the heart. The heart has four chambers: The two upper chambers are the right and left

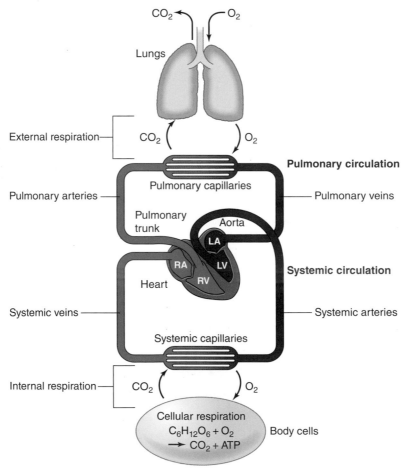

Figure 2.1 Interaction of the respiratory and cardiovascular systems.

Adapted, by permission, from D.L. Smith and Fernhall, 2011, *Advanced cardiovascular exercise physiology* (Champaign, IL: Human Kinetics), 4.

atria, and the two lower chambers are the right and left ventricles (figure 2.2). The atria receive blood from great vessels (inferior and superior vena cava and pulmonary vein), and the ventricles eject blood to the body through great vessels (pulmonary artery and aorta). The heart is functionally separated into the right side and the left side. The right ventricle pumps deoxygenated blood to the lungs (pulmonary circulation), and the left ventricle pumps oxygenated blood to the rest of the body (systemic circulation). The sides of the heart are separated physically by the interventricular septum.

The myocytes that compose the myocardium are muscle cells that contain the contractile proteins actin and myosin. Adjacent myocytes are structurally and functionally connected to each other through specialized membrane structures called **intercalated discs**. The intercalated discs contain specialized intracellular junctions (gap junctions) that allow electrical activity in one cell to pass to the adjacent cell.

As shown in figure 2.2, blood flows through the heart by passing through one-way valves that separate the atria and ventricles (atrioventricular [AV] valves) on each side of the heart and by passing through one-way valves that separate the ventricles from the aorta and the pulmonary artery. The tricuspid valve separates the right atrium and ventricle, and the mitral valve separates the left atrium and ventricle. The pulmonary semilunar valve and aortic semilunar valve (semilunar valves) permit blood to flow from the right ventricle into the pulmonary artery and from the left ventricle into the aorta, respectively. These valves open and close based on pressure differences. When pressure in the atria is greater than pressure in the ventricles, the AV valves are open and the ventricles fill with blood. When pressure in the ventricles is greater than in the atria, the AV valves are closed, and when pressure in the ventricles is greater than in the aorta and pulmonary artery, the semilunar valves are open and blood is ejected from the heart.

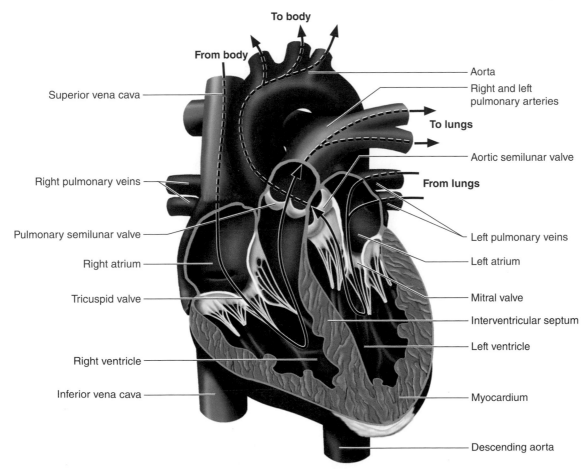

Figure 2.2   Heart structure and blood flow through the heart.

Cardiac Function

The contraction, or beating, of the heart provides the contractile force necessary to distribute blood throughout the circulatory system. The heart beats approximately 70 times per minute at rest but can increase up to approximately 200 beats/min in young adults during maximal exercise. The frequency with which the heart beats is often referred to as the **heart rate (HR)**. The amount of blood pumped from the heart with each beat is the **stroke volume (SV)**. SV averages approximately 70 ml per beat in healthy young men and can increase to about 140 ml with maximal exercise (22, 23, 24). **Cardiac output ($\dot{Q}$)** is the product of HR × SV and represents the amount of blood pumped each minute; essentially, it is a measure of blood flow through the cardiovascular system each minute. Cardiac output at rest is approximately 5 L/min, but this increases dramatically during exercise, reaching values of 25 to 30 L/min in healthy young men (22, 23, 24). Cardiac output can be increased by increasing HR, SV, or a combination of both. During exercise, both HR and SV increase to cause a large increase in cardiac output.

Key Point

During prolonged tactical activities, cardiac output must be increased and then maintained at high levels to supply working muscle with needed oxygen.

Although it is common to think of the heart as ejecting blood into the circulatory system when the heart contracts, the ability to eject blood depends on the heart filling with blood. The alternating periods of relaxation, or **diastole**, and contraction, or **systole**, allow the heart to fill with blood and then pump the blood into the circulation. Every heartbeat reflects both diastole and systole. The amount of blood that returns to the ventricles at the end of the filling period (diastole) is the **end-diastolic volume (EDV)**. The amount of blood that remains in the ventricle after the contraction period (systole) is the **end-systolic volume (ESV)**. SV is the difference between EDV and ESV (SV = EDV − ESV). It can be increased by increasing EDV (such as by increasing venous return), decreasing ESV (such as by increasing contractility), or both (24).

Conduction System

The muscle cells in the heart must be electrically stimulated in order to contract. The heart has a specialized conduction system that spreads electrical signals rapidly throughout the entire heart (figure 2.3). The electrical signal flows through the conduction system as shown in yellow in figure 2.3.

- Sinoatrial (SA) node—initiates electrical impulses. Often known as the pacemaker of the heart.

- Atrioventricular (AV) node—the signal travels from the SA node to the AV node via the internodal pathway. The electrical signal is delayed briefly (~0.1 second) at the AV node before the signal is transmitted to the ventricles.

- Atrioventricular (AV) bundle—the only connection for electrical signals between the atria and ventricles. The AV bundle is also called the *bundle of His*.

- Left and right bundle branches—carry the signal to the apex (bottom) of the heart and to the right and left ventricles.

- Purkinje fibers—the final portion of the conduction system that brings electrical signals to cardiac muscle cells throughout the ventricles. The Purkinje fibers are also called the *subendocardial conducting network*.

When thinking about how an electrical signal is generated in the heart, it is important to understand that the conduction system generates an electrical signal in the SA node (the pacemaker) that then propagates throughout the conduction system. But in a healthy person, the SA node is normally influenced by sympathetic nerve fibers (which increase HR) and parasympathetic fibers (which decrease HR). Also, once the electrical signal moves through the conduction system, it must be rapidly passed from cell to cell within the myocardium via the intercalated discs to stimulate individual myocytes to depolarize and then contract. The ability of the electrical signal to pass from one cardiac cell to the next via intercalated discs is critical to ensure that the cells contract in a coordinated way to eject blood from the ventricle. The intercalated discs create an electrical coupling of the myocytes that allows the myocardium to function as a single coordinated

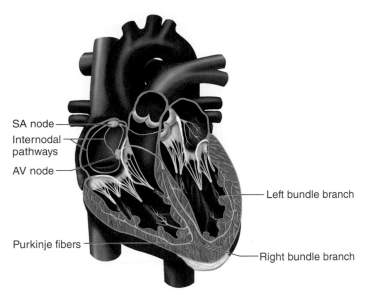

Figure 2.3   Conduction system of the heart.

unit, or functional syncytium. The atria and ventricles each contract as a unit, and thus there are two functional syncytia in the heart.

Key Point

> Withdrawal of the parasympathetic nervous system and activation of the sympathetic nervous system produce rapid increases in HR during exercise and tactical events.

Electrocardiogram

The electrical currents generated in the heart spread through the body and can be detected on the surface of the body with an electrocardiogram (ECG), as shown in figure 2.4. An ECG is a composite of all the electrical activity in the conduction system and the contractile cells of the heart. The three most distinguishable waves of the ECG are the following:

1. P wave—reflects depolarization (electrical signal) of the atria and leads to contraction of the atria.

2. QRS complex—reflects depolarization of the ventricles and leads to contraction of the ventricles. Atrial repolarization occurs during the QRS but is not distinctly seen because of the large changes in amplitude caused by the wave of depolarization spreading across the ventricles.

3. T wave—reflects repolarization of the ventricles and leads to relaxation of the ventricles.

Vascular Structure and Function

Blood vessels are responsible for distributing oxygen and nutrients to cells throughout the body and removing wastes and metabolites from active tissues. The vasculature is composed of arteries,

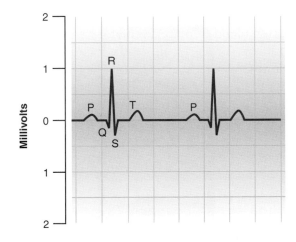

Figure 2.4   ECG tracing.

Reprinted, by permission, from NSCA, 2016, Structure and function of body systems, N. Travis Triplett, In *Essentials of strength training and conditioning*, 4th ed., edited by G. Gregory Haff and N. Travis Triplett (Champaign, IL: Human Kinetics), 14.

arterioles, capillaries, venules, and veins (figure 2.5). Each of these vessels has a specific structure that supports its particular function.

Arteries are large vessels that carry blood away from the heart to distal parts of the body. They have elastic muscular walls that permit them to accommodate the increase in blood volume and pressure when blood is ejected during systole and to recoil during diastole.

Arterioles are smaller vessels that distribute the blood to various organs. The walls of arterioles contain smooth muscle that causes **vasoconstriction** (decreased vessel diameter) when the vessels contract and **vasodilation** (increased vessel diameter) when they relax. Because of their ability to vasoconstrict and vasodilate, arterioles can exquisitely control blood flow to an organ and match blood flow to energy needs at any given moment.

Key Point

Blood-flow needs of an organ during physical activity are achieved through constriction or vasodilatation of arterioles.

Capillaries have the smallest diameter and are the most abundant vessels. They perform the ultimate function of the cardiorespiratory system—gas (oxygen and carbon dioxide) exchange between the blood and the tissue. This function is made possible by their small size, which allows them to be in close proximity to most cells of the body, and their thin walls, which allow gases and nutrients to diffuse through them.

Venules are small vessels of the microcirculation that carry blood from the capillary beds to the veins. The vessel wall of a venule contains a small amount of smooth muscle and is porous so that blood cells and fluids can move easily between the circulation and interstitial space. Veins are large, compliant vessels that carry blood back to the heart. They have elastic walls that permit them to distend and fill with blood more easily than arteries, and many have valves that prevent backflow.

As figure 2.5 shows, blood vessels carry blood to various organs. Furthermore, the circuitry that supplies the organs is in parallel, meaning that blood travels through the various circuits simultaneously. The small muscular arteries (arterioles) that determine the amount of blood supply to the organs play a vital role in distributing cardiac output to each organ based on the needs of the system. For example, by increasing the size of the arterioles for one circuit, blood flow to the stomach and liver can increase after eating without increasing blood flow to every organ. Similarly, when there is a need to dissipate heat, arterioles controlling blood flow to the skin dilate and thus blood flow to the skin increases. Of course, the most obvious example of increasing blood flow to an organ is increasing blood flow to working muscles to support exercise.

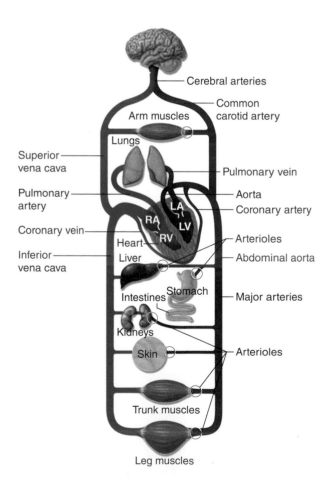

Figure 2.5 Outline of the vascular system.

Blood Pressure

Blood pressure is a major homeostatic variable that must be maintained within limits for the body to function properly. If blood pressure is too low, then blood flow is not adequate to provide needed

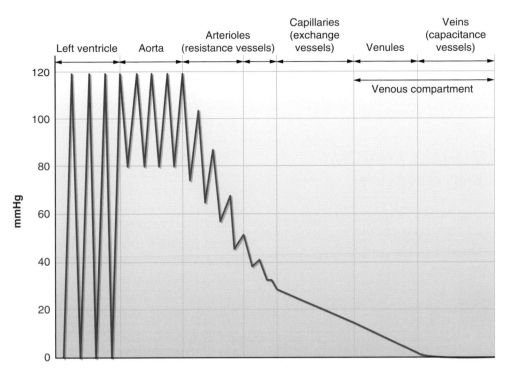

Figure 2.6 Pressure in the left ventricle and throughout the vascular system. Note the marked pressure decrease and absorption of the pulse amplitudes in the arterioles (resistance vessels).

Adapted from P-O Åstrand et al, 2003, *Textbook of work physiology: Physiological bases of exercise*, 4th ed. (Champaign, IL: Human Kinetics), 141; Adapted from Folkow and Neil 1971.

oxygen to tissues, a condition called *hypoperfusion*. On the other hand, if blood pressure is too high, it causes damage to the blood vessels that may result in accelerated disease progression or even in the rupture of a vessel (aneurysm).

Blood pressure changes dramatically throughout the vascular system (figure 2.6). It is greatest in the aorta and major arteries (such as the brachial artery) because of the force of myocardial contractions. Blood pressure in these vessels is also pulsatile because of the ability of the arteries to expand and contract. **Systolic blood pressure (SBP)** is the pressure in the arteries following contraction of the heart (systole), and **diastolic blood pressure (DBP)** is the pressure in the arteries following relaxation of the heart (diastole). DBP in the arteries does not drop to zero because the elastic recoil of the vessels against the blood in them creates pressure against the arterial wall. **Mean arterial pressure (MAP)** is the weighted average of SBP and DBP, and it represents the mean driving force of blood through the vascular system. Mean arterial pressure can be calculated using the following equation:

$$MAP = (SBP - DBP) / 3 + DBP$$

The weighted average takes into account the fact that more time is spent in diastole than in systole.

Pressure in the arterioles decreases dramatically because of their thick muscular walls. Blood pressure in the capillaries must be low in order to avoid damage to the thin-walled vessels. Blood pressure in the veins is very low because pressure has dissipated as the blood has traveled from the heart. In fact, valves in the veins along with muscular action in the legs are needed to ensure that blood from the lower body can return to the heart against gravitational force. When people are forced to stand for a long time without moving their legs (for example, soldiers), venous return is impaired. This can lead to a decrease in heart filling (a decrease in EDV), which decreases cardiac output and leads to low blood pressure and fainting.

Blood pressure is determined by cardiac output (blood flow) and resistance to blood flow in the vascular system, or **total peripheral** resistance (TPR), as shown in the following equation. This equation represents the functional relationship of the primary variables in the cardiovascular system and is fundamental to understanding cardiovascular dynamics.

$$MAP = \dot{Q} \times TPR$$

PULMONARY ANATOMY AND FUNCTION

The respiratory (pulmonary) system is responsible for bringing oxygen into the lungs, where it diffuses into the blood. In addition, it is responsible for eliminating carbon dioxide.

Respiratory Structures

The anatomy of the respiratory system is depicted in figure 2.7. The upper respiratory system consists of the nasal cavity and the pharynx, and it serves to filter, warm, and moisten the air. The lower respiratory system consists of the larynx, trachea, bronchi and bronchioles, lungs, and tiny air sacs, or **alveoli**, within the lungs. The lower respiratory system is where gas exchange occurs.

Air Exchange

Though it is possible to exert volitional control over breathing, most of the time we breathe without any conscious thought and with little effort. Breathing brings air into the lungs to support gas exchange. During exercise, breathing rate and depth increase to supply the additional oxygen that is needed for muscular contraction, and the work of breathing increases. Commonly we think of moving air in and out of the lungs as breathing; technically this is called *ventilation*, and the amount of air we breathe in 1 minute is called **minute ventilation**. Minute ventilation is equal to breathing rate multiplied by **tidal volume** (amount of air breathed with each breath).

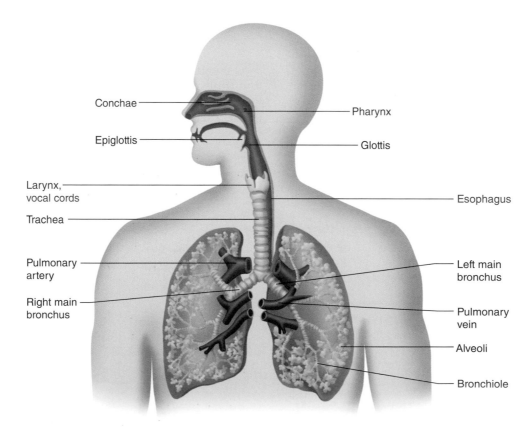

Figure 2.7 Structures of the respiratory system.

Gas Exchange

Breathing may be the most obvious function of the respiratory system, but the ultimate function is gas exchange. As shown in figure 2.1, gas exchange occurs in two places:

1. **External respiration** occurs at the level of the pulmonary capillaries, where oxygen diffuses from the alveoli into the blood and carbon dioxide diffuses out of the blood into the alveoli.

2. **Internal respiration** occurs at the level of the systemic capillaries, where oxygen diffuses out of the blood and into the cells (i.e., muscles) of the body and carbon dioxide diffuses out of the cells and into the blood.

Key Point

Gas exchange occurs in two locations in the body—the pulmonary capillaries (where oxygen diffuses from the alveoli into the blood) and the systemic capillaries (where oxygen diffuses from the blood into the working tissues, especially working muscles).

Gas exchange occurs through the process of diffusion, with each gas moving down its own concentration gradient. The partial pressure of oxygen in the alveoli ($P_{ALV}O_2$ = ~100 mmHg) is greater than the partial pressure of oxygen in the pulmonary capillaries (~40 mmHg), and hence oxygen diffuses into the blood as blood passes through the lungs (23). Venous blood that is then carried to the left side of the heart is thus fully oxygenated and has a partial pressure of oxygen of approximately 100 mmHg. Because gas exchange only occurs at the capillary level, blood flowing through the large vessels remains at constant partial pressure. Thus, as blood enters the systemic capillaries it still has a partial pressure of approximately 100 mmHg. Resting skeletal muscle has a partial pressure of approximately 40 mmHg, so oxygen diffuses out of the systemic blood into the cells. During exercise, as the cells use more oxygen, the partial pressure of oxygen in the cells decreases (to <15 mmHg) as the cells consume oxygen to produce energy (23, 26). The lower partial pressure of oxygen in the cells during exercise causes more oxygen to diffuse out of the blood and into the cells, accounting for the increased oxygen consumption seen during exercise.

ACUTE CARDIOVASCULAR RESPONSES TO EXERCISE

There are numerous cardiovascular responses to exercise. The purpose of these responses is to increase oxygen uptake so that energy can be produced to support contracting muscles.

Oxygen Consumption

The cardiovascular and respiratory systems respond to exercise in a coordinated way. The hallmark of the cardiorespiratory response to exercise is to increase the amount of oxygen that is taken into the body (by the respiratory system), transported to the cells (by the cardiovascular system), and used by the cells (through metabolism). Thus, oxygen consumption serves as an integrated measure of cardiorespiratory responses to exercise. And, because the oxygen is being used to produce energy (ATP) to do muscular work, there is a direct relationship between work performed and oxygen consumed (figure 2.8). That is to say, the more work (exercise) is performed, the more oxygen is consumed. The highest amount of oxygen that can be taken in, transported, and used during heavy muscular work is called **maximal oxygen consumption** ($\dot{V}O_2$max). $\dot{V}O_2$max is considered the best measure of cardiorespiratory fitness; however, it is not always the best predictor of performance because performance is affected by many factors.

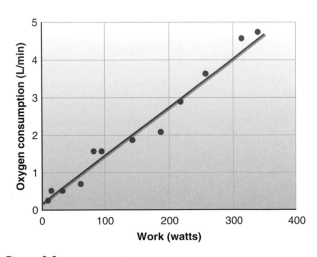

Figure 2.8   Relationship between work (exercise) and oxygen consumption.

Heart Rate

The cardiovascular system is designed to deliver oxygen and nutrients to the working tissue to remove wastes and metabolites from the working muscle. Thus, during exercise, the heart pumps more blood in order to deliver oxygen and nutrients to working muscles. Most people are aware that HR increases with exercise. In fact, HR, like oxygen consumption ($\dot{V}O_2$), generally increases linearly with increasing workload (6, 23). However, for practical reasons, exercise tests frequently use stepwise increases in workload for successive exercise stages rather than a continuously progressive workload. Thus, during an exercise test there is often a rise in HR when the workload increases followed by a leveling off of HR as the stage continues. The increase in HR is due primarily to an increase in sympathetic nervous activation that causes the SA node to depolarize more frequently. HR may increase approximately threefold during maximal exercise, from approximately 60 to 70 beats/min at rest to around 200 beats/min at maximal exercise (23).

Stroke Volume

SV, the amount of blood pumped with each beat of the heart, also increases during exercise. The increase in SV during exercise is caused primarily by two changes:

1. Increased venous return due to rhythmical contraction of skeletal muscle: Increased venous return causes an increase in EDV, which stretches the ventricles and leads to a more forceful contraction, as described by the Frank-Starling law of the heart.

2. Increased force of myocardial contraction due to sympathetic nervous stimulation: The increased force of contraction (contractility) results in lower ESV.

SV increases more during aerobic exercise than during resistance or static exercise because venous return is augmented during aerobic activi-

ties, whereas venous return is not altered greatly during resistance exercise (23). SV increases about twofold during maximal aerobic exercise: from approximately 70 ml/beat to approximately 140 ml/beat (10, 22, 23, 28). Endurance-trained individuals have a higher SV at rest, and some research suggests that they can increase their SV to a greater extent than untrained individuals can during exercise (10).

Cardiac Output

Cardiac output ($\dot{Q}$) is the product of HR and SV, and it represents the total amount of blood pumped by the heart each minute. Because both HR and SV increase during exercise, cardiac output increases greatly during exercise. Cardiac output increases linearly during exercise, reaching values that may be five to seven times greater than resting values, from about 5 L/min at rest to values of about 30 L/min at maximal exercise (10, 22, 23).

Blood Pressure

Blood pressure responds to exercise in varying ways depending upon the type of exercise. Aerobic exercise results in a relatively modest increase in SBP and little or no change in DBP in healthy adults. SBP may increase to as high as 240 mmHg during a maximal exercise test (23).

However, during heavy resistance exercise, especially if the person holds her breath (i.e., performs the **Valsalva maneuver**), both systolic and diastolic values may increase dramatically. Values of >300/180 mmHg have been observed with heavy resistance exercise (16).

Peripheral Resistance

TPR decreases dramatically during aerobic exercise. The decrease in peripheral resistance is due to widespread vasodilation in working muscle that allows more blood to be distributed to these muscles to support metabolism. Because resistance in vessels supplying working muscles decreases so dramatically, blood flow to the working muscles is greatly increased, TPR drops markedly, and blood pressure only increases modestly despite a large increase in cardiac output. On the other hand, TPR during resistance exercise does not decrease much and may even increase (13, 19). Because TPR does not drop substantially but cardiac output does increase, blood pressure is much higher during resistance exercise than during aerobic exercise.

Key Point

> Peripheral resistance decreases during aerobic exercise because vasodilation increases blood flow to working muscle.

Table 2.1 summarizes the cardiovascular responses to exercise, emphasizing the interrelatedness of the major variables.

ACUTE RESPIRATORY RESPONSES TO EXERCISE

During exercise there is an increase in carbon dioxide production and an increased need for oxygen. These changes drive the respiratory responses to exercise. Although multiple sensors affect pulmonary ventilation, the most important in regulating the response to exercise are the chemoreceptors. Chemoreceptors are located in the brain (medulla) and in the large arteries (aortic body and carotid body). These receptors are sensitive to increasing amounts of CO_2 in the blood and stimulate increased breathing to help rid the body of CO_2. The receptors also respond to decreasing levels of O_2 (23). Minute ventilation increases greatly during aerobic exercise due to an increase in breathing rate (frequency) and

depth of breathing (tidal volume). Minute ventilation at rest is approximately 5 L/min, but during maximal aerobic exercise minute ventilation often exceeds 140 L/min in trained men (23).

ACUTE ENDOCRINE RESPONSES TO EXERCISE

The endocrine system plays a central role in homeostasis and is critical in responding to stressful situations such as exercise (9). The endocrine system and the nervous system junction together in a coordinated and complementary way to maintain homeostatic balance and to respond to homeostatic disruptions, such as exercise. These two systems function so closely together that they are sometimes called the **neuroendocrine system**.

The direct link between the nervous system and the endocrine system is evident when considering the effect of sympathetic nervous stimulation. The sympathetic nerve is part of the nervous system—specifically the acceleratory nerve of the autonomic nervous system. When the sympathetic nerve is stimulated, it causes the adrenal gland to release **catecholamines** (epinephrine and norepinephrine). These hormones reinforce the neurotransmitters (e.g., norepinephrine) that are released from the sympathetic nerve to support the fight-or-flight response associated with activation of the sympathetic nervous system.

Exercise is an acute stressor; thus, it activates the sympathetic nervous system. In fact, many of the adjustments that occur in various systems of the body during exercise are in response to sympathetic nervous stimulation—that is, many of these responses are acceleratory and are associated with the fight-or-flight response. Maximal aerobic exercise results in large increases in both epinephrine and norepinephrine (9). Activation

Table 2.1　Cardiovascular Responses to Exercise

	MAP	=	$\dot{Q}$ (HR	SV)	×	TPR
Aerobic exercise	↑		↑↑	↑		↓↓
Resistance exercise	↑↑		↑↑	↔		↔

MAP = mean arterial pressure; HR = heart rate; $\dot{Q}$ = cardiac output; SV = stroke volume; TPR = total peripheral resistance; ↑ or ↓ indicates strength of response or change (↑↑ indicates greater change than ↑).

of the sympathetic nervous system increases HR, heart contractility, and breathing rate and helps to maintain blood pressure by causing vasoconstriction in vessels supplying nonworking tissue (9). Maximal resistance exercise also results in large increases in epinephrine and norepinephrine (8).

Key Point

Activation of the sympathetic nervous system plays a key role in stimulating many responses to exercise.

The hormonal system responds to exercise in order to do the following:

- Regulate metabolism: The hormonal system, along with the sympathetic nervous system, helps mobilize fuel to support energy production for the cells and helps maintain blood glucose levels.

- Regulate cardiovascular function: Hormones, along with the sympathetic nervous system, enhance cardiac function, help determine blood distribution to tissues, and help maintain blood pressure.

- Regulate adipose, muscle, and connective tissue: Hormones have a direct effect on adipose tissue and help make fatty acids available during exercise. Hormonal changes during and following exercise also play an important role in muscular adaptations to exercise.

Figure 2.9 depicts the major metabolic hormones and how they interact with various tissues (adipose, skeletal muscle, and liver) to help mobilize fuel sources and maintain blood glucose during exercise (23). This figure highlights the vast interaction of hormones and the multiple organs that must respond in a coordinated fashion to support exercise.

CHRONIC ADAPTATIONS OF THE CARDIOPULMONARY AND ENDOCRINE SYSTEMS TO EXERCISE AND HIGH-STRESS SITUATIONS

Consistent exercise training leads to chronic adaptations that allow the body to respond to the stress of exercise with less physiological

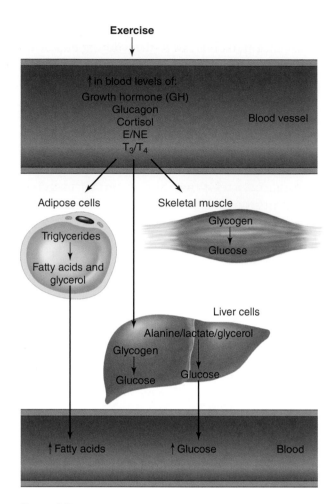

Figure 2.9 Principal hormones and their effect on fuel sources.

Reprinted, by permission, from S.A. Plowman and D.L. Smith, 2014, *Exercise Physiology for Health, Fitness, and Performance*, 4th ed. (Philadelphia, PA: Lippincott Williams & Wilkins), 638.

disruption and to perform more work (exercise). Aerobic exercise training leads to adaptations related to fuel availability and metabolic regulation such that a trained person can use energy stores more effectively to support prolonged exercise. Resistance training increases muscle mass and strengthens support structures, resulting in greater strength and power.

Maximal Oxygen Consumption

The most noted change in cardiorespiratory function with aerobic exercise training is an increase in maximal oxygen consumption ($\dot{V}O_2$max). In fact, changes in maximal oxygen consumption are considered evidence that training has improved physical fitness. Because oxygen consumption is an integrated measure of fitness, improvements in oxygen consumption reflect adaptations in the cardiovascular and respiratory systems, although cardiovascular changes are more prominent (23). Aerobic endurance training typically results in an increase of 10% to 20% maximal oxygen consumption (1) in previously untrained people (1, 23). Resistance training typically results in little or no change in maximal oxygen consumption, although circuit-type resistance training may result in modest improvements (1).

Key Point

> Aerobic endurance training results in improvements in $\dot{V}O_2$max, whereas resistance training has minimal impact on aerobic endurance.

Heart Structure and Function

Cardiac mass and the dimensions of the ventricles increase with aerobic endurance training (12, 14). Compared with an untrained person, an aerobically trained person at rest will have a lower HR, a higher SV, and a similar cardiac output (assuming body size has not changed dramatically) (23). Cardiac output remains constant at rest because the need for oxygen delivery to the body has not changed. However, the same cardiac output is achieved by a higher SV and a lower HR—thus, the cardiovascular system has become more efficient. Tracking resting HR is a convenient way to monitor improvements in fitness.

During maximal exercise, an aerobically trained person can achieve a higher cardiac output to support greater exercise levels. The increase in maximal cardiac output is achieved by a higher SV; maximal HR is relatively unchanged with exercise training (1).

Resistance training results in increased left ventricular wall and septal thickness (20, 30). Changes in SV and HR are not consistently found with resistance exercise programs (7, 31).

Vascular Adaptations

Aerobic endurance training results in increased capillary density that supports oxygen delivery to cells of the body. In addition, aerobic endurance training leads to increased diameter of blood vessels (13, 21, 25, 29). Not only does the resting diameter of the vessel increase, but the ability to vasodilate also increases. The increased ability to vasodilate reflects improved **endothelial function**. The increased endothelial function that is associated with aerobic endurance training is an important reason for the decrease in cardiovascular disease mortality and morbidity that is associated with exercise training (2, 11, 32).

Resistance training also brings about adaptations in vascular structure and function, although they are not as well studied as adaptations to aerobic endurance training. As with aerobic endurance training, adaptations in vascular function following resistance exercise are mediated by hemodynamic stimuli that influence the vessel wall (18). A recent meta-analysis found that resistance training had a positive effect on flow-mediated dilation (FMD) similar to that of aerobic endurance training, increasing FMD by 2% to 2.8%, which translates to a reduction in cardiovascular disease risk of 26% to 36% (2). Aerobic endurance training also leads to an increase in blood volume—20% to 25%—in highly trained individuals (5). Changes in blood volume occur more quickly than an increase in red blood cells, but by 1 month of training, red blood cell numbers also increase (5).

Key Point

> Both aerobic and resistance training have beneficial effects on vascular endothelium that result in improved cardiovascular health.

Respiratory Adaptations

Relatively few respiratory adaptations are associated with exercise training. The most notable change is an increase in maximal minute ventilation that is seen with aerobic endurance training. At rest, minute ventilation is unchanged, but it is achieved by a higher tidal volume and a lower breathing frequency. During maximal exercise, minute ventilation is higher following an aerobic endurance training program (33), which supports increased oxygen intake during higher levels of work. The increased maximal minute ventilation is achieved primarily by an increased maximal breathing frequency; tidal volume increases only slightly (17).

Endocrine Adaptations

Many hormones are affected by exercise training. As mentioned earlier, many of the adaptations that are seen in other systems (e.g., cardiovascular, metabolic) reflect changes in the endocrine system. Endocrine responses are greatly affected by the type of training program. In general, aerobic endurance training results in an increased sensitivity to hormones, such that a lower concentration of hormone will have the same effect after training (9, 23). Aerobic training results in a blunted exercise response to many hormones associated with activation of the sympathetic nervous system and the regulation of metabolism (15). Compared with an untrained person, an aerobically trained person will have a smaller increase in catecholamines and cortisol during the same exercise, reflecting less activation in the sympathetic nervous system and less overall stress on the system (4, 23). Other hormones involved in fuel utilization, such as insulin, glucagon, and growth hormone, are also affected by exercise training. Again, trained individuals show a dampened response to exercise compared with untrained individuals, indicating that training is associated with less physiological disruption and greater ability to meet the metabolic demands associated with exercise. Resistance training stimulates the release of many hormones, and it is thought that these hormones play a role in mediating the repair and remodeling process in the muscle that results in increased muscle mass and strength (8). Circulating levels of anabolic hormones appear to influence the magnitude of muscular adaptations (27).

CONCLUSION

Among the most noticeable responses to exercise is an increase in breathing and HR. However, there are many cardiorespiratory responses to exercise that result in an increased ability to take in, transport, and use oxygen in order to produce energy for muscle contraction. Maximal oxygen consumption is an integrated variable that reflects the combined responses of the cardiorespiratory and muscular systems, and changes in maximal oxygen consumption are the most common way to describe changes in aerobic fitness that accompany an aerobic endurance training program. Hormonal changes during exercise help coordinate many of the body's responses to exercise. Hormonal responses to exercise also provide the signal for many adaptations that occur as a result of a training program.

Key Terms

adenosine triphosphate (ATP)
alveoli
cardiac output
cardiopulmonary system
catecholamines
diastole
diastolic blood pressure (DBP)
end-diastolic volume (EDV)
endothelial function
end-systolic volume (ESV)
external respiration
heart rate (HR)
intercalated discs
internal respiration
maximal oxygen consumption ($\dot{V}O_2$max)

mean arterial pressure (MAP)
minute ventilation
myocardium
myocytes
neuroendocrine system
stroke volume (SV)
systole
systolic blood pressure (SBP)
tidal volume
total peripheral resistance (TPR)
Valsalva maneuver
vasoconstriction
vasodilation

Study Questions

1. Which part of the heart conduction system is responsible for initiating electrical impulses?

   a. SA node

   b. AV node

   c. AV bundle

   d. Purkinje fibers

2. What occurs during the T wave on an ECG?

   a. atrial depolarization

   b. atrial repolarization

   c. ventricular depolarization

   d. ventricular repolarization

3. A person is performing the Valsalva maneuver while doing heavy resistance training. Which of the following acute blood pressure changes is likely to happen?

   a. decrease in SBP, increase in DBP

   b. increase in SBP, no change in DBP

   c. increase in SBP, increase in DBP

   d. no change in SBP, increase in DBP

4. A police officer is chasing an armed suspect, and the fight-or-flight response is activated. What system of the body is initially affected?

   a. cardiovascular

   b. circulatory

   c. nervous

   d. respiratory

5. What system helps regulate metabolism, cardiovascular function, and adipose tissue?

   a. cardiovascular

   b. hormonal

   c. respiratory

   d. nervous

6. Which of the following is the best measure of aerobic fitness?

   a. cardiac output

   b. $\dot{V}O_2$max

   c. tidal volume

   d. heart rate

Chapter 3

Skeletal Muscle Anatomy and Biomechanics

Michael R. Deschenes, PhD

Raymond W. McCoy, PhD

After completing this chapter, you will be able to

- describe the components of the neuromuscular and musculo-skeletal systems;
- describe the structure and function of skeletal muscle, bone, and connective tissue;
- describe the types of muscle actions (isometric, concentric, and eccentric);
- define the roles that muscles play in movement;
- describe the principles of biomechanics;
- discuss how biomechanics affect exercise selection and execution; and
- apply biomechanical principles to exercise selection, exercise execution, and tactical job performance.

Muscle tissue, along with connective, nervous, and epithelial tissue, is one of the four major types of tissue composing the human body. Muscle tissue is versatile in its functional capacity and can be divided into three subtypes: smooth, cardiac, and skeletal. This chapter focuses on skeletal muscle tissue.

Skeletal muscle is found throughout the body and accounts for approximately 40% of the total body mass of an adult male and approximately 32% of the body mass of an adult female (10). Such a significant contribution to the body's weight indicates the importance of skeletal muscle to a person's health and ability to function in daily life, not to mention in sport and recreational activities. Not only is skeletal muscle involved in moving the body, it also is essential for digesting food (chewing, swallowing), breathing (expansion of thoracic cavity, allowing inhalation), maintaining bone health (muscular forces applied to bones promote bone density), and regulating blood glucose levels (excess blood sugar is stored in muscle as glycogen). Moreover, skeletal muscle works with other types of tissue to form vital organ systems in the body, such as the neuromuscular system and the musculoskeletal system. We will begin our discussion by focusing on the bones that skeletal muscles attach to in forming the musculoskeletal system. It is this arrangement between the muscles and bones that makes it possible for us to move not only our limbs but our entire body during physical activity.

Key Point

The physical and functional integration of skeletal bones and muscles make up the musculoskeletal system. This system enables the human body to move and perform work.

BONES AND THE SKELETON

Just as skeletal muscle works with the nervous system to form the neuromuscular system, it works with the skeleton to make up the equally important musculoskeletal system, allowing movement of the body and the performance of physical tasks that are important to tactical athletes. Skeletal muscles are joined to bones throughout the skeleton predominantly by tendons. Bones are considered living organs because, in addition to the mineral deposits that make them hard, they also contain blood vessels and nervous tissue (note that organs must be composed of more than one tissue type). In addition to its 206 bones, which are arranged to both protect vital organs and allow mobility, the adult skeleton is composed of cartilage. Unlike bone, cartilage does not feature nervous tissue or blood vessels (10); rather, it is almost exclusively made up of chondrocytes (cells that produce collagen) and a water–carbohydrate matrix. In the adult body, cartilage

- covers the ends of bones found in joints (articular),
- connects the ribs to the sternum of the rib cage (costal),
- forms the respiratory tubes carrying inhaled air into the lungs,
- gives rise to the larynx (i.e., voice box),
- composes the intervertebral discs of the spinal column,
- helps form the nose, and
- composes the external ear.

Types of Cartilage

Regardless of its location in the body, all cartilaginous tissue falls into one of three categories. The first is *hyaline cartilage*, which provides a combination of flexibility and support and is the most abundant type of cartilage in the body. Hyaline cartilage is found in articular joints, such as the knee, shoulder, and elbow, as well as the trachea, or windpipe. The second type is *elastic cartilage*, which is similar to the hyaline variety but is designed to withstand regular bending and contortion, immediately returning to its original shape. Elastic cartilage is best represented by the external ear. Finally, *fibrocartilage* is intended to withstand heavy downward pressure and stress, and accordingly it is found in the menisci of the knee joint and in the intervertebral discs of the spine (10). Everyday weight-bearing activity imparts considerable stress on those joints.

Skeletal Development

During fetal development, the skeleton gradually converts from mainly cartilage tissue to harder, more supportive bone tissue. In this process, known as **ossification**, the living cells of bone tissue, the osteocytes, secrete large amounts of extracellular matrix containing minerals such as calcium and phosphorous. Only 35% of adult bone tissue is organic, or living, tissue (mainly collagen); the remainder is composed of inorganic matter in the form of mineral salts, especially calcium phosphate (10). When secreted, the extracellular matrix arranges itself around the osteocyte in concentric rings that appear much like the rings in the trunk of a tree. These rings are referred to as *lamellae*, and the lamellae and the osteocyte combine to form the long, cylindrical osteon (also called the *Haversian system*). At the center of the osteon is the Haversian canal, which contains blood vessels that supply the osteocyte with nutrients and inorganic minerals. As bone matures, it adds osteons, thus increasing the circumference of the bone and strengthening it. The Haversian system is typically found in long bones and more specifically in the compact, or cortical, bone type that composes the shaft region, or diaphysis.

Another type of bone tissue, termed *spongy* or *cancellous*, has a honeycomb appearance and is found at the knobby ends, or epiphyses, of long bones. This is where red and yellow bone marrow are located and where red and white blood cells, along with platelets, are produced. The red marrow synthesizes each type of blood cell, while the yellow marrow produces a limited amount of white blood cells. Figure 3.1 shows the compact and spongy tissue located in long bones.

Categories of Bones

The bones of the skeleton are categorized by shape: long, short, flat, and irregular. Long bones are cylindrical and are predominantly located in the limbs and appendages. Short bones are cuboidal and are most commonly found in the wrist and ankle. A specialized type of short bone is the sesamoid bone, and its distinguishing feature is that it is embedded in a tendon. The patella or kneecap

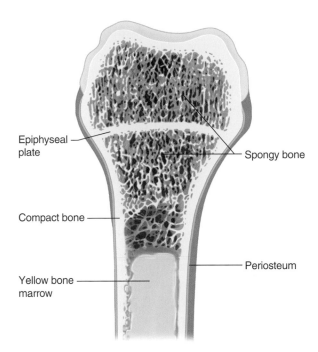

Figure 3.1 Long bone composed of both compact and spongy bone tissue.

is a sesamoid bone. Flat bones are generally thin, flat, and curved. They are best exemplified by the bones that make up the cranium, or skull. Finally, irregular bones come in various shapes and as a result do not neatly fall into any of the first three categories. The best examples of irregular bones are the vertebrae of the spinal column and hip bones of the pelvis.

Functions of Bones

Bones play a number of important roles that allow the body to function. They support the body, providing a firm framework that allows upright posture and resistance to gravity. They also serve as levers, allowing the body to perform mechanical work as well as ambulatory movement. In addition, bones protect vital, delicate tissue by encasing the brain in the skull, the spinal cord in the spinal column, and the heart and lungs in the rib cage. Bones also act as a storage depot of important minerals (e.g., calcium, phosphorous), and they promote blood cell formation (as discussed, the bone marrow is where red and white blood cells as well as platelets are produced before being released into the bloodstream) (17, 21).

Exercise-Related Bone Adaptations

Despite its relatively constant size and shape, bone tissue is not at all static; rather, it is constantly undergoing remodeling that is not obvious to the eye. This remodeling is made possible by the presence of **osteoblasts**, cells that are responsible for bone mineral deposition and thus strengthening the bone, along with **osteoclasts**, cells that reabsorb bone tissue, particularly its mineral content. If the activity of the osteoblasts exceeds that of the osteoclasts, bone build-up occurs. Conversely, if the activity of osteoclasts is greater than that of the osteoblasts, skeletal bones become thinner and weaker. Along with nutrition and the hormonal system, physical activity is a primary factor determining whether bones will undergo thickening and strengthening or thinning and weakening. Resistance exercise (weightlifting) as well as high-impact sports such as gymnastics are especially effective in improving bone mineral density and thus bone strength (5). Resistance training may be of particular value to older adults who are naturally experiencing thinning and weakening of their bones. The benefits of resistance training or high-impact sport are specific to the bones that are involved in those activities, and adaptations of the musculoskeletal system occur in unison (i.e., strong muscles lead to strong bones).

Key Point

Similar to muscle tissue, bone tissue adapts to the stresses placed upon it and becomes stronger when it is used more frequently.

SKELETAL MUSCLE

Although there are more than 600 muscles within the human body, all skeletal muscle tissue is characterized by four defining characteristics: **excitability**, or the ability of skeletal muscle to respond to electrical stimuli (i.e., impulses generated by the nervous system); **contractility**, or the capacity of skeletal muscle to shorten and generate force; **extensibility**, or the potential of muscle to stretch beyond its normal, resting length; and **elasticity**, or the ability of muscle to return to its resting length after it is stretched. These four traits

work together during dynamic movements of the body. Importantly, each one can be improved with training, meaning that skeletal muscle function is enhanced as a result of well-designed exercise training regimens (6).

Much as there are four defining characteristics of skeletal muscle tissue, during contraction muscles can play four distinct roles in the movement of the skeleton and its bony levers. The muscles serving as the principal movers of the bones during a movement are agonists, or **prime movers**. Muscles that oppose the movement generated by the prime movers are termed **antagonists**. In addition, during specific movements, muscles other than the primary movers may contribute a smaller amount of force to assist the agonists; these muscles are categorized as **synergists**. Finally, muscles called *stabilizers* perform the task of securing or stabilizing one joint so that movement can smoothly occur at another joint. Depending on the movement involved, any particular muscle may play any of these roles (i.e., agonist, antagonist, synergist, stabilizer), and the function played by any one muscle may differ depending on the movement.

As an example of how these four roles of muscle contraction come into play during a specific movement, let's examine the bench press exercise. During the bench press, the pectoral muscles act as the agonists, the anterior deltoids and triceps brachii serve as synergists, the latissimus dorsi muscles of the upper back are the antagonists, and the biceps brachii muscles perform the stabilizing function. In contrast, during seated rows, the latissimus dorsi muscles become the agonists, with the pectoral muscles acting as antagonists, the trapezius and biceps brachii muscles becoming synergists, and the gluteus maximus and lower back muscles (erector spinae) muscles becoming stabilizers. This illustrates the versatility of individual muscles when performing various movements or exercises.

Table 3.1 (page 30) displays many of the major muscles and their functions during movement. The function of the muscles during a concentric (shortening) contraction are listed. These muscles also control the opposite function listed in the table during an eccentric (lengthening) contraction. For example, the quadriceps muscles cause the knee to extend when they are contracting concentrically, such as raising the body during a deadlift. They also control the speed of knee flexion during an eccentric contraction, such as lowering the body during the deadlift.

Note that skeletal muscles are often considered groups within the body rather than individual muscles. Throughout the human body there are 13 major muscle groups, listed here in alphabetical order:

1. Abdominal muscles are located on the stomach and flex the spine. Specific muscles in this group are the rectus abdominis and transverse abdominis.

2. Biceps muscles are found on the front of the upper arm and flex the arm at the elbow joint. Specific muscles include the biceps brachii and the brachialis.

3. Calf muscles are found at the back of the lower leg. The specific muscles are the gastrocnemius, plantaris, and soleus muscles, and they extend the foot at the ankle joint.

4. Deltoids are present at the top of the shoulder joint. The three sets, or heads, of fibers that form this muscle group are the anterior (front), posterior (back), and lateral (side) heads.

5. Erector spinae muscles are found in the lower back and are used to extend the spine. Specific muscles are the iliocostalis, longissimus, and the spinalis.

6. Gluteal muscles—the gluteus maximus, gluteus medius, and gluteus minimus—make up the buttocks. This muscle group extends, abducts, and rotates the hip joint.

7. Hamstrings are composed of the biceps femoris, semitendinosus, and semimembranosus at the back of the upper leg. This muscle group flexes the leg at the knee joint.

8. Latissimus dorsi and rhomboid muscles are located in the middle of the back. The latissimus muscles pull the arms down to the pelvis, and the rhomboids (major and minor) pull the shoulder blades together at the back.

9. Oblique muscles (external and internal) are located within the rib cage on the sides of the body. When contracted, they assist in respiration by either reducing the thoracic cavity (internal obliques) during expiration or expanding the rib cage during inhalation (external obliques).

10. Pectoralis muscles comprise the pectoralis major and pectoralis minor, which are found in the upper chest. The pectoralis major helps move the upper arm (flexion, adduction, rotation). The pectoralis minor helps stabilize the scapula, or shoulder blade.

11. Quadriceps femoris, the large muscle group at the front of the upper leg, extends the leg at the knee joint. The four muscles of the quadriceps are the vastus lateralis, vastus medialis, vastus intermedius, and rectus femoris.

12. Trapezius muscles span from the middle of the spine to the base of the skull. Their main function is to move the scapula.

13. Triceps muscles are located at the back of the upper arm. When the medial, lateral, and long heads contract, they extend the arm at the elbow.

Structure of Muscle

To better understand what gives skeletal muscle its remarkable capacity to do work, we must first appreciate its structure at the cellular level. Skeletal muscle nicely exemplifies the biological tenet that form and function are tightly linked. A whole skeletal muscle comprises groups of fibers packaged together as fascicles, with each fascicle bound together by a layer of connective tissue called the *perimysium*. In turn, the whole muscle is surrounded by a layer of connective tissue called the *epimysium*, and each individual muscle cell is surrounded by a layer of connective tissue called the *endomysium*. The individual cells are called *muscle fibers* because they are long and cylindrical. Each muscle fiber comprises numerous myofibrils that are tightly packed together in a parallel arrangement extending the full length of the muscle fibers, which, in turn, typically run the full length of the whole muscle (17, 19). The relationship between myofibrils, muscle fibers, and whole muscles is depicted in figure 3.2.

Table 3.1   Function of the Major Muscle Groups of the Human Body

Joint	Muscle group	Function	Major muscles
Lower body			
Intertarsals	Inverters	Inversion	Tibialis anterior Tibialis posterior Flexor digitorum longus
	Everters	Eversion	Peroneus longus Peroneus brevis
Ankle	Plantar flexors (calf muscles)	Plantar flexion	Gastrocnemius Soleus Tibialis posterior Flexor hallucis longus Flexor digitorum longus
	Dorsiflexors	Dorsiflexion	Tibialis anterior Tibialis posterior Extensor digitorum longus
Knee	Quadriceps	Extension	Vastus lateralis Vastus intermedius Vastus medialis Rectus femoris
	Hamstrings	Flexion	Semitendinosus Semimembranosus Biceps femoris
Hip	Extensors	Extension	Gluteus maximus Semitendinosus Semimembranosus Biceps femoris
	Flexors	Flexion	Psoas major Iliacus Rectus femoris Sartorius Adductor longus
	Abductors	Abduction	Gluteus medius Gluteus minimus Tensor fasciae latae
	Adductors	Adduction	Adductor magnus Adductor longus Adductor brevis Gracilis
Pelvic girdle	Anterior	Anterior tilt	Psoas major Iliacus Rectus femoris
	Posterior	Posterior tilt	Gluteus maximus Semitendinosus Semimembranosus Biceps femoris

Joint	Muscle group	Function	Major muscles
Upper body			
Shoulder	Flexors	Flexion	Pectoralis major Anterior deltoid Biceps brachii
	Extensors	Extension	Latissimus dorsi Posterior deltoid Teres major
	Abductors	Abduction	Deltoid (all sections) Supraspinatus
	Adductors	Adduction	Latissimus dorsi Pectoralis major Teres major
Elbow	Flexors	Flexion	Biceps brachii Brachialis Brachioradialis
	Extensors	Extension	Triceps brachii Anconeus
Wrist and fingers	Flexors	Flexion	Flexor digitorum superficialis Flexor digitorum profundus Flexor pollicis longus Flexor carpi radialis Flexor carpi ulnaris Palmaris longus
	Extensors	Extension	Extensor digitorum Extensor pollicis longus Extensor carpi radialis longus Extensor carpi radialis brevis Extensor carpi ulnaris

The myofibrils are composed of muscle proteins, collectively called *myofilaments*, which are arranged in an overlapping orientation that, as we will soon see, accounts for the sliding-filament mechanism of muscle contraction (16, 17, 21). Thick filaments are composed of the protein **myosin**, a large protein, whereas the thin myofilaments feature the smaller protein known as **actin**. Upon closer examination, actin is made of two protein strands wound around each other in a double helix. Both myosin and actin are contractile filaments. The regulatory proteins called *tropomyosin* and *troponin* complement the contractile myofilaments and initiate

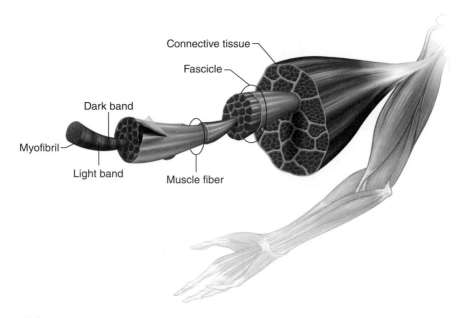

Figure 3.2   Relationship between the whole muscle, its muscle fibers, and its myofibrils.

contraction. The larger tropomyosin filament is bound to the actin, specifically within the groove resulting from the interweaving of the two actin strands, whereas troponin molecules are regularly dispersed along the tropomyosin filament. The **sarcomere**, the smallest functional unit of skeletal muscle, features the overlap of actin and myosin, which generate force, along with the presence of the necessary regulatory filaments of tropomyosin and troponin to serve as the on–off switch of the contractile activity of myosin and actin (figure 3.3).

Function of Muscle

The muscle generates force through the sliding-filament mechanism of contraction. This mechanism demonstrates how the myofilaments (myosin and actin) interact with each other to cause a twitch (a single contractile event), resulting in the muscle fiber shortening and producing force. Under resting conditions, despite their close proximity to each other, there is no physical contact between myosin and actin. More specifically, the crossbridge heads of myosin are unable to attach to binding sites on the nearby actin filaments. This is due to the fact that tropomyosin masks, or blocks, those binding sites under resting conditions. Still, even in this resting state, the crossbridge heads of myosin are energized

and ready to interact with the actin binding sites when they become exposed. Thus it is fair to say that under resting conditions, the crossbridge heads of myosin, which ultimately are responsible for muscle force production, behave much like a series of mouse traps that have been set and are ready to release their stored energy to cause contraction, but only upon the exposure of binding sites on nearby actin filaments.

Key Point

Muscle shortens when myosin and actin myofilaments slide over each other; no protein itself actually shortens.

The interaction between myosin and actin is caused by an increase in cytosolic calcium (see the next section), which binds to troponin molecules. Recall that troponin is found at regular intervals along the tropomyosin that winds around the actin molecule, blocking the binding sites. When its concentration is elevated, cytosolic calcium binds to troponin, causing a conformational shift in that molecule, which is transmitted to the tropomyosin molecule. Tropomyosin then undergoes its own conformational shift and exposes the binding sites on actin. With the exposure of the binding sites, crossbridge heads from myosin are able to attach to actin. Upon the formation of these

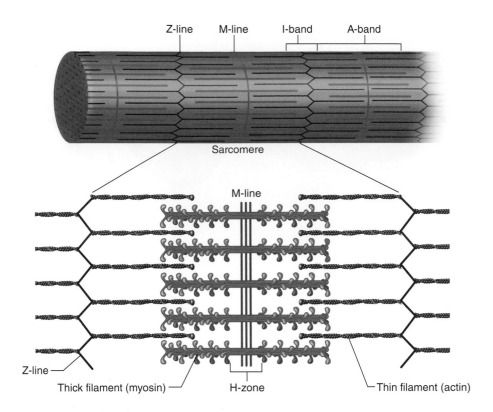

Figure 3.3   Sarcomere and its contractile filaments myosin (thick filament) and actin (thin filament). Note the degree of overlap between those two myofilaments and that the length of myosin composes the A-band (or dark band) and the length of actin determines the I-band (or light band). The H-zone is where myosin can be found without overlapping with actin. The M-line is composed of a tough, durable protein that anchors myosin in position during contraction.

actomyosin complexes, the crossbridge heads of myosin can take advantage of their energized state to release their stored energy, pulling actin along the myosin filament via the ratchet-like movement of the myosin crossbridge heads. This movement, called the *power stroke*, shortens the fiber and generates force. The amount of force generated by a contracting muscle is directly proportional to the number of actomyosin complexes formed; they are the functional units responsible for force production.

After this movement, or sliding event, has occurred, the actomyosin complex remains intact until an ATP molecule binds to the myosin crossbridge head, terminating the interaction between the myosin crossbridge head and the actin binding site. Then, with the presence of ATP on the crossbridge head, the ATPase enzyme that is always present on the crossbridge is able to hydrolyze the ATP, providing the energy needed to move the crossbridge head back to its original

position and energized state. Should any exposed actin binding site be in proximity, the crossbridge head will interact with it, causing another power stroke that further shortens the muscle fiber and produces additional force. This process repeats until cytosolic calcium levels return to resting concentrations, allowing tropomyosin to return to its normal position, where it blocks binding sites along the actin myofilaments. The sequence of events referred to as *crossbridge cycling* is portrayed in figure 3.4.

Initiation of Muscle Contraction

As stated previously, the sliding-filament mechanism responsible for muscle contraction is elicited by a sudden increase in cytosolic calcium levels. But what are the events leading to this dramatic elevation of cytosolic calcium? The source of this calcium is the **sarcoplasmic reticulum**, a large, intracellular organelle that serves as a reservoir

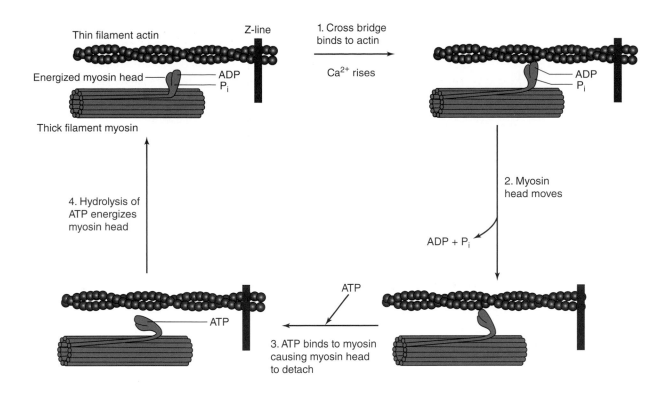

Figure 3.4   Sequential steps of myosin crossbridge cycling and the power stroke resulting in contraction and force production.

of calcium within the muscle fiber (16, 17). When a neural impulse, or electrical excitation, is delivered to the muscle fiber's surface (i.e., the sarcolemma), it travels along the sarcolemmal membrane into its T-tubules, which bring the membrane and its electrical impulse into the fiber without actually entering the internal region of the fiber (think of plastic wrap following a crevice made in a potato, following its contours while remaining on the outside of the potato). However, as the neural impulse travels into the T-tubule, it excites dihydropyridine (DHP) receptors within the T-tubular membrane. These DHP receptors are voltage sensors, and the electrical excitation of the impulse results in a conformational shift in the DHP receptors. This shift is then conveyed to the ryanodine receptors, which are in close proximity but are components of the membrane of the sarcoplasmic reticulum within the muscle fiber, making them intracellular in their location. These ryanodine receptors are calcium channels, and upon stimulation by neighboring, conformationally altered DHP receptors, these channels open, resulting in a rapid efflux of calcium from the sar-

coplasmic reticulum into the cytosol of the muscle fiber. This newly released calcium then binds to nonryanodine calcium channels on the membrane of the sarcoplasmic reticulum, causing them to open as well. This second method of calcium efflux from the sarcoplasmic reticulum is referred to as *calcium-induced calcium release* (4, 17).

When its concentration increases, cytosolic calcium binds to troponin, setting forth a series of events that exposes binding sites on actin, including the power strokes carried out by myosin crossbridge heads (i.e., sliding-filament mechanism of muscle contraction). Crossbridge cycling continues until neural stimulation of the sarcolemma discontinues, allowing calcium to be pumped back into the sarcoplasmic reticulum, thus restoring cytosolic calcium to its resting value. The process of converting the neural stimulation of the muscle fiber's external membrane to the contractile events occurring within the interior of the fiber is referred to as **excitation–contraction (E–C) coupling**, and the DHP and ryanodine receptors are essential components of this coupling process (4).

Key Point

E–C coupling enables a neural impulse to trigger a muscle twitch and force production.

Types of Muscle Action

Although we typically think of skeletal muscle contraction as a process that is characterized by muscle shortening, there are actually three types of muscle contractions, all of which result in force production (9). The first type is referred to as *concentric*, and it occurs when the force developed by the contracting muscle exceeds the load resisting movement. Accordingly, the muscle shortens and the load moves. However, when the load resisting the action of the muscle is greater than the force generated, the muscle lengthens rather than shortens. This lengthening type of contraction is referred to as *eccentric*. Both types of contractions are used in resistance training. For example, when doing biceps curls, the movement of the barbell from the starting position up to the shoulders, with the elbows in a flexed position, results from a concentric contraction. But when slowly lowering the barbell back to the starting position, where the elbows are in the extended position, an eccentric contraction occurs in the biceps brachii muscle. Finally, if the force produced by the active muscle equals the load resisting movement, it is said to be an *isometric* contraction, meaning there is no change in the length of the muscle as it exerts force.

Research has shown that, perhaps counterintuitively, the force produced by a muscle during an eccentric contraction at maximal effort is greater than that generated during an isometric contraction, which in turn exceeds that produced during a maximal concentric contraction (9). So although you may not be able to move a load in the desired direction, your muscles develop more force while lowering a weight (load) than while lifting it. Because a muscle may not shorten while it is generating force (i.e., eccentric and isometric contractions), many consider the proper term for muscle activity to be *action* rather than *contraction*, although the terms are often used interchangeably.

MUSCLE MECHANICS

In addition to the type of contraction a muscle is undergoing, other factors influence how much force, or tension, is generated by a maximally contracting muscle. For instance, how quickly the muscle is moving through its range of motion (ROM) while contracting has a major impact on how much force it will produce. This relationship is called the *force–velocity curve*. Briefly stated, the faster the rate of movement during maximal effort contraction, the smaller the amount of tension generated. Moreover, this relationship is curvilinear rather than linear; hence the term *force–velocity curve*. In other words, if there is a 25% increase in contractile velocity from a static initial position, there will not be a corresponding 25% decrease in force production. In fact, there is likely to be a decline in force far greater than 25% because decrements in force production are most precipitous when first varying from a nonmoving isometric contraction, becoming less pronounced as movement velocity increases (figure 3.5). In large part this is explained by the fact that as the speed at which the actin and myosin filaments slide over each other increases, there is a decreased probability that the myosin crossbridge heads will be able to bind to the exposed binding sites. (Think of how much more difficult it is to hit a 90 mph [145 km/h] fastball than one delivered at 60 mph [97 km/h] in baseball.) Mechanistically, this is accounted for by the fact that the fewer actomyosin complexes formed, the less tension generated by the muscle.

Another principle of muscle mechanics is called the *length–tension relationship*, shown in figure 3.6. This relationship is based on the degree of overlap between myosin and actin filaments. The most force develops when there is optimal overlap between those two contractile filaments, allowing the greatest number of actomyosin complexes to develop. Recall that it is the total number of these complexes that ultimately determines the tension generated by a contracting muscle. When the muscle is stretched beyond optimal length— interestingly, optimal length coincides with natural resting length—actin pulls away from myosin, limiting the overlap between these two myofilaments

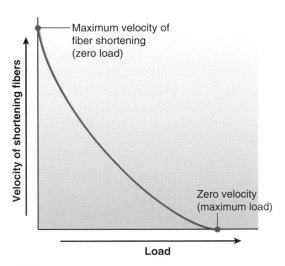

Figure 3.5 Force–velocity curve of muscle contraction. Note that the decline in force produced is not linear; decreased production is most dramatic when the rate of movement initially increases from a stationary position.

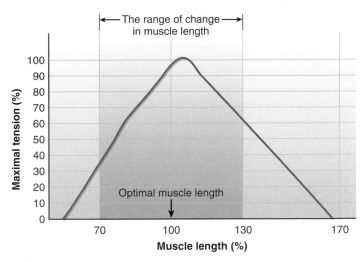

Figure 3.6 Length–tension relationship of muscle contraction. Note that peak force is produced when there is optimal overlap of myosin and actin, thus allowing the greatest number of actomyosin complexes to form.

as well the number of actomyosin complexes that can be established between them. Yet when a muscle shortens beyond optimal length, there is also a decrease in the number of actomyosin complexes that can form and thus force that can be developed (because the exposed binding sites on actin are not properly aligned with the crossbridge heads of myosin). When muscle length varies more than 30% beyond its optimal overlap between actin and myosin, whether too long or too short, the generated force drops dramatically (9, 17, 19).

NEUROMUSCULAR ANATOMY

Muscles must be stimulated to contract. The only direct stimulation of skeletal muscle tissue comes from the motor (somatic) branch of the voluntary nervous system. Thus, on many accounts it is more accurate to describe the neuromuscular system of the body and its ability to generate force. For the sake of simplicity, however, we will address specific features of skeletal muscle and its innervating motor neurons separately.

Muscle Fiber Types

A remarkable feature of the human body is its ability to perform a wide range of physical activities, from brief, powerful actions such as throwing

a grenade to long, submaximal efforts such as an extended rucksack march. Although it is the muscles' total functional capacity that makes it possible to carry out such diverse activities, the various muscle fiber types that compose the muscles are specialized to carry out specific activities.

Several methods are employed to distinguish the fiber types in human skeletal muscle, but it is generally agreed that there are three major fiber types (13, 16). For example, if cross-sections of muscle tissue are stained for the ATPase activity of myosin crossbridge heads, the three major types of fibers are referred to as *Type I*, *Type IIA*, and *Type IIX* depending on their staining intensity. On the other hand, if we distinguish fiber types according to their contractile and metabolic characteristics, we identify three major categories, referred to as *slow oxidative*, *fast oxidative glycolytic*, and *fast glycolytic*. However, the three categories of fiber types identified by these two classification schemes clearly coincide with each other. Those fibers that stain as Type I function in the same way that slow oxidative fibers do, fibers that stain as Type IIA display the contractile characteristics of fast oxidative glycolytic fibers, and fibers that stain as Type IIX show the same contractile features as fast glycolytic fibers. More recently, antibodies have been isolated (15, 18) to distinguish individual fiber types according to the specific isoform of myosin expressed by the fiber, resulting still in three major categories (Types I, IIA, and IIX). Again, although the specific variable used for categorization of fiber types might vary, the fibers themselves retain their characteristics, resulting in considerable overlap of the classification systems.

To emphasize an important point, it is the various types of muscle fibers found in our muscles that permit the body to perform such a wide array of activities. For instance, contractile activity during an endurance event is mainly assigned to the Type I, or slow oxidative, fibers, with some assistance by Type IIA, or fast oxidative glycolytic, fibers. During moderate-intensity activity (e.g., 1,500 m [1,640 yd] run), the Type IIA, or fast oxidative glycolytic, fibers mainly determine performance. Finally, during brief, maximal-intensity activities such as the 100 m (109 yd) sprint, the Type IIX, or fast glycolytic, fibers are primarily responsible for performance. Table 3.2 presents characteristics of the three fiber types.

Just as muscle fiber types are specialized to conduct certain tasks (e.g., high force but short duration, low force but long duration), whole muscles within the body sometimes have specialized tasks to perform, and the fiber types in those muscles reflect the tasks the muscles carry out. For example, the soleus (a calf muscle) functions primarily as a postural muscle, enabling us to stand upright for long periods of time, and the most abundant fiber type in that muscle is Type I, which is very fatigue resistant. However, most of the larger muscles, such as the quadriceps (thighs) and deltoids (shoulders), which take part in a variety of activities, comprise approximately equal percentages of Type I and II fibers and thus are more versatile in their activities (13).

Motor Units and Fiber Types

Muscle fibers are unable to contract until they receive an excitatory impulse from the motor system. Remember that muscle paralysis typically results from damage to the nervous system (e.g., spinal cord) rather than to the muscles themselves. Because there are far more muscle fibers in the body than there are motor neurons to innervate them, each motor neuron branches out to form numerous nerve terminal endings as it reaches the muscle. In this way a single motor neuron may innervate a multitude of fibers in a muscle (figure 3.7). The **motor unit** is defined as a single motor neuron and all the fibers that it innervates (3, 21). In large muscles, which do not require fine, complex movements, sometimes hundreds of fibers can be found in a single motor unit. In muscles that do require fine control over movements (e.g., hand muscles), perhaps only a dozen fibers form a single motor unit (3). Regardless of the size of the motor unit, all muscle fibers of that unit are the same type. In large part this is true because it is the motor neuron that determines the contractile characteristics and, by extension, the type of its associated muscle fibers.

Motor neurons also dictate the recruitment patterns of the motor units found in a given muscle. More specifically, motor neuron size determines which motor units within a muscle are most easily recruited and thus which will be the first to be

Table 3.2 Characteristics of Muscle Fiber Types

Characteristic	Type I (slow oxidative)	Type IIA (fast oxidative glycolytic)	Type IIX (fast glycolytic)
Fiber size	Small	Intermediate	Large
Capillary supply	High	Intermediate	Low
Mitochondrial content	High	Intermediate	Low
Oxidative capacity	High	Intermediate	Low
Glycolytic capacity	Low	Intermediate	High
Contractile speed	Slow	Intermediate	Fast
Contractile force	Low	Intermediate	High
Fatigue resistance	High	Intermediate	Low

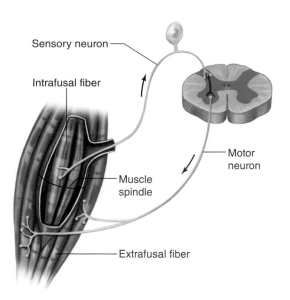

Sensory neuron

Intrafusal fiber

Muscle
spindle

Motor
neuron

Extrafusal fiber

Figure 3.7   A single motor neuron may innervate many muscle fibers in a muscle via the motor neuron.

recruited when performing a task. Smaller motor neurons are recruited first because they offer less resistance to the neural impulses generated by the motor system that initiate motor, or muscle, activity. These smaller motor neurons typically have fewer branch points and accordingly innervate fewer fibers. Moreover, the fibers innervated by small motor neurons are also smaller, generating less force, and are generally Type I, or slow oxidative, fibers. At the other end of the spectrum, the largest motor neurons are the most difficult to recruit because they offer much more resistance to neural stimulation, yet when they do respond they generate the greatest amount of force. This is due to the fact that they give rise to a large number of branch points, thus innervating a greater number of muscle fibers. In turn, these fibers are Type IIX or fast glycolytic, are large in size, and are capable of developing impressive amounts of force. As expected, motor neurons that are intermediate in size are moderately difficult to recruit and innervate a moderate number of muscle fibers, which tend to be intermediate in size and thus contractile strength. So when voluntary muscle movements are performed, smaller motor neurons are initially recruited. But if the smaller motor neurons cannot generate adequate force to perform the task, progressively larger motor neurons are called into play until the necessary amount of muscle mass

is being recruited to produce the necessary force. This is known as the **size principle** of motor unit recruitment (8).

This technique of motor unit recruitment is not the only way that we regulate the amount of force our muscles generate. Another way of progressively increasing muscle force production is called *rate coding*. In this method, the speed at which neural impulses are fired by the individual motor neuron can be increased, exciting the muscle fibers it innervates at a faster pace and resulting in greater force production by way of summation or fusion of individual twitches (see figure 3.8). In larger muscles featuring a mixed distribution of fiber types, there is interplay between the two strategies of rate coding and motor unit recruitment when trying to exert greater amounts of force (i.e., first rate coding, then recruitment, and finally a return to rate coding at maximal effort). But in smaller muscles, which tend to be more homogeneous in fiber type, it appears that rate coding is the major player in determining how much force the muscle can generate (3).

Key Point

> The neuromuscular system uses two strategies to regulate the amount of force produced in order to perform a task. One is motor unit recruitment (i.e., calling into play more motor units and muscle fibers), and the other is rate coding (i.e., how rapidly electrical impulses, or action potentials, are fired down the motor neuron to the muscle fiber it innervates).

Muscle Spindles and Golgi Tendon Organs

Along with managing rate coding and recruitment patterns, which are both voluntary strategies, regulation of muscle force production is influenced by the amount of feedback provided by neural components in the contracting muscles and associated tendons. The vast majority of fibers within any skeletal muscle are categorized as extrafusal and are designed to contract and develop force; however, all skeletal muscles also contain a small number of intrafusal fibers, which contain a capsule known as the **muscle spindle** and yield sensory feedback information concerning the

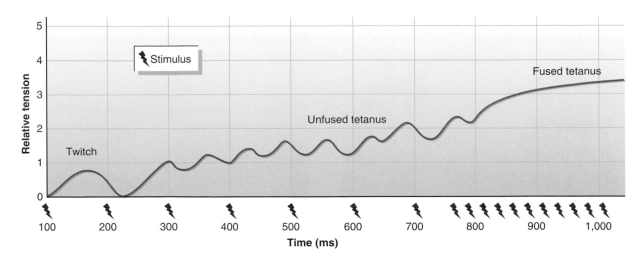

Figure 3.8 Summation of individual muscle twitches (tetanus) to produce greater muscle force.

amount of stretch experienced by the muscle. This information is then relayed to the central nervous system (CNS) so that it can adjust the amount of tension that the muscle must develop to avoid being further stretched and possibly damaged. A greater amount of weight or resistance placed upon the muscle will result in a greater degree of stretch, triggering a stronger sensory feedback signal to the CNS. The CNS reacts by eliciting a more powerful response from the muscle in order to overcome the resistance.

In addition to muscle spindles, **Golgi tendon organs (GTOs)** provide sensory feedback to the CNS so that it can elicit the proper amount of muscle contractile force to overcome the resistance placed upon the muscle. GTOs are proprioceptors that are located in the region of the tendon near the muscle's insertion point (see figure 3.9) and are sensitive to the tension exerted at the musculotendinous junction. They also play an important protective role by inducing relaxation among contracting muscle fibers, thus inhibiting excessive force production by the extrafusal fibers that may result in muscle damage.

Neuromuscular Junction

Recall that each motor unit composing a skeletal muscle features a single motor neuron and all of the muscle fibers that the neuron innervates. This implies that a message must be delivered from the nerve terminals of the neuron to the surface,

or sarcolemma, of each muscle fiber. The highly specialized synapse that enables nerve-to-muscle communication is known as the **neuromuscular junction (NMJ)**. At the NMJ, the presynaptic component features nerve terminal endings containing the vesicles (sacs) that store the excitatory neurotransmitter acetylcholine. A specialized region of the sarcolemma called the *end plate* acts as the postsynaptic component of the NMJ. The end plate is a small, swollen region accounting for less than 0.1% of the sarcolemma's entire area surrounding the muscle fiber (1), but, importantly, it expresses receptors for acetylcholine.

In the structural arrangement of the NMJ, the presynaptic acetylcholine vesicles and postsynaptic receptors are tightly coupled, with their locations mirroring each other across the synaptic cleft. In this way the release sites for acetylcholine are directly opposite from, and in close proximity to, the binding sites for that neurotransmitter. This maximizes the chance that, once released into the synaptic cleft, acetylcholine will bind to its postsynaptic receptors. Once this binding to the receptor sites occurs, channels embedded in the muscle fiber's membrane are opened, allowing an influx of sodium and an efflux of potassium. This movement of ions across the membrane elicits a localized depolarization, or electrical impulse, termed the *end-plate potential*. This local electrical charge of the end-plate region elicits an action potential that spreads throughout the entire

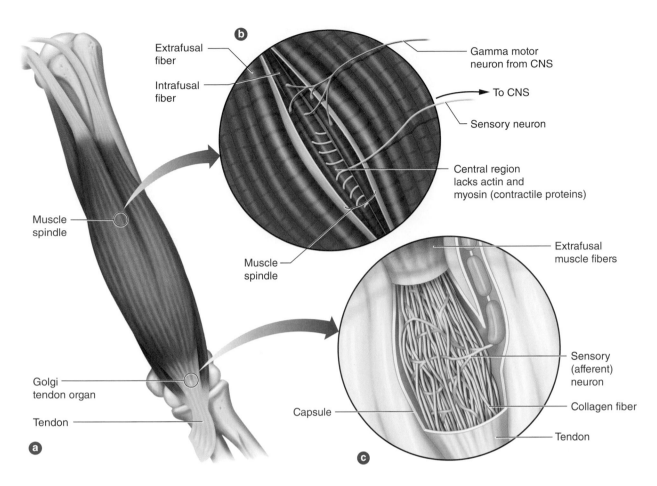

Figure 3.9 Stimulation of the Golgi tendon organ (GTO) showing muscle inhibition.

sarcolemma, exciting the whole muscle fiber. It is this excitation that is carried into the T-tubules of the fiber, triggering the E–C coupling process previously described. Thus, it is fair to say that the NMJ serves as the anchor of the neuromuscular system because it enables communication between the nervous and muscular branches of that system. Figure 3.10 illustrates the NMJ.

NEURAL RESPONSES DURING EXERCISE

As might be expected given the tight integration between the muscles and the motor neurons that form the neuromuscular system, significant neural responses or adjustments are generated during exercise. Moreover, due to the differing demands of endurance and resistance exercise, neural responses are specific to those modes of training. For example, during endurance exercise, the nervous system makes adjustments in an attempt to maintain force production and offset fatigue. A major neural response occurs by increasing the number of motor units recruited during extended submaximal exercise. More specifically, as some muscle fibers and motor units experience reductions in force production (i.e., fatigue), additional motor units, and their constituent muscle fibers, are recruited to compensate for the decreased force produced by the initial fibers. Further, as some motor units display fatigue, the nervous system activates fresh, or previously unrecruited, motor units to maintain force production, while fatigued motor units drop out, or are derecruited (11).

In addition to fatigue-related modifications to motor unit recruitment, rate coding—or the speed at which motor neurons fire impulses to muscle fibers—declines during prolonged activity, accounting for some of the fatigue noted in those

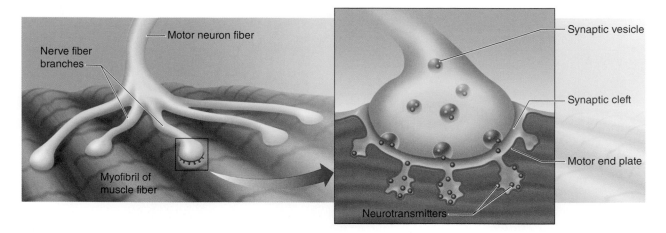

Figure 3.10 NMJ and its pre- and postsynaptic features.

active muscles (7). This change in rate coding observed in fatigued neuromuscular systems could be related to the decreased excitability of motor neuron axons that has been noted during continuous firing of electrical impulses (14). The excitability of a motor neuron's axon is related to the capacity of ATP-dependent sodium-potassium pumps to reestablish proper separation of charge across the axon's membrane between the electrical impulses traveling down the axon. During repetitive endurance activities, changes in neuromuscular transmission efficiency are also detected. This measure of neuromuscular function assesses the efficacy with which the neural impulse generated by the motor neuron is able to cross the synapse at the NMJ and excite the membrane (sarcolemma) of the postsynaptic muscle fiber. During rest, the efficiency of this nerve-to-muscle communication is about 95%. But following an extensive series of muscle contractions, this efficiency has been shown to decline to approximately 60% (2).

One particularly important neural response that takes place during resistance exercise is a great increase in the total amount of neural drive delivered to the exercising muscle so that the muscle can produce more total force (12). This permits the recruitment of a greater number of motor units and thus muscle fibers. Moreover, the rate of neural impulses delivered to contracting muscle fibers is amplified, resulting in higher force production by each muscle fiber recruited (20). Also assisting in greater force production is an elevated coordination of the agonist, antagonist,

synergist, and stabilizer muscles recruited during a movement that is mediated by improved neural communication (12).

BIOMECHANICAL PRINCIPLES

Biomechanics is commonly defined as the study of forces acting on, and generated within, a body and the effects of those forces on the tissues, fluid, or materials used for diagnosis, treatment, or research purposes (6). It is a heavily quantitative discipline that uses procedures and techniques also used in physics and engineering. Much of the forces generated by the human body during physical activities can be explained with a biomechanical analysis of the movements involved.

Lever Systems

When muscles pull on bones, they rotate a body segment around a joint. The rotational effect of the muscle action depends on the type of lever system involved. A lever system contains a lever (i.e., a body segment such as the foot, lower leg, or forearm), an axis of rotation or joint, a muscle force (generated by muscle contraction), and a resistance force (usually gravity and an object being lifted). There are three types of lever systems (figure 3.11): first class, second class, and third class (6).

1. First class: In the first-class lever system, the joint is located between the muscle force and the resistance force of gravity. Only a few examples of

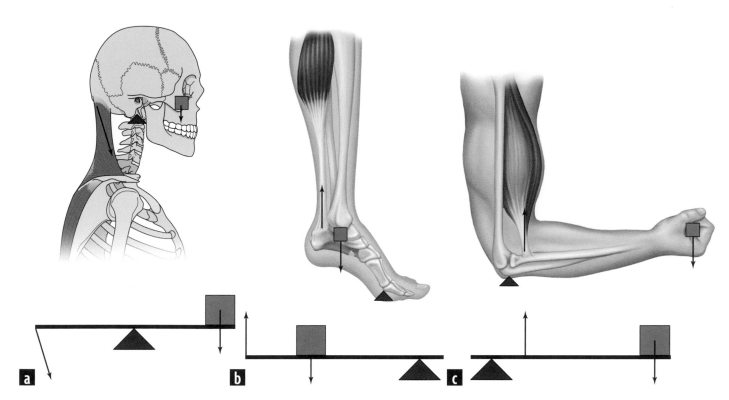

Figure 3.11 Lever systems. *(a)* A first-class lever system has the joint between the muscle force and the resistance (weight of the head). *(b)* A second-class lever system has the joint near one end and the muscle force farther away from the joint than the resistance (weight of the body). *(c)* A third-class lever system has the joint on one end and the muscle force closer to the joint than the resistance (weight of the forearm).

first-class levers can be found in the human body, such as the weight of the head on the anterior side of the cervical joints of the spine with the posterior neck muscles on the other side of the cervical joints (figure 3.11*a*).

2. Second class: In the second-class lever system, the joint is located near one end of the body segment (e.g., the arm), with the muscle force exerted farther away from the joint than the weight, or resistance (figure 3.11*b*). An example of the second-class lever system in the human body would include the body being raised up on the ball of the foot with the calf muscles and the force they exert being farther away from the ball of the foot than the weight of the body. The second-class lever system is a mechanically advantaged system because the muscle force produced is less than the weight of the body.

3. Third class: The third-class lever system is the most common one in the human body. In this system, the joint is near one end of the body segment, and the force of muscle contraction is focused at a point closer to the joint than is the weight, or resistance (figure 3.11*c*). As an example, a third-class lever system is used in a biceps curl because the elbow flexor muscles are closer to the elbow joint than the weight held in the hand. The third-class lever system is a mechanically disadvantaged system because the muscle force must be much greater than the resistance that must be overcome. This type of lever system therefore requires large muscle forces to move body segments.

Muscle Torque Versus Resistive Torque

The term *torque* refers to the rotational effect of a force around an axis of rotation (6). When a muscle force pulls on a body segment, it causes muscle torque. If the torque generated by the contracting muscle is stronger than the torque related to the resistance, the body segment will rotate about the joint. Muscle torque is calculated by multiplying the muscle force times the torque arm, which is the perpendicular distance between the joint and the muscle's line of pull. This distance is referred to as the *moment arm* or *force arm*. In figure 3.12, the muscle torque is calculated by multiplying the muscle force (100 lb [445 N]) by the force arm (0.2 ft [0.061 m]) for a muscle torque of 20 foot-pounds (27 Nm). Therefore, there are two ways to increase the muscle torque around a joint. The most common method is to increase the muscle force produced. The other method is to increase the distance between the muscle and the joint. Though the second method is mainly determined by the size of the athlete, it also varies throughout the ROM due to the changing distance between the muscle and the joint (6).

Because the body is made of levers and joints, the resistance at each joint is calculated as a resistive torque instead of weight applied in a linear direction. This resistance torque is calculated similarly to the muscle torque by multiplying the weight by the perpendicular distance between the resistance and the involved joint. This distance is often referred to as the *resistance arm*. In figure 3.12, the resistance torque is calculated by multiplying the weight of the dumbbell (10 lb [44.5 N]) by the resistance arm (1.4 ft [0.43 m]) for a resistive torque due to the dumbbell of 14 foot-pounds (19 Nm). However, the resistive torque due to the combined weight of the arm and hand (8.6 lb [38.3 N] as calculated as a percentage of the body weight of an average-sized man) must also be taken into account. This value is multiplied by the distance between the weight of the forearm and hand to the joint (0.7 ft [0.21 m]) for a resistive torque of 6 foot-pounds (8 Nm). Therefore, the total resistive torque would be the resistive torque due to the weight (14 ft lb [19 Nm]) plus the resistive torque of the forearm and hand (6 ft lb [8 Nm]) for a total of 20 foot-pounds (27 Nm).

Notice that because the muscle torque is equal to the sum of resistive torques, the opposing torques offset each other so that the forearm, hand, and dumbbell are stationary. Also note that when the arm was balanced, it took 100 pounds (445 N) of muscle force to balance the 10-pound (44.5 N) dumbbell and the 8.6 pounds (38.3 N) of the forearm and hand. With the muscle torque of 20 foot-pounds (27 Nm) and a muscle moment arm of 0.2 feet (0.061 m), the force produced by muscle is calculated to be 100 pounds, or 445 N

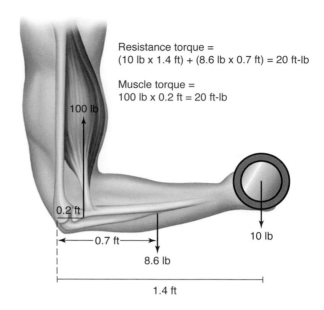

Resistance torque =
(10 lb x 1.4 ft) + (8.6 lb x 0.7 ft) = 20 ft-lb

Muscle torque =
100 lb x 0.2 ft = 20 ft-lb

100 lb

0.2 ft

0.7 ft

10 lb

8.6 lb

1.4 ft

Figure 3.12 Muscle torque and resistance torque. Muscle torque is calculated by multiplying the muscle force by the force arm, which is the perpendicular distance from the joint to the muscle force. Similarly, resistance torque is calculated by multiplying the resistance (weight) by the resistance arm, which is the perpendicular distance from the joint to the resistance.

(100 lb = 20 ft lb / 0.2 ft). The large muscle force produced relative to the smaller resistive forces is due to the fact that the body typically uses a mechanically disadvantaged third-class lever system, as previously described.

To lift as much weight as possible, it is necessary to minimize the resistance torque due to the weight by reducing the perpendicular distance from the weight to the joint (i.e., the resistance arm). This explains why first responders must keep their backpacks as close to the body as possible to minimize the resistance it presents. For example, if the responder holds the weight away from the body, the perpendicular distance from the weight to the body increases, and the resistive torque increases along with it (figure 3.13a), requiring more muscle torque to lift the weight. Conversely, when the weight is close to the body, the resistance arm decreases, so the resistive torque due the weight also decreases (figure 3.13b). This would allow the first responder to lift the weight with a lower muscle torque even though the weight itself is the same (6).

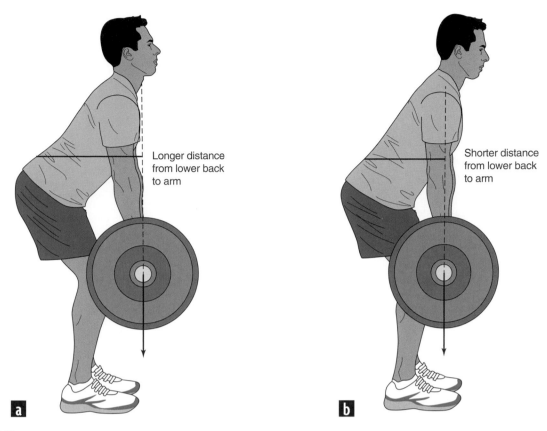

Longer distance from lower back to arm

Shorter distance from lower back to arm

a

b

Figure 3.13 Resistive torque during lifting. *(a)* The resistive torque is large when the weight is away from the body. *(b)* The same weight can have a smaller resistive torque because the weight is closer to the body.

TYPES OF MUSCLE-STRENGTHENING EXERCISES

Muscles perform many functions during exercise. Sometimes the muscles are generating force while they are stationary using isometric muscle contractions. More typically, exercise involves movements that require both concentric and eccentric muscle contractions. The following types of strengthening exercises illustrate the many ways to apply resistance to the muscles to cause them to adapt and strengthen (6, 17).

Isometric

The word *isometric* means "same length," indicating that the contracting muscle shows no movement. The muscles are actively generating force without external movement of the body or its segments. An example of an isometric exercise is pushing your hands together in front of your chest with no external movement.

Isometric muscle contraction can be found in a myriad of occupational activities: Holding a charged fire hose, maintaining proper body positions in simple tasks such as sitting or extended standing, and wearing body armor or self-contained breathing apparatus are all examples in which isometric muscular strength and endurance are essential for the tactical athlete. As such, this type of muscle contraction is utilized constantly by the tactical athlete and therefore should be considered during exercise selection. The use of planks for abdominal strengthening and maintaining proper body position during a squat exercise are examples of isometric contractions during workouts.

Isotonic

The word *isotonic* means "same tension," or force. These types of exercises include lifting weights whose resistance to the contracting muscles does not change while moving through the movement

ROM. This is best exemplified by resistance training with free weights or stacked-plate weight machines. But use of the term *isotonic* in these cases can be a misnomer because even though the weight placed on a barbell during, for example, a biceps curl does not change during the movement, the resistance to the contracting muscles does change throughout the ROM because the perpendicular distance of the resistance torque varies. Figure 3.14 illustrates how the resistance torque is low at the start of the movement because the perpendicular distance is minimized. When the weight is lifted, however, the forearm becomes horizontal and the perpendicular distance lengthens, which increases the resistance torque to the body. Although the term *isotonic* means "same tension," the resistance presented to a muscle during these contractions varies throughout the ROM. This varying resistance experienced by the contracting muscles while lifting free weights, or stacked plates on a conventional lifting machine, is the reason why variable-resistance weight machines were developed.

All tactical occupations utilize isotonic muscle contractions during their everyday activities. Whether lifting an ammo can, sandbag, or riser pack or just picking something up from the ground, isotonic muscle contractions are an integral component for the tactical athlete. Isotonic exercises are the form of resistance training that should be utilized most with the tactical athlete, because of specificity of training—that is, these exercises emulate the type of movements that are most commonly seen during everyday activities.

Variable Resistance

In variable-resistance exercises, the resistance presented to the contracting muscles by the weight training machine changes in an attempt to match the mechanics of the body so that the muscles may be maximally worked throughout the ROM. Variable-resistance training equipment can change the resistance torque that the body must overcome by altering the perpendicular distance of the resistance. In doing so, it presents the slightest amount of resistance when the muscles are at their weakest position mechanically in the ROM, and the greatest resistance is encountered

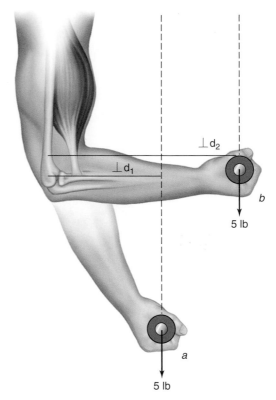

Figure 3.14   Resistive torque changes throughout the joint ROM. The resistance torque is low at the beginning of a movement *(a)* and larger when the resistance arm (perpendicular distance to the joint) increases *(b)*.

when the muscles have their greatest mechanical advantage in the ROM. In this way, sticking points during repetitions are eliminated. Variable-resistance machines accomplish this by using a pulley and cam with an axis of rotation that is not in the center of the pulley. Figure 3.15 illustrates how the perpendicular distance increases when the pulley is rotated around the cam to increase the resistive torque toward the end of the exercise.

This style of training allows (in theory) greater resistance to be elicited throughout the entire ROM; however, it may not be practical for optimization of muscular strength. Because of the many differences between individuals, the design of these machines may be less than optimal. Regardless, machine workouts can be quite effective and time efficient and thus practical for the tactical athlete. Always ensure a proper fit in every exercise machine to optimize the biomechanics of the resistance.

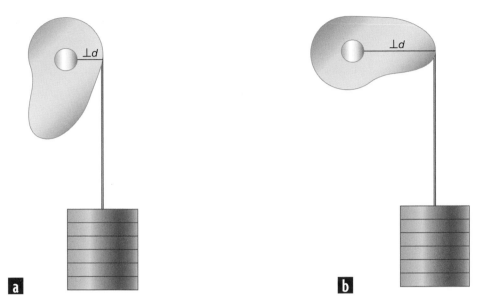

Figure 3.15 Variable-resistance exercises. Machines designed with an asymmetrical cable guide or gear will change the resistance torque to the body by changing the resistance arm (perpendicular distance to the axis of rotation). *(a)* The resistance arm is small, so the resistance torque is small. *(b)* The resistance torque is larger due to the larger resistance arm even though the weight stays the same.

Isokinetic

The word *isokinetic* means "same velocity," referring to the rate of movement through a ROM that is controlled, not the resistance on the barbell or standard weight training machine. Isokinetic exercises vary the resistance to the contracting muscles in order to maintain a constant speed of movement, and in doing so they compensate for the natural strong and weak points that exist in a ROM. Accordingly, these machines are good at measuring the amount of muscle torque the body can produce throughout an entire ROM, so they are not limited to the weakest biomechanical position, or the weak link in the chain. Examples of isokinetic training devices include the Biodex, Kin-Com, and Cybex dynamometers that are commonly used by physical therapists.

Isokinetic dynamometers are cost prohibitive for the typical strength and conditioning program and therefore not a usual component of tactical athlete training. And although a training tool that utilizes "same speed" may be a benefit in terms of controlling the rate of movement through a ROM, this type of movement is not typical in everyday activities for the tactical athlete. Movements and activities will have different speeds dependent on the joint angle and body positions. Therefore, the use of isokinetic training may lack transference (of muscular strength and power) from a biomechanical perspective. During the rehabilitation process, however, the tactical athlete might utilize an isokinetic training device rather than a stand-alone training apparatus.

Key Point

Various kinds of resistance training equipment focus on specific muscle actions (isometric, isotonic, and isokinetic). When used properly, each type effectively develops muscle strength. Considerations of how the different contractions will transfer to everyday performance of the tactical athlete should be at the forefront of exercise selection.

BIOMECHANICAL FACTORS AFFECTING MUSCLE STRENGTH

In addition to the action of a muscle, other factors contribute to the force the muscle produces. Many of the factors that determine the force generated by skeletal muscles are biomechanical, or physical, in nature. Some of these are discussed here.

Momentum

When lifting a weight at a fast speed, have you felt as if the weight continues on its own at the end of the movement natural range? This is because you have moved the weight fast enough to give it kinetic energy (energy of motion), sometimes referred to as *momentum*. Momentum is calculated by multiplying the mass of the object by the velocity of its movement. The energy of the weight due to this momentum will cause the weight to continue moving until gravity or another force stops the movement. It is important to understand momentum in weightlifting because it will change the muscle's activity during the second half of a repetition. For example, during the power clean exercise, the bar continues to rise after the initial upward pull due to its momentum, which provides time for the body to dip down to get under the bar and catch it in a crouched position. As another example of how momentum can affect exercise performance, think of doing a bench press with a light weight while exerting maximal muscle force at the fastest velocity possible. Toward the end of the movement, or repetition, the lifter must slow the momentum of the barbell by relaxing the agonist muscles of the chest (pectoralis major muscle) and perhaps even contracting the antagonist muscles of the upper back (latissimus dorsi).

Work

The mechanical definition of *work* is the amount of the force applied to an object multiplied by the distance traveled by that object. This term is useful in weightlifting when it is important to quantify the total amount of work performed during a workout. For example, if a weightlifter moved a 225-pound (1,001 N) barbell upward 2 feet (0.61 m) during each of 10 repetitions, then the total work completed during that set of 10 reps would be 4,500 foot-pounds (6,106 Nm) (225 × 2 × 10). This would be the *positive work* during the set because the applied force was in the same direction as the upward movement. But we must also account for the fact that the lifter also lowered the weight slowly to the original starting position, and as a result the lifter generated work during the negative phase of the movement. *Negative work* occurs when the movement is in the opposite direction

of the applied force. Therefore, the lifter would have completed 4,500 foot-pounds (6,106 Nm) of negative work while lowering the weight, and consequently the total work performed would be 9,000 foot-pounds (12,212 Nm). Weightlifters usually only calculate the positive work (weight training volume) when quantifying their workouts and, in most cases, they do not take into consideration the distance. This is known as volume load and would be 2,250 lb (10,010 N) in the previous example (225 lb (1,001 N) barbell × 10 reps).

Power

The term *power* is used in many ways in everyday life. However, *mechanical power* describes how fast we are able to complete the work associated with a given task (6). It is calculated as the amount of work performed per unit of time, with the units of power expressed in foot-pounds per second (ft-lb/s). For example, if a 140-pound (623 N) athlete walked up 12 10-inch (0.25 m) steps, she would have raised her body weight 120 inches (300 cm) or 10 feet (3 m). Therefore, a total of 1,400 foot-pounds (1,869 Nm) of work would have been completed. This work may have been completed in 5 seconds, thus producing 280 ft-lb/s (374 Nm/s) of power, or this same amount of work could have been done in 4 seconds, resulting in 350 ft-lb/s (467 Nm/s) of power. By producing the same amount of work in less time, more power would be generated. Alternatively, more power can be generated by doing a greater amount of work in the same amount of time. It is also possible to express power in units of horsepower (hp) by dividing the power quantified in units of foot-pounds per second by 550. This would convert the power in the previous examples from 280 ft-lb/s (374 Nm/s) to 0.51 hp or 350 ft-lb/s (467 Nm/s) to 0.64 hp. A trained weightlifter can produce about 2.5 hp for a few seconds, and an aerobically fit cyclist can produce about 0.5 hp for up to an hour.

CONCLUSION

The musculoskeletal and neuromuscular systems are major organ systems that account for a substantial portion of the human body's total mass. Skeletal muscle fulfills numerous important roles in the body, in large part by integrating with the skeletal and nervous systems to form the musculoskeletal and neuromuscular systems. But the most widely recognized function of skeletal muscle relates to its ability to contract and generate force. The broad spectrum of contractile activities that the same muscle tissue is able to conduct is quite remarkable. On a daily basis, we may rely on muscle to produce brief, powerful movements, and just minutes later we may ask those same muscles to continuously produce only mild or moderate force for an extended period time. The capacity to perform such a wide array of tasks is directly related to the structure and function of the individual muscle fibers that compose muscle tissue. More specifically, some types of muscle fibers have structural and metabolic profiles that are suited for short periods of high force produc-

tion, whereas other fiber types have size and metabolic characteristics that lend themselves to lower force production for long periods of time. It is truly impressive how these different types of fibers, with their different functional capacities, are found together in the same muscles, working together to maximize the capacity of the body to do physical work.

In this chapter, we have focused on describing skeletal and muscle structure and function, along with the principles of biomechanical analysis of movement. This information should enable the TSAC Facilitator to design effective training regimens for people in professions such as the military, law enforcement, and fire and rescue, where physical strength and fitness are essential for optimal job performance.

Key Terms

actin
antagonist
contractility
elasticity
excitability
excitation–contraction (E–C) coupling
extensibility
Golgi tendon organs (GTOs)
motor unit
muscle spindle

myosin
neuromuscular junction (NMJ)
ossification
osteoblast
osteoclast
prime mover
sarcomere
sarcoplasmic reticulum
size principle
synergist

Study Questions

1. During the eccentric movement of the biceps curl exercise, the triceps brachii acts as what type of mover?

   a. agonist

   b. antagonist

   c. synergist

   d. stabilizer

2. Which of the following skeletal muscle tissue characteristics gives the muscle the ability to stretch beyond its normal, resting length?

   a. excitability

   b. contractibility

   c. extensibility

   d. elasticity

3. The biceps femoris, semitendinosus, and semimembranosus muscles belong to which of the following major muscle groups?

   a. gluteals

   b. hamstrings

   c. quadriceps

   d. shoulder complex

4. Which of the following are the regulatory proteins of the myofilaments that are involved in the sliding filament mechanism?

   a. actin and myosin

   b. troponin and tropomyosin

   c. myosin and troponin

   d. actin and tropomyosin

Chapter 4

Physiological Adaptations and Bioenergetics

Todd Miller, PhD, CSCS,*D, TSAC-F, FNSCA

After completing this chapter, you will be able to

- identify the characteristics of the primary energy systems,
- define the training variables that can affect performance outcomes,
- describe the physiological adaptations to exercise designed to improve fitness and performance,
- discuss the volume and rate of detraining as it relates to aerobic and anaerobic capacity, and
- discuss the training requirements necessary to maintain training adaptations.

The human body is a remarkable machine, capable of tremendous feats of strength, endurance, and power. Like many machines, the body requires fuel to operate, and this fuel is contained in the food and drink we consume daily. The breakdown of food into usable energy is called *metabolism*, and the transfer of that energy within the body is referred to as **bioenergetics**. The bioenergetic pathways discussed in this chapter include the ATP-PCr system, glycolysis, and the aerobic pathway. Each of these pathways is operating to different degrees during exercise, and the capacity of each can be manipulated through training. These manipulations lead to changes in strength, endurance, power, speed, and muscle size. This chapter focuses on the operation of these biochemical pathways and training strategies for improving their performance.

BIOENERGETICS AND METABOLISM

Through the process of metabolism, chemical energy is liberated from **macronutrients** (carbohydrate, fat, and protein) in the form of the compound ATP (adenosine triphosphate). ATP provides the energy for all cellular work, and the vast majority of ATP is consumed by skeletal muscle. Indeed, skeletal muscle can be thought of as the engine that allows us to run, jump, climb, carry, drag, lift, and so on, and therefore it is the tissue where chemical energy is ultimately converted into mechanical work. Carbohydrate, protein, and fat are the three macronutrients that make up food. Normally, only carbohydrate and fat are significant sources of fuel, whereas protein is used primarily in maintaining and synthesizing muscle.

ATP-PCr, or Phosphagen, System

The immediate availability of energy to power skeletal muscle is critical during activities such as vertical jumping, short-distance sprinting, and maximal lifting. The bioenergetic pathway responsible for providing ATP during these high-intensity activities is the **ATP-PCr system** or **phosphagen system**. The ATP-PCr system resides in the skeletal muscle sarcoplasm (cytoplasm of skeletal muscle) and derives its name from the

biochemical compounds involved in the chemical reactions that produce energy: ATP and creatine phosphate (CP), also called **phosphocreatine (PCr)**. Muscle cells contain a pool of both ATP and PCr in varying concentrations, with about four to six times more PCr than ATP (16). When energy demand is high and immediate (e.g., a 40 yd [37 m dash]), ATP is rapidly broken down within the muscle to provide energy for the activity, and the ATP concentration in the muscle falls. The breakdown of ATP occurs via the actions of an enzyme called *myosin ATPase* and results in the splitting of the ATP molecule into adenosine diphosphate (ADP) and inorganic phosphate (P_i):

$$ATP \xrightarrow{\text{ATPase}} ADP + P_i$$

The removal of one P_i from the ATP molecule releases energy, which is used to power muscular work. The majority of the remaining ADP is not broken down further and does not contribute to energy provision. As the activity continues, ATP concentration within the muscle rapidly falls, and ATP must be resynthesized for the activity to continue. The cleavage of the high-energy bond in PCr liberates energy, which is used to resynthesize ADP and P_i according to the following equation:

$$ADP + CP \xleftarrow{\text{Creatine kinase}} ATP + Creatine$$

If high-intensity exercise continues, PCr is eventually depleted, and the exercise intensity must decrease. Typically, the ATP-PCr system can provide energy for short bursts of maximal activity not greater than approximately 6 seconds.

When attempting to improve performance in activities that use the ATP-PCr system as the primary energetic pathway, the principle of exercise **specificity** applies. High-intensity exercises should be chosen that require a high degree of power or force. For example, when improvement of single-effort power is the goal, as in a maximal lift in the power clean, loads should be close to maximal and only one to two repetitions should be executed for three to five sets (1). When training the ATP-PCr system, rest periods should be 2 to 5 minutes to allow for adequate resynthesis of ATP and PCr (1).

Key Point

The ATP-PCr system is important for the tactical population due to the high-intensity, short-burst activities that are often required on the job. Care should be taken to incorporate exercises, drills, and training protocols that address the ATP-PCr system.

Glycolysis

The second bioenergetic pathway involved in ATP production during exercise is **glycolysis**, also known as the glycolytic pathway. This pathway acts as the predominant source of energy during all-out efforts lasting up to about 90 seconds. Glycolysis consists of a series of chemical reactions that break down **glucose** from the blood and **glycogen** in the muscle. Fat cannot be broken down via the glycolytic pathway. Similar to the ATP-PCr system, glycolysis also occurs in the skeletal muscle sarcoplasm and involves a series of enzymatic reactions that begin with glucose or glycogen as the starting compound and end with **pyruvate** or **lactate** (figure 4.1). Glycolysis is often known as **anaerobic**, fast, or partial, glycolysis because it is the rapid, partial breakdown of glucose that occurs without the need for oxygen. The rate at which glucose is broken down in the muscle determines whether lactate or pyruvate is the primary end product of glycolysis. When exercise intensity is high and glucose is rapidly broken down, lactate is the end product.

Lactate

The breakdown of glucose in the muscle sarcoplasm produces hydrogen, much of which is shuttled into the **mitochondria** by binding to the compound nicotinamide adenine dinucleotide (NAD$^+$) to form NADH. The rapid breakdown of glucose that occurs when cellular energy demands are high causes some of this hydrogen to bind to pyruvate, resulting in the formation of lactate. Lactate production increases with exercise intensity (7, 20) and appears to depend on muscle fiber phenotype. For example, fast-twitch fibers have a greater concentration of glycolytic enzymes (2, 17) and therefore can break down glucose at a higher rate than slow-twitch fibers can. This is consistent with the significant lactate accumulation that occurs during high-intensity exercise, which is when the fast-twitch fibers are most active. Lactate concentrations in blood are a function of the rates of lactate production and clearance in the muscle. During low-intensity exercise, lactate clearance is equal to its production, resulting in stable levels of blood lactate. Both aerobic and anaerobic exercise training result in a greater ability to metabolize lactate following the cessation of exercise (5, 7), and exercise at approximately 35% of $\dot{V}O_2$max has been shown to be effective at increasing lactate clearance (figure 4.2).

Historically, lactate was thought to be a waste product of muscle metabolism that limited exercise performance. In reality, lactate provides a significant source of energy during exercise (2, 15, 23), and lactate that is not metabolized during exercise is converted back into glucose or glycogen in the liver via a process called the **Cori cycle** (figure 4.3). As lactate is produced in muscle, much of it is carried into the bloodstream and ultimately to the liver. In the liver, lactate undergoes a type of reverse glycolysis, converting back into glucose. During exercise, this glucose is typically sent back into the bloodstream, where it is carried to muscle so it can be used as fuel. When exercise ends or energy demands are low, lactate in the liver can be converted to glycogen and stored for later use.

Exercise that involves a significant contribution from anaerobic glycolysis often leads to an accumulation of lactate in the blood. The point at which the rate of lactate production by the muscles exceeds the rate of lactate clearance is the **lactate threshold (LT)**. With increasingly higher exercise intensities, a second inflection point occurs on the lactate curve. This point is termed the **onset of blood lactate accumulation (OBLA)**, and it occurs when the blood lactate concentration reaches 4 mmol/L (12, 21, 22). The LT in untrained people typically occurs at an exercise intensity corresponding to 50% to 60% of $\dot{V}O_2$max. Chronic exercise training results in a rightward shift of the lactate curve (figure 4.4, page 54), resulting in an LT that occurs at 70% to 80% of $\dot{V}O_2$max in trained athletes (3, 4). This shift is likely due to an increased ability to generate ATP aerobically, which delays the need to increase the reliance on anaerobic glycolysis for ATP production.

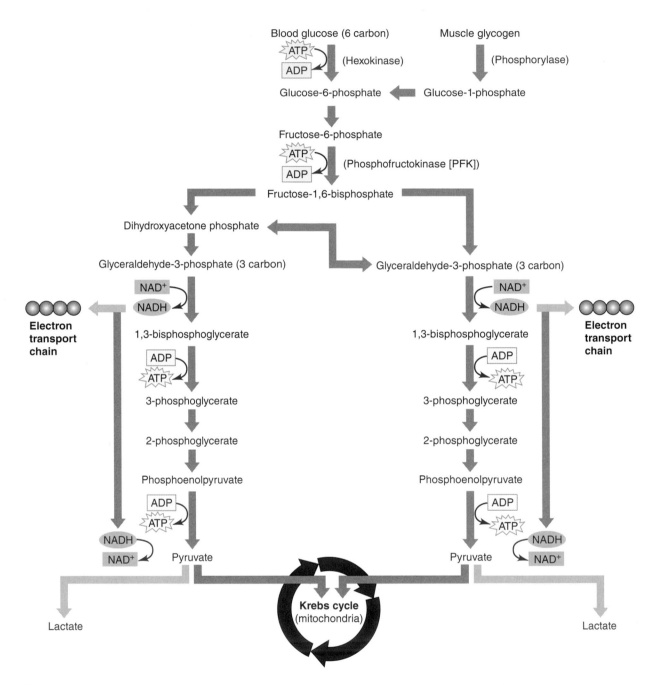

Figure 4.1 Glycolysis. The glycolytic pathway involves the enzymatic breakdown of glucose or glycogen to pyruvate or lactate.

Reprinted, by permission, from NSCA, 2016, Bioenergetics of exercise and training, T.J. Herda and J.T. Cramer. In *Essentials of strength training and conditioning*, 4th ed., edited by G.G. Haff and N.T. Triplett (Champaign, IL: Human Kinetics), 47.

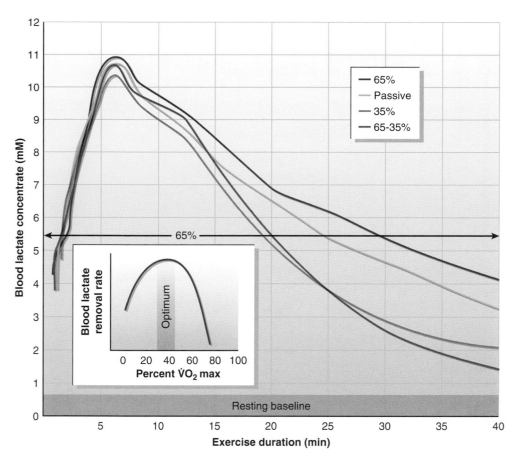

Figure 4.2 Blood lactate concentration following maximal exercise using passive recovery and active recoveries at 35%, 65%, and combination 35% and 65% $\dot{V}O_2$max. The horizontal white line indicates the blood lactate level produced by exercise at 65% $\dot{V}O_2$max without previous exercise. The bottom inset curve depicts the relationship between exercise intensity and blood lactate removal.

Adapted with permission from S. Dodd, S.K. Powers, T. Callender, E. Brooks. 1984, "Blood lactate disappearance at various intensities of recovery exercise." *Journal of Applied Physiology*, 57(5):1462. Copyright © 1984 the American Physiological Society.

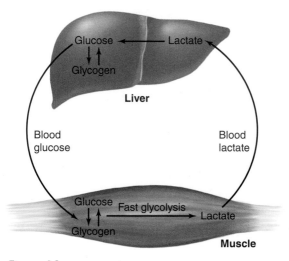

Figure 4.3 Cori cycle.

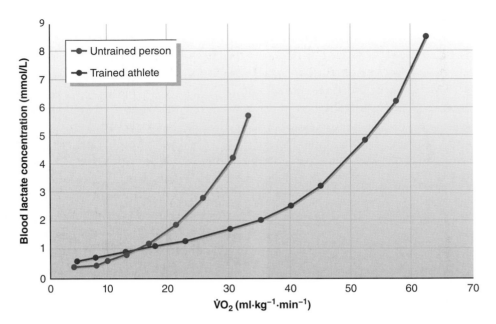

Figure 4.4   Lactate threshold and onset of blood lactate accumulation.

Reprinted, by permission, from NSCA, 2016, Bioenergetics of exercise and training, T.J. Herda and J.T. Cramer. In *Essentials of strength training and conditioning*, 4th ed., edited by G.G. Haff and N.T. Triplett (Champaign, IL: Human Kinetics), 51.

Key Point

A common goal of training is to increase the exercise intensity at which the LT occurs. This allows the tactical athlete to perform more intense work with less muscular fatigue.

Increased capacity of the glycolytic pathway is achieved through multiple-effort, high-intensity lifts, exercises, and drills. For example, interval sprinting is a popular technique that is commonly used to improve glycolytic performance. Improvements in glycolytic metabolism can occur by manipulating the sprint time or intensity, as well as the length of the rest intervals, with shorter rest periods resulting in greater overload of the glycolytic pathway (1).

Aerobic Metabolism

During exercise of lower intensity, pyruvate is the primary end product of glycolysis. The pyruvate enters the mitochondria, where it undergoes slow or complete glycolysis, resulting in the total breakdown of glucose into carbon dioxide and water. Anaerobic glycolysis only liberates about 5% of the available energy from a glucose molecule, with the remaining 95% being liberated in the mitochondria during **aerobic** metabolism. The complete breakdown of one glucose molecule yields 36 ATP, only 4 of which come from anaerobic glycolysis. The vast majority of ATP produced during exercise is done so aerobically in the mitochondria of the muscle cells. Both fat and carbohydrate are metabolized in this manner. Aerobic metabolism can be viewed as a two-step process. In step 1, hydrogen atoms are stripped from a compound called *acetyl coenzyme A*, or *acetyl-CoA*. This phase is known as the citric acid cycle, Krebs cycle, or **tricarboxylic acid (TCA) cycle**. In step 2, these hydrogen atoms are combined with oxygen in the **electron transport chain (ETC)**, which ultimately produces CO_2, H_2O, and large amounts of ATP. Because of the tremendous potential of the aerobic pathway to provide energy, the ability to supply oxygen to skeletal muscle is one of the most important factors in human exercise performance.

Tricarboxylic Acid Cycle0

Once glucose has been broken down into pyruvate in the sarcoplasm during anaerobic glycolysis, it crosses into the mitochondria and is converted into acetyl-CoA, which is the starting compound in the TCA cycle. Fat, which is broken down through a process known as **beta-oxidation**, also enters the mitochondria and undergoes conversion to acetyl-CoA. Once converted to acetyl-CoA, both lipids and glucose are metabolized identically. The TCA cycle is a series of enzymatic reactions that break down acetyl-CoA into the intermediates shown in figure 4.5. The basic operation of the cycle involves an initial chemical interaction between acetyl-CoA and oxaloacetate, which forms citrate. Following citrate, there are nine more intermediates, with the last one ending up as oxaloacetate. At this point, the cycle begins again. Only one ATP is generated with each turn of the TCA cycle; the primary goal of the cycle is to liberate hydrogen atoms from the TCA intermediates so that they can combine with NAD^+ and

FAD to form NADH and $FADH_2$. These hydrogen atoms are then shuttled from NADH and $FADH_2$ across the inner mitochondrial membrane, where they enter the ETC.

Electron Transport Chain

The ETC is a series of coupled chemical reactions that take place in the mitochondria. Hydrogen ions that have been liberated in the TCA cycle act as electron donors, passing electrons to a progressively more electronegative acceptor within the inner mitochondrial membrane. The terminal and most electronegative acceptor in the chain is oxygen, and the binding of hydrogen to oxygen produces water. The process of electron transport creates an electrochemical proton gradient between the inner and outer mitochondrial

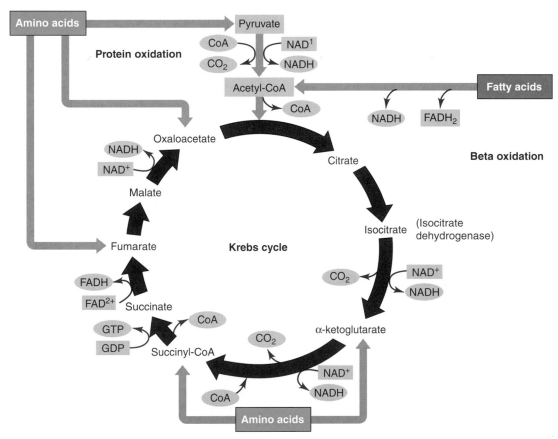

Figure 4.5 Tricarboxylic acid cycle.

CoA = coenzyme A; FAD^{2+}, FADH, $FADH_2$ = flavin adenine dinucleotide; GDP = guanine diphosphate; GTP = guanine triphosphate; NAD^+, NADH = nicotinamide adenine dinucleotide.

Reprinted, by permission, from NSCA, 2016, Bioenergetics of exercise and training, T.J. Herda and J.T. Cramer. In *Essentials of strength training and conditioning*, 4th ed., edited by G.G. Haff and N.T. Triplett (Champaign, IL: Human Kinetics), 52.

membranes, which creates the energy necessary for ATP synthesis. In short, the ETC frees up the potential energy from hydrogen, thereby moving hydrogen to a lower state of energy and harnessing that energy to synthesize ATP (figure 4.6). A popular analogy used to describe this process is that of a series of waterfalls that are used to drive paddle wheels in order to produce energy. As the water moves from a state of high potential energy to a state of low potential energy, mechanical work is performed in the form of turning the wheels.

ATP Production From Fat

The typical human being has an enormous volume of energy stored in the body in the form of fat. For example, a 165-pound (75 kg) man with a body-fat percentage of 15 would have 86,625 kcal of energy stored as fat, roughly the equivalent of 107 sticks of butter. The majority of this fat is stored as **triacylglycerols** in cells (adipocytes) that are located under the skin and

around the internal organs. A smaller amount of fat is stored inside the skeletal muscles. Fat is a major source of energy at rest and during low-intensity exercise, when oxygen demands are relatively low. As exercise intensity increases, the proportion of fat being burned progressively decreases, and the reliance on carbohydrate as fuel progressively increases.

Breakdown of fat (lipolysis) occurs under the influence of an enzyme called *hormone-sensitive lipase*, which cleaves the triacylglycerol into fatty acids and glycerol, which are then released into the bloodstream. Fatty acids then travel into the skeletal muscle mitochondria, where they are converted to acetyl-CoA through a process called *beta-oxidation*. This acetyl-CoA enters the TCA cycle and ETC as previously described. Glycerol is also delivered to the skeletal muscle, where it enters the glycolytic pathway and is converted to pyruvate. Glycerol can also be used to form glucose during times of muscle glycogen depletion, which can happen due to dietary carbohydrate restriction or exhaustive exercise (figure 4.7). Increases in aerobic capacity occur following exercise training that primarily relies on oxygen for energy production. Prolonged, low- to moderate-intensity, steady-state exercises are typically incorporated when the training goal is to increase aerobic endurance.

PHYSIOLOGICAL ADAPTATIONS TO EXERCISE

Physical exercise places a significant amount of stress on the body, and the body adapts accordingly to meet the increased physical demands. The SAID (specific adaptation to imposed demands) principle asserts that in a biological system, the adaptations that occur following exposure to some stressor (e.g., physical training) are determined by the **mode**, **intensity**, **frequency**, and **duration** of the stressor. For example, heavy resistance training will increase muscle size and strength, whereas long-term endurance training will decrease muscle size and increase the ability to resist fatigue during prolonged aerobic exercise.

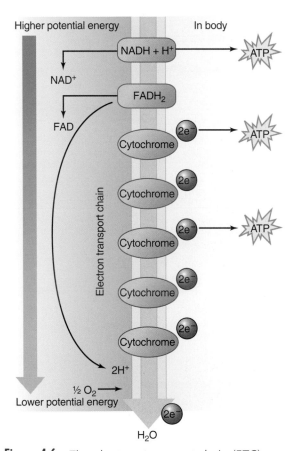

Figure 4.6   The electron transport chain (ETC).

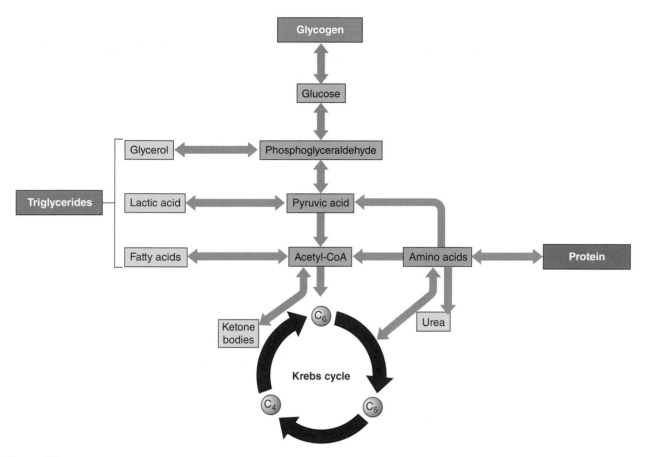

Figure 4.7 The metabolism of fat and of carbohydrate and protein share some common pathways. Note that many are oxidized to acetyl-CoA and enter the TCA cycle.

Reprinted, by permission, from NSCA, 2016, Bioenergetics of exercise and training, T.J. Herda and J.T. Cramer. In *Essentials of strength training and conditioning*, 4th ed., edited by G.G. Haff and N.T. Triplett (Champaign, IL: Human Kinetics), 54.

Key Point

Of the four training variables (mode, intensity, frequency, and duration), improvements in performance are most closely tied to intensity. Both aerobic and anaerobic activities must be performed at an intensity that is high enough to bring about the desired adaptations.

Aerobic Endurance

The ability to function aerobically at a high level relies on the ability of the cardiorespiratory system to deliver oxygen to the muscles, coupled with the ability of the muscles to utilize oxygen to produce ATP. Therefore, we can view the adaptations to aerobic exercise as those that involve both central (cardiorespiratory) and peripheral (skeletal muscle) adaptations. The metric that most often defines aerobic capacity is $\dot{V}O_2max$, which refers to the maximum amount of oxygen that the body can use in a given unit of time. Mathematically, $\dot{V}O_2max$ can be calculated according to the **Fick equation**:

$$\dot{V}O_2max = \dot{Q}\,max \times A\dot{V}O_2diff$$

where $\dot{Q}$ is equal to **cardiac output** and $A\dot{V}O_2diff$ is equal to the difference in oxygen content between the arterial and venous blood.

Because the lungs do not show a large degree of adaptation to aerobic training, we can consider the adaptations of primary importance to be those that positively affect cardiac output. Cardiac output is defined as the product of HR and SV:

$$\dot{Q} = HR \times SV$$

Increases in maximal HR or SV would lead to increases in Q̇. Following long-term aerobic training, maximal HR does not increase and may even decrease slightly (16). However, SV has a tremendous capacity for growth, and it is the primary contributing factor to an increased aerobic capacity following aerobic training. Indeed, SV has been shown to be twice as high in endurance athletes when compared with recreationally active individuals (19). Because of the increased amount of blood ejected per heartbeat following chronic endurance training, resting HR is much lower in well-trained endurance athletes. A lower HR is also seen during submaximal exercise in well-trained people. This is evident when comparing the exercise HRs of both a trained and an untrained person who are exercising at the same absolute submaximal intensity. The untrained person will generally have a much higher HR than the trained person, despite having similar cardiac outputs at a fixed workload (figure 4.8).

Due to the large increases in cardiac output that occur following chronic endurance exercise, the ability to deliver blood to exercising muscle is greatly increased. As such, both structural and biochemical changes within the muscle must occur in order for the muscle to allow for increased blood flow and oxygen extraction. Of the structural changes that occur, an increase in muscle capillarization is one of the most profound, with V̇O₂max increasing linearly as the number of muscle capillaries increases (19). In response to the chronically increased blood flow that occurs with long-term endurance training, the protein vascular endothelial growth factor (VEGF) is elevated, which causes new capillaries to form within the muscle (6). This increase in capillary number allows for an increase in blood flow through the muscle without a concomitant increase in the velocity of blood flow, which in turn allows for adequate oxygen extraction time.

A second important structural adaption to endurance exercise is a decrease in muscle fiber cross-sectional area (CSA) (1). This decrease allows for a smaller muscle area to be perfused by each capillary, and it minimizes the distance oxygen must travel to get from the capillary to the interior portion of the muscle cell. Increases in mitochondrial number and volume also result

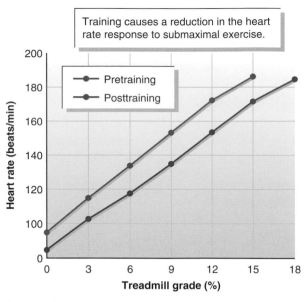

Figure 4.8 Training reduces the HR response to submaximal exercise.

Reprinted, by permission, from E.T. Howley and D.L. Thompson, 2016, *Fitness professional's handbook*, 6th ed. (Champaign, IL: Human Kinetics), 78.

from long-term aerobic training, leading to a greater enzymatic capacity of the muscle to utilize oxygen for ATP production. Adaptations to aerobic exercise are summarized in table 4.1.

Muscular Endurance

Muscular **endurance** refers to a muscle's ability to contract repeatedly against a submaximal load in a given period of time, or the ability to sustain a given submaximal force for an extended period of time. Measuring the maximum number of push-ups or pull-ups one can do in a limited amount of time is a common field technique for assessing muscular endurance. Resistance training programs that are designed to improve muscular endurance typically involve repeated muscular contractions against a relatively light load. The generalized adaptations to resistance training expressed as a function of training intensity are shown in figure 4.9 (page 60).

Muscular endurance can be expressed in absolute or relative terms. An example of a test of relative endurance would be a bench press test where people complete as many repetitions as possible with 70% of their 1RM (one repetition

Table 4.1 Physiological Adaptations to Aerobic Endurance Training

Variable	Aerobic endurance adaptations
Performance	
Muscular strength	No change
Muscular endurance	Increases for low power output
Aerobic power	Increases
Maximal rate of force production	No change or decreases
Vertical jump	No change
Anaerobic power	No change
Sprint speed	No change
Muscle fibers	
Fiber size	No change or increases slightly
Capillary density	Increases
Mitochondrial density	Increases
Myofibrillar packing density	No change
Myofibrillar volume	No change
Cytoplasmic density	No change
Myosin heavy chain protein	No change or decreases amount
Enzyme activity	
Creatine phosphokinase	Increases
Myokinase	Increases
Phosphofructokinase	Variable
Lactate dehydrogenase	Variable
Sodium–potassium ATPase	May slightly increase
Metabolic energy stores	
Stored ATP	Increases
Stored creatine phosphate	Increases
Stored glycogen	Increases
Stored triglycerides	Increase
Connective tissue	
Ligament strength	Increases
Tendon strength	Increases
Collagen content	Variable
Bone density	No change or increases
Body composition	
% body fat	Decreases
Fat-free mass	No change

ATP = adenosine triphosphate; ATPase = adenosine triphosphatase.

Reprinted, by permission, from NSCA, 2016, Adaptations to aerobic endurance training programs. In *Essentials of strength training and conditioning*, 4th ed., edited by G.G. Haff and N.T. Triplett (Champaign, IL: Human Kinetics), 121.

maximum). In contrast, a popular test of absolute endurance is the bench press test at the National Football League (NFL) Scouting Combine, where prospective NFL players complete as many repetitions as possible with a 225-pound (102 kg) barbell. Absolute endurance correlates well with muscular strength, but only when the external load being lifted is greater than 25% of the athlete's 1RM (24). Several morphological and enzymatic adaptations occur following long-term endurance training that lead to increased muscular endurance. Increases in mitochondrial size and number lead to an increased ability to utilize oxygen, thereby increasing the aerobic production of ATP at low levels of exercise intensity. Increases in the glycolytic enzymes lead to increased muscular endurance against moderate loads and increased capacity to break down glucose and glycogen. Endurance training with moderate loads also promotes an increased aerobic capacity of the fast-twitch muscle fibers, which delays fatigue during high-intensity endurance exercise.

Strength

Muscular **strength** can be defined as the maximum amount of force that a muscle or muscle group can generate at a specific velocity (14). The ability of a muscle to generate force is a function of input from the CNS and the physiological and anatomical properties of the muscle itself. Therefore, training to increase muscular strength should involve techniques that cause physical changes to the muscles, as well as enhancement of the neural pathways that innervate those muscles.

The nerves that innervate skeletal muscle are called *motor neurons*, and they are responsible for carrying signals from the CNS that tell the muscle to contract. Each motor neuron innervates a specific set of muscle fibers. A motor neuron and all the fibers that it innervates is called a *motor unit*. The number of muscle fibers innervated by a motor unit is determined by the primary role of the muscle. Relatively large muscles that are responsible for gross movements, such as ambulation, typically consist of motor units that innervate hundreds of fibers per unit, whereas small muscles that require fine motor control (such as those that move the eyes) can have motor units that consist of as few as one muscle fiber

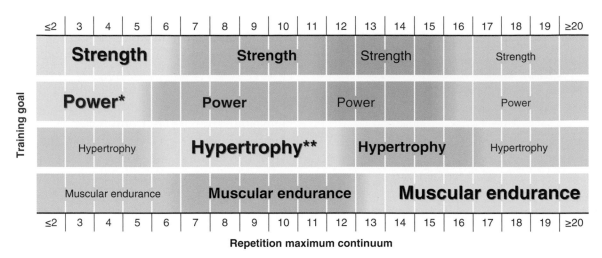

Figure 4.9 Continuum of RM ranges associated with various training goals.

*The repetition ranges shown for power in this figure are not consistent with the %1RM–repetition relationship.

**Although the existing repetition range for hypertrophy appears most efficacious, there is emerging evidence that some fiber types, depending on training status, may experience significant hypertrophy outside this range. It is too early to tell if these results would be experienced by the larger population.

Reprinted, by permission, from NSCA, 2016, Program design for resistance training, J.M. Sheppard and N.T Triplett. In *Essentials of strength training and conditioning*, 4th ed., edited by G.G. Haff and N.T. Triplett (Champaign, IL: Human Kinetics), 457.

per motor neuron. Gradations in strength within a muscle are accomplished by either increasing the number of active motor units or increasing the firing frequency of the motor units.

Neural factors are also involved during complex movements where multiple muscles or muscle groups are firing simultaneously. This intermuscular coordination is critical for maximizing strength during complex movements such as the snatch, clean and jerk, squat, and deadlift. As a general rule, the greater the complexity of the movement, the greater the role of neural factors. Therefore, the increases in strength that novice athletes see early in training are often more a result of changes in neural factors than physiological changes in the muscles themselves. This is particularly true of complex movements.

Muscular strength is often expressed as a repetition maximum (RM), with *1RM load* referring to the maximum amount of weight a person can lift only once while maintaining proper form for a given exercise. The adaptations that result from resistance training are primarily determined by the RM load used in the training. Figure 4.9 shows the RM continuum and the related adaptations at each RM range. As one might expect, maximal

strength is most improved by training at low RM loads. However, because muscle size plays a large role in strength development, it's prudent to also incorporate RM loads into a training program that help increase muscle CSA. The relationship between muscle strength and muscle CSA is shown in figure 4.10.

Key Point

Improvements in strength and power result from both neural and morphological changes. Training programs should be balanced to appropriately address both muscular and neural adaptations.

Resistance training programs for increasing strength should incorporate strategies that target neuromuscular as well as morphological adaptations. Increasing intramuscular coordination results in a greater number of motor units that can be voluntary recruited, thereby leading to greater muscle force production. Training for the purpose of maximizing intramuscular coordination should involve lifting near-maximal loads (1RM-3RM) or lifting moderate loads (10RM-12RM) to muscular failure. A submaximal load that is not lifted to failure will not recruit the fastest motor units and will

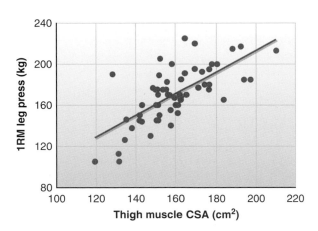

Figure 4.10 Linear relationship between leg strength and muscle CSA.

Reprinted by permission, from R. Koopman and L.J. van Loon, 2009, "Aging, exercise, and muscle protein metabolism," *Journal of Applied Physiology* 106(6): 2040-2048.

not maximize intramuscular coordination (24).

The most important morphological adaptation to resistance training with respect to increased strength is increased muscle size. This increase occurs when moderate-intensity loads (6RM-12RM) are lifted to, or nearly to, muscular failure. Lifting loads of this intensity requires a large volume of mechanical work, which leads to a high amount of muscle protein degradation. Muscle adapts to this degradation by increasing its CSA, which ultimately leads to increases in strength (24). Type II muscle fibers are the most affected by resistance training. In fact, the fast-twitch fibers of elite weightlifters are about 45% larger than those of sedentary people and endurance athletes (15).

Power

Although muscular strength plays an important role during certain tasks, muscular **power** is often a more critical factor. By definition, *power* is the rate of doing work. Work is the product of the force exerted on an object multiplied by the distance that the object travels. Mathematically, power is calculated as

$$power = work / time$$

or

$$power = force \times velocity$$

where

$$work = force \times distance$$

and

$$velocity = distance / time$$

The force × velocity relationship is one of the most important to understand when designing training programs. It is evident from figure 4.11 that when the load is high, velocity is low, and thus so is muscular power. Similarly, when movement velocity is high, the force generated by the muscle is relatively low, and thus so is the power. Maximal muscle power is usually produced when training with 30% of the maximum velocity and 50% of maximum force (24).

Power can be affected by changing either the force component or the velocity component, both of which can be manipulated through training. Programs that focus on heavy resistance training will increase muscle force production, but heavy resistance training alone is not effective at maximizing muscular power. Indeed, elite power athletes are necessarily strong, but not all elite strength athletes are powerful. As is the case with training for maximal strength, power is optimally developed when resistance training is performed with high-intensity loads. Additionally, training with moderate-intensity loads at a high velocity is equally important for increasing muscular power. Increases in muscle size lead to increases in strength, which result in an increased ability to move a load quickly, which directly leads to increases in power. Therefore, some degree of **hypertrophy** training should be incorporated when the goal is to maximize muscular power. Rate of force development (RFD) must also be trained, and this is accomplished by attempting to move heavy loads as quickly as possible. While training for RFD, the actual movement velocity of the load might be low, but the attempt to rapidly move the load is the key, because this rapidly imparts force into the implement to be moved (24). Training should also include plyometric exercises in order to maximize power (see chapter 13).

Speed

Speed can possibly be used interchangeably with *velocity* and refers to the distance a body travels per unit of time. Although speed and power are measured

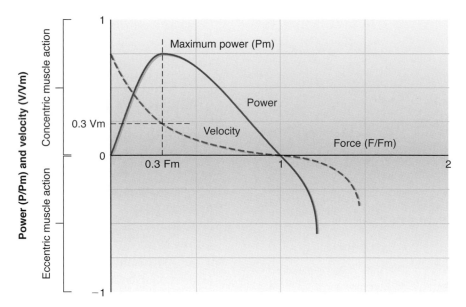

Figure 4.11   Velocity as a function of force and resulting power production and absorption in concentric and eccentric muscle actions. The greatest forces occur during explosive eccentric (lengthening) actions. Depending on the movement, maximum power (Pm) is usually produced at 30% to 50% of maximum force (Fm) and velocity (Vm).

Reprinted, by permission, from S.S. Plisk, 2008, Speed, agility, and speed-endurance development. In *Essentials of strength training and conditioning*, edited by T.R. Baechle and R.W. Earle (Champaign, IL: Human Kinetics), 460; Adapted, by permission, from J.A. Faulkner, D.R. Claflin, and K.K. McCully, 1986, Power output of fast and slow fibers from skeletal muscles. In *Human muscle power*, edited by N.L. Jones, N. McCarney, and A.J. McComas (Champaign, IL: Human Kinetics), 88.

differently and represent different values, they are related in that a high degree of muscular power is necessary to reach maximal speed quickly. Consider a 40-yard (37 m) dash, which is a common measure of speed. It is more accurate to characterize a 40-yard (37 m) dash as a test of acceleration because the person's maximal running speed may never be reached during the sprint. For example, the fastest running speed ever recorded was during a 100 m (109 yd) dash by Jamaican runner Usain Bolt in 2009. Bolt reached a maximal running speed of 27.78 miles per hour (44.71 km/h), but this speed was reached between the 60th and 80th meter of the run. Therefore, when using a 40-yard (37 m) dash to measure speed, we are referring to *average* speed over the distance, and the magnitude of the speed depends on the ability to accelerate quickly. The rate of change in velocity per unit of time defines acceleration, and it is the critical component of sprinting performance. The ability to accelerate quickly depends on the ability to rapidly transmit force from the foot into the ground, and this ability depends on lower body power. Training protocols that maximize lower body power thus should be incorporated along with specific speed training to increase sprinting performance (see chapter 13). Decreases in body fatness will also have a profound positive effect on running speed, and decreasing excess body fat is often the easiest and fastest way to improve running performance.

DETRAINING AND RETRAINING

Detraining refers to the decrease in some performance variable following a cessation in training or a decrease in volume, frequency, or intensity of training. Performance losses are specific to the type of training that decreases. For example, a reduction in aerobic endurance training will result in changes to the enzymatic and morphological properties of the musculoskeletal and cardiorespiratory systems that come about as a result of aerobic exercise. Similarly, a decrease in resistance training volume, intensity, or frequency will bring about losses in muscle size, strength, and power. Elite athletes can experience performance losses in weeks or even days following cessation of exercise (24). For example, a two-week cessation in training in male powerlifters resulted in a 12% loss of isokinetic eccentric strength and 6.4% loss of Type II muscle fiber area (13). The degree to which these decrements occur largely depends on the length of the detraining period, or the magnitude of the decrement in training volume or intensity. Long breaks in training are unhealthy and serve no useful purpose in the development of human performance. Periodization protocols are often used to eliminate long rest periods, thereby mitigating or eliminating the detraining that those rest periods often bring about.

Increases in performance that occur during retraining often occur much faster than they do when a person first begins a training program. This phenomenon supports the notion of muscle memory. It is likely that neural factors also play a major role in the ability to rapidly increase performance during retraining. The effects of detraining on some key physiological variables involved in performance are shown in figure 4.12.

The effects of detraining following cessation of resistance training are also heavily influenced by the training protocol done prior to cessation.

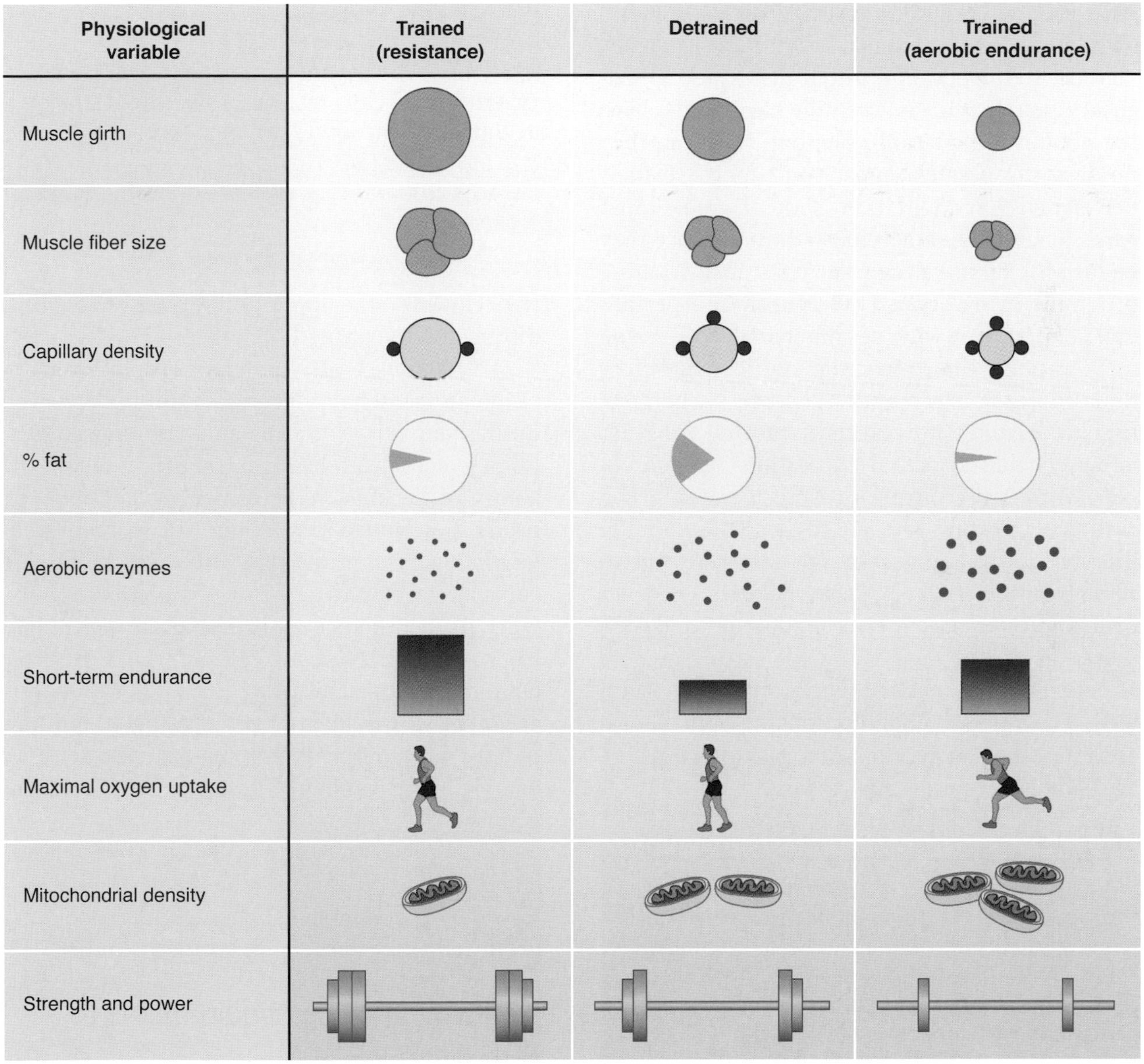

Physiological variable	Trained (resistance)	Detrained	Trained (aerobic endurance)
Muscle girth			
Muscle fiber size			
Capillary density			
% fat			
Aerobic enzymes			
Short-term endurance			
Maximal oxygen uptake			
Mitochondrial density			
Strength and power			

Figure 4.12   Relative responses of physiological variables to training and detraining.

Reprinted, by permission, from S.J. Fleck and W.J. Kraemer, 2014, *Designing resistance training programs*, 4th ed. (Champaign, IL: Human Kinetics), 298.

Gains in strength and performance that occur over a long training period tend to persist longer after cessation of training compared with gains that occur rapidly. In one study, for example, a group whose training lasted less than 2 weeks lost all strength gains nearly 40 weeks earlier than a group who trained daily over a longer period of time (8).

Time Course of Physiological and Anatomical Changes

The rate and degree to which the body adapts to strength and endurance training are highly variable and are most influenced by training intensity, volume, frequency, and initial fitness level. Sedentary people with no training experience have the greatest adaptation potential, meaning they possess the greatest capacity to increase their performance and will likely show the most rapid gains in strength or aerobic endurance once they begin an exercise program. Resistance training programs bring about both central and peripheral adaptations, with neural changes occurring more rapidly than muscular ones. In fact, the rapid increase in strength that occurs when one first undertakes a resistance training program is largely due to neural adaptations. The act of generating force during resistance training is a skill that improves as the CNS becomes better at muscle coordination and motor unit recruitment. Increases in muscle CSA also make a significant contribution to muscle force production, and such increases can be seen as quickly as three weeks after beginning a resistance training program (16). The relative contributions of both neural and muscular adaptations to resistance training are shown in figure 4.13.

Key Point

Adaptations that occur as a result of training are lost more quickly than they are gained once the training stops. The TSAC Facilitator must ensure that training frequency and intensity are adequate for increasing or maintaining improvements in performance.

Both neural and peripheral adaptations make an important contribution to muscle force produc-

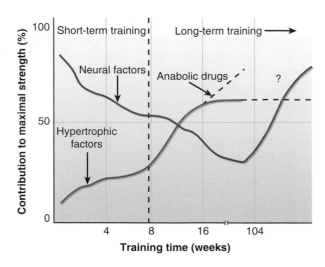

Figure 4.13 The dynamic interplay of neural and hypertrophic factors resulting in increased strength during short- and long-term training periods.

Reprinted, by permission, from S.J. Fleck and W.J. Kraemer, 2014, *Designing resistance training programs*, 4th ed. (Champaign, IL: Human Kinetics), 108.

tion. However, the upper limit of one's strength is ultimately determined by muscle CSA.

Skeletal muscle also undergoes profound adaptations to aerobic endurance training. However, unlike adaptations to resistance training, adaptations to aerobic endurance training increase the ability of the muscle to utilize oxygen for ATP production and delay fatigue during repeated, low-intensity contractions. Increases in aerobic capacity largely depend on training intensity, with greater intensities bringing on more rapid improvement. Hickson, Bomze, and Hollozy demonstrated that $\dot{V}O_2$max can increase an average of 5% in 1 week after performing 40 minutes of daily high-intensity aerobic exercise, with an overall increase of 44% following 10 weeks of training (10).

The effects of both strength and aerobic endurance training on muscle fibers are summarized in table 4.2, and table 4.3 shows adaptations that occur following aerobic endurance training.

Minimum Training Requirements to Maintain Adaptations

As is the case with adaptations at the initiation of an exercise program, the training requirements

Table 4.2   Effects of Types of Training on Skeletal Muscle

Variable	Strength training adaptations	Aerobic endurance training adaptations
Muscular strength	Increases	No change
Muscular endurance	Increases for high power output	Increases for low power output
Aerobic power	No change or increases slightly	Increases
Anaerobic power	Increases	No change
Rate of force production	Increases	No change or decreases
Fiber cross-sectional area	Increases	No change or increases slightly
Capillary density	No change or decreases	Increases
Mitochondrial density	Decreases	Increases
Stored ATP	Increases	Increases
Stored creatine phosphate	Increases	Increases
Stored glycogen	Increases	Increases
Stored triglycerides	May increase	Increases

Table 4.3   Adaptations Following Aerobic Endurance Training

Adaptation	12-month change from baseline	24-month change from baseline	Change 6 months after cessation of training
Aerobic enzymes	100%	120%	−120%
Oxidative potential of FT fibers	60%	60%	−60%
Glycogen	40%	50%	−50%
Capillary density	40%	50%	−50%
$\dot{V}O_2max$	40%	40%	−40%
Cross-sectional area of ST fibers	20%	20%	−20%

necessary to maintain a given fitness level are largely affected by one's initial fitness level. In general, well-trained elite athletes require a higher volume, intensity, and frequency of training in order to maintain their higher level of fitness. For each individual, a certain volume of training represents a stimulating load, retaining (maintaining) load, or detraining load, as shown in figure 4.14. For people with little experience, a training volume that results in increased physical fitness likely will not be adequate to increase fitness in a well-trained person. Therefore, training prescriptions must be assigned on an individual basis in order to create an adequate stimulus for improved performance.

To ensure that a person's performance is consistently improving, a program must address the concepts of overload, duration, and frequency. **Overload** refers to the fact that one must be consistently exposed to training volume, frequency, and intensity at greater-than-habitual levels. **Duration** refers to the amount of time spent in a given activity, and **frequency** refers to the number of training sessions performed over a given period of time. The frequency of resistance training necessary to maintain increases in strength depends on programmatic factors and individual differences between people. However, it has been shown that following 12 weeks of resistance training, male soccer players can maintain their strength gains with only one bout of resistance training per week (18). As a general rule, if training frequency, volume, or duration decrease, intensity should increase in order to compensate for the decrease in the other training parameters.

Because improvements in aerobic capacity are also influenced by factors such as exercise type, duration, frequency, intensity, and fitness level, it is difficult to pinpoint an exact exercise prescription for the maintenance of aerobic capacity.

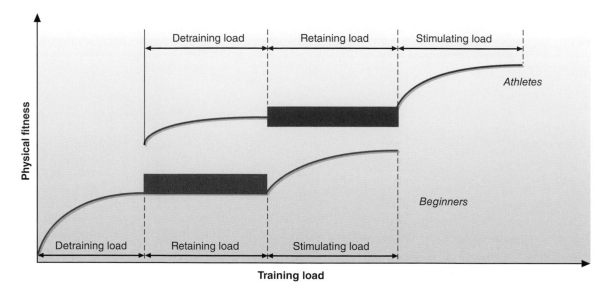

Figure 4.14 Relationship between training load (detraining, retaining, stimulating) and level of physical fitness. Rectangles indicate the neutral zones (retaining loads) corresponding to small fluctuations in the training load at which the level of fitness is basically unchanged. Note the stepladder effect, showing a change in the adaptation curve with a change in the training stimulus. A training load that leads to detraining of high-level athletes may be extremely high for beginners.

Reprinted, by permission, from V. Zatsirosky and W. Kraemer, 2006, *The science and practice of strength training* (Champaign, IL: Human Kinetics), 4.

In one study, young adults increased their $\dot{V}O_2max$ by 25% over 10 weeks of training. They then reduced their training frequency for 15 weeks while keeping intensity and duration the same. The subjects' previous gains in $\dot{V}O_2max$ were maintained with up to a two-thirds reduction in training frequency (11). However, if training intensity decreases by as little as one-third, $\dot{V}O_2max$ decreases, even if duration and frequency remain constant (9). Therefore, it appears that exercise intensity is critical in maintaining aerobic fitness.

CONCLUSION

The human body liberates energy from the macronutrients in food and fluids in the form of ATP. It does this via three main bioenergetic pathways: the ATP-PCr system, anaerobic glycolysis, and aerobic metabolism. Of these systems, the ATP-PCr provides energy the fastest, followed by glycolysis and then aerobic metabolism. The aerobic pathway is least susceptible to fatigue, followed by glycolysis and then the ATP-PCr system. Fat and carbohydrate are the primary sources of energy during exercise, whereas protein is used mainly for synthesis of skeletal muscle. Lactate (a by-product of carbohydrate metabolism) is produced during high-intensity activity and can be a significant source of fuel during exercise.

Adaptations to exercise include both central and peripheral changes. The primary structural peripheral changes that happen in skeletal muscle following chronic aerobic exercise include an increase in capillary number and a decrease in muscle CSA. There is also an increase in mitochondrial size and number, allowing for increased oxygen consumption during exercise. The most important central adaptation to endurance exercise is an increase in cardiac SV.

Chronic resistance training leads to increased strength through an increase in the ability of the CNS to recruit motor units, as well as through structural changes in the muscle. An increase in muscle size is the primary adaptation that leads to increased strength. Early on in a resistance training program, changes in strength are due mainly to neural adaptations within the CNS. The main training effects following resistance training are increases in muscle strength, power, and endurance. Which of these adaptations predominates is mainly determined by training intensity. Low RM ranges result in large increases in strength and power, moderate RM ranges result in muscle hypertrophy, and high RM ranges result in increases in muscle endurance. Muscle power is also developed by moving moderate loads quickly and by incorporating plyometric training. If intensity remains high, training adaptations can be maintained with as few as one or two training sessions per week, depending on the subject's previous training and fitness level.

Key Terms

aerobic
anaerobic
ATP-PCr system
beta-oxidation
bioenergetics
cardiac output
Cori cycle
duration
electron transport chain (ETC)
endurance
Fick equation
frequency
glucose
glycogen
glycolysis
hypertrophy
intensity

lactate
lactate threshold (LT)
macronutrients
mitochondria
mode
onset of blood lactate accumulation (OBLA)
overload
phosphagen system
phosphocreatine (PCr)
power
pyruvate
specificity
speed
strength
triacylglycerol
tricarboxylic acid (TCA) cycle

Study Questions

1. What is the primary end product of short-burst, high-intensity muscular activities?

   a. glucose

   b. acetyl-CoA

   c. triacylglycerol

   d. lactate

2. Which bioenergetic pathway provides energy for short bursts of maximal activity not greater than approximately 6 seconds?

   a. Cori

   b. glycolytic

   c. phosphagen

   d. Krebs

3. Which training variable contributes the most to improvements in performance?

   a. mode

   b. intensity

   c. frequency

   d. duration

4. How are velocity and muscular power affected when heavy loads are lifted?

   a. low velocity, low power

   b. low velocity, high power

   c. high velocity, low power

   d. high velocity, high power

Chapter 5

Basic Nutrition for Tactical Populations

Steve Hertzler, PhD, RD, LD

Amanda Carlson-Phillips, MS, RD, CSSD

After completing this chapter, you will be able to

- explain the nutritional factors affecting health and performance,
- evaluate the adequacy of a diet,
- describe nutritional strategies to optimize body composition and maximize performance and recovery,
- define the TSAC Facilitator's scope of practice regarding nutrition, and
- explain the concept of interprofessional collaboration.

Tactical athletes face many unique physical challenges as part of their job requirements. Their tasks can require considerable strength, endurance, and power. Added to the challenges of these tasks are demands imposed by factors such as sleep deprivation, extreme weather conditions, psychological stress, and extended duration of activity beyond what might be experienced by many athletes or physically active people. Maintaining optimal nutritional status is critical to coping with all of these demands. This chapter reviews nutrition information and strategies for tactical athletes to maintain the physical capacity to perform their jobs at a high level.

GUIDELINES FOR DISPENSING NUTRITION INFORMATION

TSAC Facilitators must have working knowledge of nutrition so they can answer their clients' questions. However, there are limitations to their scope of practice, which are discussed in the following section, as is information regarding referrals to registered or licensed dietitians for nutrition issues outside their scope of practice.

The question of who should provide nutrition knowledge to a tactical athlete is often a debated topic. Many strength and fitness professionals are knowledgeable about athletes' physiology, the demands of their specific activities, and the role nutrition plays in performance; however, they may not be qualified to deliver detailed nutrition information. The blurred scope of practice is due to the fact that sports nutrition is a multidisciplinary field that requires many professionals to work together. Athletic trainers, strength and conditioning coaches, dietitians, and even food service providers all must come together in order to provide the best service, information, and guidance to the athlete (28).

Scope of Practice for Nutrition

TSAC Facilitators are often asked questions regarding nutrition, be it meal planning or dietary supplementation. Though it is important for the facilitator to be educated about nutrition, there are limitations to their scope of their nutrition practice. For example, in the United States, 46 states and territories have enacted laws that regulate dietitians or nutritionists via licensure, statutory certification, or registration. **Licensure** is the most stringent of these and restricts the practice of dietetics to those meeting state requirements for licensure. Statutory certification and registration laws do not restrict the practice of dietetics, but certification does limit the use of certain titles to those meeting predetermined criteria. For complete information on which states have laws regarding dietetics and for links to individual state licensing boards, visit the website of the Commission on Dietetic Registration (www.cdrnet.org/state-licensure). In states with licensure, the RD (registered dietitian) or RDN (registered dietitian nutritionist) credential is the main prerequisite (often the additional initials LD or LN indicate that the RD is also licensed by a particular state). Thus, nutrition certifications from organizations other than the Academy of Nutrition and Dietetics (formerly known as the American Dietetic Association; www.eatright.org) typically carry no legal recognition by state dietetic licensure boards. By going to the website of each state's licensure board, one can access the specific rules and regulations for the scope of dietetics practice in that particular state.

The state of Ohio provides some excellent guidance on the types of nutrition information that people who are not licensed to provide nutrition services—such as strength coaches, personal trainers, and TSAC Facilitators—can provide to their clients. Although these guidelines were created within the context of the Ohio licensure law, they may be applicable in other states in which the licensure law is not as clearly spelled out. The guidelines specify the types of general, nonmedical nutrition information that can be dispensed by fitness professionals who are not licensed dietitians. In Ohio, these include the principles of good nutrition and food preparation, food to be included in the normal daily diet, essential nutrients needed by the body, recommended amounts of the essential nutrients, actions of nutrients on the body, effects of deficiencies or excesses of nutrients, and foods and supplements that are good sources of essential nutrients. In states with licensure, nutrition information that is prescriptive (e.g., individualized dietary recommendations with specific calorie and macro- or micronutrient targets and dietary supplements) is generally considered to be in the purview of the licensed nutrition professional. It is important to contact the applicable state licensure boards for more specific guidance on scope of practice.

Nutrition Professionals

All sports nutrition professionals should be able to answer basic nutrition questions. However, athletes with complex nutrition issues should be referred to the appropriate resource (128).

A **sports nutrition coach** is a professional who is not a registered dietitian but has basic training in nutrition and exercise science. For example, the strength and conditioning professional can act as a sports nutrition coach, providing basic nutrition education and suggestions. More complex situations in which food or nutrition is being used to treat or manage a medical condition (including a nutrient deficiency) require medical nutrition therapy and fall under the role of the sports dietitian. Sports nutrition coaches may obtain additional education by getting a sports nutrition certification.

A **sports nutritionist with an advanced degree** is a professional who works in the sports nutrition industry or conducts research in the area of sports nutrition and would therefore be able to discuss the literature on a particular topic. The sports nutritionist with an advanced degree may also choose to obtain a sports nutrition certification.

A **registered dietitian (RD)**, also referred to as a **registered dietitian nutritionist (RDN)**, is a professional who is credentialed by the Academy of Nutrition and Dietetics. RDs have met the following academic and professional requirements:

- Completion of a bachelor's degree with coursework approved by the Commission on Accreditation for Dietetics Education. Coursework typically includes food and nutrition sciences, food service systems management, business, economics, computer science, sociology, biochemistry, physiology, microbiology, and chemistry
- Completion of an accredited supervised practice program at a health care facility, community agency, or food service corporation

- Passing of a national examination administered by the Commission on Dietetic Registration
- Completion of continuing professional educational requirements to maintain registration

The RD can design individual diets based on specific nutrient requirements and can provide behavioral and dietary counseling. In addition, the RD may manage a food service operation. The RD is also usually the nutrition specialist for medical nutrition therapy.

A **sports dietitian** is an RD with specific education and experience in sports nutrition. The Board Certified Specialist in Sports Dietetics (CSSD) certification distinguishes RDs with expertise in sports nutrition from RDs who specialize in other areas of nutrition.

In summary, many people with little to no education in nutrition and exercise science or formal training refer to themselves as sports nutritionists. TSAC Facilitators should turn to dietitians or licensed nutritionists when nutritional advice exceeds their scope of practice.

Key Point

For nutrition information that is prescriptive, TSAC Facilitators should refer tactical athletes to licensed nutrition professionals with the right blend of education, experience, and credentials.

A personalized nutrition program must take into consideration the demands of the individual. Understanding the individual's goals, energy demands, and recovery needs will create a framework for the nutritional recommendations. For example, greater energy demands through increased physical activity result in the need for more calories, carbohydrate, and protein. Tactical athletes who have lower physical demands will have a decreased need for calories, carbohydrate, and protein due to less demand placed on the body. A great way to approach the nutritional needs of tactical athletes is to use the following four-step process. This process will guide the remainder of this chapter.

Step 1: Understand the demands of the tactical athlete.

Step 2: Understand basic fueling concepts.

Step 3: Within the scope of practice, create nutritional guidance for daily, or foundational, nutritional needs.

Step 4: Within the scope of practice, create nutritional recommendations to support performance and recovery.

STEP 1: UNDERSTAND THE DEMANDS OF THE TACTICAL ATHLETE

The daily energy requirements of tactical personnel are highly variable, depending on gender, body composition, activities performed, age, and environmental conditions. When thinking about the energy requirements of tactical athletes, it is necessary to have a general understanding of their basal energy expenditure, the energy demands of their training to maintain strength and endurance, and the energy demands of their job-related tasks.

Tactical athletes cannot be lumped into a single group. Just as there are a variety of positions on a football team and each player's demands are based on position, goals, and amount of time on the field and in practice, each tactical athlete's demands are based on incredibly different job functions. The functions of tactical athletes can range from tasks that require mental focus but do not have a large physical demand to tasks with a range of repeated strenuous functions that require incredible strength and endurance. Therefore, it is important to treat each athlete as an individual when it comes to thinking through nutrition needs.

The two main methods for measuring energy requirements are indirect calorimetry and doubly labeled water, which provide estimates of oxygen consumption and carbon dioxide production, respectively. Because these methods require expensive equipment and often are not practical in field settings, numerous prediction equations exist for estimating energy expenditure.

The U.S. Institute of Medicine (now known as the National Academy of Medicine) developed a set of equations for adult males and females (72). Table 5.1 provides examples of these equations for adult males and females. Using the formula in table 5.1, the estimated energy requirement for a 5-foot, 10-inch (1.78 m) male who weighs 154 pounds (70 kg), is 19 years old, and is very active would be approximately 3,551 kcal per day. Many other equations are also available, and the Harris-Benedict Equation is one that has been used for many years (table 5.1).

Table 5.1   Equations for Estimating Total Energy Requirements for Adults

	Equation
Institute of Medicine	
Men	EER = 662 − 9.53 × age in years + PA × (15.91 × weight [kg] + 539.6 × height [m])
Women	EER = 354 − 6.91 × age in years + PA × (9.36 × weight [kg] + 726 × height [m])
Harris-Benedict Equation	
Men	BEE = 66.5 + 13.75 × weight (kg) + 5.003 × height (cm) − 6.775 × age
Women	BEE = 655.1 + 9.563 × kg + 1.850 × cm − 4.676 × age

BEE = basal energy expenditure; EER = estimated energy requirement; PA = physical activity factor.

Note: PA was classified into four categories:

- Sedentary—typical daily living activities (e.g., household tasks, walking to the bus). PA = 1.00 for both males and females.
- Low active—typical daily living activities plus 30 to 60 minutes of daily moderate activity (e.g., walking at 5-7 km/h [3-4 mph]). PA = 1.11 for males, 1.12 for females.
- Active—typical daily living activities plus at least 60 minutes of daily moderate activity. PA = 1.25 for males, 1.27 for females.
- Very active—typical daily living activities plus at least 60 minutes of daily moderate activity plus an additional 60 minutes of vigorous activity or 120 minutes of moderate activity. PA = 1.48 for males, 1.45 for females.

Reprinted from Cornell University, 2000, Basal energy expenditure: Harris-Benedict equation; D. Frankenfield et al., 2005, "Comparison of predictive equations for resting metabolic rate in healthy nonobese and obese adults: a systematic review," *Journal of American Dietetic Association* 105(50): 775-789.

Studies in the military indicate that active-duty service members engaged in a variety of on-the-ground combat missions or in mountain warfare training may expend 3,500 to 7,000 kcal per day (110). A review of studies on 424 male military personnel from various units engaged in diverse missions determined that daily energy expenditures ranged from 3,109 to 7,131 kcal (mean 4,610 kcal) (135), measured over an average of 12.2 days. For 77 females studied, daily energy expenditures ranged from 2,332 to 5,597 kcal (mean 2,850 kcal) over 8.8 days. The highest energy requirements were in U.S. Marines in mountain warfare training at 2,550 m (8,366 ft) altitude at –15 °C to 13 °C (5-55 °F). Even the average daily energy requirements of these tactical athletes are greatly elevated above those of sedentary people, and meeting them can present significant challenges, especially when food availability is low or when time to eat while performing the mission is limited.

It is important to understand the amount of energy required to perform elements of specific job functions, which differs greatly among tactical athletes. Elsner and Kolkhorst (41) studied 20 firefighters who performed a series of 10 simulated firefighting tasks in full protective clothing:

1. Advancing a 41 kg (90 lb) hose off the back of a fire engine for 35 m (38 yd) and connecting to a hydrant

2. Carrying a 7.3 m (8.0 yd) extension ladder (33 kg [73 lb]) 30 m (33 yd) and extending it to a third-story window

3. Donning a self-contained breathing apparatus (SCBA)

4. Advancing two sections of fire hose (82 kg [181 lb]) from an engine to a stairwell 20 m (22 yd) away

5. Using a 5 kg (11 lb) sledge to pound on a 75 kg (165 lb) wood block and move it 50 cm (20 in.) along a concrete floor

6. Climbing three flights of stairs

7. Pulling two sections of fire hose (82 kg [181 lb]) with a rope from the ground up to a third-story landing

8. Advancing a fire hose 30 m (33 yd) through a cluttered area

9. Returning to ground level by the stairs, shoulder loading an uncharged high-rise fire hose pack (23 kg [51 lb]), and returning to the third-floor landing

10. Conducting a search and rescue to locate a 75 kg (165 lb) mannequin and drag it 30 m (33 yd)

Completion of this drill required 11.7 minutes on average. The mean $\dot{V}O_2$ was 29.1 ml·kg^{-1}·min^{-1} (8.3 METS, 62% $\dot{V}O_2$max, and firefighters reached 95% of predicted maximal HR. Excluding basal metabolism, this 11.7-minute drill required approximately 124 kcal of energy. This type of activity, extrapolated over several hours of firefighting, would result in significant energy requirements.

In addition to the daily demands of the tactical athlete's core job functions, it is also necessary to consider any exercise the athlete engages in to maintain strength and endurance, as well as any other extracurricular physical activities. Table 5.2 gives estimates for the amount of calories burned in 30 minutes from a variety of activities for a 154 lb (70 kg) adult.

Key Point

When considering the energy demands of tactical athletes, it is important to estimate their basal metabolic rate and the demands of their job function, training (strength and endurance), leisure activities, and any intermittent acute changes to their typical activity level.

STEP 2: UNDERSTAND BASIC FUELING CONCEPTS

The tactical athlete's diet should promote overall health and maximize both physical performance and recovery. Tactical athletes may perform a variety of functions with a wide range of physical and mental demands. When working with tactical athletes, it is critical to look at them as individuals and create nutritional recommendations to meet their specific needs and goals. Although tactical athletes are not playing a sport, using the evidence-based sports nutrition perspective (1, 6) will result in holistic nutrition to support a variety of demands and keep the tactical athletes at their physical and mental best.

Table 5.2   Caloric Expenditure by Type of Activity

Activity	Approximate calories per 30 minutes for 154 lb person	Approximate calories per hour for 154 lb person
Moderate physical activity		
Hiking	185	370
Light gardening or yard work	165	330
Dancing	165	330
Golf (walking and carrying clubs)	165	330
Bicycling (<10 mph)	145	290
Walking (3.5 mph)	140	280
Weightlifting (general light workout)	110	220
Stretching	90	180
Vigorous physical activity		
Running or jogging (5 mph)	295	590
Bicycling (>10 mph)	295	590
Swimming (slow freestyle laps)	255	510
Aerobics	240	480
Walking (4.5 mph)	230	460
Heavy yard work (chopping wood)	220	440
Weightlifting (vigorous effort)	220	440
Basketball (vigorous)	220	440

Reprinted from the Centers for Disease Control. Available: http://www.cdc.gov/healthyweight/physical_activity/index.html

Macronutrients

The major classes of nutrients are carbohydrate, protein, fat, water, vitamins, and minerals. Those required in larger amounts—such as carbohydrate, protein, and fat—are referred to as **macronutrients**, whereas vitamins and minerals are considered **micronutrients**. Each major class of nutrients has important physiological and metabolic aspects that relate to the health and performance of the tactical athlete.

Carbohydrate

Carbohydrate is the main energy source for high-intensity physical activity and plays a key role in meeting overall energy needs. Starch and sugar in the diet are first broken down into monosaccharides (glucose, fructose, galactose) during digestion. Then glucose molecules can either be oxidized for energy immediately or stored in long chains called **glycogen**. Glycogen is stored in the liver (75-100 g) and skeletal muscles (300-400 g) (30). Figure 5.1 shows carbohydrate and fat

usage at varying exercise intensities (percentage of maximal oxygen consumption). As exercise intensity increases, the proportion of muscular energy derived from carbohydrate increases and that from fat decreases.

Carbohydrate provides more than just energy to the body; it is also a source of fiber and additional micronutrients. Dietary fiber is important for digestive health (9, 71, 87, 95). Different types of dietary fiber have varied physiological effects in the gastrointestinal tract; therefore, it is important to include a variety of fiber sources in the diet. Some types of fiber, such as beta-glucan from oats and pectin, increase viscosity of gut contents and slow digestion, which improves blood glucose control, decreases blood lipids, and increases satiety (i.e., satisfaction) after eating. Other fibers, like the cellulose in wheat bran, improve laxation by increasing fecal bulk. Finally, prebiotic fibers, such as inulin and fructooligosaccharide, are easily fermented and may selectively increase the population of healthy, or probiotic, bacteria in the large intestine (e.g., bifidobacteria) (120).

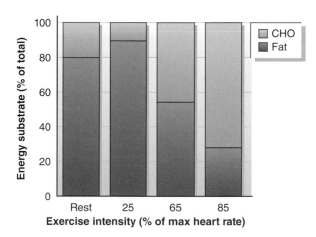

Figure 5.1 Proportions of carbohydrate and fat used for fuel at differing exercise intensities.

© 2016 from *Musculoskeletal and sports medicine for the primary care practitioner*, 4th ed., by R. Birrer, F.G. O'Connor, and S. Kane (editors), Sports nutrition and the athlete, J.M. Scott and P.A. Deuster. Reproduced by permission of Taylor and Francis Group, LLC, a division of Informa plc.

The average daily intake of dietary fiber among American adults is 21 to 23 g for males and 17 to 19 g for women (71, 145). The Institute of Medicine (71) recommends a total daily fiber AI (Adequate Intake) of 38 g for young adult males (up to age 50) and 25 g for young adult females (up to age 50). After age 50, the AI drops to 30 g for males and 21 g for females. Good sources of fiber include high-fiber cereals (bran cereals, oatmeal); whole-grain bread, rice, and pasta; fruit with skin on when applicable (pears, apples, oranges); starchy legumes (navy beans, pinto beans); vegetables (corn, peas); and nuts.

When selecting carbohydrate sources, it is important to consider the nutrient value and the intention of the carbohydrate: general energy and health or optimal performance during activity. Different types of carbohydrate are broken down at different rates, meaning that the type of carbohydrate will determine the speed at which it is digested and the corresponding **insulin** response. The slower the carbohydrate is broken down, the slower the absorption and the more gradual the insulin response. The faster a carbohydrate is broken down, the greater the insulin response and the faster the absorption. The **glycemic index (GI)** and the **glycemic load (GL)** describe the degree to which the carbohydrate in a food raises the blood glucose level (sometimes called *blood sugar level*). A GI value of 100 indicates that a food raises blood glucose to the same degree as a glucose solution. A GI value of 70 indicates that a food increases blood glucose 70% as much as the glucose solution. Foods can be classified as low GI (GI ≤55), intermediate GI (GI 56-69), or high GI (GI ≥70) (17).

The GL of food takes into account not only the GI but also the grams of carbohydrate per serving (GL = GI × g of carbohydrate per serving / 100) (17), providing a more accurate depiction of the fate of the carbohydrate in the body after ingestion. This is important because some foods might contain only a small amount of carbohydrate, and even if the GI of that carbohydrate is high, the effect on blood glucose may still be relatively small. Table 5.3 shows the GI values for some common foods.

Table 5.3 GI Values for Common Foods, Where Glucose = 100

Food	GI
White bread	75
Whole-wheat bread	74
Specialty-grain bread	48
Porridge, rolled oats	55
Porridge, instant oats	79
Cornflakes cereal	81
Corn tortilla	46
White rice, boiled	73
Brown rice, boiled	68
Spaghetti, white	49
Potato, instant, mashed	87
Potato, boiled	78
Sweet potato, boiled	63
Carrots, boiled	39
Milk	38
Ice cream	51
Fructose	15
Sucrose	65
Honey	61
Apple	36
Banana	51
Orange juice	50

Adapted from Atkinson, Foster-Power, and Brand-Miller (13).

When considering the use of the GI or GL system in meal planning for exercise performance, there are several factors to consider. First, the GI is only one piece of information about a food. For example, a baked potato has a high GI value, but it also is a nutritious food; a large baked potato (with skin) has nearly twice the potassium as a banana and is a good source of vitamin C and vitamin B$_6$ (114). By contrast, ice cream has a low GI but a high fat content. Moreover, when you combine a protein or a fat with a carbohydrate, it tends to change the glycemic effect. Therefore, it is important not to base food choices on GI or GL alone. The GI and GL are good tools for discussing the functions and features of carbohydrate but may be complicated for a tactical athlete to use in practice. Tactical athletes should get most of their carbohydrate from nutrient-dense, fiber-rich, minimally processed food, which will generally have an optimal GI or GL rating.

Protein

Protein is a macronutrient responsible for maintaining and restoring muscles, keeping blood cells healthy, providing key enzymes, and strengthening immunity. Protein has also been shown to help preserve lean muscle mass, aid in weight loss, and increase strength and endurance.

Protein serves a number of functions that support physical activity. The main roles of protein involve repairing muscle tissue that has been damaged via exercise and increasing muscle protein synthesis, which contributes to increased muscle mass and strength as an adaptation to resistance exercise. Protein can be used for energy during prolonged submaximal exercise, particularly when glycogen stores are limited, but even under these circumstances, protein only contributes up to 12% of the energy demands of exercise (42).

Food protein consists of chains of amino acids linked together via peptide bonds. During digestion, protein, which typically contains hundreds of amino acid units, is broken down into individual amino acids and mixtures of small peptides (2-10 amino acid units). Approximately 20 amino acids occur in food protein. These amino acids can be categorized as **essential amino acids (EAA)** (i.e., can't be synthesized by the body), **nonessential amino acids** (i.e., can be synthesized by the body), or **conditionally essential amino acids (CEAA)** (i.e., can't always be synthesized in amounts sufficient to meet physiological requirements). Table 5.4 lists the essential, nonessential, and conditionally essential amino acids for humans.

For the tactical athlete, maintaining muscle mass, improving strength, and enhancing recovery are often the primary considerations when it comes to protein intake. The quality of a food protein source is an important influence on the ability of the protein to support growth and development. The most common standard for protein quality at present is the **protein digestibility-corrected amino acid score (PDCAAS)** (124). A PDCAAS of 1.00 indicates that a protein is highly digestible and contains all of the essential amino

Table 5.4   Essential, Nonessential, and Conditionally Essential Amino Acids

Essential amino acids	Nonessential amino acids	Conditionally essential amino acids	Precursors to conditionally essential amino acids
Histidine	Alanine	Arginine	Glutamine/glutamate, aspartate
Isoleucine	Asparagine	Cysteine	Methionine, serine
Leucine	Aspartic acid	Glutamine	Glutamic acid, ammonia
Lysine	Glutamic acid	Glycine	Serine, choline
Methionine	Serine	Proline	Glutamate
Phenylalanine		Tyrosine	Phenylalanine
Threonine			
Tryptophan			
Valine			

Based on Institute of Medicine (72).

acids in the amounts required to support human growth and development. Table 5.5 shows the PDCAAS for various proteins. It is also important to reinforce variety and timing as tactical athletes build their nutritional day. Research has shown that including protein with each meal can help maintain lean body mass more efficiently than less frequent feedings. In addition to providing amino acids, protein can be a viable source of other performance- and health-maintaining nutrients. Fish sources like tuna and salmon are high in omega-3 fatty acids, which support the ability to manage inflammation. Eggs, besides being a great source of protein, also provide the body with choline, an amino acid shown to support brain health. Therefore, it is important to guide the tactical athlete to a variety of nutrient-diverse protein sources that are of high biological value.

Fat

Compared with carbohydrate and protein, the dietary fat requirements for physically active people typically receive little attention. However, consuming both the right types and amounts of fat is critical for physical performance, recovery from exercise, and cardiovascular health. Recommendations regarding the amount of fat consumed per day will vary depending on the type of physical activity, environmental conditions, bodyweight goals, risk factors for cardiovascular disease, and overall energy requirements. Fat is more energy dense, containing 9 kcal/g versus 4 kcal/g for carbohydrate or protein (30). This prop-

erty is especially important for tactical athletes with high energy requirements. The increased energy density of fat means that it provides a lot of food energy in a limited volume. This can be significant in situations where access to food is limited or tactical conditions do not allow much time to consume meals.

Another way in which fat differs from carbohydrate or protein is body reserves. Table 5.6 shows body stores of carbohydrate and fat for a relatively light (60-70 kg [132-154 lb]) person who is likely untrained; the body stores would be larger for heavier, trained athletes. Body reserves of carbohydrate are limited. The available carbohydrate energy from plasma glucose, liver glycogen, and muscle glycogen stores is only about 2,000 kcal (96), emphasizing the importance of consuming enough carbohydrate in the diet. There is no bodily reserve of protein that can be drawn on without potentially decreasing functional capacity. Amino acids can be drawn from muscles when intake is inadequate, but this has an undesirable effect on muscle mass and performance. Fat, on the other hand, can be readily stored. Even a reasonably lean 176-pound (80 kg) man with 15% body fat has over 100,000 kcal of stored energy available as plasma fatty acids, plasma triglycerides, adipose tissue, and intramuscular triglycerides (96). In the case of exercise performance, the issue is not the amount of fat available for fuel but rather training the body to improve the systems necessary for transporting and utilizing oxygen, which is required to use fat for energy.

Different types of fat provide different nutritional properties. **Monounsaturated fatty acids** have one double bond in the carbon chain. An example of a monounsaturated fatty acid is oleic acid (18:1), which is found predominantly in olive oil. Its double bond occurs after the ninth carbon from the omega end, and so it is referred to as an *omega-9 fatty acid* (18:1, *n*-9). Oleic acid is a key component of the Mediterranean diet and is generally considered to be a heart-healthy fat (12).

Polyunsaturated fatty acids have more than one double bond in their carbon chain. The two main types of polyunsaturated fatty acids have their first double bond at either carbon 6 (**omega-6**, or *n*-6) or 3 (**omega-3**, or *n*-3) from the omega end. Omega-6 and omega-3 fatty acids cannot be

Table 5.5   PDCAAS for Selected Foods

Food	PDCAAS
Casein	1.00
Whey	1.00
Egg white	1.00
Soy protein isolate	1.00
Beef	0.92
Pea flour	0.69
Pinto beans	0.63
Kidney beans	0.68
Wheat gluten	0.25
Peanut meal	0.52

Adapted from FAO/WHO (43); Hoffman and Falvo (64).

Table 5.6   Body Energy Stores From Carbohydrate and Fat

Energy source	Major storage form	Body stores (g)	Total body calories
Carbohydrate	Blood glucose	5	20
	Liver glycogen	100	400
	Muscle glycogen	375	1,500
Fat	Blood free fatty acids	1	7
	Blood triglycerides	8	75
	Muscle triglycerides	278	2,500
	Body fat	8,889	80,000

Adapted from Williams (152).

synthesized in the body and are therefore essential fatty acids (71). A common example of an omega-6 fatty acid is linoleic acid (18:2, *n*-6). Linoleic acid is found in large concentrations in many vegetable oils, such as corn oil, safflower oil, and sunflower oil. Common omega-3 fatty acids include **alpha-linolenic acid (ALA)** (18:3, *n*-3), **eicosapentaenoic acid (EPA)** (20:5, *n*-3), and **docosahexaenoic acid (DHA)** (22:6, *n*-3). Major sources of ALA include flaxseed oil and walnuts. Like linoleic acid, ALA is an essential fatty acid (71). To avoid essential fatty acid deficiency or imbalance, 5% to 7% of a person's energy intake should be essential fatty acids (71). Fatty fishes (e.g., salmon, mackerel, and other cold-water, high-fat fish) are good sources of EPA and DHA. Many people are familiar with the health benefits associated with omega-3 fat (e.g., lowered triglycerides, decreased heart disease risk). It is also well known that in the Western diet, the ratio of omega-6 to omega-3 fat is much higher than is desirable. The American Heart Association (AHA) recommends at least two servings of fish high in omega-3 fat (8 oz [227 g] of fish total) per week (94). The AHA also advises those with documented coronary heart disease to consume ~1 g of combined EPA and DHA per day, preferably from fatty fish, although capsules could be considered in consultation with a physician. For people with high triglycerides, the AHA recommends 2 to 4 g of combined EPA and DHA per day under the supervision of a physician (94). A key concern about the labeling of fish oil supplements is that the dose on the front of the package is stated in terms of the amount of fish oil. However, what is most important is to check the label to see the actual amounts of EPA and

DHA per dose and to verify how many capsules constitute one dose.

Saturated fatty acids, also known as **saturated fat**, tend to be solid at room temperature. Examples of saturated fatty acids include myristic acid, palmitic acid, and stearic acid. Of these fatty acids, myristic and palmitic acid tend to increase blood cholesterol while stearic does not (12, 69, 136). Animal fats, such as butter, beef tallow, and lard, and some plant fats, such as coconut oil, are especially rich in saturated fat. In its 2015 scientific report, the U.S. Dietary Guidelines Advisory Committee (DGAC) reconsidered the evidence supposedly linking high intakes of saturated fat to increased risk of heart disease.

These data weaken the case for restricting saturated fat in the diet, but the DGAC found "strong and consistent evidence demonstrates that dietary patterns associated with decreased risk of CVD are characterized by higher consumption of vegetables, fruits, whole grains, low-fat dairy, and seafood, and lower consumption of red and processed meat, and lower intakes of refined grains, and sugar-sweetened foods and beverages relative to less healthy patterns." Thus, although the DGAC lightened up a bit on the scientific evidence regarding the need to restrict saturated fat, it still acknowledged the health benefits of diets higher in fruits and vegetables and lower in saturated fat (146). The committee found strong evidence that

- reducing total fat (replacing total fat with carbohydrate) does not influence cardiovascular disease risk,

- higher saturated fat intakes relative to higher carbohydrate intakes are not associated with cardiovascular disease risk,

- replacing saturated fat with polyunsaturated fat reduces total and low-density lipoprotein (LDL) cholesterol,

- replacing saturated fat with carbohydrate reduces total and LDL cholesterol but also increases blood triglycerides and high-density lipoprotein (HDL) cholesterol, and

- replacing saturated fat with polyunsaturated fat reduces the risk of cardiovascular disease events and coronary mortality.

It is also important to consider processes that change the chemical structure of fat. For instance, the hydrogenation process (adding hydrogen atoms to unsaturated fatty acids) is used in food processing to increase the solidity of the fat and make it more resistant to spoilage (i.e., rancidity), resulting in **trans fat**. However, the nutritional disadvantages of hydrogenation include increasing the amount of saturated fat and converting some of the chemical bonds to the trans configuration. Trans fat tends to increase the level of LDL cholesterol in the blood (the bad way to transport cholesterol) and decrease the level of HDL cholesterol (the good way to transport cholesterol), which increases the risk of heart disease (71). Food labels contain information on trans fat content. There is some disagreement regarding the maximal recommendation for trans fat intake: The Institute of Medicine (71) simply recommends keeping trans fat intake as low as possible, whereas the AHA recommends obtaining <1% of energy from trans fat (94). Nonetheless, the U.S. Food and Drug Administration (FDA) no longer classifies trans fat as generally recognized as safe (GRAS), and as of June 16, 2015, food manufacturers have three years to remove it from their foods.

In summary, the differences in the chemical structure of fatty acids largely influence their biological functions. As our understanding of the role fat plays in health and performance continues to evolve, it is important to guide tactical athletes to choose a variety of fat sources from both plants and animals, with a focus on minimally processed foods rich in omega-3 fatty acids.

Fluids

Water is a macronutrient and the largest single constituent of the human body, composing about 60% of body weight. All bodily fluids are made from it, including the blood, lymph, cerebrospinal fluid, intracellular fluid, urine, and sweat. Water absorbs heat from metabolic processes, lubricates joints, serves as a medium for biochemical reactions, transports nutrients and oxygen to cells, and removes waste. The fat-free mass of the body is 70% to 75% water, while the fat mass is 14% to 40% water (74). Thus, the leaner a person is, the higher the percentage of body weight that comes from water.

Body water balance represents the difference between water gain and loss. Sources of body water gain are the intake of water (via drinking water, other beverages, and food) and the generation of metabolic water that occurs as nutrients are metabolized for energy. Body water losses include respiratory, urinary, fecal, and skin losses. For tactical athletes, the respiratory and insensible or perspiration losses are probably the most significant because of how greatly they are influenced by the environment. Respiratory water losses average 250 to 350 ml (8-12 fl oz) per day for sedentary people but can increase to 500 to 600 ml (17-20 fl oz) in active people living in temperate climates at sea level (74). If the individual is working at high altitude, respiratory water losses can increase by another 200 ml (7 fl oz) per day (74). Breathing dry air that is hot or cold contributes still more respiratory water loss, a total of 120 to 300 ml (4-10 fl oz) per day (74). Thus, tactical athletes exposed to environmental extremes while doing heavy work might lose a liter (34 fl oz) or more of water per day just via the respiratory route.

The Institute of Medicine has established AI values for total water intake of 3.7 L (125 fl oz) and 2.7 L (91 fl oz) per day for 19- to 50-year-old males and females, respectively (74). These values roughly correspond with the minimal water loss scenarios just described. It is expected that beverage intake would comprise 3.7 L (125 fl oz) and 2.7 L (91 fl oz) of the male and female AI values, with the remainder of the intake coming from water in food and the body's production of water from the metabolism of nutrients (i.e., metabolic water resulting from hydrogen protons joining with oxygen at the end of the mitochondrial respiratory chain). Table 5.7 shows the water content of selected foods.

Table 5.7   Water Content of Selected Foods

Food	Water (% weight)
Apple, raw	86
Apricot, raw	86
Banana, raw	75
Bread, white	36
Bread, whole wheat	38
Broccoli, cooked	89
Cantaloupe, raw	90
Carrots, raw	88
Cheese, cheddar	37
Cheese, cottage	79
Chicken, roasted	64
Chocolate chip cookie	4
Corn, cooked	70
Cornflake cereal	3
Crackers, saltine	4
Grapes, raw	81
Ham, cooked	70
Lettuce, iceberg	96
Macaroni, spaghetti, cooked	66
Milk, 2%	89
Orange, raw	87
Peach, raw	89
Peanuts, dry roasted	2
Pear, raw	84
Pickle	92
Pineapple, raw	86
Potato, baked	75
Squash, cooked	94
Steak, tenderloin, cooked	50
Sweet potato, boiled	80
Turkey, roasted	62
Walnuts	4

Based on Institute of Medicine (74); USDA/ARS (144).

Key Point

When considering fluid intake, it is important to evaluate both the tactical athlete's basic needs and needs associated with exercise and environment.

Based on a comprehensive review of the effects of caffeine on hydration, the Institute of Medicine concluded that caffeinated beverages count toward the requirements for total water intake (74). Its report suggested that caffeine doses >180 mg (equal to 2-3 cups of coffee) may transiently increase urinary output, but there was no evidence indicating that this would lead to a total body water deficit. Thus, it appears that moderate caffeine intake does not appreciably alter overall fluid balance, especially if caffeine is consumed in the form of a beverage. For the tactical athlete, there are also other issues to consider regarding caffeine, such as effects on physical performance, HR, blood pressure, sleeping patterns, alertness, and GI distress and stimulation. In addition, caffeine used with other ingredients (e.g., ephedra, herbs) may increase the risk of adverse events (56). These issues may govern whether or not the athlete should use caffeine, but there is not sufficient evidence to suggest that athletes should avoid moderate use of caffeinated beverages due to diuretic effects (11, 37).

With regard to alcoholic beverages, the effects on hydration and performance are largely dose-related. Shirreffs and Maughan (127) demonstrated that, in dehydrated subjects (2% loss of body weight from exercise), solutions containing up to 2% alcohol consumed after exercise did not adversely affect rehydration, but a 4% solution did. In addition, alcohol may have other adverse effects on performance, such as CNS depression, decreased power output and reaction time, and inhibition of gluconeogenesis (152). Burke et al. (24) reported that displacing carbohydrate for alcohol in the recovery period from exercise decreased muscle glycogen storage. However, the addition of alcohol to carbohydrate resulted in somewhat lower glycogen levels at 8 hours of recovery (not statistically significant) and no differences at 24 hours of recovery.

Micronutrients: Vitamins and Minerals

Vitamins and minerals have many essential functions in the body but are required in much smaller amounts in the diet compared with macronutrients (i.e., carbohydrate, protein, fat, and water). Thus, they are termed *micronutrients*. See tables 5.8 through 5.11 for a summary of vitamins and minerals, their functions, and food sources. Vitamin and mineral intake is often a function of overall energy intake. Typically, athletes consume more food than sedentary people and do not have significant problems obtaining adequate amounts of most vitamins and minerals. However, this is not necessarily the case for athletes in sports involving bodyweight restrictions or in tactical athletes who are unable to consume enough food under certain circumstances. Carbohydrate, protein, and fat are sources of energy (kcal) via their conversion to ATP, the energy currency of the cell. However, in order for this conversion to happen, many biochemical reactions must occur. Vitamins and minerals provide the **coenzymes** and **cofactors** necessary to optimize **metabolism**. Minerals also play key roles in regulating fluid balance, providing structural material for the skeleton, protecting the body from damage caused by free radicals, and serving other functions. It is beyond the scope of this chapter to discuss each vitamin and mineral in detail. However, certain nutrients or groups of nutrients, such as iron, vitamin D, and antioxidants, warrant special attention in tactical athletes.

With the ability to look at blood markers to identify deficiencies and the emergence of supplementation protocols, athletes can take a food and supplementation approach to filling any gaps they may have in their dietary intake or deficiencies that occur as a result of increased workload or lack of availability. When a tactical athlete needs a supplement, the TSAC Facilitator should call in a sports medicine physician or RD with experience in assessing and treating deficiencies and should support only products that have gone through third-party testing to ensure truth in labeling(19).

Iron

Iron is necessary for oxygen transport in the blood via its role in the oxygen transport protein **hemoglobin**. Iron is also a structural component of the **myoglobin** protein that is involved in local oxygen transfer in muscle cells. Unfortunately, iron is often low in the diets of athletes, particularly women and those who are avoiding meat (a good iron source) due to concerns about

Table 5.8 Fat-Soluble Vitamins

Vitamin	Major functions	RDA or AI for 19-50 years of age	Good sources	UL for ages 19-50 years of age
Vitamin A Preformed: retinol, retinoic acid Precursor: provitamin A carotenoids such as beta-carotene	Night vision, immune function, skin and connective tissue health, cell differentiation	700-900 mcg RAE	Preformed: butter, liver, fortified milk, cod liver oil Precursor: carrots, squash, broccoli, other dark green and yellow vegetables, orange fruits	3,000 mcg retinol
Vitamin D (cholecalciferol, ergocalciferol)	Calcium absorption from the intestine, regulation of blood calcium levels, bone health, gene regulation; acts in a manner similar to steroid hormones	600 IU or 15 mcg	Foods: fortified milk, fatty fish Sunlight exposure of the skin	4,000 IU (100 mcg)
Vitamin E (alpha-tocopherol)	Protection of lipids in cell membranes from oxidation, needed for normal reproductive function	15 mg alpha-tocopherol (22 IU from natural vitamin E [d-alpha-tocopherol] or 33 IU from synthetic vitamin E [dl-alpha-tocopherol])	Vegetable oil, sunflower seeds, mayonnaise, nuts	1,000 IU total alpha-tocopherol, 1,100 IU from sources containing synthetic vitamin E, or 1,500 IU from sources containing natural vitamin E
Vitamin K (phylloquinone from vegetables; menaquinone from bacteria)	Blood clotting, adequate carboxylation of proteins important for bone health	90-120 mcg	Green vegetables, liver; synthesized by intestinal microorganisms	ND

AI = adequate intake; IU = international units; ND = not determined; RAE = retinal activity equivalent; RDA = recommended dietary allowance; UL = tolerable upper intake level.

Based on Institute of Medicine (74); Wardlaw, Jampl, and DiSilverstro (149).

Table 5.9 Water-Soluble Vitamins

Vitamin	Major functions	RDA or AI for males and females, 19-50 years of age	Good sources	UL for males and females, 19-50 years of age
Vitamin B$_1$ (thiamin)	Coenzyme for energy metabolism; neurological functions	1.1-1.2 mg	Whole- and enriched grain products, pork products, nuts, seeds	ND
Vitamin B$_2$ (riboflavin)	Coenzyme for energy metabolism (e.g., flavin adenine dinucleotide [FAD])	1.1-1.3 mg	Whole- and enriched grain products, milk and other dairy products, mushrooms, spinach, liver	ND
Niacin	Coenzyme for energy metabolism (e.g., nicotinamide adenine dinucleotide [NAD])	14-16 mg niacin equivalents	Preformed: whole- and enriched grain products, meat, poultry, fish Precursor: amino acid tryptophan found in protein foods (60 mg tryptophan = 1 mg niacin)	35 mg
Pantothenic acid	Coenzyme for energy metabolism	5 mg	Found in a wide variety of foods	ND
Vitamin B$_6$ (pyridoxine)	Carbohydrate (glycogen) and protein metabolism (transamination reactions), heme synthesis, lipid metabolism, homocysteine metabolism	1.3 mg	Potatoes, animal protein, spinach, bananas, salmon, sunflower seeds	100 mg
Biotin	Coenzyme for carboxylation reactions (e.g., pyruvate carboxylase in gluconeogenesis pathway)	30 mcg	Found in a wide variety of foods	ND
Vitamin B$_{12}$ (cobalamins such as cyanocobalamin)	Red blood cell development and oxygen transport, nervous system functions, coenzymes involved in folate and methyl group metabolism	2.4 mcg	Animal foods, fortified cereals, other products	ND
Folate	DNA synthesis, methyl group metabolism, red blood cell development and oxygen transport	400 mcg DFE	Leafy green vegetables, fortified breads and cereals, orange juice, nuts, liver, legumes	1,000 mcg folic acid (synthetic folate used in fortification and supplements)
Choline	Neurotransmitter synthesis, homocysteine metabolism, synthesis of phospholipids in cell membranes, betaine synthesis	425-550 mg	Fish, foods containing natural phospholipids such as lecithin in soy and egg yolk; some endogenous synthesis	3,500 mg
Vitamin C	Absorption of nonheme iron; health of skin, blood vessels, and connective tissues; redox reactions in antioxidant system; hormone and neurotransmitter synthesis	75-90 mg (+35 mg for smokers)	Citrus fruits and juices, potatoes, tomatoes, cantaloupe, red and green peppers, kiwi, strawberries, broccoli, fortified foods	2,000 mg

AI = adequate intake; DFE = dietary folate equivalents; ND = not determined; RDA = recommended dietary allowance; UL = tolerable upper intake level.

Based on Institute of Medicine (74); Wardlaw, Jampl, and DiSilverstro (149).

Table 5.10   Major Minerals

Mineral	Major functions	RDA or AI for males and females, 19-50 years of age	Good sources	UL for males and females, 19-50 years of age
Sodium	Electrolyte—extracellular, cation; nerve impulse transmission; water balance and blood pressure regulation	1,500 mg*	Table salt, processed foods, condiments, sauces, soups, sport drinks	2,300 mg*
Potassium	Electrolyte—intracellular, anion; nerve impulse transmission; water balance and blood pressure regulation	4,700 mg	Baked potatoes, bananas, milk, orange juice, tomatoes, other fruits and vegetables	ND
Chloride	Electrolyte—extracellular, anion; nerve impulse transmission; water balance and blood pressure regulation; production of hydrochloric acid in stomach	2,300 mg*	Table salt, some vegetables, processed foods	3,600 mg*
Calcium	Formation of bone mineral matrix, nerve impulse transmission, cell signaling, muscle contraction	1,000 mg	Milk and other dairy products, fortified orange juice, green vegetables (e.g., broccoli, kale), calcium-set tofu, sardines	2,500 mg (mainly concerned with supplemental use vs. food)
Phosphorus	Part of bone mineral matrix, part of various metabolic compounds, regulation of acid–base balance, major ion of intracellular fluids	700 mg	Milk, meats, processed foods, soft drinks, fish	4,000 mg
Magnesium	Part of bone mineral matrix, cofactor for numerous enzymes, functioning of cardiovascular (e.g., vasodilation) and nervous systems	310-420 mg	Leafy green vegetables, nuts, seeds, chocolate, legumes, wheat bran	350 mg from supplemental magnesium (not dietary)
Sulfur	Constituent of sulfur-containing amino acids (e.g., methionine, cysteine) needed for growth, drug detoxification, regulation of acid–base balance	ND (requirement generally met if consuming adequate sulfur-containing amino acids)	Animal protein, grains	ND

AI = adequate intake; ND = not determined; RDA = recommended dietary allowance; UL = tolerable upper intake level.

*Intended more for sedentary population.

Based on Institute of Medicine (74); Wardlaw, Jampl, and DiSilverstro (149).

Table 5.11   Selected Trace Minerals

Mineral	Major functions	RDA or AI for males and females, 19-50 years of age	Good sources	UL for males and females, 19-50 years of age
Iron	Key component of hemoglobin, part of electron transport system in mitochondria, immune and cognitive functions	8-18 mg	Meats, seafood, enriched breads, fortified cereals, molasses	45 mg
Zinc	Cofactor in many enzymes, DNA function, antioxidant functions, immune function, growth and development, cell membrane stability	8-11 mg	Shellfish, meats, whole grains	40 mg
Copper	Collagen synthesis, cofactor for enzyme systems, iron metabolism, antioxidant functions	900 mcg	Cocoa, liver, beans, whole grains, shellfish	10,000 mcg
Selenium	Part of antioxidant defenses (e.g., cofactor for glutathione peroxidase), cofactor for enzyme in thyroid hormone synthesis	55 mcg	Seafood, whole-grain products (dependent on selenium content of soil), meats	400 mcg
Iodide	Component of thyroid hormones	150 mcg	Saltwater fish, iodized salt, dairy products, bread	1,100 mcg
Fluoride	Resistance of tooth enamel to decay	3.1-3.8 mg	Fluoridated water, toothpaste and fluoridated dental treatments, tea, seaweed	10 mg
Chromium	Potentiation of insulin action for blood glucose tolerance	25-35 mcg	Brewer's yeast, broccoli, whole grains, nuts, mushrooms, egg yolks, pork, dried beans, beer	ND
Manganese	Cofactor in some types of superoxide dismutase, an antioxidant; cofactor in some other enzymes	1.8-2.3 mg	Nuts, oats, beans, tea	11 mg
Molybdenum	Cofactor in enzymes	45 mcg	Beans, grains, nuts	2,000 mcg

AI = adequate intake; ND = not determined; RDA = recommended dietary allowance; UL = tolerable upper intake level.

Based on Institute of Medicine (74); Wardlaw, Jampl, and DiSilverstro (149).

saturated fat or vegetarian or vegan eating habits. Further, the demands of exercise may increase iron requirements. Exercise-induced hemolysis can increase the loss of red blood cells and hemoglobin, potentially affecting oxygen transport (112). Due to increased losses of iron in menstrual flow, iron requirements in premenopausal women (recommended daily allowance [RDA] = 18 mg) are about double those of the adult male (RDA = 8 mg) (72). Iron intake is generally positively associated with energy intake, with a typical iron intake of about 6 mg per 1,000 kcal (10). Thus, menstruating women who are restricting energy intake can have an especially difficult time meeting iron requirements. Meeting the iron RDA for women (18 mg) from diet alone would necessitate eating 3,000 kcal per day with a typical diet. Many female athletes fail to consume that amount of energy or iron.

There are several factors to consider when attempting to increase dietary iron intake. The bioavailability of iron from various food sources is influenced by the form of iron (heme versus nonheme), presence of vitamin C (for nonheme iron in particular), whether or not the person is already iron deficient, and the potential binding of iron by factors such as phytate or tannic acid (29). **Heme iron** consists of iron that is still bound to the hemoglobin and myoglobin proteins when it is ingested. This is in contrast to **nonheme iron** that might be present (e.g., iron in cytochromes, various iron salts). Absorption efficiency of heme iron from the intestine is about 25%, whereas nonheme iron is absorbed at about 17% (72). The absorption of heme iron from meat is constant and unaffected by other dietary factors. However, nonheme iron absorption is positively influenced by vitamin C, gastric acidity, and presence of heme iron (73). It is negatively influenced by iron binders such as phytate (in legumes, rice, and grains), calcium (to an extent), and tannic acid (in tea) (73). In many cases, the presence of iron binders can reduce the absorption of iron to <5% (73). This is an important consideration for those who attempt to obtain the majority of their iron from grains and vegetables. As a point of comparison, a 4-ounce (113 g) sirloin steak has 3.8 mg of iron in a highly bioavailable form. This food will provide more iron to the body than 1 cup of spinach that has 6.4 mg of iron, because the iron bioavailability from spinach is low due to iron binders (149). (See table 5.11 for other good food sources of iron.) Thus, it is important for people to know their iron status, and those who struggle to meet their iron needs from food should consider iron supplementation.

Vitamin D

Vitamin D deficiency has become relatively common. Vitamin D regulates the expression of more than 1,000 genes, is an important modulator of both inflammation and the immune response (115), plays a role in hormone production, influences neural and mental health, and affects cell turnover and regulation (108).

A recent study of 74 female soldiers (39 non-Hispanic white, 24 non-Hispanic black, and 11 Hispanic white) undergoing basic training showed that 57% of the soldiers had suboptimal vitamin D status (serum 25-hydroxyvitamin D level <75 nmol/L or 30 ng/ml) upon entry into basic training (8). By the end of basic training, 75% of the soldiers were below this cutoff. This is supported by the 2005-2006 National Health and Nutrition Examination Survey data indicating that 41.6% of U.S. adults exhibit vitamin D deficiency: The highest deficiencies are among blacks (82.1%) and Hispanics (69.2%) (48), likely due to low dietary intake of vitamin D and reduced sun exposure. Cannell et al. (27) recommend serum 25-hydroxyvitamin D levels of 50 ng/ml (125 nmol/L).

A mere 5 to 10 minutes of exposure of the arms and legs to direct sunlight can produce 3,000 IU vitamin D in the body (65). Thus, it only takes brief sun exposure to make a substantial amount of vitamin D in fair-skinned people. However, this is problematic for those who have darker skin pigments (vitamin D synthesis from the skin does not occur as readily); for those who are avoiding sunlight exposure to reduce the risk of skin cancer; for those who live in climates with winters, when there is less sun exposure; or for those who live at higher latitudes (north of the 37th parallel; roughly equivalent to Richmond, Virginia, or San Francisco, California) (60).

Tactical athletes should understand their vitamin D status. If a vitamin D deficiency exists, correct it from a general health perspective, even if this correction does not improve athletic performance.

Antioxidants

Antioxidants are important nutrients that defend the cells from potentially harmful levels of free radicals. **Free radicals** are molecules that contain one or more unpaired electrons in their outer orbital and are thus unstable. They naturally occur in the cells of the body, and their production increases during exercise. In order to achieve a more stable configuration, the free radical steals electrons from neighboring victim compounds. This alters the biological function of the victim compound and can convert it to a free radical, initiating a chain reaction that can progress to the point of causing significant cell damage. In order to control the activity of free radicals, the body has developed a number of enzymatic and nonenzymatic defense systems. These defense systems can donate electrons to the free radical, stabilizing it. Enzymatic systems in the cells include enzymes such as superoxide dismutase, glutathione peroxidase, and catalase. Minerals such as zinc, copper, manganese, and selenium are important cofactors for these enzymes. Vitamins such as vitamin E, vitamin C, and the vitamin A precursor **beta-carotene** are mainly involved in nonenzymatic systems. Therefore, several nutrients play a role in the body's defense mechanisms.

Powers, Nelson, and Larson-Meyer (115) indicate that dietary intake and baseline nutritional status are likely to be important modifiers. Moreover, if a person has suboptimal or deficient intakes of these nutrients, supplementation could be helpful. This is a significant point to consider for tactical athletes, who may be under stressful conditions for an extended period of time, as opposed to sport athletes, who have more control over diet, intensity, and duration of training. For example, Wood et al. (155) fed a nutritional formula containing a blend of antioxidants, structured lipids, and other nutrients to soldiers in the Special Forces Assessment and Selection (SFAS) school who were undergoing rigorous training and sleep deprivation. The subjects in the control group had a difficult time maintaining adequate intakes of vitamin E, folate, and magnesium and experienced a decline in immune status compared with the specialized formula group. The group who consumed the specialized nutrition formula saw improvements in several markers of immune status compared with the control group during this stressful time.

It is clear from the scientific evidence that diets high in fruits and vegetables offer numerous health benefits from naturally occurring antioxidants. It is difficult to mimic the effects of diets high in fruits and vegetables using supplements due to the unique combination of nutrients found naturally in food; however, for athletes with a low intake of vegetables and fruits (sometimes due to the lack of availability of these foods), it is important to consider supplementation to fill in the gaps of the diet. Research has shown that antioxidant supplementation has performance benefits for those who present deficiencies, including improved performance due to lessened fatigue, decreased exercise-associated muscle damage, and improved immune function. But high-dose supplementation of isolated antioxidant nutrients is not recommended and could even impair the adaptation to exercise (115); therefore, a balanced supplement covering a wide range of nutrients is recommended. As with all supplementation recommendations, it is best to leave the recommendations up to the sports medicine team or RD.

Key Point

Although research indicates certain trends in vitamin and mineral deficiencies in specific populations, it is important to think of each tactical athlete as an individual and recommend a dietary analysis and blood analysis to identify any micronutrient deficiencies.

STEP 3: PROVIDE NUTRITIONAL GUIDANCE

Although it is necessary to understand and respect scope of practice, it is also critical that TSAC Facilitators understand general nutrition concepts, provide general nutrition information, and act as conduits to nutrition professionals should the need be out of the facilitator's scope of practice. In 1997, the Institute of Medicine began publishing a series of reports, known as the **Dietary Reference Intakes**

(DRI), to establish recommended nutrient intakes. The DRI represent an extension of the **Recommended Dietary Allowance (RDA)** and comprise four categories (72):

1. *Estimated Average Requirement (EAR):* Refers to the average daily nutrient intake that is estimated to meet the requirements of half of the healthy individuals in a particular life stage and gender group.

2. *Recommended Dietary Allowance (RDA):* Refers to the average daily nutrient intake that is sufficient to meet the nutrient requirements of nearly all (97%-98%) healthy individuals in a particular life stage and gender group.

3. *Adequate Intake (AI):* Refers to the recommended average daily intake based on observed or experimentally determined approximations or estimations of nutrient intake by a group (or groups) of apparently healthy people that is assumed to be adequate; used when an RDA cannot be determined.

4. *Tolerable Upper Intake Level (UL):* Refers to the highest average daily nutrient intake level that is likely to pose no risk of adverse health effects to the general population. As intake increases above the UL, the potential risk of adverse effects may increase.

DRI were established for water, vitamins, minerals, carbohydrate, protein and amino acids, fat and fatty acids, dietary fiber, and cholesterol. Another concept presented within the DRI reports for macronutrients (e.g., carbohydrate, protein, fat) is the **Acceptable Macronutrient Distribution Range (AMDR)**, which highlights the recommended intakes of these nutrients as a percentage of daily energy intake. For adults, the AMDR is 45% to 65% of energy from carbohydrate, 10% to 35% of energy from protein, and 20% to 35% of energy from fat (72). To determine your DRI for all the nutrients, go to http://fnic.nal.usda.gov/interactiveDRI.

Military personnel often have different nutrient requirements than those of the general population. For example, warfighters may have a high level of physical exertion in either hot or cold climates and thus have greater needs for energy, fluids, electrolytes, carbohydrate, fat, and protein compared with a sedentary person. The same is true for police, firefighters, and other tactical personnel. As such, the U.S. military has established a modified version of the DRI. Though similar in many respects to the DRI, there are important differences, such as larger energy requirements (depending on duty), increased protein requirements, elevated sodium and fluid needs (again, based on environmental conditions), and some alterations in mineral requirements (e.g., potassium, magnesium, zinc). The **Military Dietary Reference Intakes (MDRIs)** are found in Army Regulation 40-25 (39). Table 5.12 summarizes these requirements. Carbohydrate and fat are not listed in the summary table but are discussed elsewhere in the document. The MDRIs are used to determine the nutrient composition of military rations, in particular the MREs (Meals, Ready to Eat). Each MRE provides approximately 1,250 kcal (roughly one-third of the energy requirement), 51% carbohydrate, 13% protein, 36% fat, and one-third of the MDRIs for vitamins and minerals (143).

Daily Carbohydrate Needs

Daily carbohydrate recommendations vary depending on the metabolic carbohydrate tolerance of the tactical athlete, the type of activity associated with the athlete's job function, specific exercise requirements, and phase of training. It is important to match carbohydrate intake with carbohydrate requirements. Often, the very-high-carbohydrate diets specified for athletes have been designed with the endurance athlete in mind. However, those who perform tasks shorter duration and higher intensity may not be as dependent on maintaining muscle glycogen stores.

- Daily carbohydrate needs for strength athletes, for instance, might range from 1.8 to 3.2 g carbohydrate per pound of body weight (4-7 g/kg body weight) (25, 131). This translates into 308 to 539 g carbohydrate per day for a 170-pound (77 kg) person.

- For athletes involved in endurance exercise, carbohydrate needs are likely to be higher, from 3.6 to 5.5 g per pound of body weight

Table 5.12 MDRI Recommendations for Calories, Carbohydrate, Protein, Fat, and Fluids

Activity level and energy source	Recommendation	Example for a male (moderate activity)	Amount needed during activity in heat or at altitude	Example for a female (moderate activity)	Amount needed during activity in heat or at altitude
Energy (kcal/day)					
General routine		3,250		2,300	
Light activity		3,000		2,200	
Moderate activity		3,250		2,300	
Heavy activity		3,950		2,700	
Exceptionally heavy activity		4,600		3,150	
Carbohydrate	50%-55% of kcal	406-447 g/day	—	288-316 g/day	—
Protein	91 g/day (range 63-119 g/day)	—	—	72 g/day (range 50-93 g/day)	—
Fat					
Weight maintenance or job with higher physical activity	≤35% of kcal	≤126 g/day	—	≤89 g/day	—
Weight loss or job with lower physical activity	≤30% of kcal	≤108 g/day	—	≤75 g/day	—
Fluids	1 qt (1 L) of beverage per 1,000 kcal expended	3.25 qt/day (3 L/day)	4-6 qt/day (4-5 L/day)*	2.3 qt/day (2 L/day)	4-6 qt/day (4-5 L/day)*

*Under conditions of high sweat loss, activity beyond 3 hours, or poor nutritional intake, a carbohydrate-electrolyte beverage may be needed as part of these fluid requirements. Recommendation for carbohydrate-electrolyte beverages are carbohydrate from sugar or starch at 5 to 12 g per liter, 230-690 mg sodium per liter; and 78-195 mg potassium per liter.

Adapted from Army Regulation 40–25 BUMEDINST 10110.6 AFI 44-141, Nutrition Standards and Education. Available: http://armypubs. army.mil/Search/ePubsSearch/ePubsSearchDownloadPage.aspx?docID=0902c851800103f0

(8-12 g/kg body weight) (25). This translates to 616 to 924 g per day for the 170-pound (77 kg) athlete. The high end of the carbohydrate range for the endurance athlete would probably apply just to short periods of carbohydrate loading prior to competition, while the lower end of the range might represent more typical training intakes.

Table 5.13 shows the carbohydrate content of some common foods.

Daily Protein Needs

The protein needs of tactical athletes will likely be considerably higher than those of inactive people. During exercise, there is increased oxidation of amino acids, especially branched-chain amino acids, for energy. This is particularly true when glycogen stores are depleted. Under these circumstances, up to 12% of the energy cost of activity can be met by protein (42). Further, extra protein is needed to repair muscle protein that has been damaged due to exercise. Finally, tactical athletes must often perform in environments where access to appropriate amounts of carbohydrate (and food in general) is limited. When carbohydrate is low in supply, there is increased **gluconeogenesis** (i.e., conversion of amino acids to glucose). Thus, carbohydrate spares protein (both exogenous and endogenous) from being oxidized for energy.

The protein requirements for tactical athletes depend on intensity of workload, overall energy and carbohydrate intake, and gender. Table 5.14 describes the daily recommended protein intakes for tactical athletes. During stressful conditions, protein requirements could be higher than these

Table 5.13   Foods Providing 25 to 30 g Carbohydrate

Food	Amount
Fruit	1 piece (large)
Fruit juice	1 cup (8 fl oz)
Cereal	1 cup (8 fl oz)
Baked potato	1 (large)
Milk	2 cups (16 fl oz)
Dried beans, cooked	2/3 cup (5.3 fl oz)
Rice or corn	1 cup (8 fl oz)
Winter squash	1 cup (8 fl oz)
Tomato juice	2 1/2 cups (20 fl oz)
Sport drink	2 cups (16 fl oz)
Energy bar	1/2 to 1 (depending on brand)
Energy gel	1 packet

Based on American Diabetes Association/Academy of Nutrition and Dietetics (5); Pennington (114).

numbers, especially if combined with low intake of energy and carbohydrate. An upper limit to how much protein a tactical athlete might require is unknown. Somewhat higher intakes have proven safe and beneficial for some athletes, and protein requirements should be individualized as much as possible.

It is important for the tactical athlete to consume protein at frequent intervals throughout the day to ensure adequate levels of circulating amino acids for muscle repair and growth. Protein consumed in the postexercise period and before bedtime could be important for fostering anabolism (21, 90, 119, 148).

In general, safety concerns regarding high-protein diets for healthy, active people have been largely exaggerated by health care professionals and the media. One source of confusion arises regarding the definition of a high-protein diet. For the purpose of this chapter, a high-protein diet constitutes a daily protein intake of 2.0 g/kg (0.9 g/lb) body weight or more, which is over double the present RDA of 0.8 g/kg (0.4 g/lb) body weight for adults (71). There is no evidence that protein intake at that level is associated with adverse health effects in healthy, active people with normal liver and kidney function (26). In people with some degree of renal compromise or liver disease, the advice of a health care professional should be sought regarding the appropriate amount of protein.

Key Point

Given the definition of a high-protein diet as a daily intake of 2.0 g/kg (0.9 g/lb) body weight, there is no evidence that protein intake at that level is associated with adverse health effects in healthy, active people with normal liver and kidney function.

Another concern that has been expressed is that high-protein diets may reduce bone density. However, there is no evidence that people on high-protein diets have lower bone mineral density, reduced bone strength, or accelerated bone loss (57, 93). In fact, protein helps strengthen bone, mainly by enhancing the collagen portion of bone that helps to increase its tensile strength (62). Thus, there is no reason to think that daily protein intakes of up to 2.0 g/kg (0.9 g/lb) body weight would adversely affect bone health as long as the intake of calcium and other nutrients important for bone health is adequate.

The main concern regarding high-protein diets is the increased water requirement that could result from urinary excretion of nitrogenous waste (e.g., urea) from oxidation of excess protein (88). For this reason, it is sensible to avoid greatly exceeding protein requirements. For most tactical athletes, a daily protein intake of up to 2.0 g/kg (0.9 g/lb) body weight probably would not greatly exceed their protein requirements. This concern

Table 5.14 Recommended Daily Protein Intakes for Tactical Athletes

Level of activity	Protein intake	Sample daily protein intake for a 170 lb (77 kg) person
Low to moderate activity	0.4-0.5 g/lb (0.8-1.0 g/kg) body weight	68-85 g
Vigorous activity (aerobic endurance or strength exercise)	0.5-0.6 g/lb (1.2-1.4 g/kg) body weight	85-136 g
Vigorous activity plus insufficient carbohydrate or calorie intake	0.7-0.9 g/lb (1.5-2.0 g/kg) body weight	119-158 g

Adapted from Human Performance Resource Center (68).

also highlights the importance of adequate fluid intake.

Daily Fat Needs

Previously, recommendations for fat intake in athletes, which correspond well with the MDRI, were that 20% to 35% of total energy should come from fat (7). In the most recent guidelines (1), the lower cut point of 20% of energy from fat was retained, but no upper limit on fat was established. This may be due to the fact that the nutrient requirements of athletic activities can vary, and athletes often experiment with dietary macronutrient compositions to improve performance. However, people who are less active, have high blood lipids, are overweight, or have other cardiovascular risk factors may wish to obtain no more than 30% of energy from fat. Tactical athletes in cold environments or with food volume restrictions, however, might want to aim for 35% of energy from fat or more.

One difficulty with expressing recommendations as a percentage of energy from fat is that this does not coincide with how the fat content of food is reported on food labels, which is in grams per serving. Thus, it is important to be able to convert between the two systems. For example, for a person who requires 2,700 kcal per day, how many grams of fat should be consumed to obtain 30% of energy from fat? To answer this question, first multiply the 2,700 kcal by 0.30 (the decimal equivalent of 30%) to get the number of kcal from fat, which turns out to be 810. Now divide the 810 kcal from fat by 9 kcal/g (the energy density of fat) to get the number of grams of fat per day, which comes to 90 g. A shortcut for determining the fat allowance in grams per day, which only works when 30% of energy is the desired fat goal,

is to simply divide the overall energy requirement by 30. Translating from a desired percentage of energy from fat to a recommended number of grams per day is helpful because food labels will make more sense. If tactical athletes understand that their daily fat need is 90 g, it is much easier to see that a food with 30 g fat per serving (e.g., a fast food burger) will use one-third of that day's fat allotment. When it comes to saturated fat, the AHA recommends less than 7% of energy from saturated fat (94), although 10% of energy from saturated fat might be a more realistic goal. Therefore, for people requiring a total daily fat intake of 90 g, the saturated fat intake should be no more than 30 g (10% of energy).

A number of books and online resources provide information on the content of fat and other nutrients in food. One of the best and most reliable is the USDA Food Composition Database (www.nal.usda.gov/fnic/foodcomp/search).

In summary, tactical athletes should aim to obtain 20% to 35% of their energy from fat. They should moderate saturated fat intake and avoid or keep trans fat intake low. The remainder of fat should be composed of a variety of healthy monounsaturated (e.g., olive oil, canola oil) and polyunsaturated fat, with an emphasis on increasing the ratio of omega-3 to omega-6 fat. Fish oil supplements may be advisable for certain people because of their cardiovascular benefits and less potential for inflammation (see chapter 7).

STEP 4: CREATE NUTRITIONAL RECOMMENDATIONS TO SUPPORT PERFORMANCE AND RECOVERY

One of the most significant sports nutrition discoveries of the last 25 years or so has been the concept of **nutrient timing**. With some understanding of the physiology of exercise and body systems in general, it becomes possible to learn not just what to eat but also when for best performance and recovery. (Again, TSAC Facilitators must stay within their scope of practice when providing nutrition information.) The pre- and postexercise periods are especially important for both performance and recovery.

Considerations for the Preexercise Meal or Snack

The preexercise or preactivity meal or snack primes the body with the nutrients it needs. In the preexercise period, there are several considerations:

- Gastrointestinal tolerance
- Fluids for hydration
- Overall energy (kcal) content and carbohydrate availability
- Fat and protein intake
- Possible inclusion of caffeine

Gastrointestinal tolerance is a major issue in athletes. Physical activity tends to divert blood flow from the intestine to the extremities, so digesting large meals can be difficult during this time. It is paramount to avoid adverse gastrointestinal symptoms for obvious reasons.

There are several strategies for designing preexercise meals to improve tolerance during exercise (2, 16, 30, 123):

- Avoid large amounts of dietary fiber, and be aware of foods that are solely fructose based and prepackaged foods (e.g., bars) that contain sugar alcohols.
- Keep the fat content low to avoid slowing gastric emptying.
- Allow a time interval between the meal and the exercise that is appropriate for digesting the size of the meal.
- Include a moderate amount of protein, again to avoid slowing gastric emptying.
- Keep calorie and carbohydrate levels high enough to provide energy for exercise but low enough to facilitate gastric emptying.

On the other hand, it has been suggested that a high insulin response to a preexercise feeding may be detrimental to performance due to the inhibitory effects of insulin on fat oxidation. The general consensus is that a lower GI preexercise feeding (typically 45 minutes to 3 hours before exercise) is associated with lower blood glucose and insulin responses and with higher levels of free fatty acids and fat oxidation during exercise compared with the higher GI feeding (103). Despite the clear metabolic effects of low versus high GI preexercise feedings, there is considerable disagreement among studies regarding improvement of performance. Some studies have reported benefits in performance with a low versus high GI preexercise feeding, whereas others have shown no effects (103). Given the uncertainty in the scientific literature, tactical athletes should consider what meals are tolerated best, whether carbohydrate is to be consumed during exercise, what type of exercise performance is required, the length of time between eating and exercise, and what food choices are available in making the best decisions for preexercise feeding.

Performance Nutrition: Fluid and Electrolyte Considerations

Preventing dehydration is critical for the tactical athlete because it can cause deterioration of both cognitive and physical performance. The Institute of Medicine presented reviews of the scientific literature on the effects of **dehydration** on cognitive and physical performance (mainly endurance exercise), showing that a 2% loss of body weight or more in a short time due to fluid loss can significantly impair performance (74). Although these effects of dehydration have been recognized for some time, athletes often fail to totally replace fluid losses even when they have access to water or other beverages during exercise (53). There are no clear reasons why athletes stop drinking before fully replacing fluid losses. The main goal is to prevent any more than a 2% loss in fluid, but overdrinking (i.e., weight gain during exercise) should also be avoided in order to prevent **hyponatremia**, or excessive dilution of sodium in the plasma. Thirst can serve as a signal to increase water intake, but the thirst response is not perfect (3). Therefore, drinking according to a regimen rather than the thirst response might be helpful in certain circumstances. A fluid plan that supports most physical activity is 0.4 to 0.8 L (14-27 fl oz) per hour, although this should be customized to the environment, tolerance, and individual sweat rate. Finally, tactical athletes should consider the temperature of their beverage. Cold beverages have been shown to help maintain or reduce core temperature, resulting in improved performance in hot environments (3).

It is important to consider all the factors that influence fluid losses in a drinking schedule. There have been multiple cases of ultra-endurance athletes (e.g., 100-mile [161 km] run participants) who developed life-threatening hyponatremia due to drinking excessively on a schedule (107). Risk factors for this type of hyponatremia include

- slow running speed (i.e., less intensity),
- cool and less humid environmental conditions that make fluid losses considerably less than expected,
- overconsumption of beverages (e.g., 50–50 dilution of soda with water) that have low sodium content, and
- inadequate urination due to failure of the fluid regulatory mechanisms.

Electrolytes are ions in the blood that help regulate fluid balance (see the section on minerals for more information). Electrolyte losses through the skin and sweating are highly variable and depend on physical activity intensity and duration, heat, humidity, clothing, and acclimatization to exercise. Insensible perspiration losses are approximately 450 ml (15 fl oz) a day for the average adult (72). With regard to perceptible skin sweat losses during exercise, water loss can range from 0.3 to >2 L (10-68 fl oz) per hour (72). Urine volume typically ranges from 1 to 2 L (34-68 fl oz) per day, depending on hydration status, and gastrointestinal fluid losses (i.e., fecal losses) are 100 to 200 ml (3-7 fl oz) a day (72). Thus, an estimate of total water losses under minimal conditions (temperate climate, 2 hours of activity at a sweat rate of 0.5 L [17 fl oz] per hour) might be approximately 3.6 L (122 fl oz) a day. Under more extreme conditions (hot or cold air, elevated altitude, 2 hours of exercise at a sweat rate of 1.5 L [51 fl oz] per hour, and 8 hours of activity at a sweat rate of 0.3 L [10 fl oz] per hour), total water losses might be 8.5 L (287 fl oz) per day or higher. To replace these losses, the military rule of thumb of about 1 quart (1 L) of fluid intake per 1,000 kcal expended is a good estimate, given that the fluid losses described here would probably be associated with daily energy expenditures of 3,600 and 8,500 kcal for minimal and extreme conditions, respectively. In addition, fluid intake can come from multiple beverages, not just water. Many people misinterpret guidelines for overall water intake from all sources as simply the amount of drinking water needed per day. However, beverages other than water can provide a portion of the total water requirement.

Sodium and other electrolytes play a key role in regulating water balance during exercise. Sweat contains 920 to 1,840 mg sodium and 1,065 to 2,485 mg chloride per liter (98). Other electrolytes, such as potassium at 156 to 312 mg per liter, are much lower in magnitude and relatively easy to replace via the diet. Because sweat is hypotonic with regard to sodium, blood sodium levels most often rise during active periods of sweat loss. As such, there is usually no need to replace sodium in order to avoid low blood sodium levels (i.e., hyponatremia) during exercise; however, there are exceptions. Athletes who have not acclimatized to exercise in the heat often have larger sodium concentrations in their sweat versus those who have acclimatized (3). A lack of acclimatization combined with the presence of clothing and gear that increase the need for sweating in the heat can rapidly accelerate sodium losses in tactical athletes. Excessive losses of sodium and fluid could increase the risk of muscle cramping, hyponatremia, and heat illness in these circumstances. The same is true for prolonged endurance events, in which athletes may have difficulty replacing enough sodium over time or may have entered the race with poor electrolyte levels. The sodium content of most commercially available sport drinks generally does not exceed 120 mg per 8 ounces (237 ml), which may be too low to adequately replace sodium in these individuals (144). It may be beneficial in these cases to use a beverage with a higher sodium concentration than a typical sport drink.

Key Point

The sodium content of most commercially available sport drinks generally does not exceed 120 mg per 8 ounces (237 ml), which may be too low to adequately replace sodium in people who are salty sweaters, heavy sweaters, or prone to cramping. Therefore, explore electrolyte-replacement beverages, powders, or tabs with more than 200 mg sodium per 8 ounces (237 ml).

As previously mentioned in this chapter, sports nutrition commonly teaches that athletes should avoid caffeinated beverages to minimize their diuretic effect. However, a number of studies have challenged the notion that caffeine adversely affects water balance or thermoregulation during exercise (11, 37). The research suggests that doses of caffeine up to 6 mg/kg (4 mg/lb) body weight do not have a significant impact on thermoregulatory responses and that the impacts on urine volume and flow and sweat are not likely to have a significant effect on 24-hour fluid or electrolyte balance. The effects of exercise tend to blunt the potential diuretic effect of caffeine. Therefore, if caffeine has a positive impact on performance for a particular tactical athlete, it can have an ergogenic effect in combination with an appropriate fueling and hydration strategy.

Performance Nutrition: Recovery After Exercise or Activity

Upon the completion of physical activity, the tactical athlete should start the recovery process to replenish glycogen (refuel), stimulate protein synthesis (rebuild), and correct fluid loss (rehydrate). The immediate postexercise period (within 60 minutes of finishing activity) is a critical window for delivering nutrients to the body because glucose and amino acid transporters are upregulated in muscle, insulin sensitivity of the muscle cells is enhanced, and the inhibitory effects of exercise on anabolic hormones and muscle protein synthesis pathways have subsided (75, 76). The more frequently a tactical athlete is active, the more important the recovery window becomes. Some research has shown that if athletes are meeting their macronutrient needs and are only active one time per day, they may be able to

recover through a normal diet; however, for many tactical athletes, nutrient intake varies. Therefore, creating a routine around recovery nutrition is a great strategy to ensure the athlete does not suffer from underrecovery, which could eventually lead to overtraining symptoms.

Early (immediately after exercise) versus late (at least 3 hours after exercise) consumption of carbohydrate and protein resulted in better protein synthesis (91) and muscle hypertrophy in response to resistance training (33). It appears that at least 10 g protein and 8 g carbohydrate postexercise are needed to stimulate the desired effects on muscle glucose uptake and muscle protein synthesis (91). However, additional research suggests that consuming 20 g protein after resistance exercise results in maximal muscle protein synthesis (104). Thus, an intake of at least 20 g protein immediately and 2 hours after exercise is recommended.

The ratio of carbohydrate to protein in Ivy et al. (77) was almost 3:1, whereas the ratio from Cribb and Hayes (33) was closer to 1:1 (34.4 g carbohydrate and 32 g protein consumed pre- and postexercise vs. morning and evening). Although certain products may claim to have the ideal ratio of carbohydrate to protein, the truth is that the optimal ratio has yet to be determined, and it may vary depending on whether maximal muscle glycogen synthesis or muscle protein synthesis is the primary goal of the athlete. A general approach is that the greater the intensity of the activity, the greater the need for glycogen recovery. As for protein, obtaining enough leucine to stimulate protein synthesis is the core driver for recovery; 2.0 to 2.5 g of leucine tends to stimulate signaling pathways that promote muscle building (18).

Recovery Nutrition: Focus on Carbohydrate Type

Foods with differing GI values may have benefits depending on when they are consumed relative to exercise. For example, in the immediate postexercise period it is important to get nutrients into the muscle cells as soon as possible to promote protein synthesis and rebuild glycogen stores. High GI carbohydrate stimulates large blood glucose and insulin responses (133), and a high level of insulin helps drive amino acids and glucose into the muscle cells. Given that low muscle glycogen levels can be a limiting factor for intense physical activity, ensuring that tactical athletes have enough carbohydrate both daily and in the recovery period can be beneficial, especially for those with multiple bouts of physical activity each day. Moreover, taking into consideration speed of carbohydrate delivery using higher GI carbohydrates is a beneficial strategy to achieve glycogen restoration (22).

Recovery Nutrition: Focus on Protein Type

Similar to the GI concept for carbohydrate, different types of protein also have different rates of digestion and release of amino acids into the circulation. Much research has focused on the two major subfractions of dairy protein—whey and casein. **Whey protein** is a soluble and rapidly digested protein, causing a spike in plasma amino acids within 1 to 2 hours of digestion that then quickly dissipates (15). **Casein protein**, on the other hand, is digested more slowly, and the postprandial rise in plasma amino acids is more moderate and sustained than for whey protein (15). Both casein and whey are high-quality proteins based on their PDCAAS values, but it has been suggested that their different rates of digestibility may have implications for the timing of protein ingestion and effects on muscle protein synthesis and breakdown.

Because of its rapid digestibility and high leucine content, whey protein stimulates muscle protein synthesis more so than casein when consumed in the immediate postexercise period (67, 113, 134, 151). By contrast, casein has a greater impact on inhibiting protein breakdown (15, 34), probably due to its slower release of amino acids into the circulation. As the result of such studies, many strength athletes use isolated protein sources at different times of day, such as whey protein in the immediate postexercise period and casein before bedtime.

However, interpreting the research on this issue is complex. When comparing isolated sources of protein such as whey and casein, a number of methodological issues with study design cloud interpretation of the data (15, 35, 86, 118, 140):

- Standardization based on total amount of protein versus leucine content of the protein
- Differential effects of whey and casein in older versus younger subjects
- Time frame over which muscle protein synthesis is measured
- Whether whole-body versus muscle protein synthesis is measured
- Limitations of measuring muscle protein synthesis alone versus measuring muscle protein balance (net of protein synthesis and breakdown)

Recent studies of a blend of 25% whey protein isolate, 25% soy protein isolate, and 50% sodium caseinate have shown levels of postexercise muscle protein synthesis equivalent to that of whey protein alone (116, 117).

Given the uncertain state of the science on protein digestibility rates and the effects on muscle protein synthesis and balance, there is no consensus regarding the optimal feeding of an isolated protein type at a particular time of day (26). At present, it appears that the more important consideration is to get adequate amounts of high-quality protein throughout the day, including the postexercise period, consuming blends of slow-, intermediate- (e.g., soy), and fast-digesting protein frequently (111).

During sleep, hormones that increase the potential for muscle growth (e.g., growth hormone, insulin-like growth factor) are elevated (36, 51, 105). Thus, protein consumption before bedtime can help supply amino acids during this important growth period. A source of casein (e.g., milk, cheese, cottage cheese, supplemental form) can be helpful during this time because of its slower digestion and more sustained amino acid release into the blood. Protein consumed at other times of day is also important for functions such as preventing hunger and minimizing protein breakdown, so it is important not to neglect protein during these times either. A recommendation is to consume 0.3 g of high-quality protein per kg of bodyweight (0.14g/lb) every 3-5 hours over multiple meals (1), with one of those times being the postworkout period. The amount at each feeding depends on the individual's protein need. See table 5.15 for the protein content of various foods.

Table 5.15   Protein Content of Selected Foods

Food	Serving size	Protein content (g)
Extra-lean ground beef, pan browned, well done	3.5 oz (100 g)	28.0
Cottage cheese, 1% fat	1 cup (226 g)	28.0
Chicken breast without skin, roasted	1/2 breast (85 g, or 3 oz)	26.7
Salmon, Atlantic, wild, cooked by dry heat	3 oz (85 g)	21.6
100% whey protein (third-party tested)	1 scoop	~21
Tofu, raw, firm	1/2 cup (124 g)	19.9
Greek yogurt, flavored	6 oz (170 g)	14-18 (depending on flavor)
Milk, skim	1 cup (245 g)	8.4
Yogurt, 1% fat, flavored	1 cup (227 g)	8.1
Peanut butter, creamy or crunchy	2 tbsp (32 g)	8.0
Cheese, part-skim mozzarella	1 oz (28 g)	6.9
Soy milk	1 cup (240 g)	6.6
Egg, boiled, hard or soft	1 large (50 g, or 1.75 oz)	6.3
Egg substitute	1/4 cup (60 g)	6.0
Chili beans, canned	1/2 cup (127 g)	6.0
Peas, green, frozen, boiled	1/2 cup (80 g)	4.1

Based on Pennington (114).

Key Point

> Consistent recovery nutrition is an important part of the adaptation process. When tactical athletes have more than one bout of activity per day, it is critical to use a personalized, targeted recovery approach to ensure glycogen restoration and muscle recovery.

The sidebar titled "Postexercise Recovery Meals" includes some ideas for postexercise meals. For a summary of all recommendations for a male tactical athlete who is 170 pounds (77 kg), see table 5.16.

PROVIDING GUIDANCE ON ENERGY BALANCE AND NUTRITION TOOLS

The intention of this chapter is to provide TSAC Facilitators with the background, context, and information to be able to answer basic questions about nutrition. The facilitator should point the tactical athlete to a qualified nutrition professional when a specific, personalized plan is needed.

Nutritional Strategies for Fat Loss and Lean Mass Gain

Many tactical athletes may determine that they would like to alter their body composition or that the demands of their position require some type of adjustment. When guiding a tactical athlete through this process, ensure that the timing of this adjustment is thoughtful and that the athlete has the energy to maintain high levels of performance while achieving the body composition goals.

Energy Excess: Fat Loss

For people who are above their desirable body weight and wish to lose excess body fat, it is important to set realistic goals. The energy content of 1 pound (0.5 kg) of **adipose tissue** (i.e., body fat) is approximately 3,500 kcal (149). Thus, 1 pound (0.5 kg) of extra body fat indicates that energy intake has exceeded energy expenditure by 3,500 kcal. The reduction of body fat can be achieved by a combination of reducing energy intake and increasing energy expenditure. In general, exercise alone is not sufficient to cause significant weight loss (40); rather, it is most critical in the maintenance of weight loss that has occurred. With regard to energy intake, the main concern is finding a level of energy intake that is low enough to reduce body fat but at the same time is achievable and practical for the individual. Restricting energy intake too severely can lead to excessive hunger and relapses of poor eating behaviors. A reasonable goal is a total negative energy balance of 500 kcal per day, which would

Postexercise Recovery Meals

Option 1 (645 calories, 94 g carbohydrate, 25 g protein, 20 g fat, 3.8:1 carbohydrate:protein)

- 1 regular bagel
- 2 tbsp (32 g) peanut butter
- 8 oz (237 ml) 1% low-fat chocolate milk
- 1 oz (30 g) seedless raisins

Option 2 (627 calories, 93 g carbohydrate, 39 g protein, 11 g fat, 2.4:1 carbohydrate:protein)

- 2 cups (473 ml) flavored soy milk plus 3 heaping tsp (30 g) soy protein isolate
- 4 graham cracker squares
- 1 medium apple

Option 3 (380-510 calories, 72-76 g carbohydrate, 21-25 g protein, 3-8 g fat, 2-3:1 carbohydrate:protein)

- 1 scoop high-quality, third-party-tested 100% whey protein
- Ice cubes (optional)
- 2 medium bananas

Can be made into a smoothie in a blender.

Table 5.16 Nutrient Recommendations for a Male Tactical Athlete Weighing 170 Pounds (77 kg)

Timing	Carbohydrate	Protein	Fat	Fluid
Daily (general recommendations)	• 3-5 g/kg body weight per day (low activity levels/skill based) • 5-7 g/kg body weight per day (general training) • 7-10 g/kg body weight per day (high training levels)	1.2-2.0 g/kg body weight per day (higher needs for those who are more active or consuming lower amounts of carbohydrate)	20%-35% of daily needs	• 2.7 L (91 fl oz) per day (women) • 3.7 L (125 fl oz) per day (men)
Preexercise	• 1 hour prior = 0.5 g/kg body weight • 2 hours prior = 1 g/kg body weight • 3 hours prior = 1.5 g/kg body weight • 4 hours prior = 2 g/kg body weight	0.15-0.25 g/kg body weight	No specific recommendation	17-20 fl oz (503-591 ml) of water or sport drink 2-3 hours before exercise and 10 fl oz (296 ml) 10-20 min before physical activity
During exercise	If exercise duration is beyond 60 min or of extreme intensity, 30-60 g carbohydrate an hour	No specific recommendations	No specific recommendations	0.4-0.8 L (14-27 fl oz) per hour
Postexercise	0.8-1.2 g/kg body weight	0.3-0.4 g/kg body weight	No specific recommendations	1.25-1.5 L (42-51 fl oz) for every kg of fluid lost

Based on M.N. Sawka et al. 2007. "American College of Sports Medicine position stand. Exercise and fluid replacement," *Medicine and Science in Sports and Exercise* 39: 377-390.

theoretically result in the loss of 1 pound (0.5 kg) of body fat per week. This energy deficit of 500 kcal per day could be made up of a reduced dietary intake of 300 to 400 kcal and 100 to 200 kcal of physical activity. This strategy might work well for those who are not very fit to begin with. In most cases, a total daily energy deficit greater than 1,000 kcal is not recommended because it is unachievable over the long term.

Another technique that might help with reducing energy intake is to eat frequent, small meals (five or six per day). Contrary to popular belief, this type of meal pattern has not been shown to increase metabolic rate (85). However, it may help to manage hunger so that the tactical athlete does not eat excessive amounts of food at a particular time. Finally, it is critical that tactical athletes preserve their lean body mass while decreasing their body fat. Maintaining a higher level of protein intake—2.3 g/kg (1.0 g/lb) versus 1.0 g/kg (0.5 g/lb) body weight per day—during times of energy restriction helps to retain muscle mass while losing body fat (102).

Lean Muscle Mass Gain

Some tactical athletes will wish to gain weight. Under most circumstances, the majority of the weight gain should be from lean tissue and not fat mass, although there may be times when gaining some body fat is desirable (e.g., insulation during cold exposure). In general, some increase in energy intake will be required, but it is difficult to set an absolute energy target. Some dietary supplements, such as creatine, can help to increase muscle mass and yet are noncaloric (20). However, creatine alone does not increase mass. Creatine provides metabolic support to short, explosive movements; therefore, it supports physical adaptation through training. Also, a positive energy balance of 500 kcal per day (the reverse of the scenario for weight loss) would lead mainly to a gain of 1 pound (0.5 kg) of body fat per week. It still may be a reasonable target but needs to be within the context of an exercise program. The best advice in these situations is multifactorial:

- Ensure that an appropriate exercise program is in place for the tactical athlete.
- Verify that protein intake is consistently meeting the established requirements.

- Ensure that calorie and protein needs are being met. Quantity should not overshadow quality. The inclusion of nutrient- and energy-dense foods will ensure the athlete maintains health and performance while increasing lean body mass. Increase the energy density of the diet (i.e., more energy in less volume).
  - More frequent meals (five or six per day) may be helpful to consume an appropriate amount of food.
  - As stated previously in this chapter, fat has 9 kcal/g, whereas protein and carbohydrate each have 4 kcal/g. Thus, fat is more energy dense than carbohydrate or protein.
  - Water content also influences the energy density of food. For example, raisins have an energy density of 3.0 kcal/g, whereas grapes have an energy density of 0.67 kcal/g.
  - Adding milk powder to casseroles and soups can add protein and calcium.
  - Adding 100% whey protein powder or soy protein to foods like oatmeal or smoothies can help tactical athletes meet their protein needs.
- Opt for a higher ratio of carbohydrate to protein in the postworkout period (3:1 or 4:1).
- Under the guidance of a qualified nutrition professional, dietary supplements (e.g., creatine) can be helpful during certain training phases. (See chapter 7 on supplements.)

Low Energy Availability and the Female Athlete Triad

Energy availability is dietary energy intake minus exercise energy expenditure (4). Consistent low energy availability has been shown to result in low energy and underrecovery. A possible warning sign is if energy intake is less than 30 kcal/kg fat-free mass (4). Low energy availability is a key component of the female athlete triad that can lead to impaired bone health and increased risk of osteoporosis and fractures. Each component of the female athlete triad exists on a continuum ranging from the normal or optimal state to a clinical condition, as shown in figure 5.2.

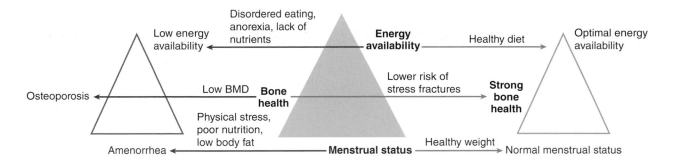

Figure 5.2 The female athlete triad and energy availability.

Helping Tactical Athletes Evaluate Their Nutrition

Giving tactical athletes guidance on what the science recommends is a great step toward helping them reach their nutritional goals, but many may benefit from exposure to various tools that will give them some autonomy as they evaluate their nutritional practices. A number of military-specific tools have been developed to support and guide the tactical athlete, with two of the most prominent being the following:

www.health.mil/Military-Health-Topics/
Operation-Live-Well/Focus-Areas/Nutrition

www.navyfitness.org/nutrition

One simple approach to promote nutritional adequacy is to focus on achieving the recommended number of servings from the various food groups. The U.S. Department of Agriculture (USDA), in collaboration with other agencies, has established the ChooseMyPlate.gov website to provide information on the number of servings that are recommended from the various food groups. One convenient feature of this site is the Super-Tracker for calculating the recommended number of servings per food group based on individual needs. As an example, the SuperTracker calculated the daily recommended number of servings for a 25-year-old, 175-pound (79 kg) male who is 5 feet, 10 inches (1.78 m); engages in more than 60 minutes of physical activity per day; and requires 3,200 calories per day. The results were 10 ounces of grains, 4 cups of vegetables, 2.5 cups of fruits, 3 cups of dairy, 7 ounces of protein, and 11 tea-spoons of oil. The resulting graphical printout defines amounts of individual foods that count as a serving from each food group. This system has replaced the Food Guide Pyramid, although there are still some links to older Food Guide Pyramid materials. There are a total of five food groups on the ChooseMyPlate.gov site (grains, fruits, vegetables, dairy products, and protein foods), along with information on oils and empty calories.

Another feature on the site is a search function in which one can look up combination foods such as tacos or spaghetti and see how many servings from each food group the combination food contains. Multiple other tools on the site are helpful as well, including information for kids, pregnant and breast-feeding women, and people who want to lose weight. Figure 5.3 illustrates the MyPlate concept.

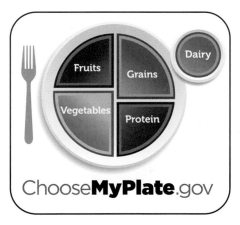

Figure 5.3 Sample plate with recommended portion sizes from the food groups.

USDA's Center for Nutrition Policy and Promotion. choosemyplate.gov

The ChooseMyPlate.gov site encourages people to meet the recommended number of servings from each food group as a way to ensure adequate intakes of essential nutrients. The site also lists a recommended maximum amount of empty calories to limit the amount consumed per day. This promotes high nutrient density, in which the diet provides a high level of nutrients relative to the amount of energy.

Related to the food group concept is the **exchange list** system developed by the Academy of Nutrition and Dietetics and the American Diabetes Association (ADA). In this system, foods are classified into exchange groups as starches, fruits, milk, sweets and desserts, nonstarchy vegetables, meats and meat substitutes, fats, or alcohol. Within each exchange group, the portion size of each food is standardized to provide the same macronutrient content. For example, a starch exchange counts as 15 g carbohydrate, 0 to 3 g protein, 0 to 1 g fat, and 80 kcal. A starch exchange could be a slice of bread or half of an English muffin, among many other choices. Booklets (now titled *Choose Your Foods*) that detail the types and amounts of foods and beverages that count as particular exchanges are available at www.nhlbi.nih.gov/health/educational/lose_wt/eat. Printed copies of these exchange list booklets can be purchased at www.eatrightstore.org. For details on how to use the exchanges, see the previously mentioned website from the National Heart, Lung, and Blood Institute (NHLBI).

Interprofessional Collaboration

Although it is useful for TSAC Facilitators to enhance their knowledge of nutrition in order to respond to general nutrition questions, it is also important to know when to refer a client to a licensed dietetics professional for more specific advice. This is especially true when a medical issue such as type 1 diabetes, celiac disease, or food allergies and intolerances has been identified. In addition, some RD practitioners have achieved an additional board certification to practice sports dietetics in particular, the Certified Specialist in Sports Dietetics (CSSD; www.cdrnet.org/certifications/board-certification-as-a-specialist-in-sports-dietetics).

TSAC Facilitators should identify a network of nearby RDs for referral when necessary. The websites of the Collegiate and Professional Sports Dietitians Association (CPSDA; www.sportsrd.org) and the Academy of Nutrition and Dietetics (www.eatright.org) and its dietetic practice group (SCAN) dealing with sports, cardiovascular, and wellness nutrition (www.scandpg.org) all have features to help people locate RDs in their area.

CONCLUSION

TSAC Facilitators are often the first, and perhaps only, fitness professionals their clients consult about nutrition. The information in this chapter provides a foundation for answering these types of questions. In addition, the USDA, the Institute of Medicine, and the Academy of Nutrition and Dietetics provide a number of online and print resources that TSAC Facilitators can use to help clients achieve their nutrition and fitness goals. For complex nutrition questions, design of prescriptive diets, or clients with significant medical concerns (e.g., diabetes, food allergies and intolerances), referral to an RD is advisable for the safety of the client and to avoid potential liability issues for the fitness professional.

Key Terms

Acceptable Macronutrient Distribution
   Range (AMDR)
adipose tissue
alpha-linolenic acid (ALA)
antioxidants
beta-carotene
casein protein
coenzymes
cofactors
conditionally essential amino acids (CEAA)
dehydration
Dietary Reference Intake (DRI)
docosahexaenoic acid (DHA)
eicosapentaenoic acid (EPA)
electrolytes
essential amino acids (EAA)
exchange list
free radicals
gluconeogenesis
glycemic index
glycemic load
glycogen
heme iron
hemoglobin
hyponatremia

insulin
licensure
macronutrients
metabolism
micronutrients
Military Dietary Reference Intake (MDRI)
monounsaturated fatty acids
myoglobin
nonessential amino acids
nonheme iron
nutrient timing
omega-3 fatty acid (*n*-3)
omega-6 fatty acid (*n*-6)
polyunsaturated fatty acids
protein digestibility-corrected amino acid
   score (PDCAAS)
Recommended Dietary Allowance (RDA)
registered dietitian (RD), or registered
   dietitian nutritionist (RDN)
saturated fatty acid, or saturated fat
sports dietitian
sports nutrition coach
sports nutritionist with an advanced degree
trans fat
whey protein

Study Questions

1. Which of the following is the first step to address the nutritional needs of tactical athletes?

  a. Understand basic fueling concepts.

  b. Understand the demands of the tactical athlete.

  c. Within the scope of practice, create nutritional guidance for daily, or foundational, nutritional needs.

  d. Within the scope of practice, create nutritional recommendations to support performance and recovery.

2. Which of the following activities creates the greatest energy expenditure?

  a. running 10 mph (16 km/h)

  b. bicycling 16-19 mph (25.7-31 km/h)

  c. soccer (general)

  d. boxing (sparring)

3. As exercise intensity increases, how does the proportion of muscular energy used from carbohydrates and fats change?

  a. decreased carbohydrates, increased fats

  b. decreased carbohydrates, decreased fats

  c. increased carbohydrates, decreased fats

  d. increased carbohydrates, increased fats

4. Which of the following is an essential amino acid?

  a. alanine

  b. leucine

  c. asparagine

  d. serine

Chapter 6

Tactical Fueling

Maj. Nicholas D. Barringer, PhD, RD, CSCS,*D, CSSD
Maj. Aaron P. Crombie, PhD, RD

After completing this chapter, you will be able to

- describe nutritional needs in general and the unique nutritional needs of tactical athletes,
- describe nutritional strategies that optimize body composition and maximize physical performance and recovery in tactical scenarios,
- describe signs, symptoms, behaviors, and performance variations associated with obesity and altered eating habits and disorders, and
- analyze case-specific and problem-centered scenarios for tactical fueling.

The opinions or assertions contained herein are the private views of the authors and are not to be construed as official or reflecting the views of the Army, the Department of Defense, or the U.S. Government.

Fire and rescue personnel, law enforcement officers, military members, and other tactical athletes have similar fueling needs dictated by occupational conditions and requirements (68). Tactical athletes typically must perform demanding physical tasks while under load, which may include specialized clothing and **personal protective equipment (PPE)**, such as body armor or SCBA; while exposed to environmental hazards (e.g., smoke, fire, combat); and while subjected to environmental extremes such as heat, cold, altitude, and arduous terrain. These tasks are often further complicated by aggravating factors such as energy and sleep deficits, which can affect both cognitive and physical performance (29, 41, 53). Tactical athletes may be similar to sport athletes in that they have increased nutritional requirements to support training and events. However, tactical athletes may not have the benefit of time to prepare, refuel, and recover, and thus they may suffer consequences in task performance and personal risk if plans are not put in place to facilitate recovery. Performing tasks in such extreme conditions and under load dramatically affects energy expenditure, and prolonged operations (e.g., long patrols, military engagements, work–rest cycles in fighting wildfires) will influence the quantity and quality of tactical athletes' nutritional intakes (5, 6). Furthermore, thought must be given to logistical constraints that will affect food variety, quantity and quality, and availability, especially in instances of combat and disaster relief, where the local infrastructure may be disrupted. The tactical environment yields unique conditions that affect the nutritional requirements of people operating in such a setting, even for short periods of time.

NUTRITIONAL NEEDS OF TACTICAL ATHLETES

Guidance for recommended nutritional intakes are provided for U.S. military members in the **Military Dietary Reference Intakes (MDRI)** in joint publication Army Regulation 40-25 on nutrition standards and education (1). This publication references U.S. Army Research Institute of Environmental Medicine (USARIEM) Technical Note TN 00/10 (8), which provides the rationale for MDRIs, using median weights for males (79

kg [174 lb]) and females (62 kg [137 lb]), based on the Dietary Reference Intakes (DRIs) (see chapter 5). In turn, the MDRIs are used to develop the **Nutritional Standards for Operational and Restricted Rations (NSOR)**, which are criteria that rations must meet if they are to be the sole source of nutrition for military personnel for prolonged periods of time. The NSOR are designed to be used when planning troop feeding in a field setting (8). However, these reference ranges are based on coverage for large groups of people, and specific recommendations should be tailored based on the individual's anthropometrics, intensity and duration of workload, and performance environment.

Currently there are no published recommendations for nutritional needs specific to tactical athletes outside the military. The primary goal is meeting the tactical athletes' overall energy needs and achieving **energy balance** to facilitate maintenance of lean body mass. The operational environment will alter recommendations for specific **micronutrient** needs, as discussed later in the chapter. Note that fire and rescue and law enforcement may have prolonged periods with no sustained operations, during which recommendations consistent with their training schedules will be appropriate. Dietary intake during downtime or between missions or calls should be similar to the intake of athletes in the off-season. These off-cycle diets should provide sufficient energy and protein to maintain a desirable body composition and support lean mass maintenance or gain, and the majority of fat should be unsaturated. Recommendations must also include consuming plenty of fruits, vegetables, and whole grains from a variety of foods to ensure micronutrient needs are met. See chapter 5 for general nutrition recommendations, including ChooseMyPlate.gov. Again, dietary plans should be individualized based on the athlete's fitness, performance, and **body composition** goals. If the athlete is coming off a prolonged mission and has lost lean mass, those deficits should also be addressed with small energy surpluses to support weight gain. Military tactical athletes may also have periods of recovery, but these are usually supplemented with training.

Total daily energy expenditure (TDEE) has been observed in excess of 4,500 kcal per day in U.S. Army Ranger training (75), over 5,000 kcal per day during U.S. Army Special Forces training (43, 45, 75), and over 4,500 kcal per day in firefighting scenarios (19). Limited data are available for law enforcement personnel. Energy needs are typically higher during missions and must be adequate to support training requirements, but they can vary considerably. Maintenance of energy balance is necessary for preserving body and muscle weight, sparing muscle breakdown, maintaining glycogen stores, and sustaining work and power output and attenuation of muscle fatigue (4, 9, 83). Energy requirements increase with intensity of physical activity and in cold and hot versus temperate environments:

- Cold: 35 to 68 kcal/kg body weight per day
- Hot: 40 to 75 kcal/kg body weight per day
- Temperate: 32 to 63 kcal/kg body weight per day

However, energy consumption in arduous environments is often decreased (6). In addition, as energy needs and intakes increase, so do requirements for the micronutrients (described in chapter 5) involved in energy metabolism.

NUTRIENT REQUIREMENTS OF TACTICAL ATHLETES UNDER VARIOUS CONDITIONS

The human body must maintain homeostasis with regard to body temperature and hydration, and ideally it should maintain energy balance as well. For tactical athletes, maintenance of lean mass and physical and cognitive performance is also required. All of these factors are tied to both survivability and performance of tactical tasks under stressful conditions. Normal core body temperatures range from 36.5 to 37.5 °C (97.7-99.5 °F) and can rise as high as 41 °C (106 °F) during extreme physical activity and febrile conditions. Body temperatures above 40 °C (104 °F) can result in impaired thermoregulation, which can lead to heat injury and stroke (13), permanent brain damage, and ultimately death. Likewise, cold temperatures (depending on percent body fat) can result in shivering; impaired coordination, speech, and cognition; loss of consciousness and thermoregulation; and ultimately death (73).

Performing in these conditions, and adapting or acclimatizing to environmental stressors such as heat, cold, altitude, and terrain, rely on maintaining optimal nutritional status and nutrient intake. Optimal nutrition facilitates maintenance of hydration status, accrual (during training) and preservation (during prolonged or multiple operations) of lean mass, and peak cognitive performance, and it mitigates the balance of inflammatory responses and reduces the risk for nutritional deficiencies. Without adequate energy, protein, and micronutrient intakes, tactical athletes who must perform tasks for prolonged periods may suffer decreased performance in tactical tasks, which could result in life-threatening situations.

Nutritional intake must meet training and mission needs, support lean mass accrual, facilitate rapid recovery, and account for potential imbalances (prolonged unavoidable energy deficit). Furthermore, many tactical athletes are held to specific body composition standards (military, law enforcement) or standards associated with optimal performance of tactical tasks. Nutrient needs are dictated by the training and operational environment, mission tasks, and nutrition products available for consumption.

Key Point

Match the appropriate macronutrient and micronutrient recommendations to the tactical athlete's mission.

Nutrient Needs During Environmental Challenges

The human body can acclimate to environmental stress (heat, cold, hypoxia) through metabolic and physiological adaptations (perspiration volume and rate, shivering, vasodilation and vasoconstriction), but suboptimal nutrition can affect these responses. A common theme among all environmental extremes is an increase in energy expenditure. This increase is secondary to the extremes themselves (heat, cold, altitude) and to performing work under such conditions. Hot environments are associated with ambient temperatures above 30 °C (86 °F), cold environments are below 0 °C (32 °F), and high-altitude environments are above 3,050 meters (10,000 ft) (5, 6). In hot environments, higher energy expenditure is a result of increases in ventilation and sweat gland activity (6). For the tactical athlete, physiological responses to cold may not be as pertinent because specialized clothing is usually worn, but the added weight of clothing plus movement in conditions typical of cold environments (e.g., over ice, through snow) increase energy expenditures. At altitude, decreases in the partial pressure of oxygen and humidity affect physiological responses; combined with the likelihood of operating in rugged terrain, they contribute substantially to energy expenditure (5).

Environmental extremes also increase requirements for fluids and in some cases micronutrients (30, 34, 37, 48, 55, 60). Also common in these types of environments are a lack of appetite and decreased availability and consumption of food and fluids; coupled with increases in energy and nutrient requirements, they compound the problem and can create significant energy deficits (30, 34). If not corrected through appropriate nutritional intake, this can lead to loss of lean mass, depleted muscle glycogen, and decreased fine motor coordination, physical performance, and work capacity (5).

Fluid and Electrolyte Needs

Fluid needs can be estimated based on the body weight and energy intake of the person (typically 1 ml or 0.03 fl oz per kcal), therefore accounting for increases in energy requirements that certain environmental conditions present. Dry body weight taken before and after events can indicate weight loss due to fluids and therefore help gauge replacement. The box "Mission Hydration" summarizes the recommendations of the Academy of Nutrition and Dietetics and the American College of Sports Medicine (ACSM) (64).

Depending on the environment, fluid needs may increase at rest and during work. In a hot environment, fluid replacement (as opposed to fuel) is the priority, and adequate intakes are required to minimize fatigue and prevent heat-related injury. Failure to replace fluids adequately will compromise thermoregulation because a reduction in blood volume may decrease sweat rates and limit evaporative cooling (51, 67). With acclimatization, sweat rate and plasma volume increase, the onset of sweating (threshold) begins at a lower core temperature, and resting and exercising core temperature and HR are lower (5, 6, 21).

Cold environments also increase fluid needs. However, they often promote a decreased thirst sensation and cold-induced diuresis, which can led to inadequate fluid intakes and excessive fluid losses (39, 44).

Altitude poses similar problems with maintaining fluid homeostasis. At altitude the humidity is lower, and individuals will experience fluid losses from hypoxia-induced increases in ventilation and diuresis, which are further imbalanced by reduced intakes secondary to poor thirst sensation and possible decreased availability of fluids (34, 48). Although energy needs are greatly increased at altitude, given the reduced oxygen availability and physiological stress placed upon the body, carbohydrate is preferred over energy-dense fat (30), which requires oxidative metabolism. The hypoxic environment will increase lipid peroxidation of unsaturated fatty acids in cell membranes (including red blood cells), and adequate polyunsaturated fat and supplementation with antioxidants, particularly vitamin E, may help offset this free radical damage (7, 15). Over several days to even weeks, the body also adapts to hypoxemia with increases in hematopoiesis to increase hemoglobin concentration

Mission Hydration

- Before mission: Consume 5 to 7 ml (0.2-0.24 fl oz) per kcal of water or sport drink 4 hours before.
- During mission: Consume enough fluid to limit dehydration to <2% loss of body weight.
- After mission: Consume at least 450 to 675 ml (15-23 fl oz) for every 0.45 kg (1 lb) of body weight lost.

Sodium

The *2015-2020 Dietary Guidelines for Americans* recommends a sodium intake of 2,300 mg for men and women between 18 and 50 years of age (2). This equates to 1,000 to 1,300 mg per 1,000 kcal for those with a relatively sedentary lifestyle. However, increases in ambient temperature and sweating increase sodium losses, even with acclimatization, and thus increase overall needs. As environmental temperatures and energy expenditures rise, overall energy intake should increase, including a corresponding increase in sodium intake. Sodium is often replaced through fluids, and the recommended sodium concentration in fluid-replacement beverages ranges from 20 to 50 mmol/L (46-115 mg/dl) (67, 70). Sometimes this is insufficient, so eating "small amounts of salty snacks or sodium-containing foods at meals will help to stimulate thirst and retain the consumed fluids" (67).

Table 6.1   Recommended Daily Protein Intakes for Various Activity Levels

Activity level or conditions	Grams per pound body weight	Grams per kilogram body weight
Low to moderate activities include sitting quietly or engaging in light exercise such as a brisk walk, yoga, hiking, or softball.	0.4-0.5	0.8-1.0
Endurance training is vigorous exercise that challenges the aerobic system, such as running, cycling, swimming, and sports such as basketball or racquetball.	0.5-0.6	1.2-1.4
Strength training involves resistance exercise such as weight training, lifting heavy objects, and use of resistance bands. Typically the goal of muscle building is to increase lean body mass without gaining fat, so it's important to eat right and maintain energy balance.	0.6-0.8	1.4-1.7
High energy demands combined with insufficient calories require greater intakes.	0.7-0.9	1.5-2.0

Reprinted from Human Performance Resource Center, from the Consortium for Health and Military Performance (CHAMP). http://hprc-online.org/nutrition/files/ProteinRequirementsTable.pdf

and therefore the oxygen-carrying capacity of the blood; new red blood cells can be seen within four to five days (37). The erythropoietic adaptation to altitude depends on iron stores, and although additional iron may not be necessary in males, females and those who are iron insufficient or deficient would benefit from supplemental iron up to four weeks before going to high-altitude environments.

Protein Needs

Protein intake must be high enough to support rigorous training, including resistance training. The percentage of energy provided from protein may be higher during periods of unavoidable and prolonged energy deficit. Strenuous military training has shown decreases in whole-body protein balance, increases in protein flux and breakdown, and large energy deficits (14, 44, 58). Investigators have also found that ingesting twice the amount of protein in the daily **Recommended Dietary Allowance (RDA)** of 0.8 g/kg body weight during rigorous training may help preserve lean mass (14, 57-59). Recommendations for protein in athletes vary based on the type of training and athletic goals, with aerobic sports and activities receiving recommendations of 1.2 g/kg body weight (0.6 g/lb) per day and up to 1.7 g/kg body weight (0.8 g/lb) per day for strength-based sports (64). These guidelines are appropriate for tactical athletes, but 2.0 g/kg body weight (0.9 g/lb) may be needed during periods of energy deficit to maintain muscle mass and therefore physical performance (58). (See table 6.1.)

Carbohydrate Needs

Carbohydrate requirements increase concomitantly with increases in energy needs. Following are guidelines for daily intake based on activity levels:

- 3 to 5 g/kg body weight (1.4-2.3 g/lb) for light training <60 minutes per day
- 5 to 7 g/kg body weight (2.2-3.2 g/lb) for moderate-intensity training 60 minutes per day
- 6 to 10 g/kg body weight (2.7-4.5 g/lb) for moderate- to high-intensity endurance exercise 1 to 3 hours per day
- 8 to 12 g/kg body weight (3.6-5.5 g/lb) for moderate- to high-intensity exercise lasting 4 to 5 hours per day (66)

Note that 600 to 650 g may be the most amount of carbohydrate that can be used for glycogen replacement (18) and may result in gastrointestinal distress (20), so absolute amounts need to be considered.

In extreme conditions such as high altitude, increased carbohydrate intake is recommended. Additional carbohydrate supplementation has demonstrated ergogenic benefits (55, 60).

Micronutrient Needs

Micronutrient needs are often associated with increases in oxidative metabolism (see chapter 4). With a balanced diet, increases in energy intakes result in increases in micronutrient intakes. However, the tactical environment and prolonged operations may make increased intakes of nutrients more difficult. Increased cellular damage from the environment, stress, and heavy work output may also require modifications to recommended nutrient intakes, especially when it comes to antioxidant intakes.

Calcium and Vitamin D

Calcium is required in adequate amounts to reduce risk for stress fractures during basic military training and other strenuous tactical training, especially for people who are unaccustomed to regular physical training. Increased perspiration during exposure to hot environments (including when acclimatized) will increase losses of sodium, chloride, potassium, calcium, magnesium, and iron (79). However, if nutritional intake is sufficient to meet overall energy needs, a well-balanced diet should replace these losses.

Vitamin D is a vitamin of particular interest to the tactical athlete; recent research has demonstrated a high prevalence of insufficiency and deficiency in this population (23, 77, 82). Because vitamin D supports bone health (31), and blood levels of vitamin D have been significantly associated with muscle mass (25), strength (26), and testosterone (80, 81), sufficient levels may be needed to optimize performance. To maintain adequate levels, the Endocrine Society recommends that adults consume 600 IU per day of vitamin D (33, 65), although 1,500 to 2,000 IU per day may be required to consistently achieve sufficient levels (32).

Iron

Poor iron status is associated with decrements in both cognitive and physical performance. Following basic military training, iron status has been shown to deteriorate in both males and females, but to a greater extent in females (47, 84). Iron supplementation in female military trainees showed attenuation in this decline when compared with nonsupplemented controls (47, 84).

Female athletes especially are at risk of poor iron status, primarily due to menstrual losses coupled with lower overall dietary intakes compared with men. Although iron supplementation is effective at improving iron status, supplements may result in gastrointestinal irritation, nausea, and even constipation (3). Therefore, adequate iron intakes are best achieved through dietary sources (see the box "Dietary Sources of Iron").

Iron is obtained from heme and nonheme sources (78). Plants and iron-fortified foods contain nonheme iron only, whereas meat, seafood, and poultry contain both heme and nonheme iron. Heme iron is the preferred source, and makes up approximately 40% of the iron present in meat. Nonheme iron should be consumed with a source of vitamin C (e.g., citrus fruits, strawberries, peppers, tomato products, potatoes, cabbage) to improve absorption (74). A mixed diet including heme iron and vitamin C may be the best method for meeting daily iron needs. Iron recommendations for military personnel in high-altitude environments are likely good guidelines for other tactical athletes operating at altitude, again with the preferred source being iron-rich foods to prevent iron overload and gastrointestinal side effects. These high-altitude recommendations are 15 mg of iron daily for men and 20 mg for women, whereas the RDA is 8 mg for men and 18 mg for women (62).

Dietary Sources of Iron

- Legumes (lima beans, dried beans, kidney beans)
- Dried fruit (raisins, prunes, dried apricots)
- Eggs (including yolk)
- Iron-fortified cereals
- Oysters and other shellfish
- Poultry and red meat (beef, lamb, pork) (78)

Nutrient Needs During Deployment and Shift Work

Deployment and shift work are realities for the tactical athlete and can negatively affect sleep, physical performance, cognition, and immune function (42). Besides practicing good sleep, nutritional strategies may help reset the circadian rhythm (28). Some research has shown consuming a high-glycemic meal within 4 hours of bedtime may improve sleep-onset latency compared with a low-glycemic meal (28). Timing is critical; a high-glycemic meal 1 hour before bed has been shown to disturb sleep (56). Consuming a high-protein diet, avoiding a high fat intake, and taking in around 1 g of tryptophan (the amount found in 10 oz or 284 g of turkey) may also improve sleep onset and quality (28). Melatonin may serve as an alternative to pharmaceutical interventions to promote sleep (17). Employing optimal nutritional strategies in conjunction with good sleep hygiene can mitigate the deleterious effects of deployment and shift work on performance.

Operating on a Caloric Deficit for Prolonged Periods

Nindl and associates have documented the negative consequences of operating in a prolonged caloric deficit (53). At the U.S. Army Ranger School, soldiers experiencing 1,000 kcal deficits per day for eight weeks lost 13% body mass, with 6% being fat-free mass (4). The soldiers also experienced a drop in physical performance, with a 16% decrease in jump height, 21% decrease in explosive power, and 20% loss in maximal lift strength (53). Similarly, Sharp and colleagues (69) reported a 3.5% decrease loss in fat-free mass, 4.5% loss in $\dot{V}O_2$max, and 4.9% loss in explosive power but no significant change in vertical jump and lifting strength after a nine-month Afghanistan deployment (58). Such data are not available for tactical athletes within the civilian sector, but similar consequences might be expected.

One of the proven strategies to counter energy restriction and mitigate the associated lean mass losses and performance decrements during prolonged tactical operations is to increase protein intake. The Center Alliance for Dietary Supplement Research (CADSR) and the U.S. Army Medical Research and Materiel Command (USAMRMC) consensus statement recommends a protein intake of 1.5 to 2.0 g/kg body weight (0.7-0.9 g/lb) per day for periods of substantial exertion with inadequate caloric intake (57).

Coping With Unpredictable Access to Food and Water

Due to operational demands and unpredictable missions, tactical athletes need to be prepared to maintain their fueling at any given moment. One simple way to meet nutritional needs is to carry a protein-rich bar (19) or other whole foods such as nut butters or boiled eggs as a snack. Being prepared is critical. One study of 387 Marines found that a snack bar consisting of 8 g carbohydrate, 10 g protein, and 3 g fat led to fewer medical visits and heat exhaustion cases compared with controls receiving either no snack bar or a snack bar with identical carbohydrate and fat grams without protein (22). Having a nutritionally balanced snack available at all times can mitigate the consequences of missing a meal (59).

Although fat intake is usually not a concern because most tactical situations requiring restriction are not long enough to warrant concerns about a deficiency, the type of fat consumed is important. In particular, linoleic acid and omega-3 fatty acids are beneficial (27). **Omega-3** fatty acids, specifically, **eicosapentaenoic acid (EPA)** and **docosahexaenoic acid (DHA)**, are of interest to the tactical athlete because their availability may be limited in tactical situations and prepared snacks (62). Several medical and nutrition experts recommend supplementation as the most efficient means of increasing EPA and DHA in the tactical athlete (21). Although no recommendations are yet available for the tactical athlete, ways to increase EPA and DHA in the diet of the warfighter are being explored (50). Industry and the military are looking for ways to increase the availability of foods high in omega-3 fatty acids by enhancing the omega-3 content of various foods, including chicken, baked goods, milk, and eggs.

Hydration is also a concern during unexpected and unplanned missions because of the negative effects even mild **dehydration** can have on cognitive function, mood, and marksmanship (24, 76). Given that 1 quart (1 L) of water weighs 2 pounds (1 kg), the total weight of the load to be carried by tactical athletes may limit the amount of water carried. Nolte and colleagues (54) recommended a minimum volume of 300 ml (10 fl oz) per hour for soldiers undergoing a 16 km (10 mi) rucksack march when the temperature was only 24.6 °C (76.3 °F) (68). Fluid intakes for wildland firefighters are somewhat higher during work in hot environments (up to 39 °C [102 °F]) and will likely range from 300 to 1,000 ml (10-34 fl oz) per hour depending on the ambient temperature (40, 61). See the previous box on mission hydration for guidance. Planning for extra water via air drops or using known safe water sources in the area with the appropriate prophylactics such as iodine tablets are other ways to circumvent carrying the extra weight.

Key Point

> Establish a nutrition and hydration plan before the mission and an alternative plan in case the mission goes long so the tactical athlete remains fueled regardless of the situation.

Tips to Help Tactical Athletes Meet Their Nutrient Requirements

In the sport world, athletes train for competitive events. In the tactical world, a competitive event would be analogous to an operation, and thus preparations should be made within this context. An operation could be any event from chasing a criminal to responding to an emergency call, patrolling a crowd on a hot day, or engaging in wildfire suppression. Considerations should be made for refueling during, between, and after operations. Tactical athletes should plan for periods where they can refuel and rehydrate in order to maintain euhydration and replenish glycogen stores. For example, military personnel on dismounted patrols should plan for meals after completing patrols as well as fueling during patrols as appropriate. Long periods of time with poor access to nutrition or fluids should be anticipated with planning to mitigate the effects.

The nutritional goals prior to beginning an event or operation are primarily to ensure that the tactical athlete is euhydrated (i.e., a normal state of body water content) and has optimal fuel stores (muscle and liver glycogen). Glycogen stores depend on sex, diet, lean mass, and the training status of the tactical athlete. Typically, 300 to 400 kcal of glycogen are stored in the liver and 1,200 to 1,600 kcal are stored in the muscles. Much like exercise, the type, duration, and intensity of activities performed during an operation will determine **macronutrient** needs, but the general recommended macronutrient content of the diet is

- 45% to 65% carbohydrate,
- 15% to 35% protein, and
- 20% to 35% fat (64, 66).

With longer activities, there is greater reliance upon blood glucose (liver glycogen) and free fatty acids as energy sources, but short-term, high-intensity activities may be dispersed in the larger scope of the operation, and these activities will increase utilization of intramuscular energy stores (glycogen and intramuscular fat). Following an event or operation, the nutritional goals are to replenish glycogen stores, provide adequate protein to repair damaged tissue, and rehydrate.

Before the tactical athlete leaves the police station, firehouse, or wire for a mission, a meal or a shake containing 40 g carbohydrate, 20 to 25 g protein, and adequate fluid should be consumed. For hydration purposes, the tactical athlete should be weighed before the mission begins.

During missions lasting multiple hours, the tactical athlete should consume 30 to 60 g carbohydrate per hour in whatever form the athlete prefers (e.g., gels, bars, beverages, high-carbohydrate foods) along with fluids. At the end of the mission, the tactical athlete should reweigh and consume 16 to 20 fluid ounces (473-591 ml) for every pound (0.5 kg) of weight lost (67, 70). The tactical athlete should consume a meal or supplement containing 60 to 80 g or more of carbohydrate (depending on mission length) and 20 to 25 g protein (depending on body size and composition).

The optimal carbohydrate-to-protein ratio is 1:1 to 4:1. However, this refers to high-quality carbohydrate and protein to replenish muscle glycogen rather than an isocaloric high-carbohydrate drink (69). Protein recommendations are based on research demonstrating that 20 to 25 g achieves maximal protein synthesis (52). Carbohydrate recommendations are based on an estimated oxidation rate of approximately 1 g per minute (35). Although these recommendations are based on research, the reality on the ground will dictate fueling strategies; the goal is to get as close to the recommendations as possible rather than worrying about precise macronutrient intake. The strenuous nature of the mission and body composition of the tactical athlete should also be considered. The recommendations in table 6.2 are based on vigorous operations.

Case-Specific Tactical Scenarios

The following case studies illustrate the need to consume fluids and snacks to sustain physical and cognitive function in tactical situations. A common scenario is when an operation is unexpectedly long. Whether it is a military mission that suddenly is extended, EMS personnel responding quickly to a mass casualty incident, or police officers in a standoff, tactical athletes may become nutritionally compromised if they don't plan ahead. Other scenarios include environmental challenges and shift work. Not planning for adequate nutrition can negatively affect performance. It is imperative that tactical athletes not only learn how to fuel adequately before the mission but also have a plan such as a paced snack or extra fluids in case the mission goes longer than anticipated.

CASE STUDY
Mission Extended

The original mission was supposed to be 6 hours in Southwest Asia but turned into a 36-hour mission. The tactical athletes completed a 2 km (1 mi) movement to target (infiltration) and movement away from target (exfiltration) in a mix of hilly and urban terrain. It was 40 °C (104 °F) in the sun and 35°C (95 °F) in the shade. Each tactical athlete was carrying at least 100 fluid ounces (3 L), one oral rehydration salt pack, and one MRE ration. When the mission was extended, air supply dropped an additional 6 L (203 fl oz), two to three gel packs, and one MRE per person. The lesson learned is always plan for a longer mission.

CASE STUDY
Firefighting in the Heat

A firefighter was responding to a house fire in July in Texas, and the temperature was 38 °C (100 °F). The TSAC Facilitator had learned early on that planning for adequate nutrition and hydration was critical to keep firefighters healthy and mission ready. Based on the TSAC manual, the facilitator had established the following plan:

- Have firefighters monitor their urine color to maintain a clear to light yellow color while at the firehouse or coming on shift.
- Plan a high-carbohydrate meal with 10 to 20 g protein and 20% or less calories coming from fat.
- Plan for cool beverages and popsicles to aid in hydrating and lowering core temperature when recovering from firefighting or cycling in and out of the fire.
- Have firefighters weigh themselves when they return to the firehouse and consume 16 to 24 fluid ounces (473-710 ml) for every pound (0.5 kg) of fluid lost.

The firefighters followed the TSAC Facilitator's advice and remained adequately fed and hydrated despite the heat.

NUTRITION-RELATED CONDITIONS AND CHRONIC DISEASES OF TACTICAL ATHLETES

Tactical athletes face the same nutrition-related chronic diseases as the general population:

Table 6.2   Mission Fueling

Nutrient	Before mission	During mission	After mission
Carbohydrate	≥40 g	30-60 g per hour	60-80 g
Protein	20-25 g	No recommendation established	20-25 g
Fat	No trans fat, ≤10% saturated fat	No trans fat, ≤10% saturated fat	No trans fat, ≤10% saturated fat

Based on Jeukendrip and Gleeson (35); Moore et al. (52); Rodriguez, Di Marco, and Langley (64).

obesity, altered eating habits and disorders, diabetes, and coronary artery disease (10, 38, 63). The good news is that intake of food with a higher nutritional quality is associated with lower risk for chronic disease, so strategies to combat these nutrition-related conditions are available (16). The Nutritional Quality Index (NQI) is a ranking system that quantifies food's nutritional value to calories per serving. The TSAC Facilitator still must be aware of the signs, symptoms, and performance variations associated with nutrition-related conditions and chronic disease, as well as prevalence in each tactical athlete population, and refer athletes to an RD or a licensed nutritionist.

Key Point

All nutrition-related conditions and chronic diseases should be referred to the appropriate medical provider, RD, or RDN.

Obesity

The tactical athlete is not immune to the growing obesity epidemic. The *2011 Health Related Behaviors Survey of Active Duty Military Personnel* reported an obesity rate of 12.4% across all U.S. services, with a rate per service of

- 15.8% for the Army,
- 14.9% for the Navy,
- 4.9% for the Marine Corps,
- 9.7% for the Air Force, and
- 10.5% for the Coast Guard (10).

Obesity rates for police officers—based on abdominal measurements with ≥102 inches (259 cm) for males and ≥88 inches (224 cm) for females—have been reported at 27.1% based on a 70-person

sample by Baughman and associates (11, 76, 77). High rates of obesity based on **body mass index (BMI)** have been reported in firefighting communities (36, 71). This is concerning not only because of performance and physiological health concerns but also psychological concerns; obesity is associated with serious psychological distress in both men and women (72). When BMI is used in conjunction with either waist circumference or percent body fat, the rates of obesity change (36).

BMI is an index derived from weight and height or weight in kilograms divided by height in meters squared. Individuals are then classified as having a normal BMI (18.5-24.99), overweight BMI (25.0-29.99), or obese BMI (>30.0) (56). However, BMI is not appropriate for muscular people because it will inaccurately label them as overweight or obese. For this reason, it is best to assess both BMI and waist circumference or percent body fat to accurately identify tactical athletes who are obese (36).

Altered Eating Habits and Disorders

A survey of 76,476 U.S. service members reported the overall rate of eating disorders at 3.1%, with 2.9% in male service members and 4.3% in female service members (63). Data on eating disorders in firefighters and police are limited, but eating disorders should still be considered when working with all tactical athletes because posttraumatic stress disorder (PTSD) has been associated with eating disorders (49). Given the negative impact of altered eating habits and disorders on the tactical athlete's health and performance, early identification of signs and symptoms is imperative. A good position paper on altered eating habits and disorders in the tactical athlete is the *National Athletic Trainers' Association Position Statement: Preventing, Detecting, and Managing Disordered*

> ## Risk Factors of Coronary Artery Disease
>
> Look for the following risk factors in tactical athletes:
>
> - Age (>40 for men, >45 for women)
> - Sex (males at higher risk)
> - Family history of coronary heart disease, smoking, hypertension, diabetes, obesity, unhealthy cholesterol levels, low physical activity levels, and accumulation of abdominal fat (82)

Eating in Athletes (12). A TSAC Facilitator should refer anyone with an eating disorder to a qualified expert such as a physician, RD, or behavior health specialist.

Some signs, symptoms, behaviors, and performance variations associated with altered eating habits and disorders are as follows (12):

- Dehydration
- Muscle cramps
- Extreme weight fluctuations
- Fatigue beyond what is normally expected from training
- Fear of weight gain

Coronary Artery Disease Risk Factors Associated With Dietary Choices

Coronary artery disease causes 45% of deaths among firefighters while they are on duty (38). Even more concerning is that the odds of death from coronary artery disease was highest (12.1 to 136) during fire suppression (38). Experiencing a cardiovascular event while subduing a fire not only puts the firefighter's life in greater danger but also the lives of the other firefighters and possibly the people they are trying to save.

CONCLUSION

Appropriate fueling and hydration are imperative for the tactical athlete's optimal performance. The TSAC Facilitator must consider the missions, environments, and physiology of their athletes and make recommendations appropriate to the setting and within the TSAC Facilitator's scope of practice. Most fueling recommendations for tactical athletes are derived from various sports, so be aware of emerging research using tactical athletes that either verifies or changes current practices. The biggest difference in fueling the tactical athlete versus the typical sport athlete is the unexpectedness variable; for instance, the end of a game or match is predetermined, whereas a mission often is not. Although overtime is a possibility in most sports, it is typically measured in minutes, whereas for the tactical athlete overtime could be measured in hours or even days. Thus, it is essential the tactical athlete is adequately fueled before the mission, that a nutrition plan is in place to maintain fueling for the duration of the operation even if that is unknown, and a recovery nutrition plan has been agreed upon to optimize recovery for the next mission.

Key Terms

body composition
body mass index (BMI)
dehydration
docosahexaenoic acid (DHA)
eicosapentaenoic acid (EPA)
energy balance
macronutrient
micronutrient

Military Dietary Reference Intake (MDRI)
Nutritional Standards for Operational and
  Restricted Rations (NSOR)
omega-3 fatty acid
personal protective equipment (PPE)
Recommended Dietary Allowance (RDA)
total daily energy expenditure (TDEE)

Study Questions

1. Which of the following body temperatures creates the most potential for impaired thermoregulation?
   a. 36.5 °C (97.7 °F)
   b. 37.5 °C (99.5 °F)
   c. 38.3 °C (101 °F)
   d. 40 °C (104 °F)

2. During missions lasting multiple hours, how much carbohydrate should a tactical athlete consume per hour?
   a. 20-25 g
   b. 30-60 g
   c. 80-120 g
   d. 130-150 g

3. A tactical athlete is in strenuous field training in which prolonged periods of energy deficit occur. Which of the following is the primary reason a daily protein intake of 2 g/kg body weight (0.9 g/lb) is needed?
   a. increase lean muscle mass
   b. maintain physical performance
   c. decrease body fat percentage
   d. improve aerobic capacity

4. At least how much fluid should be consumed by a tactical athlete for every pound (0.5 kg) of weight lost during a mission?
   a. 10 fl oz (296 ml)
   b. 16 fl oz (473 ml)
   c. 23 fl oz (680 ml)
   d. 32 fl oz (946 ml)

Chapter 7

Ergogenic Aids

Abbie E. Smith-Ryan, PhD, CSCS,*D, FNSCA, FISSN
Colin D. Wilborn, PhD, CSCS, ATC
Eric T. Trexler, MA, CSCS, CISSN

After completing this chapter, you will be able to

- describe the limitations of regulating dietary supplements,
- identify the approaches to risk stratification of dietary supplements,
- explain the methods of use and potential benefits and risks of common performance-enhancing supplements,
- describe the process for reporting an adverse reaction to a dietary supplement, and
- recognize and discuss the signs and symptoms of ergogenic aid abuse.

The use of dietary supplements is increasingly common among sport athletes, tactical athletes, and the general population, resulting in a multibillion-dollar global supplement industry. Although some nutritional supplements may offer benefits for tactical personnel, consumers should be aware of the regulation, oversight, and effects of supplements and their manufacturers, packers, and distributors to avoid consuming products that may have inaccurate labeling or contain banned or deleterious ingredients.

REGULATION OF DIETARY SUPPLEMENTS

In the United States, the **Food and Drug Administration (FDA)** regulates a broad spectrum of products, including food products, drugs, biologics, and medical devices. The FDA is also responsible for regulating finished dietary supplements and dietary ingredients contained in such products. In 1994, the U.S. Congress passed legislation that defined the term **dietary supplement**, with important legal implications for the regulation of these products. As a result of this legislation, dietary supplements are viewed as a distinct class of products under the foods umbrella and are therefore subject to regulations that differ from those of drugs, conventional foods, and food additives. The FDA is the agency responsible for taking action against any adulterated or misbranded dietary supplements being marketed and sold. The FDA also collates adverse event reports from all supplements and manufacturers. A brief review of the legislative history of supplement regulation helps to clarify the roles and responsibilities of the FDA.

Legislative History of Supplement Regulation

The first legislation for dietary supplement regulation in the United States was the Food, Drug, and Cosmetic Act of 1938. Under this legislation, dietary supplements were largely subject to many of the same regulatory standards as other food products and drugs. In 1973, new regulations were enacted to clarify the regulation of vitamin and mineral supplements, with restrictions on the potency and combinations of vitamin and mineral supplements that could be sold. These regulations were controversial and ultimately negated by the Proxmire Amendment in 1976. The Nutrition Labeling and Education Act of 1990 set new guidelines for the nutrition labeling requirements for food, which also pertained to dietary supplements. This legislation established guidelines for labeling nutrient content, along with establishing guidelines and procedures relating to health-related label claims. These guidelines were enacted for food products, but the Dietary Supplement Act of 1992 delayed the application of many guidelines to dietary supplements. This delay was intended to allow Congress and the FDA more time to consider a number of regulatory issues pertaining to dietary supplements before enforcing the new guidelines. Two years later, new legislation largely restructured the regulatory oversight of dietary supplements and clarified the roles of regulatory agencies.

Dietary Supplement Health and Education Act

The Dietary Supplement Health and Education Act (DSHEA) was passed by Congress in 1994. This legislation defined *dietary supplement* as a product taken by mouth that contains a dietary ingredient intended to supplement the diet. Such dietary ingredients may include vitamins, minerals, herbs or other botanicals, amino acids, dietary substances used to supplement the diet (such as enzymes or tissues from organs or glands), or a concentrate, metabolite, constituent, extract, or combination of these ingredients. Further, a dietary supplement is intended to be orally ingested as a pill, capsule, powder, tablet, or liquid, and it must be clearly labeled as a dietary supplement rather than a conventional food product. Prior to DSHEA, dietary supplements were generally regulated in a manner similar to other food products. This legislation designates dietary supplements as a distinct category of foods and distinguishes them from food additives, which has important implications for how they are regulated.

Current guidelines require that all manufacturers of dietary supplements register their facilities with the FDA. However, manufacturers can market and sell a supplement without notifying the FDA or offering evidence of safety or efficacy, provided that the supplement contains dietary ingredients that were sold in a dietary supplement in the United States prior to October 15, 1994. For supplements containing any new dietary ingredients, the manufacturer must present sufficient evidence to the FDA that the new ingredient is reasonably expected to be safe, unless the ingredient has been recognized as a food substance that is present in the food supply without chemical alteration. In the case of new dietary ingredients, this evidence must be provided at least 75 days before marketing the product. Current guidelines require all companies that manufacture, package, label, or store dietary supplements that are held or distributed in the United States to comply with **Current Good Manufacturing Practices (CGMPs)**. These CGMPs are intended to protect consumers by ensuring the purity, quality, and composition of dietary supplements. In addition, current guidelines state that supplement manufacturers and distributors must investigate and report any serious adverse event reports they receive (figure 7.1). A serious adverse event results in death, a

life-threatening experience, hospitalization, permanent impairment, or medical intervention (30).

Key Point

Dietary supplements and dietary ingredients are regulated by the FDA, but products can be marketed and sold without notifying the FDA if using ingredients that were sold prior to 1994.

The Federal Trade Commission (FTC) primarily regulates supplement advertisement, whereas FDA guidelines regulate the labeling of dietary supplements. These guidelines state that companies must label their product in a manner that clearly designates the product as a dietary supplement and provides information regarding the net contents and each dietary ingredient in the supplement. Labels may contain **structure/function claims**, which describe how a supplement may affect the normal structure or function of the human body and the means by which this structure or function is affected. Labels can also contain claims pertaining to general well-being and the prevention of nutrient deficiency, provided that the label also

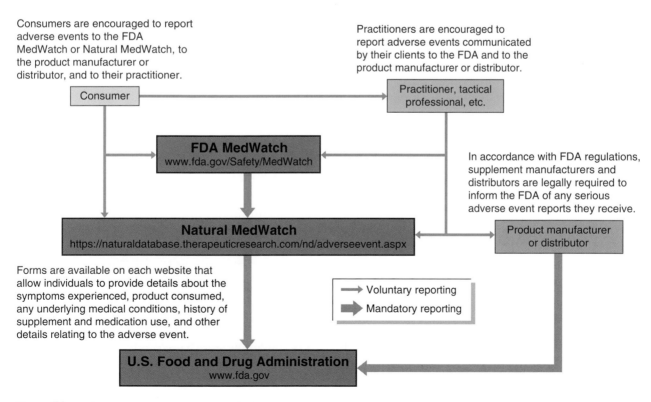

Figure 7.1 Adverse event reporting with dietary supplements (30).

contains information regarding the prevalence of that deficiency in the United States. Companies must submit a notice to the FDA within 30 days of marketing a product with any of these claims on the label and must be able to substantiate that the claims are not misleading, but companies do not need FDA approval to print such claims on product labels. As such, labels must also bear the following disclaimer: "This statement has not been evaluated by the Food and Drug Administration. This product is not intended to diagnose, treat, cure, or prevent any disease." Once a dietary supplement hits the market, the FDA is responsible for taking action against companies that manufacture or distribute supplements that violate current guidelines.

Third-Party Review of Supplements

Although the FDA has authority to order product recalls and take action against noncompliant manufacturers and distributors of dietary supplements, the FDA is typically not able to identify noncompliant products until after they have been marketed and sold. Thus, dietary supplements containing adulterants or contaminants may be purchased by consumers before the FDA can demonstrate that a supplement is unsafe or in violation of federal guidelines to restrict the sale or consumption of the supplement. Multiple recent studies have documented cases in which over-the-counter dietary supplements have been adulterated with banned or unapproved stimulants (21, 22), anabolic steroids and related compounds (20), or pharmaceutical drugs (20, 28). As a result, a number of companies have emerged to perform independent third-party testing to verify or certify the purity of dietary supplements. By limiting supplement consumption to products that have been tested by a third party, tactical athletes can greatly reduce their risk of adverse events or failed drug screens as a result of dietary supplementation.

Current supplement certification programs are offered by companies such as NSF International, Informed-Choice, U.S. Pharmacopeia, Consumer Lab, and the Banned Substances Control Group (BSCG). Companies that manufacture and distribute supplements can voluntarily (and for a cost) submit their products for independent verification and certification from these companies; upon approval, these products will bear a logo on the product label to demonstrate that they passed inspection. Tactical personnel should be advised to carefully inspect the label of any potential supplement purchase and seek out products that bear logos indicating third-party certification from a reputable company.

Third-party testing can take a number of forms:

- **Certification of manufacturing facilities:** This process generally includes a full (paper or electronic and physical) audit of the manufacturing facilities, including personnel, equipment, operating procedures, and records kept by the facility, to ensure that the facility complies with CGMPs and is free of contaminants. Facility certification typically includes return visits, whereby the certifying body performs periodic visits to ensure that the manufacturer maintains compliance with CGMPs while enrolled in the certification program.

- **Certification of raw ingredients:** Companies that distribute raw ingredients for use in a wide range of supplements can voluntarily enroll to have their ingredients certified. This certification generally involves a third-party company testing the ingredients for identity, purity, strength, and quality. The testing typically aims to verify that the ingredient is prepared and handled according to CGMPS, matches the identity and purity that are claimed, is free of contaminants, and is free of banned substances.

- **Certification of finished dietary supplements:** For this certification, third-party companies generally inspect a facility to ensure CGMP compliance. They then test the finished product to ensure that it meets label claims (including identity and purity of ingredients), is free of contaminants, and is free of banned substances.

To ensure that compliance is maintained for certified facilities, raw ingredients, or finished products, companies must generally agree to periodic follow-up testing for as long as they remain enrolled in the program and claim to be third-party certified. Any certification labels should be closely inspected to determine what types of certification and product testing were performed. Logos may indicate that the manufacturer's facility was voluntarily audited and inspected to ensure CGMP compliance, that the product was tested for banned substances and adulterants, or that the product was tested to verify the contents of listed ingredients. The exact testing and certification procedures can vary among third-party testing organizations, but the consumption of certified products can significantly reduce the risk of consuming deleterious or banned substances in dietary supplements, thereby reducing the risks of adverse events and positive drug screens.

ANTI-DOPING AGENCIES AND DIETARY SUPPLEMENT RESOURCES

A number of national and international agencies are charged with preventing doping in athletics. These agencies often oversee drug testing programs and provide educational materials to athletes. Information on dietary supplements is typically included in these educational materials, which are largely applicable to sport athletes and tactical athletes alike.

World Anti-Doping Agency

The **World Anti-Doping Agency (WADA)** is an independent organization that sets international standards regarding doping in athletic competition. The WADA prohibited substance list is recognized and used by various sport federations around the world (113), including the International Olympic Committee (IOC). Because many countries lack strict rules governing the manufacturing and labeling of dietary supplements, WADA urges athletes to practice caution regarding the use of dietary supplements. WADA does not offer independent testing of dietary supplements, nor does it certify manufacturers, facilities, or products for use in sport.

U.S. Anti-Doping Agency

The **U.S. Anti-Doping Agency (USADA)** is the national anti-doping organization in the United States. This organization also urges consumers to practice caution when considering dietary supplements, because supplements can reach store shelves before the FDA is aware of adulterants, undeclared ingredients, or other compliance issues. Similar to WADA, USADA does not offer independent testing or certification of dietary supplements. In addition to providing a list of red flags indicating that a dietary supplement may be at increased risk of containing a deleterious or banned ingredient, USADA maintains a list of high-risk products that can be readily accessed by interested consumers (107). (See the list of educational resources near the end of the chapter.)

Government Resources

A number of free government resources are available to help increase awareness and provide information about dietary supplements. The **Human Performance Resource Center (HPRC)** was established by the U.S. Department of Defense (DoD) in 2009. The goal of the HPRC is to gather and disseminate fitness, wellness, and performance-oriented information to warfighters and their families. The DoD and HPRC have collaborated on a joint initiative called **Operation Supplement Safety (OPSS)**, which is an educational campaign to inform current and retired warfighters and their families about the benefits and risks of dietary supplements and how to go about using dietary supplements when necessary. The OPSS website is a comprehensive resource that provides information about third-party certification, red flags, and other ways to evaluate the risks of supplements; military drug testing; FDA oversight of the supplement industry; reporting of adverse events; and links to outside resources to assist in evaluating products and ingredients. Though HPRC and OPSS are directed toward warfighters, their content typically applies to a wide range of tactical athletes who face similar physical demands and drug screenings.

OPSS advises tactical personnel to review dietary supplements cautiously before consuming them. It provides information regarding supplement risk stratification, supplements that may be beneficial to warfighters, and a list of products to avoid (see the box titled "Educational Resources" toward the end of this chapter). The HPRC directs consumers seeking unadulterated dietary supplements to the NSF Certified for Sport list. Recommendations for supplements to avoid can be found in the OPSS list of high-risk dietary supplements. Altogether, the HPRC offers a variety of educational resources across a range of media platforms to provide tactical athletes with information to help identify potentially beneficial supplements and avoid supplements that pose undue risks for adverse health effects or failed drug screens.

Additional agencies providing beneficial information include the Office of Dietary Supplements (ODS), Dietary Supplement Label Database (DSLD), FDA, and National Center for Complementary and Integrative Health (NCCIH). Specifically, ODS provides information regarding dietary supplements as well as an overview of the decision-making process for supplement use. The DSLD provides an extensive database of supplements with the facts panel, origin of ingredients, label claims, and company contact information for each supplement. The FDA provides information for consumers, as well as details regarding adverse event reporting. Finally, the NCCIH provides general information mostly related to herbs and minerals.

RISK STRATIFICATION OF SUPPLEMENTS

Dietary supplements should be evaluated based on their risk stratification. Specifically, the potential benefits and risks should be identified before using an ingredient or product. A number of available resources (see the list of educational resources near the end of this chapter) can be used to help formulate the risk stratification for each ingredient of interest.

Identifying the Risk

Before purchasing, ingesting, or recommending a dietary supplement, consumers and practitioners should evaluate the potential risks and benefits of the supplement. To identify potentially beneficial supplements, peer-reviewed literature should be critically reviewed to determine if a given supplement is likely to yield benefits considering the characteristics of the individual or population consuming it and to determine the specific performance or health outcomes. When benefits are likely, they must be weighed against the cost and potential risks of supplementation. A number of common supplements that may benefit tactical personnel are discussed later in this chapter. Tactical personnel should certainly avoid any supplements that list banned substances on the product label. It may also be valuable to identify whether the product has been tested or verified by a third party (see the list of educational resources near the end of the chapter). A list of companies and products with safety concerns is published at the USADA website: www.supplement411.org. To minimize the risk of consuming supplements that are contaminated or contain undeclared banned ingredients, it may also be prudent to avoid other products from companies that manufacture supplements with banned ingredients. For general guidelines, see the box titled "Tips for Avoiding High-Risk Dietary Supplements."

The process of risk stratification is complicated by differences in chemical nomenclature, meaning a single compound can be identified by numerous names. For example, 1,3-dimethylbutylamine

---

Tips for Avoiding High-Risk Dietary Supplements

To avoid high-risk dietary supplements, do not use these types of products:

- Products with vague proprietary blends listed on the label (a proprietary blend does not list all amounts of ingredients)
- Products that make unrealistic claims, such as "Gain 16 pounds (7 kg) of muscle mass in 12 weeks"
- Products that are hormonal (e.g., testosterone boosters, estrogen blockers, aromatase inhibitors)
- Products containing ingredients written in nomenclature similar to steroids (may contain a series of numbers and suffixes that end in –ol, –one, or –ene, among others)

has multiple names and may be listed on product labels as DMBA, 2-amino-4-methylpentane citrate, 4-amino-2-methylpentane citrate, 4-amino methylpentane citrate, Amperall, AMP, AMP citrate, 4-AMP citrate, or 4-methyl-2-pentanamine. A recent study identified this compound in multiple dietary supplements (22), and the FDA issued a statement that it fits the criteria of a new dietary ingredient. However, DMBA has not gone through a formal approval process, and tactical athletes should avoid supplements containing it. Similarly, beta-methylphenethylamine (BMPEA) has been identified in dietary supplements (19) but has not undergone formal approval as a new dietary ingredient and may be listed as up to 14 different names.

Risk stratification should involve independently determining the potential risk (low, moderate, or high) of consuming a supplement, along with the potential for benefit. Any supplement deemed as high risk should be avoided, regardless of its potential for benefit. An ideal supplement has high potential for benefit and low risk; however, in some instances one might consume a supplement that has moderate potential for benefit and low risk or high potential for benefit and moderate risk. When possible, tactical personnel should seek help from qualified practitioners to assist with risk stratification and decisions pertaining to the use of certain dietary supplements.

High-Risk Anabolic Supplements

Orally ingested anabolic compounds have long been associated with increased risks of adverse events and failed drug screens. Consumers can typically identify these products by the way they are marketed—as legal steroid alternatives, designer steroids, prohormones, steroid precursors or derivatives, or potent testosterone boosters. In addition, such products often list ingredients written in steroid-like nomenclature—they generally include a series of numbers and suffixes that end in *–ol*, *–one*, or *–ene*, among others. The fraudulent marketing of oral prohormones and designer steroids as dietary supplements became so widespread that the Designer Anabolic Steroid Control Act was signed into law in December 2014. This legislation demonstrated a focused effort to ban a number of common ingredients and improve the enforcement of laws pertaining to this class of banned substances.

Despite this new legislation, consumers must be proactive in avoiding banned anabolic substances that may be illegally present in dietary supplements. As shown by Cohen et al. (20), banned substances, including steroid-like anabolic compounds, can be found in dietary supplements purchased online or over the counter long after they've been banned or recalled by the FDA. The risk of purchasing adulterated supplements could be even higher when buying from online sources. Web-based retailers pose additional challenges to the agencies that enforce U.S. laws regarding supplement sales. These challenges include jurisdiction issues regarding international transactions, greater anonymity of online entities, the ability to rapidly change website content, and challenges identifying the physical location of online retailers and their inventory. Online retailers, especially those that are internationally based, may be less likely to comply with FDA guidelines and CGMPs, less likely to conduct inspections of manufacturing facilities that supply their ingredients or products, and more likely to distribute supplements manufactured by disreputable companies. These high-risk anabolic products are described in more detail later in this text.

Key Point

A risk stratification should be performed before using dietary supplements. This includes evaluating the benefit-to-risk ratio. A number of resources can be used to evaluate this ratio, including this chapter and the list of educational resources near the end of the chapter.

COMMON PERFORMANCE-ENHANCING SUBSTANCES: POTENTIAL BENEFITS, RISKS, AND SIDE EFFECTS

Data suggest that a majority of tactical athletes (85%) report current supplement use. However, knowledge among this group is low, with 75%

gaining information from popular press magazines, 55% from friends and colleagues, and 31% from the Internet (54). Although supplement consumption is high, popular media do not recognize that a variety of dietary supplements on the market have yet to be evaluated in human research, and most ingredients and supplements have failed to demonstrate positive benefits with low risk. Specifically, a number of common ingredients do not produce any positive effects on performance, body composition, cognition, or overall health. In contrast, only a few ingredients and products have either demonstrated continual positive benefits in active populations or have a mix of positive or no effects, providing potential support for use in a tactical setting. Evaluating the risk-to-benefit ratio is important when making supplement choices; with many ingredients, consumption may result in ergolytic or negative effects on health and performance. Financial considerations are also important; higher priced goods are not always associated with greater effects. Common ingredients consumed by tactical personnel, as well as ingredients that have ergogenic potential with low risk, have been outlined in this section and summarized in table 7.1. This list is not meant to be comprehensive; instead, it provides information on ingredients that have the best risk-to-benefit ratio or that are most commonly consumed.

Amino Acids

Supplemental amino acids fall into three categories: nine **essential amino acids (EAA)**, three **branched-chain amino acids (BCAAs)**, and eight **conditionally essential amino acids (CEAA)**. EAAs are amino acids the body cannot manufacture that must be consumed in the diet. The nine EAAs are histidine, isoleucine, leucine, lysine, methionine, phenylalanine, threonine, tryptophan, and valine. Leucine, isoleucine, and valine collectively compose approximately 30% of total muscle protein content. BCAAs are found in high concentration in whey protein (26% BCAA), milk (21%), meat, fish, eggs, and other quality protein sources. Although they are readily available in dietary sources, BCAAs are in high demand as the primary amino acids oxidized during exercise (especially aerobic exercise), with protein con-

tributing <20% to the total energy requirements (82). Amino acids are fundamental for protein synthesis.

CEAAs are typically produced endogenously, but during severe stress (e.g., illness, burns, injury) their production may not be sufficient to meet demands. The CEAAs include arginine, cysteine, glutamine, tyrosine, glycine, ornithine, proline, and serine. The beta form of the nonessential amino acid alanine (beta-alanine) has been thoroughly studied as an ergogenic aid and specifically evaluated in tactical personnel. It is described in the next section.

Research in typical training environments has demonstrated that all nine EAAs are required for optimal protein synthesis; specifically, pre- and postexercise consumption of amino acids may enhance uptake and availability of amino acids for protein synthesis. Tipton and colleagues (103) demonstrated a significant additive effect of combining EAA supplementation before and after a resistance training bout compared with resistance training alone, resulting in improved muscle protein balance over a 24-hour period. Furthermore, combining EAAs with carbohydrate before an exercise training session has been shown to improve protein synthesis to a greater extent than when consumed after exercise (62, 69).

As summarized in table 7.1, research investigating BCAA supplementation before, during, and after exercise has demonstrated augmented protein synthesis and reduced protein degradation, ultimately enhancing recovery time (11, 67). BCAA doses ranging from 4 to 15 g have demonstrated a decrease in muscle breakdown and an increase in muscle building (87). Additionally, BCAA supplementation (7.5 g) may also enhance central fatigue and mental performance during prolonged exercise (10). BCAAs may conceivably enhance performance in endurance athletes by enabling them to train at higher intensities while maintaining mental focus. This may be of particular interest for tactical athletes facing strenuous physical and mental demands.

CEAAs do not directly stimulate muscle protein synthesis, but two of the most common CEAAs, arginine and glutamine, may have a beneficial role during periods of stress. Although these two amino acids are widely used in sport supplements,

Table 7.1 Dietary Supplements Commonly Used by Tactical Athletes or With Scientific Support for Use

Ingredient	Serving size	Function	Side effects	Benefit	Risk
Amino acids	3-20 g	↑ protein synthesis, ↓ DOMS (62, 69)	None	Moderate	Low
Anabolic-androgenic steroids (AAS)	Supraphysiological	↑ protein synthesis, ↑ strength (9, 40)	See text (acne, ↑ blood pressure, gynecomastia, clitoromegaly, and so on)	High	High (illegal)
Arginine	2-9 g (UL 20 g daily)	↑ blood flow, nitric oxide (6)	Diarrhea	Low	Low
Aromatase inhibitors	Supraphysiological	↓ estrogen, ↑ testosterone (37, 60)	Unknown	Moderate	High (illegal)
Beetroot or pomegranate extract	500 ml (17 fl oz) of juiced beets 2.5 h preexercise; 500-1,000 mg 30 min preexercise	↑ blood flow (6, 104)	Hypotension, beeturia (i.e., reddish urine)	Moderate	Low
Beta-alanine	6.4 g daily in four divided doses (loading); 3.2 g daily (maintenance)	↑ carnosine, maintains pH (105)	Paresthesia (tingling)	Moderate	Low
Beta-hydroxy-beta-methylbutyrate (HMB)	1 g three times daily (3 g daily)	↓ protein breakdown, ↑ protein synthesis (70, 73)	None	Moderate	Low
Branched-chain amino acids (BCAAs)	6-14 g daily in 3:1:1 leucine:valine:isoleucine ratio	↑ protein oxidation, ↓ DOMS (6, 87)	None	Moderate	Low
Caffeine	200-400 mg daily	↑ energy, mood, endurance (27, 52, 105)	↑ blood pressure, HR, restlessness, headaches, ↓ focus, sleep, mental acuity	Moderate-high	Low-moderate
Creatine	4-6 g daily or 20 g daily in four divided doses for loading	↑ energy/ATP, neuroprotection (15, 47)	Minor weight gain with loading	High	Low
Dehydroepiandrosterone (DHEA)	50-1,600 mg	↑ sex hormones (testosterone/estrogen) (73, 110)	Unknown	Low	High (illegal)
Erythropoietin (EPO)	Supraphysiological	↑ red blood cells (78)	Blood thickening	Low-moderate	High (illegal)
Glutamine	5-45 g daily	↑ recovery, immune function (14, 31)	High ammonia levels	Low	Low
Growth hormone (GH)	Supraphysiological	↑ protein synthesis, strength (34, 114)	Unknown	Low	High (illegal)
Melatonin	0.5-3 mg (starting with a lower dose is recommended)	Improves sleep (86)	Daytime sleepiness, headaches, fatigue	Moderate-high	Low (but high for pilots)
Multivitamin	Once daily	Supplements diet with vitamins and minerals (54)	None	Moderate	Low
Omega-3 fatty acids	1-2 g of EPA and DHA (in a 2:1 ratio)	↑ cell structure, mood, recovery (5)	Blood thinner	High	Low
Protein powder	Variable	↑ protein synthesis and strength (68)	None	High	Low

Serving size is listed as commonly reported within the literature.

ATP = adenosine triphosphate; DOMS = delayed onset muscle soreness; UL = Tolerable Upper Intake Level.

their role is minimal during healthy conditions. Specifically, **arginine** is the direct precursor to nitric oxide, which is a potent vasodilator, thereby potentially improving circulation and blood pressure (7). Arginine is also important for normal physiological function, and it has been reported to help maintain lean body mass, improve wound healing, and stimulate GH when dietary intake is low or metabolic rate is high (e.g., wounds, injury, surgery) (65, 112). Overall, although arginine may be an effective vasodilator, it has little effect on performance in healthy people (7).

Glutamine is the most abundant amino acid in the body and is found in a number of popular supplements for recovery and immune function. The glutamine–immune function hypothesis is based on a decrease in glutamine levels following intense training, eventually leading to a suppressed immune system. Although the majority of available studies do not demonstrate a direct effect of oral glutamine supplementation to improve immunity, glutamine may play a positive role indirectly (15). Several independent reviews of the literature have all come to similar conclusions: glutamine supplementation for various clinical conditions (e.g., critically ill and septic patients, multiple-trauma patients, postsurgical patients) may require high doses (20-30 g per day) for a sustained period of time (consumed immediately upon injury and continuously thereafter) to be effective in influencing net protein balance and immune function (15, 31). However, with exercise studies, supplementation amounts have ranged from 150 mg (23) to 5 g (71) to >20 g (61). Currently, the appropriate amount for athletes, and in particular tactical athletes, is uncertain (5, 18).

In summary, for amino acid supplementation, the risk is low and the benefit is moderate for muscle protein synthesis and delayed onset muscle soreness (DOMS). Consuming EAAs before and after training likely assists in stimulating muscle protein synthesis. Further, consumption of EAAs or BCAAs during exercise, especially endurance exercise, may result in reduced soreness and improved recovery, with more support for the use of EAAs. Based on the available evidence, if EAAs are used to enhance the effects of training and to improve recovery, 3 to 20 g per day could be consumed in combination

with carbohydrate 30 minutes preexercise and within 1 hour postexercise. Of particular note, animal protein sources and protein powders are excellent sources of EAAs and include BCAAs, making protein one of the best options for EAAs. BCAA supplementation is most effective between 7 and 15 g, with a UL of about 35 g daily for an average-weight male (500 mg/kg body weight). BCAA and CEAA supplementation is not likely to produce significantly greater effects compared with consuming all EAAs.

Beta-Alanine

Beta-alanine is a non-proteinogenic amino acid that is produced endogenously in the liver. Humans also consume beta-alanine through foods such as poultry, beef, pork, and fish. The ergogenic properties of beta-alanine are limited; however, beta-alanine has been identified as the rate-limiting precursor to carnosine synthesis (39) and has been consistently shown to increase levels of carnosine in human skeletal muscle. Carnosine is a metabolic buffer within skeletal muscle and plays a direct role in maintaining pH during high-intensity exercise. Beta-alanine has become a universal ingredient, found in a variety of sport nutrition products. However, it is commonly used ineffectively with only one dose. It must be consumed daily (4-6 g in divided doses) for about four weeks.

Though the science supports beta-alanine as an effective ingredient for improving performance in a variety of populations, establishing its benefits requires further research. Theoretically, increasing skeletal muscle carnosine levels through chronic training or beta-alanine supplementation would improve the ability to buffer hydrogen ions and maintain pH, thereby improving anaerobic performance. In addition, like creatine, described later, individual responses to beta-alanine supplementation vary widely. High responders may increase muscle carnosine by 55% and wash it out at 3.5% per week, with a relatively complete washout at 14.6 weeks (3). In contrast, low responders only increase muscle carnosine by 15% and washout at 2.5% per week, with a complete washout in 6.5 weeks. Thus, the impact of beta-alanine when consumed daily for about four weeks varies from person to person. Theoretically, increasing skeletal muscle carnosine levels through chronic training or beta-alanine supplementation should improve the ability to buffer hydrogen ions and maintain pH, thereby improving anaerobic performance.

A variety of studies have evaluated the performance effects of beta-alanine in a range of athletes, including tactical groups. Research demonstrates that daily supplementation of 4 to 6 g of beta-alanine for two to four weeks may improve exercise performance lasting 1 to 4 minutes (105). Beta-alanine supplementation may be advantageous in tactical athletes, potentially attenuating fatigue, enhancing neuromuscular performance, and reducing oxidative stress (90-93). The use of beta-alanine has been evaluated in military personnel, demonstrating improvements in peak power and marksmanship, as well as a limited and variable response to cognitive performance (44). On the other hand, an expert panel that reviewed the use of beta-alanine in military personnel concluded that there was insufficient evidence to recommend its use by military personnel (55). More research is needed to determine which tasks are consistently improved with supplementation.

Most importantly, the risk of beta-alanine supplementation is low and the benefit is moderate (105). Paresthesia (tingling), typically in the face, neck, and back of hands, is the most widely known side effect of beta-alanine and is commonly experienced when large single boluses (>800 mg) are consumed. These larger doses are often found in multi-ingredient supplements and result in greater excretion rates. Additionally, using a sustained-release formula, which is now the most common form of beta-alanine on the market (CarnoSyn), reduces the tingling side effects. To date, there is no evidence to suggest that this tingling is harmful. Although not all individuals will experience paresthesia, it is typically dose dependent, with higher doses resulting in greater side effects. Currently, no safety data exist on the long-term use of beta-alanine (i.e., >1 year).

In conclusion, beta-alanine supplementation (3.2-6.4 g per day) for at least 28 days appears to significantly elevate intramuscular carnosine levels and enhance performance in both trained and untrained people by maintaining the intra-muscular pH. The most recent data suggest that, when combined with high-intensity training, beta-alanine may enhance training volume and quality, leading to improvements in both aerobic and anaerobic performance. More notably, beta-alanine may help improve marksmanship, peak power, 50 m (55 yd) casualty carry, and lean body mass under periods of intense training; however, more tactical-specific research is needed.

Beta-Hydroxy-Beta-Methylbutyrate

Beta-hydroxy-beta-methylbutyrate (HMB) is a natural metabolite of the essential amino acid leucine and may play an important role in the prevention of protein breakdown and upregulation of protein synthesis, especially in stressful physiologic situations (70, 73). Specifically, HMB may regulate enzymes responsible for muscle tissue breakdown. A meta-analysis substantiated the use of HMB as an effective sport supplement, detailing its effect on improved strength and lean mass in anaerobic and aerobic training. It was further reported to spare muscle protein catabolism and to speed recovery (70, 73).

HMB has demonstrated a positive effect on lean body mass during resistance training in untrained people, especially under periods of stress (e.g., untrained, lack of calories, high training volume) (76, 77). Though HMB has been shown to be an effective anti-catabolic supplement, its use in trained people has yet to demonstrate any consistent benefits (58). It has been proposed that trained people may need a higher dose to demonstrate the anti-catabolic effect, but more research with this population is necessary (70). In tactical environments with high energy expenditure; heat, cold, or altitude exposure; and low-calorie intake, HMB may provide benefits by reducing muscle breakdown and augmenting protein synthesis.

In summary, HMB supplementation appears to work best for those who are untrained or in the process of altering their training program and want to lessen the associated muscle soreness and damage. Based on the available evidence, 3 g per day is recommended for three to five weeks when starting a new program or under periods of stress (70, 73). To date, there are no reported side effects from using HMB. However, due to the cost it would likely not be beneficial for everyday training in a very fit population. Instead, the risk-to-benefit ratio would be more appropriate during periods of high volume or high stress (low sleep, low calories, high training volume). More work is required in tactical environments.

Caffeine

Caffeine is one of the most widely used supplements in the world, especially among tactical groups (see the box titled "Key Points About Caffeine"). It is a central nervous system (CNS) and metabolic stimulant used to reduce feelings of fatigue and to restore mental acuity (48). Many studies have demonstrated the exercise performance–enhancing effects of caffeine (52). The traditional hypothesis is that caffeine increases the levels of fight-or-flight chemical messengers, including epinephrine and norepinephrine, which promote fat utilization and result in the sparing of intramuscular glycogen. Furthermore, there are strong data to support the use of caffeine for enhancing mood, vigilance and focus, energy, and marksmanship—all important components of tactical performance (64, 102).

The benefits of caffeine have been repeatedly shown, especially in military personnel. The Committee on Military Nutrition Research and the Food and Nutrition Board have accepted that 150 mg of caffeine will increase endurance and physical performance among military personnel. Additionally, a dose of 200 mg has been shown to improve focus and vigilance during a shooting task, despite 72 hours of continuous sleep depriva-

tion (102). Also, successive caffeine intake (four 200 mg doses over 24 hours) in the late evening and early morning aided in maintaining cognitive function over a three-day period with minimal sleep (51). In addition, caffeine may help tactical athletes by positively influencing their psychological state and altering their pain perception. Research has shown caffeine supplementation to result in reduced rating of perceived exertion (RPE) during constant load exercise (27), which may translate to improved training volume and thresholds during military tasks.

The risk of caffeine at appropriate doses is low, while the benefits are high. However, it is suggested that athletes take an initial dose of 3 mg/kg body weight to test for caffeine sensitivity. The overconsumption of caffeine from a variety of sources, such as chewing gum with coffee, soda, and blended supplements, causes adverse effects in tactical personnel, so care should be taken to assess all caffeine sources. Of interest to tactical personnel, cycling from high to low (or no) caffeine intake may increase physiological sensitivity.

Creatine

Creatine is an organic compound that is synthesized in small amounts within the body from the amino acids arginine, methionine, and glycine. Creatine can also be obtained through exogenous sources, from foods that are high in protein, such as fish and beef (12). Approximately 95% of all creatine stores in the body are found in skeletal muscle, with numerous studies demonstrating

---

Key Points About Caffeine

- Doses of 200 mg consumed 30 to 60 minutes before exercise appear to be most effective for physical and mental performance (27, 52).
- Caffeine may enhance fat oxidation and spare carbohydrate, which may improve performance.
- Evidence suggests that a beneficial effect from caffeine can be achieved with a dose of 1.4 to 4.0 mg/lb (mg/0.5 kg) body weight. This would equate to 266 to 760 mg for a 190-pound (86 kg) person.
- Overconsumption of caffeine can result in negative side effects (see table 7.1).
- To date, the largest amount of caffeine ingested by tactical personnel in controlled studies was 800 mg (consumed in four divided doses of 200 mg) over a 24-hour period, with no adverse effects in caffeine-naive and caffeine-habituated Special Forces personnel (51).

an increase in intramuscular creatine concentrations through supplementation (16). The rationale for augmenting creatine levels is based on initial energy substrate use during the onset of exercise and because creatine acts as an energy buffer to help maintain pH. As previously described (see chapter 4), the ATP-PCr system is always the first to supply energy during exercise, yet PCr is depleted at an extremely rapid rate. Creatine supplementation enhances ATP availability by increasing muscle PCr storage, improving performance in high-intensity, short-duration exercise (12).

Creatine is one of the most widely used ingredients among military personnel, with few to no adverse effects reported (42). Based on decades of work, creatine monohydrate has been reported to be one of the most effective ergogenic aids available in terms of increasing intense exercise performance and lean body mass when combined with exercise (16). Additionally, recent literature suggests additional benefits for preventing traumatic brain injury and injuries, as well as improving bone health and neuromuscular function (17, 42, 80, 94, 99). Furthermore, despite what the popular press reports, creatine monohydrate may act as an agent to improve or maintain hydration and thermoregulation, thereby preventing muscle cramps and dehydration (95).

Creatine monohydrate is the most commonly studied form of creatine, and it's arguably the most bioavailable and effective (47) in terms of intense exercise performance and lean body mass when combined with exercise (16). As mentioned, creatine is also one of the ingredients most widely used by military personnel. Although few side effects have been noted (42, 47), one well-known side effect is an increase in body mass (weight gain). Another less known and less common side effect is an increase in anterior compartment pressure: Creatine supplementation (6 days of 20 g per day loading followed by 28 days of 5 g per day) abnormally increased compartment pressure in the lower leg both at rest and after 20 minutes of running relative to a placebo (79). Creatine supplementation should stop immediately if this occurs.

The safest way to use creatine is to take 3 to 5 g per day for 28 to 30 days. Research has shown that it takes approximately 28 days for muscle creatine stores to return to presupplementation levels after discontinuing the supplement. In contrast, the quickest method of increasing muscle creatine stores may be to consume approximately 0.3 g/kg body weight per day of creatine monohydrate for at least three days, followed by 3 to 5 g per day thereafter to maintain elevated stores. Creatine loading may be used when there is a quick need to enhance PCr availability (i.e., quick deployment); however, it is not necessarily the safest or best way. Although creatine supplementation has been shown to dramatically increase the amount of creatine stored in skeletal muscle, people respond differently to creatine ingestion, and high and low responders have been reported (24, 35, 101, 106). Marked responses have been noted in people with normally low muscle creatine stores (e.g., vegetarians), whereas minimal increases have been noted in those with high initial levels. However, even if initial creatine levels are high, a number of other benefits related to protection against traumatic brain injury (80) and thermoregulation (95) may result. More importantly, there is no evidence of detrimental effects of supplementation with creatine monohydrate (42, 47). To date, the only reported side effect in some individuals is minor weight gain, which subsides after one to two days of supplementation.

The addition of carbohydrate or carbohydrate and protein to a creatine supplement appears to increase muscular retention of creatine, although the effect on performance may not be greater than using creatine monohydrate alone (16). Creatine monohydrate supplementation has a relatively high potential benefit and a low risk profile when appropriate doses are used. However, caution should be taken when consuming creatine in multi-ingredient products; dosing may vary, and initial evidence suggests creatine combined with caffeine may cause upset stomach in some people (38).

Multi-Ingredient Workout Blends

Multi-ingredient pre- and postworkout supplements have become increasingly popular, with formulations that include various ingredients, such as creatine, caffeine, BCAAs, whey protein, nitric oxide precursors, and single amino acids (53, 74, 75, 89, 96, 97). A number of these ingredients have been evaluated individually (reviewed previously in this chapter), but potential synergistic and combinatory effects should be evaluated in the multi-ingredient blend. A few packaged products have been evaluated, but caution should be taken when choosing or consuming a multi-ingredient preworkout supplement blend. These supplements may have ingredients that are efficacious, but they may not be included in efficacious doses or cannot be taken just one time for an effect. Also, the use of a multi-ingredient product increases the risk of consumption of a banned ingredient or an ingredient with unknown effects.

Of the few multi-ingredient products that have been evaluated within research, some have been shown to improve muscular endurance (33, 41), running time to exhaustion (111), and power output (33). Some studies documented improvements in subjective feelings of energy and focus (97, 111), whereas others (33) did not. When taken for four to eight weeks, multi-ingredient preworkout supplements have been shown to increase strength (53, 97), power output (74), and lean mass (75, 96). However, the risk of these products is moderate and the benefit is moderate. To reduce the risk, blended products that have been tested by a third party (e.g., NSF International, Informed-Choice, BSCG) should be chosen over those without testing. A better approach is to choose single efficacious ingredients (e.g., creatine, caffeine, beta-alanine, amino acids) or preworkout blends that have only a few recognizable ingredients and that have previously been studied in humans. Common side effects from some pre- and postworkout blends include increased HR, nausea, diarrhea, and dizziness. These side effects generally come from consuming unknown doses, as well as effects from combined ingredients.

Multivitamins

Vitamins and minerals are the most frequently consumed dietary supplement among tactical personnel (54). Unlike other supplements, vitamins and certain minerals are considered essential for their roles in normal physiological function. Due to the high demands of training and other physiological demands, supplemental nutrient intake may be important in this population. The Institute of Medicine Committee on Optimization of Nutrient Composition of Military Rations for Short-Term, High-Stress Situations recommends that nutrients be provided through whole foods first and then supplemented with fortified foods and dietary supplements (46). A multivitamin dietary supplement might be included in this strategy. However, to date, there is little information on the dose and frequency for these supplements to be efficacious. Despite the lack of direct data, adverse effects of multivitamins are low in tactical personnel. The risk-to-benefit ratio of multivitamin use is low to moderate, with few risks and moderate benefit. Care should be taken when individuals are consuming a number of fortified foods with additional multivitamin intake and blended or multi-ingredient supplements; often each of these products contains 100% of the total daily values required. Additionally, the ingestion of multivitamins with multiple doses throughout the day requires further evaluation because they typically contain other unknown ingredients. A once-per-day multivitamin holds little risk.

Omega-3 Fatty Acids

The potential benefits of long-chain omega-3 fatty acids **eicosapentaenoic acid (EPA)** and **docosahexaenoic acid (DHA)** have continued to gain attention, especially in the tactical world. EPA and DHA are essential nutrients that can be synthesized from alpha-linolenic acid (ALA); however, humans are unable to synthesize ALA, making it necessary to consume either ALA or EPA and DHA through the diet. Only fish and fish oils contain EPA and DHA, which are incorporated into the wall of each cell in the body. Note that plant-based sources of omega-3 (via ALA) have very low conversion rates to EPA and DHA, rendering them ineffective sources of omega-3 fatty acids (72).

The potential benefits of omega-3 fatty acids range from enhancing neuroprotection, cognition, and mood to reducing inflammation, cancer, and cardiovascular disease risk (63, 85). No studies have examined their effect on performance, but it has been suggested that omega-3 fatty acids might mitigate DOMS (85). Most relevant for tactical personnel may be the potential effects of omega-3 fatty acids as an intervention to reduce the effects of traumatic brain injury.

Omega-3 supplementation is of interest, but food sources should be the first line of effort. A daily intake of 3 g per day of omega-3 fatty acids is generally regarded as safe according to the FDA (30). This serving size has also been suggested specifically for military personnel (36). Although one side effect of omega-3 supplementation is antithrombosis or increased bleeding (6), at doses of 3 g daily, there appears to be no increased risk for bleeding (6, 19). Tactical personnel can easily consume the amount needed through food without a concern for risk.

Key Point

The omega-3 fatty acids EPA and DHA are essential fatty acids and can only be made by the human body in limited amounts. Fish and fish oil are the preferred sources of omega-3 fatty acids; intake of plant-based sources of ALA may not be sufficient to generate the needed amounts of EPA and DHA.

Protein

Due to the physical demands of military and tactical training, it is not surprising that protein powders are commonly used supplements in this population. The use of supplemental protein in tactical personnel may yield improvements in body composition, lean body mass, strength, and muscle soreness. Although protein powders are generally recognized as safe, there are a variety of protein types and quality levels. Special attention should be paid to the type of protein because it can affect digestion, absorption, recovery, and muscle protein synthesis. Whey protein continues to be one of the better protein types in terms of bioavailability and effects. There are various types of whey:

- **Whey protein concentrate (WPC)** is found in most whey protein powders and contains 60% to 70% total protein by volume, with the remaining 30% to 40% made up of lactose and lipids. WPC is the most common form of whey due to its lower cost and added flavor from carbohydrate and fat.
- **Whey protein isolate (WPI)** contains at least 90% total protein and very little lactose, making it an ideal choice for people with lactose sensitivity. Isolates are gaining popularity because they have zero carbohydrate, they have an improved taste, and there is a growing literature on their positive effects on muscle size and recovery (26, 45); however, they are more expensive.
- **Whey protein hydrolysate (WPH)** is partially or predigested protein that is touted for its faster absorption rates and more efficient utilization. However, currently the science supports equal results when comparing WPI and WHP in humans (45).

A separate class of milk protein is just milk, which has a growing body of evidence to support its use, especially postexercise (84). Milk has a unique blend of fast-acting whey and sustained-releasing casein, providing a prolonged anabolic response. It contains a number of ingredients that help with recovery: carbohydrate to help restore muscle glycogen; electrolytes (sodium, calcium, potassium, and magnesium) to replenish what's lost in sweat; B vitamins, which are essential in metabolism; and vitamin D. People searching for nonmilk protein may consider rice, pea, and hemp proteins. To date, evidence shows rice protein has some positive effects in comparison to whey. However, the amount of leucine seems to mediate the results: More rice protein (35 g) is needed to obtain 3 g of leucine (compared with 25 g of whey protein), which initiates and maintains muscle protein synthesis (26, 49).

Overall, protein powders have a low risk-to-benefit ratio, but food sources are still preferred when possible (68). However, the type of protein may make a large difference when it comes to side effects, such as gas and upset stomach.

Nitric Oxide Stimulators

Nitric oxide stimulators are often used to increase blood flow and indirectly influence performance (4). Given their importance in producing nitric oxide, arginine and citrulline supplements have been investigated in a number of studies (7, 100). The research with arginine has not shown positive effects on performance. Additionally, although evidence suggests that L-citrulline does not improve exercise performance, citrulline malate has been shown to improve repetitions to fatigue.

It is not known if nitric oxide production is the mechanism underlying these results. Nonetheless, nitric oxide stimulators may increase blood flow and are found in a number of preworkout supplements.

More recently, natural sources of dietary nitrate, such as beetroot and pomegranate extract, have been studied as precursors of nitric oxide. Beetroot has been shown to improve performance and reduce the oxygen cost of exercise (7). Further, the ergogenic effect of beetroot does not appear to apply exclusively to untrained populations (59). Pomegranate extract is a highly concentrated source of dietary nitrate and polyphenols, and it has been shown to enhance blood flow and high-intensity exercise performance (104). Natural sources of dietary nitrate have repeatedly yielded more positive effects on blood flow and performance than arginine or citrulline. Additionally, few to no side effects have been documented with these ingredients.

Evidence does not support significant improvements in general health or performance from citrulline or arginine supplementation. The risk for arginine and citrulline is low, but the benefits are also low. Using more natural ingredients, such as beetroot and pomegranate, to stimulate nitric oxide also has a low risk but moderate benefit.

ILLEGAL PERFORMANCE-ENHANCING SUBSTANCES

A wide range of people, from sport athletes and TSAC Facilitators to bodybuilders and figure athletes, use performance-enhancing substances. These substances are purported to

- increase metabolism,
- mimic hormones,
- increase muscular development through protein synthesis,
- increase fat loss,
- aid in recovery of energy systems, and
- enhance immunity (32, 81).

If these substances are not classified as a drug or they are not making health claims, then they do not require premarket approval by the FDA.

However, that does not mean they will not trigger a positive test for an illegal substance, putting the TSAC Facilitator at risk of suspension or loss of employment. Thus, it is important to outline two classes of these substances: those that are illegal and those that are banned by organizations such as the National Collegiate Athletic Association (NCAA), IOC, and WADA.

Anabolic-Androgenic Steroids

Anabolic-androgenic steroids (AAS) have been used to enhance athletic performance for decades. These steroids are a synthetic derivative of the male sex hormone **testosterone**, which is responsible for male sex characteristics and increases in muscle size via increased protein synthesis. Testosterone is produced in the gonads and derived from cholesterol.

Exogenous or supplemental testosterone has been shown to have many positive effects that are tempting to athletes of all kinds. The most prevalent of these is muscular size and strength. Several studies have demonstrated increases in lean mass in a variety of populations, including older men (29), younger men (8), bodybuilders (109), and strength-trained athletes (50). Although AAS may lead to water retention, contributing to weight gain, the overall consensus is that it is due to lean mass accretion. However, the changes in lean mass are highly dose dependent (88).

The current literature supports the notion that increases in lean mass will increase performance (40). The most notable of these performance increases has been seen in markers of strength. More than two dozen studies have shown AAS to be effective at increasing strength (8, 29, 40). Others have shown similar findings in just three to four weeks of administration. A review of the available literature determined that strength changes are between 5% and 20% of baseline strength (40).

These strength and body composition changes are desirable for many athletes. However, the use of AAS is associated with several significant side effects (9). Although few studies have evaluated these side effects, the androgenic properties of AAS are mostly responsible. The androgenic part is what gives males their primary sex characteristics.

Increases in endogenous testosterone lead to more free testosterone or estrogen, which causes the following side effects in men (81):

- Male pattern baldness
- Adult acne
- Gynecomastia (growth of breast tissue in men)
- Increased blood pressure
- Testicular atrophy
- Decreased sperm count
- Impotence

Female-specific side effects include the following:

- Menstrual irregularities
- Masculinization
- Clitoromegaly

Long-term AAS abuse is also associated with liver damage and psychological changes such as aggression and depression. The risk associated with unprescribed use of AAS is high, and the benefits do not outweigh the risk.

Growth Hormone

Growth hormone (GH) or somatotropin is released from the pituitary gland. Two hormones act in concert to increase or decrease GH output from the pituitary gland: **somatostatin** and **growth hormone–releasing hormone (GHRH)**. Somatostatin acts on the pituitary to decrease GH output, whereas GHRH acts on the pituitary to increase GH output. GH has been shown to respond naturally to most exercise modalities, including running, resistance exercise, and cycling (56). GH is paramount for a variety of physiological actions, including decreased glycogen synthesis, decreased glucose utilization, increased amino acid transport, increased protein synthesis, and increased fatty acid utilization. However, the response of GH to exercise is highly variable. The release of GH depends on intensity, load, rest, and volume of exercise. It appears that high- or moderate-intensity activity and short rest periods elicit the greatest GH response to resistance training (57). Previous reports suggest that a threshold intensity of exercise must be reached before a significant increase in GH can be

detected; the type of exercise may also play a role in GH secretions (98). For example, treadmill running (use of both arms and legs) has demonstrated a greater GH response than cycling (legs only).

Little research has been done on the effects of human growth hormone (HGH) supplementation in athletic populations; most research suggests there is no athletic advantage to taking HGH. Although some studies in the last 10 years have demonstrated an increase in whole-body protein synthesis (43), other data suggest that combining HGH supplementation with resistance training does not result in greater benefits than resistance training alone (114). Clearly, some controversy exists as to whether HGH is an effective performance-enhancing substance. The greatest application of HGH continues to be in children of short stature, not athletes, yet it remains a common drug in athletic populations (34). It appears that use of HGH is increasing in athletic populations despite the uncertainty of its benefits (34). The risk of supplemental HGH for athletic use is unknown and may not provide any benefit. Importantly, HGH is on the WADA list, so it is banned by most major sport and doping organizations.

Erythropoietin

Erythropoietin (EPO) is a hormone secreted by the kidneys that increases the rate of red blood cell production. Recombinant EPO is most commonly used by endurance athletes to increase the oxygen-carrying capacity of the blood by stimulating red blood cell production. Previous data have shown increases in hemoglobin from greater red blood cells, resulting in an increased ability to utilize oxygen during exercise ($\dot{V}O_2$max) and improve exercise performance. Despite the general link between hemoglobin and oxygen delivery, there is no definitive evidence that increasing hemoglobin as a result of EPO or varied altitude training will improve oxygen delivery or performance (78). The side effects of EPO are consistent, with increases in hematocrit concomitantly increasing blood viscosity and thus increasing the risk of thrombosis, which is further exacerbated when dehydrated. Other reported side effects include hypertension and headaches (9). EPO is banned by most major sport and doping organizations.

Testosterone Boosters

A number of so-called dietary supplements on the market are promoted as testosterone boosters. A **testosterone booster** inhibits aromatase, an enzyme involved in the conversion of testosterone (an androgen) to estradiol (an estrogen) (37). With this in mind, aromatase inhibition can have two potentially favorable outcomes in males. First, aromatase inhibition can decrease the amount of estrogen produced and minimize the unwanted physiological effects. The second outcome is increased testosterone (i.e., testosterone booster) because of decreased estrogen conversion. Aromatase inhibition may also prevent the development of gynecomastia as a result of AAS use. Due to the function of blocking estrogen, these agents are unlikely to have any effects in women. A few over-the-counter aromatase inhibitors have been evaluated, with results demonstrating increased bioavailability of testosterone (60, 83).

However, a number of side effects, including increases in estrogen and decreases in testosterone following cessation of intake, may arise. Additionally, side effects similar to those of testosterone and AAS may result. These products should not be used unless under the direction of a physician. Some over-the-counter or online supplements may contain varied amounts of active ingredients, illegal drugs, and fillers, which could exacerbate the side effects. The risks of using over-the-counter testosterone boosters greatly outweigh any possible benefit.

Prohormones

Prohormones are precursors to steroids that have been shown to increase muscle size, strength, and recovery as well as nitrogen retention and protein synthesis within the muscle. Prohormones include dehydroepiandrosterone (DHEA), androstenedione, 4-AD, 1-AD, nordiol, and other analogs. Selective androgen receptor modulators (SARMS) are also popular types of prohormones that are used frequently. With prohormone supplementation, androgen conversion is limited due to an enzyme-dependent reaction that occurs in the muscle and liver to facilitate the conversion of prohormones to anabolic steroids. Furthermore, prohormones are readily aromatized into estrogen compounds, which likely cause an increase in fat mass and severely deter natural testosterone production. Although clinical studies on prohormones are scarce, one small study with 10 participants showed no anabolic or ergogenic effects with 344 mg per day of norandrostenedione (224 mg) and norandrostenediol (120 mg) over an eight-week period of prohormone supplementation (108). Most studies indicate that prohormones do not affect testosterone, and some may actually increase estrogen levels (13, 37, 81). Although touted anecdotally, prohormones have little to no application in performance. Prohormones are steroid-like compounds, so most athletic organizations have banned their use. Use of dietary supplements that contain prohormones could result in a positive drug test for anabolic steroids. The majority of these substances are illegal and are banned by WADA, the NCAA, the NFL, and most major sport leagues. The benefits of prohormones are low, and the risks are moderate to high.

Dehydroepiandrosterone (DHEA)

Dehydroepiandrosterone (DHEA) is a steroid produced naturally by the adrenal glands that serves as a precursor to the sex hormones testosterone and estradiol. The conversion of DHEA to estradiol would not be advantageous for athletes in light of its anabolic effect on fat cells (i.e., increased fat cell size). However, the conversion of DHEA to testosterone may have performance-enhancing effects. Although testosterone is a potent anabolic hormone that promotes skeletal muscle protein accrual, DHEA supplementation (100 to 150 mg per day for up to four weeks) has not shown an effect on testosterone in young men (14, 25). It appears DHEA may be more effective for the elderly, who have physiologically low levels (73, 110). The benefits for the tactical athlete appear to be low, and because DHEA is on the WADA prohibited list, it poses a high risk.

DHEA Derivatives

A number of DHEA derivatives are on the market, some of which include **7-keto-DHEA**, **19-nor-DHEA**, and others. Supplement claims include preservation of lean body mass as well as improvements in bone mineral density, insulin resistance, liver thermogenesis (which increases calorie burning), cognition, and immunity. Although rat studies have shown that supplementation elicits a thermogenic effect, the limited human studies indicate no anabolic or lipolytic effects (13). The potential benefit of DHEA derivatives is low and the risk is high.

SIGNS AND SYMPTOMS OF ERGOGENIC AID ABUSE

Illegal performance-enhancing substances are associated with a litany of side effects and problems. As mentioned previously, most of the signs and symptoms are substance specific. Most negative effects of AAS, GH, and blood doping (EPO) are reversible if use is discontinued. However, there may be permanent ill effects if abuse continues (81).

AAS use is related to a long list of signs and symptoms. Long-term studies of the effects of AAS on morbidity and mortality are almost nonexistent, so the literature usually focuses on acute effects. The signs and symptoms of AAS use fall into six categories (13, 40, 81):

1. Cardiovascular: decreased HDL (good cholesterol), increased LDL (bad cholesterol), increased blood pressure, and increased risk of heart attack (2, 32)
2. Musculoskeletal: abscesses, tendon ruptures, and premature growth plate closure
3. Endocrine: infertility, gynecomastia, testicular atrophy, enlarged clitoris, male pattern baldness, and excessive hair growth (66)
4. Psychological: mania, depression, aggression, mood swings, rage, and delusions
5. Hepatic: liver damage and cancer (1)
6. Skin: acne, fluid retention, and cysts

The use of AAS has been strongly associated with heart attacks and strokes, although little scientific evidence supports this report (13). AAS also slows or even stops endogenous production of testosterone, which leads to testicular atrophy and requires testosterone replacement therapy.

Educational Resources

A variety of educational resources are available to help evaluate the risks and benefits of dietary supplements. It is important to consult these resources due the rapid turnover of new products, formulas, and companies.

- U.S. Anti-Doping Agency (USADA) High-Risk Dietary Supplement List, a highly valuable resource that discloses ingredients found in specific products that are not listed on labels: www.supplement411.org
- World Anti-Doping Agency (WADA) 2016 Prohibited List: http://list.wada-ama.org
- Informed-Choice registered product search: www.informed-choice.org
- Consumer Lab: www.consumerlab.com/results/index.asp
- FDA Safety Alerts and Advisories: www.fda.gov/Food/RecallsOutbreaksEmergencies/SafetyAlertsAdvisories/
- Dietary Supplement Labels Database: www.dsld.nlm.nih.gov/dsld
- Human Performance Resource Center (HPRC) Dietary Supplements Classification System: http://hprc-online.org/dietary-supplements/dietary-supplement-classification-system-1
- HPRC Operation Supplement Safety (OPSS): http://hprc-online.org/opss
- National Center for Complementary and Integrative Health (NCCIH): http://nccih.nih.gov/health/atoz.htm
- Office of Dietary Supplements (ODS) Dietary Supplement Fact Sheets: http://ods.od.nih.gov/factsheets/list-all

Reports indicate that AAS abusers may see swings in mood and aggression (13, 40), and aggressive behavior is one of the more obvious signs of abuse. Rapid weight gain is another sign of AAS use. Some types of AAS are associated with weight gain of 15 to 20 pounds (7-9 kg) in just four to six weeks. The side effects of GH may be similar; however, its effectiveness is still in question. It is difficult to identify signs and symptoms of abuse aside from those mentioned. However, it is important to be in tune with athletes under training supervision—asking questions, talking about regimens, and inquiring about dietary supplement use.

CONCLUSION

Dietary supplementation is a common practice among tactical athletes, and certain dietary supplements may yield benefits. Due to the post-market regulation of dietary supplements, TSAC Facilitators should be knowledgeable about how to help tactical athletes perform risk stratifications of supplements before using them. TSAC Facilitators must also know when to bring in a performance dietitian. The educational resources provided in this chapter, and by various anti-doping agencies, will help tactical athletes to avoid certain red flags or supplements on high-risk lists and to determine whether products have undergone independent third-party certification or verification. Tactical personnel should avoid purchasing or consuming supplements marketed for weight loss, preworkout, or bodybuilding (containing prohormones or designer steroids); some products are marketed as legal steroid alternatives and contain ingredients with nomenclature very similar to illegal steroids.

Key Terms

anabolic-androgenic steroids (AAS)
arginine
beta-alanine
beta-hydroxy-beta-methylbutyrate (HMB)
branched-chain amino acids (BCAAs)
caffeine
conditionally essential amino acids (CEAAs)
creatine
Current Good Manufacturing Practices (CGMPs)
dehydroepiandrosterone (DHEA)
dietary supplement
docosahexaenoic acid (DHA)
eicosapentaenoic acid (EPA)
erythropoietin (EPO)
essential amino acids (EAA)
Food and Drug Administration (FDA)

glutamine
growth hormone (GH)
growth hormone–releasing hormone (GHRH)
Human Performance Resource Center (HPRC)
Operation Supplement Safety (OPSS)
prohormone
7-keto-DHEA
somatostatin
structure/function claims
testosterone
testosterone booster
U.S. Anti-Doping Agency (USADA)
whey protein concentrate (WPC)
whey protein hydrolysate (WPH)
whey protein isolate (WPI)
World Anti-Doping Agency (WADA)

Study Questions

1. Based on its name, which of the following substances is likely to be a steroid-like compound?
   a. anadrol
   b. AMP citrate
   c. pentanamine
   d. methylpentane

2. Which of the following is a branched-chain amino acid?
   a. lysine
   b. histidine
   c. isoleucine
   d. threonine

3. Which of the following describes the role of HMB?

   a. increase levels of carnosine

   b. increase red blood cell concentration

   c. improve muscle protein catabolism

   d. prevent protein breakdown

4. Which of the following foods contain the lowest amount of omega-3 fatty acids?

   a. herring

   b. salmon

   c. mackerel

   d. peanut butter

Chapter 8

Testing and Evaluation of Tactical Populations

Maj. Bradley J. Warr, PhD, MPAS, CSCS

Patrick Gagnon, MS

Dennis E. Scofield, MEd, CSCS,*D

Suzanne Jaenen, MS

After completing this chapter, you will be able to

- identify the types of performance tests for evaluating tactical athletes,
- explain the purpose or rationale for selecting performance tests for tactical athletes,
- administer performance test protocols safely and effectively,
- evaluate the results of performance tests, and
- describe how to use performance test results for tactical populations.

The opinions or assertions contained herein are the private views of the authors and are not to be construed as official or as reflecting the views of the Army or the Department of Defense.

Tactical personnel operate in civil crises, emergencies, and combat—all of which may involve lifting, carrying, dragging, crawling, jumping, sprinting, and running. Therefore, **physical preparedness** is a key priority for tactical athletes. *Physical preparedness* can be defined as a state of optimal health and having the physical ability to perform technical, tactical, and physically demanding job requirements (52) (figure 8.1). Appropriate testing tools that quantitatively measure fitness and work capacity are commonly used to determine job suitability, and achieving a passing score on a **physical assessment** is one of the foremost prerequisites for a tactical occupation. Assessments should be based on job-specific physical requirements (identified through job task analyses) and provide an indication of job suitability. Physical assessments also measure overall fitness (i.e., muscular strength and endurance, body composition, aerobic capacity) and identify health-related risk factors (e.g., cardiovascular disease, high blood pressure). In short, physical assessments measure health status, physical preparedness, and job suitability for employment in tactical occupations.

Key Point

Physical assessments should measure the ability to perform a specific task and should help determine job suitability.

HISTORY OF FITNESS TESTING IN TACTICAL OCCUPATIONS

Physical assessments have evolved as a result of developments in scientific research, equipment loads, operational environments, and doctrine. Current fitness tests for tactical populations are summarized in appendix tables 8.1 to 8.6 near the end of the chapter, and sources for current test protocols are listed in appendix table 8.7, also near the end of the chapter.

Military

Over the last century, the U.S. Army's physical training and evaluation has undergone numerous revisions aimed at improving soldiers' physical

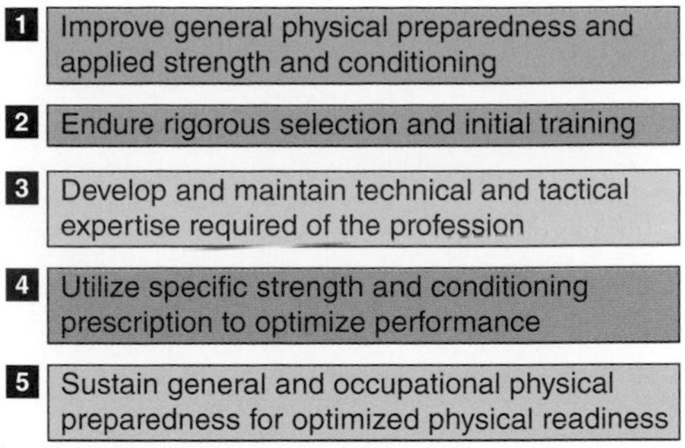

Figure 8.1 Development of the tactical athlete.

Adapted from Scofield and Kardouni (46).

preparedness. After World War I, the Army recognized that fitness tests were necessary to determine whether soldiers were physically prepared for battle and that activities such as group games, wrestling, and hand-to-hand combat were necessary adjuncts to the callisthenic exercises used at the time (39). As a result, minimum physical standards were established for a physical fitness test (PFT) that included the 100-yard (91 m) dash, running broad jump, 8-foot (2.4 m) fence climb, hand-grenade throw, and obstacle course. In 1946 the PFT changed to include pull-ups, squat jumps, push-ups, sit-ups, and a 300-yard (274 m) run (3). Because the PFT was not mandatory after basic combat training, the physical achievement test was added in 1957 as a tool for commanders of combat units to evaluate their unit's physical readiness. The physical achievement test consisted of a 75-yard (69 m) dash, triple jump, 5-second rope climb, 150-yard (137 m) man carry, and 1-mile (1.6 km) run (4). The 1973 field manual (FM) 21-20 published the Army Physical Evaluation Test (APET), which consisted of 15 exercises that were either included or excluded in seven physical evaluations (5). In 1980, the U.S. Army implemented the APFT, a three-event physical fitness test (push-ups, sit-ups, and 2 mi [3 km] run), and in 2020 the APFT was replaced with the six-event Army Combat Fitness Test (ACFT).

In addition to the United States, other countries have remodelled their military fitness testing and evaluation. In 1972 the Canadian Forces (CF; also known as the Canadian Armed Forces [CAF]), adopted a version of the Cooper aerobic test (i.e., running 1.5 mi [2.4 km] as fast as possible for running 1.5 mi [2.4 km] as fast as possible for time) (6). The CF also tested muscular endurance by including push-ups, bent-knee sit-ups, and chin-ups. In 1979 the CF adopted a new fitness test, the CF Exercise Prescription (EXPRES), that included push-ups, sit-ups, trunk forward flexion, and handgrip strength. In the late 1980s the CF EXPRES included minimum physical fitness scores based on age and gender to reflect research conducted in response to the Canadian Human Rights Act of 1977 (6, 22). The purpose of this act was to ensure that federal employers managed all personnel fairly and indiscriminately. In 2010 a new fitness assessment concept was proposed, Fitness for Operational Requirements of CAF Employment (FORCE), to test the mission readiness of personnel using battle simulation tasks (41). In 2012, the final FORCE assessment was approved and consisted of a sandbag lift, an intermittent loaded shuttle run, 20 m (22 yd) rushes, and a sandbag drag. There is ongoing research to further modify the FORCE protocol so that it remains operationally relevant and compliant with the Canadian Human Rights Act (41). Other countries, such as Australia, Singapore, and New Zealand, have modified their military fitness testing and evaluation in accordance with combat requirements (8, 9, 16).

Fire

The 1974 NFPA (National Fire Protection Association) Standard 1001 published minimum physical fitness requirements for entrance into fire service (where duties are primarily structural) (36). This test involved the following:

1. Running 1.5 miles (2.4 km) in under 12 minutes
2. Twenty-five bent-knee sit-ups in 90 seconds
3. Five pull-ups
4. Walking a beam (20 ft [6 m] long by 3-4 in. [8-10 cm] wide) while carrying 20 pounds (9 kg) of hose without falling off
5. Ten push-ups
6. Lifting and carrying 125 lb (57 kg) for 100 feet (30 m) without stopping
7. Lifting and moving a 15-pound (7 kg) weight, alternating from outside the left foot to the waist to outside the right foot, 14 times in less than 35 seconds

In 1997, the U.S. Fire Service Joint Labor Management Wellness-Fitness Initiative developed the Candidate Physical Ability Test (CPAT) (2) to measure a candidate's ability to perform critical firefighting tasks (2). The CPAT continues to be used by most U.S. firefighting departments. Further review of physical testing was conducted in 1998 by the U.S. Air Force to help determine which test battery the Department of Defense Firefighter Physical Fitness Program should adopt (37). This comprehensive review provided a list of firefighting tasks that had been published by previous authors.

In 2015 the NFPA issued an updated version of NFPA 1583, Standard on Health-Related Fitness Programs for Fire Department Members, which superseded the 2008 version. The first edition of this document, published in 2000, provided a comprehensive health and fitness resource for firefighters and an adjunct to NFPA 1582, Standard on Comprehensive Occupational Medical Program for Fire Departments (27). The NFPA 1583 standard contains recommendations for an annual physical fitness assessment (PFA) that can be administered to incumbent firefighters, as well as a prequalification tool before attempting the physical performance assessment (PPA) (27). The PFA measures general fitness parameters (aerobic endurance, muscle endurance, muscle strength, flexibility, body composition, and anaerobic endurance) and consists of the following tasks: victim rescue, forcible entry and ventilation, hose advance, stair climb with load, hoisting, and carry evolution (27).

Law Enforcement

In 1883, the Pendleton Civil Service Reform Act was approved by the U.S. Congress, establishing a civil service commission to develop competitive examinations regarding the fitness of civil service applicants (1). Although the Pendleton Act was directed at federal employees, it was the first law to recognize the utility of fitness assessments in the candidate selection process. Over the last 40 years, physical ability testing protocols in the United States and Canada have had to comply with legislation protecting people from discriminatory hiring practices (21, 25). As a result, physical ability tests are required to be objective, to reflect physical demands observed in the field, and to use nondiscriminatory minimal standards. An overview of the U.S. Federal Law Enforcement Physical Efficiency Battery (PEB), a pre-employment physical fitness test, can be found in appendix table 8.5 near the end of the chapter.

Occupational task analyses of law enforcement in various countries have shown many similarities in the work capacity of occupational tasks (13). Of the various tests that evaluate occupational fitness, the Physical Abilities Requirement Evaluation (PARE) developed by the Royal Canadian Mounted Police is a legally defensible test that directly reflects activities observed during a task analysis (13). Coupling occupational fitness with general fitness tests may be ideal to assess occupational performance and health.

TYPES OF PERFORMANCE TESTS

The physical assessment battery selection process should take into consideration variables such as the test population, time, equipment, resources, and the specific information that is to be gleaned from the tests. When preparing for and administering performance tests, the intended goals of the testing should be determined. TSAC Facilitators should know in advance what population they are interested in and what information they want to gain from the test. The following sections describe the types and goals of testing, as well as other considerations for specific populations.

Goals of Fitness Testing for Tactical Athletes

Occupational task performance shapes outcomes on the job for the individual and the team, underscoring the importance of measuring both general health and fitness and the physical ability to complete tasks. Components of a fitness assessment include a health screening, evaluation of general fitness, and evaluation of the fitness attributes required for occupational performance. This information will indicate physical preparedness

and appropriate training for improving physical deficiencies. Periodic fitness assessments thereafter are used to measure progression, check for recovery status or fit-for-duty status, recognize achievement, and provide motivation for future improvement or maintenance. Moreover, fitness tests may instill positive psychological states through performance goal setting, fostering personal growth, optimizing physical performance, reducing anxiety, and increasing motivation and confidence (20).

Occupational Readiness

Valid fitness tests are best developed after completing a needs analysis of the tactical occupational specialty. Test selection should be carefully determined after observing and analyzing job-specific physical demands (e.g., casualty evacuation, ladder climb, material handling and lifting). The rationale for this is that although a general fitness test may provide information about physical characteristics (e.g., aerobic and muscular endurance), it does not necessarily predict occupational readiness (49). For this reason, analyzing job-specific physical demands is imperative to developing a valid occupational readiness test. Minimum scores for safe task execution should also be established during this process. Most organizations have minimum cutoff scores. It is not the TSAC Facilitator's role to establish those scores, but the facilitator can design training programs for tactical athletes that lead to improved performance of fitness tests.

General Fitness Assessment

Health-related fitness norms are widely available in most countries and are often developed for a variety of populations. Standard scores derived from these tests can be useful and even provide motivation. For example, the U.S. National Collegiate Athletic Association (NCAA) or National Football League (NFL) population norms from various fitness tests can be used in setting goals for individuals. However, these tests are developed for specific athlete populations and thus may not reflect specific occupational physical demands or measure critical aspects of performance. Nevertheless, a variety of fitness tests have been developed to measure general health status, and these can be useful for both an overall health assessment and to establish personal goals.

As discussed, fitness assessments provide quantitative data reflective of health status and operational readiness. Testing should include validated measures of the major components of physical fitness (i.e., aerobic and muscular endurance, muscular strength, muscular power, flexibility, agility, and body composition) that indicate physical health and identify health-related risk factors (28). Aerobic endurance and body composition, for example, are strong independent predictors of chronic disease such as heart disease and diabetes. These tests can be important screening tools for preventive health care and career longevity.

Additional fitness components, such as muscular strength and endurance, have previously been correlated with tactical job performance. In 2004, Rhea and Alvar (43) reported results from a study examining the correlation between the occupational demands of firefighters and physical fitness measures that could then be used to develop appropriate physical training programs. They found that firefighting job performance significantly correlated ($p < 0.05$) with total fitness ($r = -0.62$), bench press strength ($r = -0.66$), handgrip strength ($r = -0.71$), bent row endurance ($r = -0.61$), bench press endurance ($r = -0.73$), shoulder press endurance ($r = -0.71$), squat endurance ($r = -0.47$), and 400 m (437 yd) sprint time ($r = 0.79$). In addition, body fat has been found to be one of the best predictors of physical performance while wearing versus not wearing body armor among military personnel (44), and it has been negatively correlated with $\dot{V}O_2max$ ($r = -0.44$), squat jump ($r = -0.45$), standing long jump ($r = -0.67$), and various sprint tests ranging from 5 to 20 m (5-22 yd) ($r = -0.42$ to -0.53) (51).

Administering an appropriate battery of physical tests that accurately reflect occupational physical requirements will provide the quantitative data used for the development and prescription of the strength and conditioning program.

Physical Characteristics

Military, law enforcement, and fire and rescue personnel must be fit for duty and ready to perform a myriad of physically demanding tasks. The physical requirements often span the spectrum from aerobic capacity to muscular strength and power. For example, police on a prolonged foot pursuit will require optimal aerobic capacity, whereas casualty evacuation may require muscular power.

In 2013, the NSCA TSAC program sponsored the second Blue Ribbon Panel on Military Physical Readiness: Military Physical Performance Testing, which brought together 20 experts on the subject (7). Though not an official military panel, the experts recommended a number of **predictive field tests** to assess physical characteristics in the military. Table 8.1 provides a sample of these recommendations.

Aerobic endurance is the ability to exercise large muscle groups at a level somewhere between moderate and high intensity for more than a few minutes. It is typically measured as the amount of oxygen consumed per kilogram of body weight in 1 minute (34). An example of this type of activity might include carrying a loaded rucksack for multiple miles as quickly as possible. This not only requires the muscles of the lower extremity to work on moving the body forward, but it also requires the upper extremity and core muscle groups to stabilize the load while the arms are swinging. Although muscular endurance is intimately involved with this task, providing adequate

Table 8.1 Physical Characteristics and Predictive Field Tests

Physical characteristics	Predictive field tests
Muscular strength	Handgrip dynamometer, pull-up, incremental dynamic lift, push-up
Muscular endurance	Push-up, burpee (squat thrust), squat
Muscular power	Standing broad jump, vertical jump, medicine ball throw
Aerobic fitness	Running tests, beep test
Agility	300 yd (274 m) shuttle run, T-test agility drill
Flexibility	Functional movement screen, sit and reach, Y-balance

Adapted from NSCA, 2013, *NSCA's 2nd Blue Ribbon Panel on Military Physical Readiness: Military Physical Performance Testing.*

oxygen to the working muscles also requires adequate cardiorespiratory function.

The most precise test for measuring aerobic fitness is gas analysis (using open-circuit spirometry to measure the gas exchange between oxygen and carbon dioxide in the airway) during maximal aerobic exercise (e.g., running, biking). Although this method is accurate, it requires the administrator to have a high level of technical competence, is best performed in a controlled environment, requires individualized testing, and can be cost prohibitive. Other field-expedient methods can be used to closely predict aerobic fitness, but they must be performed with maximal physical effort. Running tests of distances from 1.5 to 3 miles (2.4-4.8 km) continue to be used by military and paramilitary organizations to predict aerobic fitness (see appendix table 8.4 near the end of the chapter).

Muscular strength is the maximum amount of force that can be generated by a muscle or muscle group (34). The most accurate method of determining muscular strength is performing a 1RM lift. Although this is the most accurate test for strength, it can be time consuming and difficult with untrained participants. A properly performed 1RM includes multiple warm-up sets with 3- to 5-minute rest periods between sets. The starting weight of the first set should be approximately 50% of the predicted 1RM, and subsequent sets should increase by 4 to 9 kg (9-20 lb) for upper body exercise and 14 to 18 kg (31-40 lb) for lower body exercise (34). Alternative methods of predicting muscular strength include using the handgrip dynamometer (12, 24) and deriving a 1RM from a multiple RM set (e.g., 3RM). Prediction tables for specific lifts have been published to help test administrators determine strength. Tests of muscular strength for tactical populations are shown in appendix table 8.2 near the end of the chapter.

Muscular endurance is the ability of a muscle or muscle group to repetitively perform work for an extended period of time (34). Most military and paramilitary occupations involve activities that require muscular endurance. Tasks such as a repetitive box lift (e.g., loading ammunition containers) and foot march require muscle endurance (18, 55). To test muscular endurance, military and paramilitary organizations generally use tests that measure the maximal number of repetitions of exercise such as the push-up or sit-up that can be performed in a standardized length of time (e.g., 2 minutes). The test ends either when the participant reaches volitional fatigue or the time for the test has ended (see appendix table 8.1 near the end of the chapter).

Muscular power can be described as the rate of work per unit of time, making it a function of strength and speed (34). Whereas muscular strength is the maximal amount of force generated, muscular power is influenced by the rate at which strength can be expressed. For example, dragging an injured or unconscious person to safety as quickly as possible is a common task in military and paramilitary occupations. This task not only requires the strength to lift a portion of the victim's body weight but also the ability to move the victim quickly to safety. One method to test muscular power uses an isokinetic machine (Wingate test), but it can be cost prohibitive. Field-expedient tests such as the standing broad jump and medicine ball put have been correlated with lower body and upper body power, respectively (26).

Flexibility is the ability to move a joint through the entire ROM (34). Flexibility tests should be performed to assess the ability to meet specific occupational demands (12, 45). A well-known example of a lower back and lower extremity flexibility test is the sit and reach (see appendix table 8.6 near the end of the chapter). The sit and reach provides a useful index of flexibility and requires limited equipment, skill, and instruction (53).

Agility is the ability to change movement speed and direction. An example of agility is a police officer or soldier moving laterally while being fired upon. This requires rapid starting and stopping, as well as body direction and postural changes. Agility can be tested using predictive field tests such as the Illinois agility test (see appendix table 8.3 near the end of the chapter). The Illinois agility test requires the participant to start in the prone position, rise to stance, and sprint for 10 m (11 yd) before making the first change of direction. The subject then sprints another 10 m before running between cones in a slalom fashion. After running through the cones, the subject sprints 10 m, changes direction, and finishes with final sprint of 10 m (11 yd) (11).

Key Point

When designing a job-specific physical assessment, the components of physical fitness should be considered during the job task analysis. These include aerobic and muscular endurance, muscular strength and power, flexibility, and agility.

Criticality of Physical Attributes

Daily duties may require either frequent or infrequent use of specific physical characteristics in response to imposed demands. A deployed foot soldier may frequently carry heavy loads for long distances. A police officer might have to conduct a foot pursuit, and a firefighter may have to drag an incapacitated victim to safety. Although they may only perform these tasks infrequently over the course of a career, it is imperative that they be able to do so at any time due to the critical nature of the task. Because all job-specific tasks are essential regardless of performance frequency, maintaining the ability to perform them is critical; this is known as **criticality** of physical attributes (38).

Physical Characteristics Versus Skill

When selecting or developing a battery of tests to assess physical characteristics or predict occupational suitability, the skill required to complete the test must be considered. It may not be ideal to use a test that could be influenced by a skill resulting from repetitive training. For example, repetitively lifting and loading large rounds of ammunition may demonstrate muscle endurance, but a certain level of expertise, technique, and training may be required to effectively handle these ammunition rounds repetitively. A push-up also demonstrates upper body muscular endurance, but it requires less skill than handling large rounds of ammunition and can be learned after a brief demonstration; therefore, the results of the test would not be clouded by prior skill level.

Tests Based on Work Demands and Training Status

Task-simulation tests can be useful tools to assess job suitability (e.g., CPAT). Task or job simulations tend to have strong face validity, meaning that participants performing the test understand the purpose and believe that the test measures their ability to do the job (29, 38). Predictor tests, such as push-ups, may not directly measure task performance but may predict potential to succeed at related tasks (14, 35). The task-simulation approach requires careful analysis of the method for determining cutoff scores (minimal standards), which are discussed later in this chapter. When the task simulations and their standards are valid predictors of the job, it becomes easy to assess readiness for the job or address any deficiencies by targeting areas that seem to be weaker in the task performances. Task-simulation tests can be resource intensive, requiring specific equipment and facilities. Additionally, they may require a certain level of skill or training, as previously discussed.

Exercise Prescription

Although probably not a primary consideration for establishing a physical fitness testing program for a group or an occupation, fitness tests can be used to establish baseline performance measures, set goals, and develop exercise prescriptions. Subsequent tests can then serve as a monitoring system for programming.

Applicants Versus Incumbents

The goal of **applicant** fitness testing is to select workers with the physical capacities required to complete specialized training or to safely complete the major job tasks without undue risk of injury to self or others. Military and paramilitary organizations often use standardized physical assessments to determine an applicant's physical capacity in relation to the demands of the occupation. Outcomes from standardized fitness tests may result in a distinct classification of pass or fail, or they may be absolute scores that are then used to rank order. Regardless of the outcome, for legal and ethical reasons, physical assessments administered to applicants must be linked to job requirements. Applicant testing may be composed of fitness tests based on the important fitness requirements for job performance that utilize similar movement patterns and demands from **job-simulation tests (JSTs)**, which replicate important tasks as determined by a thorough job analysis. If JSTs are used, it is critical that skills that may be learned during occupational training are not incorporated in applicant screening.

For example, it would be unfair to administer a test that requires a firefighting applicant to wear a self-contained breathing apparatus (SCBA) because it is a skill that an applicant may or may not possess prior to job training. However, given that wearing SCBA is a job requirement for firefighting, the test could require carrying a SCBA to determine if the applicant is able to perform this aspect of the job. Evidence-based preselection or prescreening physical training programs can be developed to prepare the applicant for a fitness test or occupational training.

The goal of **incumbent** testing is to ensure that personnel maintain the physical fitness necessary to perform essential job tasks and that they can perform the tasks safely and effectively. Incumbent testing may be composed of general fitness or JSTs. JSTs are the preferred method for evaluating incumbents because they reduce the potential for errors that can occur when using results from a general test to predict job performance. If JSTs are used, it is important to ensure that incumbents have an opportunity to practice the test, become familiar with the task order, overcome any learning effect associated with the test, and determine the best approach for maximizing performance.

Job-Specific Simulations Versus Fitness Test Batteries

Table 8.2 highlights the main differences between JSTs made up of task simulations and fitness-component test batteries that are composed of validated, widely accepted, field-expedient fitness tests. In some cases, logistical considerations, legal obligations, or financial constraints might dictate the choice of test.

Validity and Reliability

The accuracy—that is, the validity and reliability—of testing protocols needs to be established. **Validity** may be determined through construct validation, content validation, or a combination thereof.

Construct validation involves statistical comparison of the physiological demands of critical job tasks to the physiological demands measured during the testing protocol (23). This comparison ensures that the testing protocol measures what it claims to be measuring and not other skills or abilities. Examples of physiological demands may include oxygen consumption and HR. The assistance of statisticians may be useful; they can run a variety of statistical tests to determine

Table 8.2 Pros and Cons of Physical Assessment Tests

Test	Pros	Cons
Job-simulation test (JST)	• Has high face validity • Relationship between test and job components is easily understood by the workforce • Applied standard is typically age and gender neutral • Permits trade-offs between workers' strengths and weaknesses • Facilitates training for the job versus training for the test	• Skill and fitness may be confounded • May be a learning curve associated with performance, requiring workers to practice test before being evaluated • More difficult to base exercise prescription on test results • Assesses operational capabilities versus health-related fitness • Assumes that job components are represented in their appropriate proportions in the simulation
Fitness-component test	• Has construct validity • Protocols recognized by scientific community as both reliable and valid • Protocols universally recognized and accepted • Measures important fitness constructs • Normative data used for test results facilitate exercise prescription • Results can be linked to healthy behaviors	• Tests are twice removed from the job • Individual test results tend to have limited predictive power • Relationship between test and job components not easily understood by the workforce • Applied standard is typically age and gender stratifies • Leads to training for the test versus training for the job

Adapted, by permission, from J. Bonneau, 2001, Evaluating physical competencies fitness related tests, task simulation or hybrid. In *Bona Fide occupational requirements: Proceedings of the consensus forum on establishing Bona Fide requirements for physically demanding occupations*, edited by N. Gledhill, J. Bonneau, and A. Salmon (Toronto, On, Canada: York University), 23-36.

the strength of the relationship between the physiological requirements of a job task and the fitness test performance.

Content validity uses Likert scale ratings provided by experienced incumbents that compare the likeness of the test components with the job components (23). Tests with high content validity replicate the distances moved, weights of equipment lifted and carried, and heights of lifts and are performed in gear typically worn on the job.

Fitness testing uses a battery of protocols recognized by the scientific community as both reliable and valid, and it measures important fitness constructs such as aerobic endurance, muscular strength, muscular endurance, power, agility, flexibility, and balance. The test–retest **reliability** of JSTs needs to be determined before implementation. Because JSTs are a type of physical assessment, physical fitness should be the only factor influencing performance. Therefore, if individuals perform the JST on consecutive days, their score should not significantly change, because their fitness level should not significantly change unless there is some influence of fatigue and soreness that results from the testing itself. In order to ensure the test is valid and reliable, a statistical comparison of test–retest scores may be completed.

Key Point

Test validity is achieved when the test assesses the desired physical characteristic. When a test is reliable, one would expect the participant to achieve similar results on repeated tests when performed under similar conditions.

Alternative Tests for Injured or Restricted Individuals

In most instances, applicants must perform an initial screening exam as it is designed. There are no alternative tests based on an individual's specific physical limitations. However, some organizations allow incumbents to take an alternative physical assessment because of physical limitations, such as an injury or illness diagnosed by a medical provider. Under these circumstances, the medical provider may recommend an alternative exam. Examples of alternative exams are provided in the appendix tables near the end of

the chapter. Although these exams are different from the original exams, they test the same physical characteristic.

For example, let's say an incumbent is unable to run due to an injury of the lower extremity. Based on the recommendation of a medical provider, the incumbent may be asked to perform a test on a stationary bike in lieu of a test that requires running. Although both tests evaluate muscular and aerobic endurance, the stationary bike does not result in the high impacts to the lower extremities and spine that are associated with running. It is not the TSAC Facilitator's responsibility to determine who should be allowed to take an alternative exam. However, it is reasonable to expect the TSAC Facilitator to administer the alternative exam in accordance with the organizational protocol.

TESTING PROCEDURES

Fitness testing and JSTs indicate health status, identify health-related risk factors, and help predict job performance. Appendix table 8.7 near the end of the chapter lists resources that include testing protocols.

Guidelines for Testing Based on Order, Equipment, Personnel, and Time

Order of testing, equipment, personnel, and time limitations must be considered when determining the feasibility of a physical assessment. Following are guidelines for each factor.

Order of Testing

Ideally, each test participant will complete the physical assessment battery in the same order and environment. If testing permits, a climate-controlled environment, such as a gymnasium, may be preferred. This eliminates the potential influences and variations of weather and testing surfaces. Test order and rest periods also need to be planned in advance. Standardization of test order not only eliminates the possibility of an advantage between participants but can also maximize performance from a physiological standpoint. The NSCA recommends the following test order (34):

1. Nonfatiguing (e.g., vertical jump, sit and reach)
2. Agility (e.g., T-test)
3. Maximum power and strength (e.g., 1RM bench press)
4. Sprint (e.g., 40 yd [37 m] sprint)
5. Muscular endurance (e.g., push-up)
6. Fatiguing anaerobic capacity (e.g., 300 m [328 yd] run)
7. Aerobic capacity (e.g., 1.5 mi [2.4 km] run)

Equipment Requirements

Although there are many state-of-the art devices that offer high precision, reliability, and accuracy, the financial burden or requirement for space may make them prohibitive. Under conditions of limited resources, field-expedient tests using equipment that is readily available or portable may be preferred.

Personnel Requirements and Qualifications

Planning must account for the number of personnel required to administer the assessment in a safe and professional environment. The training and capabilities of the test administrators also should be considered when selecting tests. A facilitator would not want to select tests that are beyond the technical capacity of the test administrators because this could result in erroneous test scores. Additionally, all personnel conducting the test should be capable of administering it in similar fashion. Under ideal circumstances, a participant's test scores should be reliable and independent of the test administrator (i.e., scoring and grading should be standardized with minimal intra- and intergrader variability). This can be accomplished by selecting tests that are simple to administer, providing standardized instruction to the test administrators, and preparing the administrators with training and rehearsals.

Time Requirement

Time limitations can create significant challenges. Consideration needs to be given to the length of time that each test requires, number of participants that will be tested, amount of rest between physical tests, optimal time of day for testing, and additional work or training requirements in the days before and after testing. It would not be fair to participants to conduct physical testing in the immediate days following a period of physically rigorous work or training.

Safety Considerations

Conducting a risk assessment before the testing day can help identify safety risks and mitigation measures. Variables such as temperature (heat or cold), terrain, equipment, supervision, water, and first aid can factor into testing procedures. To mitigate potential risks, the facilitator should ensure that participants are appropriately dressed for the weather, the time of day of testing is optimal based on anticipated conditions, testing site selection is considered, equipment is inspected for proper function, ample water is available, additional personnel are available for administration and supervision, and appropriate medical supplies and expertise are available in the event of an injury.

Health Screening

Most governing bodies for fitness professionals have adopted some form of health screening questionnaire. The level of detail varies greatly among questionnaires, and many include disclaimers about the inherent risks of performing a fitness assessment that may require participants to exert themselves at an intensity higher than normal. Some organizations may even recommend monitoring pre- and posttest vital signs (e.g., resting HR, blood pressure) and have adopted industry-recognized indications that preclude people from being physically tested until after approval by a physician.

Participant Instructions

Standardized test instructions and demonstrations should be prepared as a script, and they should be read and demonstrated to all test participants in a similar fashion. This ensures that every participant receives the same instructions and demonstration in an effort to prevent variation and bias between test participants or testing sessions. Demonstrating what constitutes completion of the test is recommended. This demonstration can even be followed by examples of incorrect performance techniques as long as everything is standardized.

Warm-Up and Cool-Down

All physical fitness assessments should include warm-ups and cool-downs to optimize results and reduce the risk of injuries. Warm-ups should be dynamic and progressive, and they should target muscle groups as well as ROMs that will be stressed during the fitness evaluation. Not only do warm-up activities increase HR and blood flow to the muscles in preparation for testing, but they also allow test administrators to make an informal assessment of the participants' proficiency and ease of movement (56). On the other hand, cool-downs lower HR progressively to prevent potential consequences of maximal exertion. The cool-down period not only allows for HR recovery, but it also is an opportunity for the TSAC Facilitator to observe participants for distress or injury as opposed to immediately sending them home or back to their unit lines once the test is complete.

Test Termination Criteria

While performing laboratory physical fitness testing, various **test termination** criteria can be used to maximize participant safety. When conducting testing with large groups, applying strict test termination criteria is more complicated, but all administrators should know and follow the criteria. Common sense must also prevail, and test administrators should use their judgment to stop people before they injure themselves either from incorrect technique or from overexerting themselves to a point where coordination or balance are affected. It is better to err on the side of caution rather than allowing participants to incur an injury because they continued the test. Any physical fitness test protocol should be accompanied by standard operating procedures that clearly define the test administrator's responsibilities with regard to not only test termination but administration of the entire protocol.

Key Point

Tests should be terminated if the participant is at risk of injury due to incorrect technique or overexertion. TSAC Facilitators should always remain conservative in their judgment to terminate a test.

Guidelines for Testing Frequency Within the Training Program

The purpose of testing often dictates the **test frequency**. If the physical test is for entrance into a profession or school, it is likely to be performed one time per participant, but it will have to be administered as often as the demand requires (e.g., testing for selection, testing during a specialized training course).

If the purpose of testing is to demonstrate maintenance of fitness or physical preparedness to perform a job, participants may need to complete the tests quarterly, semiannually, or annually. This requirement, along with participant availability and logistical support requirements associated with test administration, must be considered when planning for testing over the course of the year. Test administration should also be synchronized with the operations tempo and the periodization of physical training. It is not ideal to conduct readiness testing during peak operations because participants' scores may not reflect their optimal ability due to physical fatigue, soreness, or sleep deprivation (19). Similarly, test administration should align with ongoing physical training programs. Ideally, testing is performed to establish baseline fitness levels at the beginning of periodized training and then again at the conclusion in an effort to measure program effectiveness and the participant's effort (42).

Psychological and Motivational Techniques

Most tactical athletes share the common trait of wanting to serve and protect others, but not all have the same beliefs or motivations regarding their personal fitness or even the need for fitness at all to do their job. As practitioners in this field, we encounter the entire spectrum, from the highly fit and dedicated individuals whom we almost need to hold back, to the sedentary ones who require convincing to move at least a few times a week. Self-determination theory (SDT), developed by Deci and Ryan in 1985 (15), is a broad framework for the study of human motivation. SDT is a way of framing motivational studies, a formal theory that defines the roles of intrinsic and extrinsic motivation in behavior and performance. Conditions supporting the individual's experience of autonomy, competence, and relatedness are said to lead to the highest levels of motivation and engagement for activities, including enhanced performance and persistence. To be sure, some people are intrinsically motivated; they gain pleasure simply from participating or performing. These people strongly believe that fitness is important, and they will exercise no matter what. On the other end, some people require some level of external motivation in order to adhere to a training program or attain optimal physical performance (17).

Deci and Ryan (15) refer to three types of regulation of extrinsic motivation: external, introjected, and identified. The first category is the person who is less likely to exercise or perform on a test unless there is some kind of pressure or reward unrelated to fitness, such as a financial reward. For example, some organizations give money or financial credits for attaining a milestone on their annual fitness test. The second category will be motivated by a form of social recognition such as a T-shirt, pin, or medal stating their achievements on the fitness test. Military organizations around the world have used this type of reward in one form or another. Finally, the last category is people who require a valuable outcome from performing well on the fitness test—a reward that is directly related to the behavior. In a tactical population where fitness is valued, a good performance on the annual test may result in points toward a possible promotion, which is a reward that is highly valuable and related to the behavior.

In any case, for rewards to be effective, they must be achievable and meaningful to the targeted population (32, 54). If rewards benefit only an elite few, they will likely not produce the desired outcome. Some people simply will not push themselves to perform at their best because they are so far from the goal that their chances of achieving it are almost nonexistent. One way to motivate these individuals is to ensure that they are part of a group and that their individual performance, even if marginal, can positively influence the group's overall performance. For example, in a fire hall, the various shifts could be placed in a competitive scenario where the best group average gets some extra leave or vacation time. In that case, even those who are least fit are motivated to do their best because they don't want their performance to prevent their group from getting that leave time, and they will also benefit from the leave time themselves. This approach is based on the Köhler effect, where individuals work harder when included in a group than when working alone (30, 31).

The Canadian Armed Forces (CAF) have designed an incentive program based on many of these principles. When CAF members take the FORCE evaluation, their performance is plotted on a graph that compares them with their age and gender counterparts. Based on how well they performed, they can achieve a bronze, silver, gold, or platinum level. Each level has its own reward, ranging from points on their annual performance appraisal geared toward promotion, to material rewards such as T-shirts and gym bags, to a performance pin to wear on their uniform at the platinum level. This pin is given to 0.1% of the population, so the value of this reward is not diluted—not just anyone receives it. In addition, the Royal Canadian Navy, Canadian Army, Royal Canadian Air Force, and other commands have instituted a group reward system whereby all individual performances are aggregated into a group structure unique to the command. The group with the highest average on the FORCE evaluation is then officially recognized by the commander (50).

EVALUATION OF PERFORMANCE TEST RESULTS

Results from the fitness test or JST should be clearly documented. They should also be available for appropriate personnel to review.

Recording Results

Both hard-copy and electronic databases of results should be maintained by the test administrator. The hard copy is an efficient and inexpensive way to record results during the testing, and the electronic database is useful for tracking averages and temporal changes in test scores among individuals or the group.

Whether the test results are used for tracking participants' ability to fulfill the demands of their occupation or simply for health reasons, all results should be recorded in a database. A physical performance database can provide departments or groups with valuable information on the status of their team or population as well as help to answer recruiting questions, assess efficacy of fitness programming, look at physical profiles of successful candidates on certain courses, and analyze injury rates based on performances on various components of the fitness test battery. Management of performance data is discussed in greater detail in chapter 22.

When organizations invest resources in physical fitness evaluations, they expect the results of those investments to lead to positive impacts on the workforce and its productivity or, in the case of tactical populations, operational readiness. Therefore, organizations must be able to compile fitness results and report on them in such a way that will satisfy the leadership of the organization. Fitness reports can address a multitude of questions, reporting on fitness status, improvements from one testing cycle to another, fitness levels related to injuries or sick days, and occupational capabilities. Reporting to the chain of command or the leadership is also critical whenever individuals fail to meet the minimum requirements of the assessment in accordance with organizational guidelines. Reporting failures ensures visibility of potential operational liabilities that should be addressed. In tactical populations, a weak individual quickly becomes the limiting factor in team effectiveness and in extreme cases can cause mission failure or loss of life.

Protecting fitness performance data is imperative. This type of data includes personal and medical information, and it is not for wide dissemination. In the United States, medical data obtained during screening and testing may fall under the Health Insurance Portability and Accountability Act of 1996 (HIPAA), and precautions should be taken to protect this information. The appropriate personnel may review this data; any medical information or test results may be subject to review only by certain people (10). Organizational security policies should also be enforced in order to protect the information contained in the database. Individual data are as important to protect as the aggregate of group data; both can pose a threat to operational security by providing valuable information on unit strengths and weaknesses

as well as operational readiness. Reports that are published should be declassified to mitigate risk to the organization.

Normative and Descriptive Data

A crucial step in implementing a physical fitness test is establishing a **minimally acceptable standard**. Setting standards results in a cutoff score that classifies applicants or incumbents into two groups: those who meet the standard and those who do not. Because standards should not be arbitrary, and given the complexity and legalities associated with setting standards, professionals in the development of standards should be consulted. As previously stated, TSAC Facilitators do not establish minimal standards, but they may be involved in the process. Additionally, any applicable Equal Employment Opportunity Commission (EEOC) guidelines must be considered. Examples of minimally acceptable standards for fitness tests are provided in appendix tables 8.1 to 8.6 near the end of the chapter.

In the **normative reference approach**, an incumbent's performance is described in relation to a normative sample, and the standard is set using a statistical procedure. In the statistical analysis method, the level of acceptability in the performance of the test item is typically established by setting the standard at the mean plus 1 standard deviation (1SD) (68.3% of the population would meet the standard), the mean plus 2SD (95.4% of the sample would meet the standard), or the mean plus 3SD (99.7% of the sample would meet the standard) (38).

In the **ratings of performance method**, which is typically used for JSTs, incumbents may be requested to observe the JST performed at various paces (e.g., mean performance time, mean + 1SD, mean + 2SD, mean + 3SD) and determine the minimal acceptable pace for completing the test in a safe, efficient, and reliable manner (48). Given that the variable of interest is work capacity, people who complete a JST in the fastest time are considered to have a greater work capacity than those who take longer to complete the same JST. It is therefore possible to rank performance by time taken to complete a JST. Timed performance tests are often influenced by technical and systemic variability. Technical variability can be minimized in the test design by ensuring a consistent testing location, ambient temperature, time of day, and task calibration. Variability may be introduced by the participants and can occur when participants learn the test and develop pacing strategies. The physical conditions of the individual participant (e.g., sleep, fatigue, nutrition, hydration) also may affect JST performance from day to day (34).

Adverse Impact Analysis (Age, Gender, and Ethnicity)

Using fitness standards to predict occupational readiness may generate unintentional barriers for an individual, resulting in either direct or adverse impacts. **Adverse impact** can be defined as the circumstance in which a group of differences in performance relative to common standards results in a disproportionate failure rate in a subgroup (22). If an adverse impact is present, the standard must either be justified or reexamined. The effect of imposing tests and standards on subgroups of incumbent workers must be considered because any adverse impact on a minority group may be cause for legal action and grievance by an employee (47). Testing one's ability to perform an occupational task to a standard as opposed to a predictive removes the possibility of adverse impact because the occupational task is absolute, meaning neither gender nor age has bearing on whether the person is able to complete the task.

Although adverse impact statistics play a critical role, there are no clear legal guidelines in Canada for determining the performance of a subgroup as disproportionate and causes of adverse impact on that subgroup. However, in the United States, the Uniform Guidelines on Employee Selection Procedures determine adverse impacts using the four-fifths rule or the 80% rule (22, 25). If the passing rate for a subgroup (e.g., females) is less than 80% than the group with the highest passing rate (e.g., males), then an adverse impact for females exists. The 80% test is calculated by dividing the passing rate of a subgroup on a particular standard by the passing rate of the majority group (highest success rate). Any value less than 80% shows an adverse impact.

Adverse impact does not necessarily equate to discrimination, and discrimination can only be determined in a legal context. Typically, adverse impact based on gender can be traced to (a) male and female differences in aerobic fitness, muscular strength and endurance, and body composition; (b) incongruence between current physical fitness levels and job demands; (c) lack of experience with manual material handling; and (d) employment in a nontraditional occupation where training is delivered by males (40). This latter point is important to keep in mind because males and females may approach task performance differently. For example, males performing a forcible entry may swing a sledgehammer like a baseball bat, with a close grip near the end of the handle, whereas females may swing the sledgehammer with a choke grip, with their hands closer to the head of the sledgehammer. Both techniques are acceptable so long as the standard is met.

USE OF PERFORMANCE TEST RESULTS

Performance test results can be used to analyze trends, strengths, and weaknesses. Relying on a well-structured fitness performance database allows an organization to analyze results not only for each testing session or cycle but also over extended periods of time for the group and individuals. Tracking trends in performance parameters can generate much interest from various stakeholders within a group or even outside the organization. Performance data can demonstrate what types of training may be more effective than others, where a group's strengths lie, and areas where more or different training may be required to ensure operational readiness and optimize mission success. In large organizations, data related to units, formations, location, environmental conditions (e.g., temperature, altitude, humidity), or trade or specialty (e.g., military occupation, SWAT, rescue) can lead to changes in training practices, modalities, or conditions to best suit the needs of the group. Some trends are difficult to identify unless the data reveal them in a report or simply in a telling graph.

Use of Test Results to Design or Modify Training Programs

Fitness test and JST outcomes can identify physical strengths and weaknesses, which can then be used for exercise prescription. Aerobic endurance, muscular strength, muscular endurance, power, flexibility, and agility exercise can be emphasized more or less depending on where test scores lie on a standardized scale. Prescribing appropriate exercise without this data can overlook specific components of fitness that need improvement and would benefit from individual program prescription.

Goal Setting to Optimize Operational Readiness

One drawback of fitness-component tests (presented in table 8.2 previously) is the fact that people tend to prepare for what they are tested on. So if the test is a distance run combined with push-ups or a 1RM bench press, incumbents will dedicate a significant amount of training time to those tests. At first glance, it's what we want; the goal is for them to increase their physical performance. But training specificity ultimately disadvantages our operators, police officers, and firefighters if it does not prepare them for the rigors of their job. Unfortunately, law enforcement officers, soldiers, firefighters, and EMS technicians seldom have to run a long distance completely unloaded or lift a heavy load only once during the course of a shift. The exercise prescription that is generated from the fitness test results must address the true demands of the occupation to avoid developing really fit individuals but with the wrong function, much like training an offensive lineman using a triathlon program. In ideal conditions, the fitness test reflects the occupational rigors.

The concept of the tactical athlete has become more widely accepted in many organizations, and the principles used with high-performance athletes have certainly transitioned into the tactical environment. Nevertheless, there are significant differences between the tactical athlete and high-performance athlete in any sport (46). Tactical athletes do not have the luxury of peaking once or twice during a year. They often have to maintain an optimal level of operational readiness year-round because their job requires them to be able to perform on any given day without knowing how long or how hard the task will be. Training programs must adequately challenge all of the physical attributes and energy systems. Knowing that tactical athletes often work with external loads and require good mobility and agility, muscular endurance, and core strength, the test results should provide some indication of the goals to set for groups or individuals within the group based on the mission or occupational demands.

Guidelines for Coaching Tactical Populations to Reach Required Standards

The most important objective of the TSAC Facilitator is to ensure personnel are physically prepared to perform occupational tasks. Physical readiness is often determined by evaluating metrics calculated from a select battery of fitness tests. Typically, this is done by comparing an individual's fitness test scores with established minimum cutoff scores. For example, an organization may have a physical requirement to run a minimum distance in 12 minutes or perform a minimum number of push-ups in 2 minutes. When personnel fail to meet physical standards, the TSAC Facilitator must design and implement physical training programs aimed at the occupational tests.

Understanding and Addressing Failures

Fitness tests and JSTs are tools to identify personnel fitness status, job readiness, and suitability. Occasionally, failing part or all of a test will occur at times, and appropriate personnel actions are taken. People slip under the standards for numerous reasons, and understanding the causes of these failures should influence the training intervention chosen to get them back in physical condition to meet their job demands. Being physically active is a behavior that can fluctuate over time or during various stages of life based on family, work, or other commitments. Injuries and illnesses may also contribute to not achieving the desired level of fitness to serve at full capacity. No matter what the causes are, it is imperative for the tactical athlete to take action and for TSAC Facilitators to help the athlete return to full serving capacity.

Scope and Content

Based on the cause of the failure, a remedial program can be more or less prescriptive. It can also include components other than regular workouts to address the fitness issue, such as weight management classes, nutritional counseling, and smoking cessation clinics. People who fail fitness standards may not like to be physically active or may have little motivation to improve. Hence a one-size-fits-all remedial program may not be effective. Successful remedial programs tend to be individualized, multifaceted, and inclusive of other fitness and health professionals.

Supervised Versus Self-Supervised

In military settings, remedial training is often delivered in group settings and is directly supervised by a qualified instructor or some other directing staff. In other instances, personal training options may be offered to tactical athletes based on their availability, their work schedules, and costs to the individual and organization. Depending on the cause of the failure, self-supervised physical training may be the most appropriate approach. Examples may be when a person is returning to regular training after a sedentary period due to injury recovery or when the cause of failure is linked to something specific. On the other hand, benefits can also be realized from appropriate supervision. Supervision provides the opportunity for education and accountability (33).

CONCLUSION

Physical fitness testing is a valuable tool for assessing health status, health-related risk factors, job readiness, and suitability. A job analysis should be completed before selecting the testing battery to help ensure that the tests are accurately assessing the intended objectives. Testing can involve general fitness tests, JSTs, or a combination of the two. The recorded test scores need to be compared with appropriate standardized cutoff scores, they should be managed both on paper and electronically, and they should be secured. Deficiencies identified from the tests can be used for goal-directed exercise prescription.

Key Terms

adverse impact
aerobic endurance
agility
applicant
criticality
flexibility
incumbent
job-simulation test (JST)
minimally acceptable standard
muscular endurance
muscular power

muscular strength
normative reference approach
physical assessment
physical preparedness
predictive field tests
ratings of performance method
reliability
test frequency
test termination
validity

Study Questions

1. As part of a physical fitness battery, a tactical athlete is tested on the number of push-ups performed in 2 minutes. What muscular attribute is being assessed?

   a. endurance

   b. strength

   c. power

   d. speed

2. Which of the following tests measures muscular strength?

   a. 3RM squat

   b. vertical jump

   c. 300 yard (274 m) shuttle

   d. beep test

3. Which of following is the correct order of testing for a physical fitness battery?
   a. 300 m (328 yd) run, 40 yd (37 m) sprint, T-test, 1RM bench press
   b. 40 yd (37 m) sprint, 1RM bench press, 300 m (328 yd) run, T-test
   c. 1RM bench press, T-test, 300 m (328 yd) run, 40 yd (37 m) sprint
   d. T-test, 1RM bench press, 40 yd (37 m) sprint, 300 m (328 yd) run

4. What type of extrinsic motivation is driven by receiving social recognition in the form of a medal or T-shirt stating the accomplishment?
   a. participatory
   b. external
   c. introjected
   d. identified

Appendix Table 8.1   Muscular Endurance Tests: Minimum Standards for a 22-Year-Old

Organization	Push-ups		Sit-ups		Sandbag lift (20 kg [44 lb])	Kneel–stand test
	Men	Women	Men	Women		
U.S. Army	42	19	50	50		
U.S. Navy	37	16	46	46		
U.S. Marine Corps	NA	NA	50*	50*		
U.S. Air Force	42	33	38	18		
U.S. Immigration and Customs Enforcement (ICE)	15	15				Initial 10 position changes of kneel–stand test must be completed in 25 s followed by 2 min of kneeling then to standing
Canadian Armed Forces (CAF)					30 reps	
UK Ministry of Defence	34	13	40	40		

NA = not tested.

*Crunches.

Appendix Table 8.2   Muscular Strength Tests: Minimum Fitness Standards

Organization	Pull-ups or flexed arm hang		Bench press		Sandbag drag (100 kg [220 lb])
	Men	Women	Men	Women	
U.S. Marine Corps	3 reps or 15 s	3 reps or 15 s	NA	NA	NA
U.S. Federal Law Enforcement Training Center (FLETC)	NA	NA	75th percentile (1RM ≥128.2% of body weight)	75th percentile (1RM ≥66.1% of body weight)	NA
Canadian Armed Forces (CAF)	NA	NA	NA	NA	20 m (22 yd)
Bundeswehr (German armed forces)	5 s	5 s	NA	NA	NA

NA = not tested or not applicable.

Appendix Table 8.3   Agility and Power Tests: Minimum Fitness Standards

Organization	Illinois agility test		20 m (22 yd) intermittent loaded (20 kg [44 lb] sandbag) shuttles	4 × 20 m (22 yd) rushes	11 × 10 m (11 yd) shuttle run
	Men	Women			
U.S. Federal Law Enforcement Training Center (FLETC)	16.27 s	18.31 s	NA	NA	NA
Canadian Armed Forces (CAF)	NA	NA	400 m (437 yd) < 5:21 min	51 s	NA
Bundeswehr (German armed forces)	NA	NA	NA	NA	60 s

NA = not tested or not applicable.

Appendix Table 8.4 Cardiorespiratory Endurance: Minimum Fitness Standards for a 22-Year-Old

Organization	1 km (0.6 mi), 1.5 mi (2.4 km), 2 mi (3 km), or 3 mi (5 km) run		6.2 mi (10 km) cycle ergometer or bicycle test		100 m (109 yd), 450 m (492 yd), 500 yd (457 m), or 800 yd (732 m) swim		2 km (1 mi) or 2.5 mi (4 km) walk	
	Men	Women	Men	Women	Men	Women	Men	Women
U.S. Army	16:35 min[c]	19:36 min[c]	24:30 min	25:30 min	20:30 min	21:30 min	34:30 min	37:00 min
U.S. Navy	13:30 min[b]	15:30 min[b]			13:00 min[f] or 12:50 min[e]	14:30 min[f] (450 m [492 yd] ≤ 6:35)		
U.S. Marine Corps	28 min	31 min	NA	NA	NA	NA	NA	NA
U.S. Air Force	13:36 min[b]	16:22 min[b]	NA	NA	NA	NA	16:16 min[g]	17:22 min[g]
Bundeswehr (German armed forces)	6:30 min[a]	6:30 min[a]	NA	NA	4 min (battle dress uniform)[d]	4 min (battle dress uniform)[d]	NA	NA
UK Ministry of Defence	11:15 min[b]	14:00 min[b]	NA	NA	NA	NA	NA	NA

Organization	12 min ergometer or elliptical machine	5 min step test	6 km (4 mi) loaded (15 kg [33 lb]), 12.8 km (8.0 mi) loaded (15-25 kg [33-55 lb]), or 3 mi (5 km) loaded (45 lb [20 kg]) march	Multistage fitness test	
				Men	Women
U.S. Navy	Caloric conversion to 1.5 mi (2.4 km) time score				
U.S. Immigration and Customs Enforcement (ICE)		Step up and down on a 16 in. (41 cm) step at a rate of 96 steps per min for 5 min			
Bundeswehr (German armed forces)	NA	NA	60 min[h]	NA	NA
UK Ministry of Defence	NA	NA	Max time of 2 hr but not less than 1:55 hr[i]	Level 9 lap 6	Level 7 lap 3

NA = not tested or not applicable.

[a]1 km (0.6 mi) run; [b]1.5 mi (2.4 km) run; [c]2 mi (3 km) run; [d]100 m (109 yd) swim; [e]450 m (492 yd) swim; [f]500 yd (457 m) swim; [g]2 km (1 mi) walk; [h]6 km (4 mi) loaded (15 kg [33 lb]) march; [i]12.8 km (8.0 mi) loaded (15-25 kg [33-55 lb]) march.

Appendix Table 8.5 Combat or Operational Abilities Tests

Organization	Test name	Events	Standards
U.S. Marine Corps	Combat Fitness Test (CFT)	• 800 yd (732 m) movement to contact course[a, b, d] • Ammunition can lift[c] • 300 yd (274 m) shuttle run[a, d] • Maneuver under fire course[a]	Movement to contact: 4:13 min Ammo can lift: 33 reps Maneuver under fire: 3:58 min
International Association of Fire Fighters (IAFF), International Association of Fire Chiefs (IAFC)	Candidate Physical Ability Test (CPAT)	• Stair climb[a, b, d] • Hose drag[c] • Equipment carry[b, c] • Ladder raise and extension[c] • Forcible entry[a, c] • Search and rescue[a] • Ceiling breach and pull[a, c]	Maximum time to complete the test is 10:20
National Wildfire Coordination Group (NWCG)	Work capacity tests • Pack test • Field test • Walk test	• 3 mi (5 km) hike with 45 lb (20 kg) pack[b, d] • 2 mi (3 km) hike with 25 lb (11 kg) pack[b, d] • 1 mi (1.6 km) walk with no load[d]	• 45 min (arduous work) • 30 min (moderate work) • 16 min (light work)
U.S. Federal Law Enforcement Training Center (FLETC)	Physical Efficiency Battery (PEB)	Obstacle course with the following: • Climb a 7 ft (2 m) slanted wall[a, c] • Climb a horizontal rope suspended 12.5 ft (3.8 m) above the ground[c] • Traverse a horizontal rope 20 ft (6 m)[a, c] • Jump a ditch measuring 6 ft (2 m) wide and 12 in. (30 cm) deep[a] • Run or walk across a 30 ft (10 yd) beam without falling off[a] • Jump or climb over two 4 ft (1.2 m) walls[a, c] • Cross a horizontal ladder suspended 8 ft (2.4 m) above the ground[a] • Crawl through a simulated covert[a] • Climb a 20 ft (6.1 m) vertical ladder[c] Also includes the following tasks: • Lift and carry at least 50 lb (23 kg) unaided[c] • Tread water for 20 min without a flotation device[b, d] • Tread water for 20 min using personal clothing as a flotation device[b, d] • Climb and drop from a 7 ft (2.1 m) ladder suspended over water[a, c]	Physical performance requirements are specific to each FLETC training program and thus may vary depending on the course a student is enrolled in
UK Ministry of Defence	Operational Fitness Tests (OFTs)	OFT 1: Load—15 kg (33 lb) Part 1—2.4 km (1.5 mi squad march Part 2—2.4 km (1.5 mi) individual effort	Part 1: 18 min Part 2: 15 min
		OFT 2: Load—50 kg (110 lb) Part 1—500 m (0.3 mi) squad march Part 2—2.4 km (1.5 mi) individual effort	Part 1: 7.30 min Part 2: 15 min
		OFT 3: Load—25 kg (55 lb) 4.8 km (3 mi) squad march	Not less than 38:30 min but less than 39 min
		OFT 4: Load—20-30 kg (44-66 lb) Part 1—6.4 km (4 mi) squad march at 10.40 min/km Part 2—1.6 km (1 mi) squad march	Part 1: 17 min/mi Part 2: not less than 12:30 min but less than 13 min Total time: 1:21 hr
		OFT 5: Load—25-35 kg (55-77 lb) 16 km (10 mi) squad march (3.2 km/h) with 2 × 1 min stops per km with personnel crouched on one knee	Total time: 5 hr (3.2 km/h)
		OFT 6: Load—20-30 kg (44-66 lb) 40 km (24.9 mi) squad march over 2 days • Day 1: 20 km (12.4 mi) • Day 2: 20 km (12.4 mi)	Day 1: 20 km (12.4 mi) in under 3:30 hr Day 2: 20 km (12.4 mi) under 3 hr
		Representative military tasks (completed during OFTs): • Casualty drag, 30 m (33 yd) grassy surface)[c] • 2 m (2 yd) wall climb on obstacle courses[a, c] • 35 kg (77 lb) ammo can lift (1 m [1 yd] × 5) in 2 min[b, c] • 2 × 20 kg (44 lb) jerrican carry 150 m (164 yd) in 1:40 min[b, c]	Same requirements for both men and women

[a]Power and agility; [b]Muscular endurance; [c]Muscular strength; [d]Cardiorespiratory endurance

Appendix Table 8.6   Body Fat and Flexibility: Minimum Fitness Standards for a 22-Year-Old

Organization	% body fat		Sit and reach	
	Men	Women	Men	Women
U.S. Army	22	32	NA	NA
U.S. Navy	23	34	NA	NA
U.S. Marine Corps	18	26	NA	NA
U.S. Federal Law Enforcement Training Center (FLETC)	11.19	19.96	21.5 in. or 54.6 cm (75th percentile)	23.2 in. or 58.9 cm (75th percentile)

NA = not tested or not applicable.

Appendix Table 8.7   Testing Resources

Organization	Test	Equipment	Reference
U.S. Army	*Army Combat Fitness Test (ACFT)	(See the URL reference for the specific equipment for each of the six tests)	FM 7-22 www.army.mil/acft/
U.S. Navy	Physical Fitness Assessment (Navy PFA)	2 timers or stopwatches Clipboards for each scorer Black pens for each scorer 25 yd (23 m) or 50 yd (46 m) swimming pool Treadmill Elliptical trainer Stationary bicycle	OPNAVINST 6110.1J www.public.navy.mil/bupers-npc
U.S. Marine Corps	Physical Fitness Test (USMC PFT)	Pull-up bars 2 timers or stopwatches Clipboards for each scorer Black pens for each scorer	MCO 6100.13
	Combat Fitness Test (CFT)	2 timers or stopwatches Clipboards for each scorer Black pens for each scorer Cone markers Tape measure 30 lb (14 kg) ammo cans Red or yellow utility flag Dummy grenades Sandbags	MCO 6100.13
U.S. Air Force	Air Force Fitness Assessment	2 timers or stopwatches Clipboards for each scorer Black pens for each scorer	Air Force Instruction 36-2905, 21 October 2015
International Association of Fire Fighters (IAFF), International Association of Fire Chiefs (IAFC)	Candidate Physical Ability Test (CPAT)	2 timers or stopwatches Clipboards for each scorer Black pens for each scorer 50 lb (23 kg) vest 2 × 12.5 lb (6 kg) weights StairMaster StepMill 200 ft (61 m) of double-jacked 1.75 in. (44 mm) hose marked at 8 ft (2 m) and 50 ft (15 m) past the coupling at the nozzle Automatic nozzle—6 lb (± 1 lb) or 3 kg (± 0.5 kg) Two 55 gal (208 L) drums secured together, with bottom drum filled with water or other ballast for weight Rescue circular saw—32 lb (± 3 lb) or 15 kg (± 1 kg) Chainsaw—28 lb (± 3 lb) or 13 kg (± 1 kg), blades guarded, fluids drained, spark plugs removed Tool cabinet 55 gal (208 L) weighted drum Two 24 ft (7 m) aluminum ground ladders Pivoting bracket for ladder raise Retractable safety lanyard for ladder raise Attaching brackets for ladder raise Forcible-entry machine 10 lb (5 kg) sledgehammer Toe box Search maze 165 lb (75 kg) mannequin (unclothed) Mannequin harness Device for ceiling breach and pull 6 ft (2 m) pike pole	Fire Service Joint Labor Management Wellness-Fitness Initiative Candidate Physical Ability Test, 2nd Edition

(continued)

Appendix Table 8.7 *(continued)*

Organization	Test	Equipment	Reference
National Wildfire Coordination Group (NWCG)	Work capacity test	2 timers or stopwatches 45 lb (20 kg) packs (pack test) 25 lb (11 kg) packs (field test) Safety vests Route markers Distance markers (1 mi [1.6 km] and midpoint) Vehicles (e.g., bicycle, all-terrain) to monitor participants Radios and cell phones Scale	NWCG 310-1 standards for wildland firefighters NFES 1109 www.nwcg.gov/pms/pubs/pubs.htm
U.S. Federal Law Enforcement Training Center (FLETC)	Physical Efficiency Battery (PEB)	2 timers or stopwatches Clipboards for each scorer Black pens for each scorer Cone markers Measuring tape Sit-and-reach measuring device Single fulcrum bench Weight bar Free weights Confidence course	FTC-TMD-01 (10/2015) www.fletc.gov/physical-efficiency-battery-peb
U.S. Immigration and Customs Enforcement (ICE)	Preemployment physical fitness test	2 timers or stopwatches Clipboards for each scorer Black pens for each scorer 16 in. (41 cm) step Metronome (96 steps/min)	www.ice.gov/doclib/about/offices/ero/pdf/dro_pft_faqsheet.pdf
Canadian Armed Forces (CAF)	Fitness for Operational Requirements of CAF Employment (FORCE)	2 timers or stopwatches Clipboards for each scorer Black pens for each scorer 8 × 20 kg (44 lb) sandbags Measuring tape Cone markers 3 m (3 yd) strap Carabiners 2 m (2 yd) high wall 10 kg (22 lb) plate Scale Blood pressure cuff and stethoscope	FORCE Program Operations Manual www.cg.cfpsa.ca/cg-pcOttawa/EN/
Bundeswehr (German armed forces)	Basic Fitness Test	2 timers or stopwatches Clipboards for each scorer Black pens for each scorer 15 kg (33 lb) backpack 50 m (55 yd) swimming pool 400 m (437 yd) track Pull-up bar Measuring tape Cone markers	www.kampfschwimmer.de/234/?lang=en www.reservisten.bundeswehr.de
UK Ministry of Defence	Annual Fitness Test	Safety vehicle Water First aid Reflective marching vests White and red lights Timers or stopwatches for each scorer	TP0066 - MATT 2
	Operational Fitness Tests (OFTs)	Safety vehicle Water First aid Reflective marching vests White and red lights Timers or stopwatches for each scorer 2 m (2 yd) high wall 35 kg (77 lb) ammo cans 20 kg (44 lb) jerricans	

*The Army believes FULL implementation of the ACFT may start as early as March 2022.

Chapter 9

Development of Resistance Training Programs

Nicholas A. Ratamess, PhD, CSCS,*D, FNSCA

After completing this chapter, you will be able to

- define general concepts of resistance training program design;
- discuss the various modalities (traditional and new) in resistance training;
- describe the needs analysis process for tactical populations;
- design a resistance training program with the components of exercise selection, order, intensity, volume, rest interval, repetition velocity, and frequency;
- discuss the rationale for circuit and metabolic training for tactical populations; and
- apply the principles of progressive overload, specificity, and variation in tactical populations.

Resistance training is a method of conditioning in which an individual works against a wide range of resistance loads to enhance health, fitness, and performance (41). Resistance training is a fundamental modality for military personnel, SWAT teams, special operations forces, law enforcement officers, firefighters, and rescue first responders. The importance of resistance training for tactical athletes has long been recognized. For example, although basic training by military personnel improves several fitness components, the improvements are more comprehensive and substantial when weight training is included (see table 9.1) (71-73, 90). Metabolic, neural, muscular, connective tissue, endocrine, and cardiovascular changes take place that contribute to increases in muscular strength, power and speed, hypertrophy, endurance, athletic performance, balance, and coordination (35, 59).

Tactical strength and conditioning programs prepare the individual for prescreening fitness testing, basic training and occupational instruction, and fitness maintenance and improvement while on the job. Fitness improvements enable the tactical athlete to perform job-related tasks with superior precision, efficiency, and outcomes. The U.S. Army's approach to strength and conditioning focuses on improving muscle strength, aerobic and anaerobic endurance, and mobility (86). Fundamental skills such as sprinting and running, striking, swimming, rolling, climbing, crawling, squatting and lunging, pushing and pulling, jumping, landing, vaulting, throwing, and carrying are emphasized in military strength and conditioning programs. The goal of such programs is to prepare soldiers to march long distances with heavy combat gear; fight effectively in combat; drive vehicles through rough terrain; employ hand grenades; assault, run, and crawl for long distances; jump over obstacles and out of trenches; climb ropes, walls, and other barriers; and lift and carry heavy objects (including wounded soldiers) for long periods of time, often in warm temperatures in nutrition- and sleep-deficient states (86). Improvements in health- and skill-related components of fitness via resistance training can improve fighting ability and tolerance of stressful conditions (36, 50).

Comprehensive training for tactical athletes may include the integration of resistance training with plyometric, speed, agility, flexibility, and aerobic training and the training encountered by participation in the occupation (50). The precise balance of training modalities is essential to optimize performance and reduce the risk of overtraining and injury. Tactical athletes concurrently performing high-intensity resistance training and aerobic training with high frequency increase the risk of attenuating muscle strength and power gains (34). This incompatibility can be alleviated by instituting appropriate training cycles and allowing more recovery between training sessions during concurrent training. This has applications to military personnel, who perform significant amounts of aerobic and anaerobic training, mostly in the form of bodyweight exercise and calisthenics (20). The importance of **weight training** (resistance training with free weights, machines, or similar equipment) was noted early on by DeLorme and Watkins (17), who examined the benefits of weight training in injured soldiers returning from World War II. Using weight training to optimize strength gains in tactical athletes is critical to meeting occupational demands (36).

Key Point

Comprehensive training for tactical athletes may include the integration of resistance training with plyometric, speed, agility, flexibility, and aerobic endurance training and the training encountered by participation in the occupation.

Resistance training includes several exercise modalities designed to progressively overload the human body. The source of resistance varies but may include body weight, manual (self-applied or partner) resistance, water, stretchable bands or tubing, sport-specific devices, free weights, machines, medicine balls, suspension devices, balance equipment, and special implements (59). A resistance training program consists of variables that, when manipulated, provide a stimulus for adaptation. The importance of manipulating the acute program variables for optimal improvements was noted by Dr. William Kraemer and now serves as the basis for scientific resistance

Table 9.1 Selected Studies Examining Resistance Training in Tactical Athletes

Authors	Subjects	Training	Results
Schiotz et al. (74)	22 Army ROTC men	• RT: 4 days/week, 10 weeks, 9 exercises • CL-PER: 50%-105% 1RM, 1-8 sets × 1-30 reps • NP: 80% 1RM, 4-8 × 6-20 reps • Running: 4 days/week	• CL-PER: ↓ % body fat; ↑ 1RM SQ, BP, push-ups, sit-ups; ↓ rucksack run time • NP: ↑ 1RM SQ, push-ups; ↓ rucksack run time
Roberts et al. (69)	115 firefighter recruits, mostly men	• RT: 2-3 days/week, 16 weeks, 9 exercises • CL-PER: 70%-90% 1RM, 3 sets × up to 12 reps • Endurance training: 40%-60% 1RM • CV training: 65%-90% predicted max HR, 20-30 min/day; job-specific activities 20-30 min/day	↑ $\dot{V}O_2$max, # of push-ups, max grip strength, LBM; ↓ fat mass
Kraemer et al. (37)	35 active-duty Army soldiers	• RT: 4 days/week, 12 weeks, UP • Strength work: 4-5 sets × 5RM-10RM, 2-3 min RI • Hypertrophy work: 2-3 sets × 10RM-25RM, 1 min RI • Aerobic training: 4 days/week, 2 days 70%-80% $\dot{V}O_2$max, 2 days 400-800 m (437-875 yd) intervals • 4 groups: TB+ET, UB+ET, TB, ET	• TB: ↑ # of push-ups and sit-ups, VJ • TB+ET: ↑ # of push-ups and sit-ups, VJ; ↓ loaded 2 mi (3 km) run time • UB+ET: ↑ # of push-ups and sit-ups; ↓ loaded 2 mi (3 km) run time • ET: ↑ # of sit-ups, ↓ loaded 2 mi (3 km) run time • 6%-23% greater push-up and sit-up performance when RT was added to ET
Kraemer et al. (33)	82 untrained women	• CL-PER RT: 6 months, 3 days/week • TP: 3 sets × 8 exercises, 3RM-8RM (more for abs), 2 min RI • UP: 3 sets × 7-8 exercises, 3RM-8RM (more for abs), 2 min RI • TH: 3 sets × 8-9 exercises, 8RM-12RM (more for abs), 30-90 s RI • UH: 3 sets × 7-8 exercises, 8RM-12RM (more for abs), 30-90 s RI • FT: BW exercises, plyometrics, partner resistance, 6-20 reps, 1 min RI • Aerobic training–only group	• 1RM SQ: ↑ TP, TH, FT • 1RM BP: ↑ TP, TH, UP, UH, FT • 1RM HP: ↑ TP only • Jump power: ↑ TP, TH, FT • BP throw: ↑ TP, TH, UP, UH, FT • SQ reps: ↑ TP, TH, UP, UH, FT • 1RM box lift: ↑ TP, TH, UP, UH, TH • Box lift reps: ↑ all groups • Push-ups and sit-ups: ↑ TP, TH, UP, UH, FT • 2 mi (3 km) run time: ↓ all groups
Knapik (31)	13 female soldiers	• RT: 14 weeks, 3 days/week, 10 exercises, 3 × 10 reps (up to 13 on the last set) • Running 2 days/week	• ↑ 1RM of 6 exercises • ↑ floor lifting strength and repetitive lift reps
Marcinik et al. (45)	43 Navy men 87 Navy men	• 10 weeks of either aerobic + calis. or aerobic + CRT at 40% or 60% 1RM, 3 days/week • 8 weeks of either aerobic + calis. or aerobic + CRT (15 exercises) at 70% 1RM, 3 days/week	• Upper and lower body dynamic strength and endurance ↑ only in aerobic + CRT • Upper and lower body dynamic strength and endurance ↑ in aerobic + CRT
Marcinik et al. (46)	22 Navy women 115 Navy female recruits	• 10 weeks of aerobic + CRT at 60% 1RM • 10 weeks of either aerobic + calis. or aerobic + CRT at 40 or 70% 1RM, 3 days/week	• Dynamic strength and endurance ↑ • Aerobic + CRT at 70% ↑ dynamic strength and endurance more than aerobic + calis. and aerobic + CRT at 40%
Santtila et al. (71-73)	72 male military recruits	• All subjects—military training, 300 hr, 8 weeks • ST group—added total body RT 2-8 sets × 30%-100% 1RM CL-PER 3 days/week to military training • ET group—added 60-90 min of aerobic training 3 days/week to military training	• All groups ↑ $\dot{V}O_2$max 8.5% to 13.4% • ET and ST ↑ isometric leg extension strength by 9% to 13%; military-only training group did not change • All groups ↓ 3 km (2 mi) loaded combat (~14.2 kg [31.3 lb] added or 19% of body mass) test run time: ST—12.4%, ET—11.6% vs. 10.2% ↓ with military-only training • ET and ST groups ↑ isometric arm extension strength by 13.9% and 11.8% • Only ST group ↑ max RFD of arm extensors by 28.1%
Williams et al. (90)	52 male and female British Army recruits	• 10 weeks of basic training + RT, ET, circuit training, and sports • RT: total body 2 days/week, 3-4 sets × 75%-100% of 6RM, 1 min RI	• 8%-19% ↑ in material handling (max box lifts, lift and carry tests, loaded marching, incremental dynamic lifts to 1.45 m [1.6 yd]) performance • Many ↑ greater than basic training alone

(continued)

Table 9.1 *(continued)*

Authors	Subjects	Training	Results
Peterson et al. (54)	14 firefighter trainees	• 9 weeks of RT using CL-PER or UP, 3 days/week, total body RT + ballistic and plyometric exercises • Workouts: hypertrophy/endurance (5-9 sets × 65%-85% 1RM, 90 s RI), strength (3-75 sets × 75%-100% 1RM, 2-4 min RI), power (2-6 sets × BW to 75% 1RM, 2-5 min RI)	↑ BP & SQ 1RM, power output, & performance (equipment hoist, hose pull, stair climb, crawl, drag, sledgehammer), jump ability with several ↑ greater in UP than CL-PER
Harman et al. (20)	32 civilian men	• 8 weeks (5 days/week) of either Army standard physical training (e.g., BW push-ups, sit-ups, pull-ups, lunges, sprints) or weight training (2 days/week) + sprints, hikes, and agility (3 days/week) • Weight training—4 circuits of 3 exercises (e.g., BP, row, pulldown, step-up, pull-up) performed for 2-3 sets each	• Improved 3.2 km (2 mi) with load run/walk time, 400 m (437 yd) run time (with load), obstacle course time, simulated casualty recovery time, 30 m (33 yd) rush time, sit-up and push-up reps, 1RM SQ and BP, jumping ability • Both groups similar ↑ except for sit-ups and obstacle course run (better improvements with Army training)
Pawlak et al. (53)	20 male firefighters	12 weeks—2-3 days/week, circuits with 10-15 reps/exercise (push-ups, sit-ups, BW squats, lunges) + 20 min CV exercise	↑ ability to complete standard firefighting tasks, handgrip strength, ↓ % body fat, BMI, RHR

RT = resistance training; CL-PER = classic periodization; NP = nonperiodized; UP = undulating periodization; 1RM = one repetition maximum; SQ = squat; BP = bench press; CV = cardiovascular; HR = heart rate; $\dot{V}O_2$max = maximal aerobic capacity; LBM = lean body mass; RI = rest intervals; FT = field training; TB = total body resistance training; TH = total body hypertrophy; TP = total body strength/power; ET = aerobic endurance training; UB = upper body resistance training; UH = upper body hypertrophy; UP = upper body strength/power; VJ = vertical jump; calis. = calisthenics; RFD = rate of force development; BW = body weight; HP = high pull.

training program design (36). There are many ways to design effective resistance training programs while adhering to general training guidelines. Program design should be specific to the goals and needs of the tactical athlete and should first begin with the needs analysis.

NEEDS ANALYSIS

The **needs analysis** consists of answering questions based on the tactical athlete's goals and desired outcomes, assessments, limitations on workout frequency and duration, equipment availability, health and injury status, and occupational physiological demands. Tactical occupations are physically demanding. A well-designed, progressive resistance training program can benefit tactical athletes preparing for basic training or maintaining physical conditioning for active duty. The U.S. Army uses a three-phase training system consisting of initial conditioning, toughening, and sustaining phases following principles of precision, progression, and integration (86). During basic training, recruits must be prepared for calisthenics, sprint and distance running, combat training, marching, obstacle course navigation (involving climbing and agility tasks), engagement skills, marksmanship, and load-carriage

tasks (23). Current military personnel are often required to carry loads that are heavier than those used in the past (32).

Key Point

> The needs analysis consists of answering questions based on goals and desired outcomes, assessments, limitations on workout frequency and duration, equipment availability, health and injury status, and occupational physiological demands. It is a critical component of designing tactical strength and conditioning programs.

Law enforcement officers need muscle strength, power, endurance, flexibility, speed, and agility during hand-to-hand combat, apprehension and pursuit of suspects, self-defense, weapons carrying and use, and emergency response. Similar to military careers, the occupation involves periodic lifting and handling of heavy objects, dragging, running and sprinting, climbing, overcoming obstacles, jumping, stair-climbing, squatting, kneeling, and crawling. In some cases the events may be prolonged until the situation has been resolved. The restraining of suspects involves all components of self-defense, such as grappling, using joint locks, striking, punching, kicking, blocking, pushing and twisting, using takedowns and throws, carrying, applying handcuffs, and using weapons (13). Similarly, corrections officers require these fitness components to subdue and break up fights between inmates, escort uncooperative prisoners, lift and carry prisoners, search cells, and pursue inmates during escapes (26).

SWAT teams require advanced firearm, physical fitness, and tactical maneuvering skills and are responsible for extended law enforcement duties, such as situations involving hostages, barricaded hostile environments, clearing of dangerous areas, riots and crowd control, illegal drug operations, and terrorist situations where deadly force may be needed (13). SWAT teams typically use tactical gear that adds mass and provides resistance to motion while they secure perimeters, enter structures, and assist in moving injured people. One study showed that SWAT officers ranked high in bench press strength but displayed a wide range of values for core strength, power, and aerobic capacity (58). Thus, a tactical strength and conditioning program targeting muscle strength, power, endurance, flexibility, and aerobic fitness is needed to meet the occupational tasks and hazards.

Firefighters require muscular strength and endurance, power, flexibility, and aerobic endurance. Commons tasks include carrying equipment; raising ladders; pulling, hoisting, and climbing stairs with hoses; dragging victims; forcibly entering buildings with a sledgehammer or axe; performing ceiling breach and pulls with a pole; and searching for victims (2). Some of these tasks are short (e.g., forcible entry, raising a ladder), and some require extensive endurance because they may be performed for long periods of time (e.g., carrying loads, hoses, or victims). Protective equipment may range in mass to up to 25 kg (55 lb) (69). Some firefighting tasks include lifting and carrying objects up to 36 kg (79 lb) or more, pulling objects up to 62 kg (137 lb), and working with objects in front of the body weighing up to 57 kg (126 lb) (44). Performing firefighting tasks may yield HR values of 150 to 188 beats/min (14) and peak oxygen consumption of 41.5 to 43 ml·kg^{-1}·min^{-1} (with a mean of 23 ml·kg^{-1}·min^{-1}) (18, 40). HR values can range between 85% and 100% of the maximum predicted HR and remain high throughout the course of fighting the fire (44). Sounding the alarm may increase HR an average of 47 beats/min, and an increase in HR of at least 30 beats/min may be observed while firefighters are on the truck (7). Thus, understanding the occupational requirements is critical to developing a strength and conditioning program for firefighters.

Testing

Testing and evaluating tactical athletes is a critical component of the needs analysis and is covered in detail in chapter 8. Tactical athletes may have to undergo periodic testing and evaluation of physical and occupational performance. Most tactical occupations require preemployment fitness screening tests to determine if the person possesses the necessary physical attributes to perform the job. Once the tactical athlete is on the job, testing serves many purposes, including

- identification of strengths and weaknesses,
- evaluation of progress,
- identification of training load and intensity, and
- assessment of tactical athletic talent.

Military personnel may undergo routine physical testing involving selected tests of aerobic and local muscle endurance, power, and agility (23, 50). Resistance training (alone and in combination with aerobic training) and bodyweight calisthenic training improve multiple parameters of the Army's physical or combat fitness test (16, 37). Each state has its own physical requirements and fitness criteria for entry into the police academy. Often, timed push-up, step-up, sit-up, pull-up, vertical or broad jump, 1.5-mile (2.4 km) run, sit-and-reach, and bench press tests are included as part of a fitness testing battery (83). Firefighter ability tests such as the CPAT consist of assessments such as stair-climbing, dragging a hose, carrying equipment, raising and extending a ladder, and performing forcible entry, search and rescue, and ceiling breach and pulls (83). Other law enforcement and military branches may use other fitness assessments (e.g., shuttle runs, sprints, swim tests) as well (83). Body-fat percentage and specific conditioning traits indicate success rates in passing physical fitness tests (16). Resistance training programs are partly designed to correct weaknesses based on evaluation scores. A properly designed resistance training program can prepare the tactical athlete to excel during periodic testing.

Injury Prevention

The needs analysis includes evaluating the use of resistance training for injury prevention. Stress fractures, anterior knee pain, ankle sprains, plantar fasciitis, and low back pain are common overuse injuries encountered during high-volume running and load carriage (23). Poor physical conditioning and high body-fat percentage are associated with a higher rate of injury in military personnel (23). The physical stress of load carriage has long been associated with reduced performance and unnecessary injuries or ultimately death (32). The method of load carriage is important (e.g., double packs, pack frames, hip belts, vests, yokes). Load carriage is associated with greater risk of blisters, foot pain, low back pain, lower limb stress fractures, and knee pain (32). Common injuries in firefighters are sprains and strains in the shoulders, knees, and lower back, usually resulting from excessive forces encountered while operating in awkward body positions or from overexertion (2). The most common injuries in law enforcement personnel include sprains, strains, and soft tissue tears, followed by contusions, lacerations, and to a lesser extent broken bones, puncture and gunshot wounds, and burns (12). These injuries mostly occur while arresting subjects, conducting investigations, and chasing subjects on foot; in vehicular accidents; and, to a lesser extent, while training and doing other physical activity (12).

RESISTANCE TRAINING PROGRAM DESIGN

The training of tactical personnel mirrors the training of athletes in some respects because both professions require peak physical conditioning for success. The resistance training program is a composite of several variables: exercise selection and subsequent muscle actions used, exercise order and workout structure, intensity, volume,

rest intervals between sets and exercises, repetition velocity, and training frequency.

Key Point

The resistance training program is composed of several variables, including exercise selection and subsequent muscle actions used, exercise order and workout structure, intensity, volume, rest intervals between sets and exercises, repetition velocity, and training frequency.

Exercise Selection

Exercise selection refers to all of the exercises in the resistance training program. The selected exercises play a significant role in the transfer of muscle strength, power, and endurance from training to job performance. Exercise selection is affected by several factors, including the targeted muscle actions, size and number of muscle groups targeted, goals of the program and of each exercise, equipment availability, source of resistance, posture and body positioning, widths of grip and stance, unilateral versus bilateral exercises, and the intent to isolate muscle groups or target specific movements with resistance. Thus, a large number of exercises can be performed.

Key Point

Each exercise variation should be treated as a separate exercise. Any change in position or equipment will result in a different direction of stress on the body and amount of weight lifted and may necessitate a change in the number of repetitions performed.

Muscle Actions

Fitness gains are specific to the muscle actions performed. Dynamic motions consist of **concentric muscle actions** (muscle-shortening actions) and **eccentric muscle actions** (muscle-lengthening actions). **Isometric muscle actions** (static contractions) are also important. Strength is greatest during eccentric muscle actions, and thus strength and hypertrophy improvements are greatest when eccentric actions are emphasized; loaded eccentric muscle actions are more conducive to muscle damage (35). Isometric strength depends on ROM but is less than maximal eccentric strength and greater than maximal concentric strength (35).

Isometric muscle actions exist in many forms during resistance exercise, including stabilizer muscle contraction to maintain posture and stability, brief pauses between eccentric and concentric actions, gripping or support tasks, and the primary contraction type of certain exercises. Tactical athletes need sufficient isometric strength to perform occupational tasks such as loading and carrying, gripping, climbing, transporting victims, handling weapon recoil, restraining subjects during arrest, and engaging in hand-to-hand combat. Because concentric force production is lowest of the three muscle actions, oftentimes resistance training targets loading appropriate based on maximal concentric strength. Exercises such as planks and leg lift holds are predominantly isometric and strengthen core muscles. Exercises such as the farmer's walk and sandbag carry require the tactical athlete to isometrically contract for grip and postural support and are specific to occupational tasks.

Sufficient eccentric strength is also important. Some tactical maneuvers involve significant eccentric muscle strength (e.g., landing from jumps, grappling, climbing). Heavy eccentric training can be used in the form of heavy negatives (e.g., lowering heavy weights), forced negatives from a partner during eccentric phases, and unilateral negatives (e.g., performing a two-limb machine exercise concentrically but performing the eccentric phase with one limb). Tactical athletes have been known to perform exercises such as negative pull-ups in order to increase strength to augment regular pull-up performance (83). Note that a higher level of lifting competency is needed for heavy eccentric training versus traditional approaches.

Exercise Classifications

Exercises are generally classified as single or multiple joint. **Single-joint exercises** target one joint or major muscle group, whereas **multijoint exercises** target more than one joint or major muscle group (81). Single-joint and multijoint exercises are effective for increasing muscle strength, endurance, and hypertrophy. Multijoint exercises are more complex and are most effective for increasing

strength and power because of the greater loading used (35, 59). In addition, multijoint exercises may have greater transfer of training effects to tactical performance (10). Some exercises are **closed chain kinetic exercises**, where the distal segments are fixed, and some are **open chain kinetic exercises**, where the distal segment freely moves against loading. In comparison, moderate to high relationships exist between closed chain multijoint exercises and jump performance (10), indicating a greater potential role for multijoint exercises in improving performance.

Multijoint exercises may be classified as basic strength or total body exercises. **Basic strength exercises** (squat, bench press) involve at least two major muscle groups, whereas **total body exercises** (Olympic lifts and variations) involve most major muscle groups of the body and are the most complex exercises (35). These exercises are effective for increasing power because they require rapid force production and fast body movements (81).

Combination exercises are a trend in strength and conditioning to increase the metabolic response. These exercises involve combining two or more exercises into one sequential movement pattern for a series of repetitions. They may be performed by combining Olympic lifts and variations (clean from the floor, front squat, and push press to finish) or non-Olympic lifts (lunge with torso rotation, squat rotational press, push-up and renegade row, lunge and press, and thruster). Combination exercises are primarily used to increase muscular endurance and hypertrophy; strength training effects are secondary. Exercises that stress large muscle groups increase the metabolic demands and provide a potent stimulus for physiological adaptations.

Core and Assistance Exercises

Core exercises recruit one or more large muscle areas, involve multiple joints, and are a priority when selecting exercises because of their application to athletics (81). For the tactical athlete, core exercises consist of large muscle mass, multijoint exercises that improve strength and power. Often they are performed early in a workout to optimize performance. **Assistance exercises** strengthen smaller muscle groups or movements secondary to the core exercises (81). Tactical resistance training programs should consist of both core and assistance exercises (81).

Corrective Exercises

Some single-joint and multijoint exercises may be considered corrective. **Corrective exercises** target muscle groups that are prone to strength or length imbalances via adaptation or dysfunction. Imbalances could lead to joint dysfunction and altered movement patterns, thereby increasing the likelihood of overuse injuries and pain (52). Some muscles, such as the pectoralis minor and major, psoas group, hamstrings, and anterior neck flexor muscles, are more prone to shortening, whereas the gluteus maximus and medius, rhomboids, mid- to lower trapezius, and multifidus are more prone to lengthening (52). The resulting effects have been termed **upper cross syndrome** and **lower cross syndrome**, leading to postural imbalances such rounded shoulders and anterior pelvic tilt or hip flexion (52). In addition, weak core, hip abductor and external rotator, and gluteus maximus muscles are related to higher incidences of ankle and knee injuries, hamstring strains, and low back pain (52). Corrective exercises (plus myofascial release and flexibility exercises) can help correct postural deficits, restore neuromuscular function, and correct imbalances (15). These exercises can be included in warm-ups, cool-downs, and during the main lifting segment of the workout. The U.S. Army recommends performing 5 to 10 reps of some of these exercises for the core, shoulder, and hip musculature each day directly after warming up for other conditioning activities (86).

Unilateral and Bilateral Exercise Performance

Another consideration in exercise performance is unilateral (one arm or leg) versus bilateral (two arms or legs) exercises. Training unilaterally increases muscle strength in both trained and untrained limbs (48). Training bilaterally may increase the ability to produce maximal force simultaneously on both sides, thereby reducing the bilateral deficit known to exist in lesser-trained populations (39). Unilateral exercises require greater balance and stability compared with bilateral exercises. Performing a unilateral dumbbell exercise (with one dumbbell using asymmetric loading) requires the trunk muscles to contract intensely to maintain proper posture in order to offset the torque produced by unilateral loading. Often tactical athletes may face occupational situations that involve asymmetric loading, and the athletes must contract their muscles intensely to maintain postural control during normal locomotion (e.g., carrying a heavy load on one side of the body while walking, running, or ascending or descending steps or a ladder). Thus, including unilateral exercises and asymmetric loading in the resistance training program may be beneficial. Note that when the lifter is supporting a weight on one side, the next set should stress the opposite side so muscle balance occurs as both sides are trained equally. Asymmetric loading can be used bilaterally in multiple ways via specialized implements and exercises such as partner carries.

Resistance Training Equipment

Exercises may use a variety of resistance training equipment, such as free weights (barbells, dumbbells, and associated equipment), body weight, suspension devices, manual (self-applied, partner) resistance, stretchable bands or tubing and springs, sport-specific devices, machines, kettlebells, medicine balls, weighted vests and backpacks, balance equipment (stability balls, BOSU balls, wobble boards, and balance discs), implements (chains, sandbags and heavy bags, kegs, tires, sledgehammers, sleds, pulling ropes and battling ropes, thick bars, and strength competition equipment such as farmer's walk bars, backpacks, logs and log bars, super yokes, stones and stone-lifting devices), occupational equipment (ladders, mannequins, and hoses), and water (aquatic resistance training). Each mode of resistance has unique qualities.

Body Weight The human body is the most basic form of resistance for exercises such as body-weight squats, lunges, push-ups, pull-ups, dips, reverse dips, sit-ups, crunches, leg raises, and hyperextensions. Conditioning drills such as rope and wall climbing, obstacle navigation, and calisthenics also use body weight as the main source of resistance. Bodyweight training is a staple of tactical strength and conditioning (20, 51). Other conditioning modalities, such as aerobic training, speed, agility, and plyometric training, also use body weight as a source of resistance. Control of one's body is critical to tactical performance (50), so bodyweight exercises are paramount to tactical strength and conditioning. A progressive 12-week bodyweight training program consisting of push-ups, pull-ups, and sit-ups has been shown to increase lean tissue mass in addition to improving endurance in each exercise (16). Bodyweight exercises can be made more difficult by changing grip and stance width, leverage, or cadence or by using one versus two arms or legs. For example, adding a lateral crawl to a push-up can increase

metabolic demand and energy expenditure (64). Performing the burpee exercise yields oxygen consumption and energy expenditure values in excess of values for several traditional resistance exercises (64). These data provide a scientific rationale for inclusion of several bodyweight exercises in metabolic conditioning programs. Table 9.2 presents some common bodyweight exercises in tactical resistance training.

Free Weights and Machines   Training programs also consist of free weight and machine-based exercises. **Free weights** require the tactical athlete to control and move the weight freely in any

Table 9.2   Sample Bodyweight Exercises for Tactical Athletes

Upper body	Lower body	Trunk or core	Total body
Pull-up + variations	Squat (various stances and arm positions)	Leg raise (bent and straight legs)	Squat thrust, burpee (with or without push-up)
Alternating-grip pull-up	Lunge and reverse lunge + variations	Side-lying leg raise	Jumping jacks
Pull-up with heel hook	Single-leg squat	L-hang and isometric leg raise	Army crawl
Negative pull-up	Single-leg Romanian deadlift	Ab crunch and variations	Bear crawl
Muscle-up, kipping	Reverse leg curl	Flutter kicks	Crab walk
Flexed arm hang	Duck walk	Sit-up + variations	Rope climb
Pull-up hang	Glute squeeze	Knee-up + variations	Climbing (wall, fence)
Dip	Prone hip extension	Plyo leg raise	Mountain climber
Reverse dip	Clam shell	Twisting knee-up	Wheelbarrow
Push-up + variations	Prone windshield wipers	V-up	Planche + progressions
Push-up with lateral crawl	Supine bridge + variations (1 and 2 legs)	Reverse trunk twist	Front lever
Handstand push-up	Single-leg tuck	Plank and side plank with limb motion + variations	Human flag
Walking on hands	Walking Spiderman with overhead reach	Windmill	Superman
Plank-up	Lying hip abduction and adduction	Bend and reach	Quadruped
Neck bridging	Lunge with posterolateral reach	Ab rollout	
Inverted row		Press-up	
Forearm wall slide			
Prone shoulder press			
Prone internal and external rotation			
Prone scapular circuit (I-, T-, Y-, L-, and W-raises)			
Scapular wall slide			

These exercises may also be loaded with weights in addition to body weight. Muscle groupings are generalized; thus, several exercises listed may stress additional muscle groups as well.

direction. Several types of **machines** (specifically designed for resistance training) exist, including free-form cable pulley, plate-loaded, variable-resistance, hydraulic resistance, and pneumatic resistance machines, that allow for quick and easy change of loads. Free weights and machines both have several advantages and disadvantages (59). Free weight exercises may pose a slightly greater risk of injury because they require the lifter to maintain body stability and displacement of the resistance, whereas machines assist in stabilizing the body and resistance movement. With free weight exercises, the tactical athlete must control repetition velocity, and the movements are more similar to occupational movements compared with the movements of machine-based exercises. It has been suggested that free weights require greater coordination and muscle stabilization than machines because free weights must be controlled through all spatial dimensions whereas machines generally involve uniplanar control (85). Both free weights and machines are effective for increasing strength. Free weight training leads to greater improvements in strength assessed with free weights, and machine training results in greater performance on machine tests (11). Several exercises, including the Olympic lifts and variations, are performed with free weights and cannot be adequately performed with machines (85). Some exercises (e.g., leg extension, lat pulldown) are difficult to perform with free weights, so machines are a better alternative; in addition, a lifter may not need assistance from a spotter when performing machine-based exercises. Free weights allow the desired ROM (and greater hand and foot placement possibilities), whereas some machines can be restrictive.

Balls Medicine balls are weighted (1-30 lb [0.5-14 kg]) rubber or leather balls of various sizes that are used for general resistance training, calisthenics, and plyometric exercises. Rubber medicine balls are useful because they bounce and can be thrown safely, minimizing the risk of injury and damage. Stability balls are inflatable and come in many sizes (30-85 cm [12-33 in.]). They target core musculature because stabilizer muscles must contract to a greater extent than they would during a similar movement in a stable environment in order to keep the trainee from rolling. The loading used with stability balls is lower compared with stable equipment such as a bench or the floor due to the positive relationship observed between body stability and the maximum resultant force applied to a weight (4, 47). BOSU balls resemble stability balls with the exception that the bottom is flat. Instability training with stability and BOSU balls, in addition to other devices such as wobble boards and balance discs, helps increase balance, coordination, and activity of stabilizer muscles (8).

Elastic Bands and Chains Elastic bands provide variable resistance. Resistance increases as the band stretches further, and different bands provide different levels of resistance. Bands are light, portable, and can be added to free weight exercises (such as the bench press, deadlift, and squat) to create variable resistance. Chains may be used in a similar manner (19). A segment of the chain rests on the floor at the low end, so the athlete only has to support and lift a fraction of the weight. Less chain weight is supported by the floor during bar ascent, forcing the tactical athlete to produce more tension. Chains also oscillate, which increases the stability requirement. They are mostly used for multijoint exercises such as the squat and bench press. Chains can be used solely for resistance for certain exercises. For example, chains can be wrapped around the arms, shoulders, and neck for resistance during exercises such as push-ups, dips, and pull-ups and during various running drills.

Strength Implements **Strength implements** have increased in popularity and offer great benefits to the tactical athlete. Implements provide a different stress than free weights—they are unbalanced, and gripping may be difficult (19). *Kegs* are fluid-filled drums that weigh 9 to 14 kg (20-30 lb) to more than 136 kg (300 lb). Fluid movement within the keg increases the balance requirement via asymmetric loading. *Kettlebells* have handles that allow them to swing freely. Leverage changes and more rotation occur, placing greater strength demands on hand and forearm musculature. *Logs* or *log bars* allow weights to be added to each side and may be filled with water to add resistance. Large logs can be used for a one-sided clean and press (where the tactical athlete lifts one side of the log while the other side remains on the ground). *Thick bars* can enhance grip training for pulling exercises because they are usually 2 to 3 inches (5-8 cm) in diameter. *Weighted vests* or *backpacks* can be loaded with weights and used for many drills, including sprint training, plyometrics, rucking, and specific tactical maneuvers. *Farmer's walk bars* allow the tactical athlete to grasp a heavy weight and walk or run with it for a specified distance. A *super yoke* also allows the tactical athlete to carry heavy weight during walking, which may resemble an occupational load-carrying task.

Tires from trucks and heavy equipment are used for end-to-end flipping. Tires come in a variety of sizes and are often lifted for multiple repetitions as quickly as possible. The motion translates to several tactical maneuvers, such as heavy-object manipulation and hand-to-hand combat. There is also a potent metabolic effect (21) that assists in improving muscle endurance. Smaller tires can be used as resistance in running and carrying drills and can be used in partner grappling drills. Tires may also serve as a target for sledgehammer training. Swinging sledgehammers stresses core and grip musculature. *Sledgehammers* come in various sizes ranging from 8 to 20 pounds (4-9 kg) and are used for vertical, horizontal, and diagonal swings. *Sandbags* range from light to over 100 pounds (45 kg) and provide unbalanced resistance. *Heavy bags* (punching bags) are beneficial for combat and rescue training because they mimic an opponent or victim and can be thrown or lifted in multiple directions. *Stones* of various sizes (10-300+ lb [5-136+ kg]) can be lifted to various heights or used for carrying tasks and loading medleys.

Ropes are used for multiple purposes, such as climbing, pulling, and suspension training, and have been important in tactical resistance training. *Battling ropes* are around 50 to 100 feet (15- 30 m) long and 1 to 2 inches (2.5 to 5.0 cm) thick and are used mostly for wave training. The length and diameter of the ropes, as well as the velocity and amplitude of the waves, are thought to govern exercise intensity. Waves are generated via multiple movement patterns as the ropes are anchored at a fixed point. A large number of exercises can be performed, such as single- and double-arm waves, and several others can be performed when using various postures (standing, kneeling, lunging, squatting) and when integrated with other modalities such as plyometric drills and footwork agility (e.g., lateral shuffles, hops). Battling ropes are used to increase strength and endurance, and they provide potent metabolic and cardiovascular responses that are greater than those provided by traditional resistance exercises performed for three sets of 10 repetitions with 2-minute rest intervals (64).

Sleds provide resistance to primarily linear movements and are loaded with weights for pushing (from low and high body positions) or pulling (with a harness). Although sleds have been used extensively for speed training, sleds loaded with heavier weights have been used to increase strength and power during horizontal pushing and pulling movements. The loading depends on several factors, including training goals, movement velocity, and amount of friction between the sled and the surface. Maddigan and colleagues (42) compared maximal sled loading for 10 steps per leg with a 10RM barbell squat and reported that sleds loaded with 124% of 10RM loading were equivalent to squat performance. These data indicate that sleds can be loaded with more weight than can be used in the squat when strength and metabolic conditioning (not maximal speed development) are the goals. Sled training also provides the tactical athlete with a large metabolic response (21) that could be used for endurance training.

Numerous exercises are beneficial to tactical athletes. Tables 9.2 and 9.3 depict just a few of the exercises that can enhance strength and power, hypertrophy, endurance, core strength, tactical occupational performance, and combat skill. Tactical athletes should include unilateral and bilateral single-joint and multijoint (free weight, bodyweight, and machine) exercises into their resistance training programs, with emphasis on multijoint exercises for maximizing muscle strength, size, power, and endurance (81). Exercise variation is critical and can be included in the periodized program design. Most studies examining resistance training in tactical athletes included 6 to 10 exercises per workout and more in some cases when circuit training programs were used (see table 9.1).

Exercises may be altered by changing posture, hand and foot position and width, unilateral versus bilateral motion, and direction; adding an isometric component; and using BOSU balls, DBs, KBs, MBs, SBs, sandbags, bands, chains, machines, TRX, and other implements and resistance devices. Muscle groupings are generalized; thus, several exercises may stress additional muscle groups as well.

Exercise Order Within Workout Structures

Exercise order refers to the sequence of exercises performed. Acute lifting performance and rate of strength increases during resistance training are affected by the sequence of exercises. Exercises performed early in the workout generate higher repetition numbers and weight lifted because less

Table 9.3   Sample Resistance Exercises for Tactical Athletes

Upper body	Lower body	Trunk or core	Total body
Bench and chest press + variations	Back and front squats + variations	Renegade bar rotation	Power clean + variations
Incline/decline press + variations	Lunge (multidirection) + many variations	DB T-rotation	High pull
Flys + variations	Split squat	Wheelbarrow drag	Power snatch + variations
Bent-over row + variations	Lateral squat	Turkish get-up	Push press
Renegade DB row	Box squat + variations	MB/slam ball wood chop	Renegade clean and press
Lat pulldown + variations	Step-up + variations	Russian twist	Deadlift + variations
Sledgehammer swing	Jump squat	SB exchange	Bear-hug deadlift (bag)
Low pulley row	Overhead squat + variations	Cable rotation	Sandbag rotational deadlift
Shoulder press + variations	Overhead lunge + variations	Squat rotation press	Battling rope circuit
Shoulder scaption	Good morning	Sit-up and press	Tire flip
Shoulder internal/external rotation + variations	Leg press	SB rollout	Sled push/drag
Hyperextension press	Back extension/glute-ham raise		KB swing
Shrug	Reverse hyperextension		Sandbag/keg carry
Upright row	Prone bent-knee hip extension		Partner carry/drag
Lateral raise	SB leg curl		Sandbag/sled drag
Front raise	Leg curl		Farmer's walk
Curl + variations	Leg extension		Super yoke walk
Preacher curl	Toe raise + variations		Thruster
Triceps extension + variations	Ankle dorsiflexion		Heavy bag throw
Triceps pushdown + variations	Glute rope pull		DB loading medley
DB jab/uppercut/cross/hook	Hip thrust/bridge + variations		
Four-way neck	Wobble board/BOSU squat		
DB rotation press	Band-resisted step-up, walk, lateral shuffle		
Shoulder-to-shoulder press	Hip adduction and abduction (lying, standing)		
KB side press			
Wrist and reverse wrist curls			
Wrist roller			
Plate grab and pinch grip			
Pullover			

DB = dumbbell; KB = kettlebell; MB = medicine ball; SB = stability ball.

fatigue is present; exercises performed later in the workout may be more affected by fatigue. Priority may be given to the most goal-specific structural exercises early in a workout. Often these are multijoint exercises that stress large muscle groups. Performance of multijoint exercises declines when these exercises are performed later in a workout (82) or directly following exercises that stress similar muscle groups (61). Although several sequencing strategies can be used, general recommendations give priority to core exercises during strength and power training (81). Goals of the training program, in addition to goals of each exercise, help determine the appropriate exercise order.

Training Goals and Exercise Order

Common goals of resistance training include improved muscle strength, power, hypertrophy, muscular endurance, and motor performance (81). The goals of resistance training reflect the needs analysis of the tactical athlete. The most stringent sequencing guidelines are seen when strength and power are the major training goals. Motor performance (i.e., tactical athletic skills) sequencing is similar to strength and power sequencing. The reason for this stringency is that strength and power are best trained with minimal fatigue. This allows the tactical athlete to lift maximal loading, perform the maximal number of repetitions per loading scheme, and utilize the highest quality of repetition effort (power output), thereby eliciting several neuromuscular adaptations leading to optimal strength and power improvements (81).

High-intensity endurance (the ability to maintain high levels of force production over an extended period of time) and power endurance (the ability to maintain high power output over time) are different goals and can be trained with numerous sequencing strategies. For high-intensity and submaximal local muscular endurance training, the tactical athlete needs to train, in part, in a fatigued state. Muscular endurance is enhanced in several ways, but an effective strategy is training to and beyond exhaustion coupled with short recovery periods. Muscle hypertrophy is multifactorial; that is, a tactical athlete striving to increase muscle hypertrophy needs to target both mechanical and metabolic factors contributing to growth (75). Mechanical factors relate to the mechanotransduction of tissue loading (i.e., high forces and rates of force development, motor unit recruitment, muscle lengthening and accentuated eccentric muscle actions, increased activation of protein synthesis pathways integrated with hormonal responses and growth factor upregulation) consistent with principles of strength and power training (75). Metabolic factors relate to tissue hypoxia and metabolic stress (i.e., increased activation of protein synthesis pathways via hormonal responses and growth factor upregulation in response to occluded blood flow) consistent with principles of muscle endurance training (75). Thus, many sequencing strategies are effective (81).

Workout Structure

Sequencing guidelines depend upon the structure of each workout. Workout structures include total body workouts, upper and lower body split workouts, and muscle group split routines. Goals, time and frequency of training sessions, occupational demands, and personal preferences may determine which structure is optimal for the tactical athlete.

Total Body Workouts   Total body workouts use exercises that work all major muscle groups. These workouts include traditional and circuit resistance training. Many sequencing methods can be used depending on whether the exercises stress a few muscle groups (where several exercises are used to target the entire body) or total body exercises. Most studies examining resistance training in tactical athletes have used total body traditional (31, 33, 37, 69-73, 90) and circuit (20, 45, 46, 71-73, 90) resistance training workouts and modified upper and lower body split workouts (33, 37, 74). Total body workouts tend to be popular, especially when targeting functional performance, because many tactical maneuvers involve total body efforts.

For strength and power training, the following sequencing guidelines are recommended (81):

1. Perform large muscle mass core exercises before small muscle mass exercises.

2. Perform multijoint exercises before single-joint, isolation exercises.

3. For power training, perform Olympic lifts (sequenced from most to least complex) before basic strength lifts (most complex are snatch and related lifts followed by cleans and presses).

4. Rotation of upper and lower body exercises or opposing (agonist–antagonist or push–pull) exercises is an option when a total body workout is used. Exercises targeting different muscle groups can be staggered between sets of other exercises to increase time efficiency.

Multijoint exercises are given sequencing priority because they are most effective for increasing strength and power (81). Isolated, small muscle mass exercises may promote isolated muscle fatigue that could limit multijoint exercise performance. Alternating exercises (agonist–antagonist or push–pull) appears to help recovery, preserve or augment performance, and maintain efficiency (6, 61, 81). Large muscle mass exercises (e.g., squats) have been shown to augment the metabolic responses to smaller mass exercises (e.g., bench press) when the small mass exercise follows the large mass exercise in sequence (63). Thus, a number of sequencing strategies can be prescribed. Exercise sequencing can change as exercises are added to or removed from a training cycle. The aforementioned recommendations attempt to maximize performance of core exercises, but some exceptions may exist based on training priorities. For example, some exceptions include warm-ups and cool-downs where exercise sequencing is not a primary concern due to the low to moderate intensity and volume used. In addition, if an exercise needs to be prioritized, then it can be performed earlier in sequence.

For muscular endurance and hypertrophy training, fatigue is critical for inducing adaptations, and a number of sequencing strategies may be used. These strategies may follow basic strength/power guidelines previously mentioned for sequencing or use different strategies (e.g., small before large muscle mass exercise, single-joint before multijoint exercises) to improve conditioning. For example, a technique called *preexhaustion* requires the lifter to perform a single-joint exercise first to fatigue a muscle group before performing a multijoint exercise. Perfor-

mance decrements may be observed (less weight and repetitions) (5, 87), so this technique targets muscular hypertrophy and endurance, with limited strength training effects. Tactical training to improve occupational performance appears most effective when strength/power sequencing strategies are followed (31, 33).

Upper and Lower Body Split Workouts Upper and lower body split workouts divide upper and lower body exercises into different workouts. However, some modified upper and lower body split workouts entail training certain upper body muscles one workout and lower body muscles plus some different upper body or core exercises on another day, or they may entail training upper body muscles only. This structure is beneficial when traditional resistance exercises are included. However, it is difficult to use this structure when tactical athletes include total body and functional movement exercises in their workouts.

For strength and power training, the following sequencing guidelines are recommended (81):

1. Perform large muscle group exercises before small muscle group exercises (e.g., squat before bench press).

2. Perform multijoint exercises before single-joint exercises (e.g., barbell lunge before leg extension).

3. Rotation of opposing exercises (push–pull) may be performed (e.g., bent-over row paired with bench press).

Some exceptions to these guidelines may exist based on training priorities. TSAC Facilitators may choose to prioritize certain exercises or focus on trainee weaknesses; for example, a small muscle mass exercise may be performed before a large muscle mass exercise if the small mass exercise is prioritized to strengthen a weakened area. Numerous sequencing strategies may be used for muscular endurance and hypertrophy training, including those recommended for strength and power training.

Muscle Group Split Routines Muscle group split routines include exercises for specific muscle groups during a workout. This type of structure is used by people who want to maximize muscle hypertrophy, such as bodybuilders. The rationale is to target only one or two major muscle groups per workout with several exercises at various angles using multiple loading and repetition schemes to induce high levels of fatigue. The relatively long recovery period between workouts (i.e., muscle groups are not directly trained again for at least 72 hours) is thought to maximally stimulate muscle growth (59).

For strength and power training, the following sequencing guidelines have been recommended for muscle group split routines (81):

1. Perform multijoint exercises before single-joint, isolation exercises.

2. Perform large muscle mass exercises before smaller muscle mass exercises (if more than one major muscle group is trained during the workout).

3. Perform high-intensity exercises before low-intensity exercises (heaviest to lightest).

Some exceptions may exist based on training priorities and the goals of each exercise. Likewise, numerous sequencing strategies may be used for muscular endurance and hypertrophy training based on the TSAC Facilitator's priorities for the athlete.

Intensity

Intensity describes the amount of weight lifted or the complexity of the exercise and is interdependent on all other program variables, including volume, rest intervals, frequency, and repetition velocity. Resistance training intensity can be increased by using a higher relative percentage of the person's 1RM, increasing weight within an RM zone, or adding an absolute amount of weight to an exercise. Increasing relative percentage is common in periodized training programs, especially for structural exercises such as the Olympic lifts, squat, deadlift, and bench press. Training within an RM zone requires an increase in repetitions with a specific weight until a target number is reached. Then weight is added while repetitions are reduced to the starting value (e.g., 8RM-12RM zone). The most practical way to increase loading is by increasing the weight in absolute amounts. The tactical athlete's maximal strength does not need to be known. Rather, when the loading becomes easier to lift, an absolute amount is added

for progression. All methods of increasing intensity are effective for improving fitness and can be used in multiple ways (depending on the exercise) for tactical resistance training. However, caution should be used during simultaneous progression of multiple variables (59).

Strength Training

Gains in muscle strength can be seen with light loads (45%-50% of 1RM) in novice lifters, but heavier loads (≥80%-85% of 1RM) are needed to increase maximal strength in advanced trainees for structural multijoint and several single-joint exercises (35). Heavy weights are needed to maximize motor unit recruitment, and optimal recruitment of fast-twitch motor units is needed to maximize strength (36). A meta-analysis has shown that 60% of 1RM produces the largest strength effects in novice lifters, and 80% to 85% of 1RM (for six repetitions or less) produces the largest effects in trained lifters (66). Light to moderate intensities (60%-80% of 1RM) can be effective for increasing strength in large muscle groups when accompanied by high lifting velocities (59). Low to moderate intensities for some corrective exercises may be preferred, especially when training scapular, rotator cuff, and spinal muscles, as well as some core muscles. Closed chain exercises performed on one leg or arm are more intense than on two legs or arms because a greater percentage of body weight must be sustained by limited muscle mass. Therefore, light to moderate loads may be preferred for such exercises. With heavier weights comes lower repetition number and vice versa. The number of repetitions performed relative to the percentage of 1RM depends on the exercise and the level of muscle mass involvement.

Tactical athletes require a spectrum of intensities for optimal strength training. The intensity should be based on the training goals and the specific training phase. Intensity and volume prescription are most effective when a periodized approach is used (81). Periodized resistance training is most effective for increasing muscle strength and tactical occupation performance (33, 37, 54, 69-73). The tactical athlete should include specific training cycles within the yearly training plan that target specific fitness components, although occupational demands can often be a challenge.

For strength training, it is recommended that tactical athletes train with loads corresponding to 60% to 70% of 1RM for 8 to 12 repetitions initially and advanced tactical athletes cycle training loads of 80% to 100% of 1RM to maximize muscular strength (35, 81). Each exercise should be treated as a specific entity with its own goal and an intensity that matches the goal. A workout may consist of varying intensities even if the goal is peak strength or power. For example, during a strength phase the tactical athlete may be performing the squat at 90% of 1RM but may be performing a rotator cuff exercise at a lower intensity. The inclusion of strength training entails heavy weightlifting for some exercises.

Power Training

Training for maximal power requires a mixed strategy. Because peak power is the product of force and velocity, both components must be trained. This requires a spectrum of intensities. Moderate to heavy loads are needed to increase maximal strength (the force component), whereas low to moderate intensities performed at fast lifting velocities are needed to maximize rate of force development (35). Peak power for ballistic exercises such as the jump squat and bench press throw occurs at intensities ranging from 0% (body weight) to 30% of 1RM (10, 24) and 70% to 80% of 1RM for the Olympic lifts (29). Ballistic resistance exercise is different from traditional resistance exercise because the deceleration phase during propulsion is eliminated by maximally accelerating the load via jumping or releasing the weight. Ballistic resistance training increases maximal strength and can augment upper body strength gains when added to traditional resistance training (43). For power training, the NSCA recommends loads of 80% to 90% of 1RM for single-effort events (1-2 repetitions) and loads of 75% to 85% for multiple-effort events (3-5 repetitions) (81). Olympic lifts and variations are also recommended, using periodized intensities of 30% to 85% of 1RM (or heavier) depending on the training goals, phase, and experience of the tactical athlete. Additionally, the tactical athlete may train for power with other modalities, including plyometric, speed, agility, anaerobic interval, and tactical performance drills.

Hypertrophy Training

A positive relationship exists between muscle size and strength potential (27). Thus, hypertrophy (size) is a contributing factor to strength, power, and performance improvements. Heavy loads in combination with moderate and light loads are effective for increasing muscle hypertrophy. Heavy loads stress mechanical growth factors, whereas moderately heavy loads stress metabolic growth factors. The 6RM to 12RM loading zone (67%-85% of 1RM) has generally been regarded as a hypertrophy zone that elicits an optimal combination of mechanical and metabolic growth-inducing responses (35), and it has been frequently targeted by bodybuilders. However, recent studies have shown similar muscle hypertrophy gains between this range and heavy weight training (78). Thus, moderate and heavy loading both appear to increase muscle size. Lower intensities yielding 12 to 15 repetitions or more can increase muscle hypertrophy, presumably through metabolic stress (76). Thus, tactical athletes may require a spectrum of intensities to maximize hypertrophy in a periodized manner (35, 76). Hypertrophy training may be viewed as a blend of strength and endurance training to maximize the mechanical and metabolic stresses leading to tissue growth. For tactical athletes whose goal is hypertrophy, the NSCA recommends training with loads corresponding to 67% to 85% of 1RM for 6 to 12 repetitions in a periodized manner (81).

Muscular Endurance Training

Local muscular endurance training is a necessity for the tactical athlete. Several occupational tasks performed by tactical athletes require high levels of submaximal and maximal muscular endurance (see the Needs Analysis section earlier in this chapter). Strategies for endurance training with traditional resistance training involve performing sets to and beyond exhaustion, progressively increasing repetition numbers with a given load, using high-repetition sets, and reducing rest intervals in between sets (35), but they depend on scheduled occupational activity as well. For local muscular endurance training, the NSCA recommends using ≤67% of 1RM for ≥12 repetitions. (81). Set duration may be the prescription tool for some exercises (e.g., isometric exercises such as the plank and flexed arm hang, implement drills such as sledgehammer swings). In this case, the total set duration can be increased, or intensity can be increased (e.g., using a weighted vest during the plank, swinging a slightly heavier hammer) while using a constant set duration for muscle endurance training. Modern tactical conditioning programs have used various metabolic training strategies, where multiple modalities are integrated within each workout, intensity and volume are moderate to high, rest intervals are short (circuit training), and each circuit may progressively decrease time to completion (see discussion later in this chapter).

Training Volume and Volume Load

Training volume is the number of sets times the number of repetitions, whereas **volume load** is calculated by multiplying the load lifted by the number of sets times the number of repetitions. Manipulating training volume or volume load is accomplished by changing the number of exercises per session, the number of repetitions per set, the number of sets per exercise, or the loading. There is an inverse relationship between volume and intensity such that volume should be low when intensity is high.

Training Volume and Goals

Strength training is synonymous with low to moderate training volume because a low to moderate number of repetitions is performed per set for structural exercises. Hypertrophy and muscle endurance training are synonymous with low, moderate, and high intensity and moderate to high volume. Volume load is modestly related to muscle hypertrophy changes in women and highly related to strength increases in men and women (55). Training volume may vary considerably. Current volume recommendations for strength and endurance training are one to three sets per exercise by novice lifters and multiple sets with systematic variation of volume and intensity by intermediate and advanced lifters (81). A dramatic increase in volume is not recommended when intensity is high. Not all exercises need to be performed with the same number of sets, and the emphasis of higher or lower volume is related to program priorities, training status, and type of modality.

The number of sets performed per exercise and workout depends on variables such as intensity, frequency, nutritional intake, and recovery. Most volume training studies compared single- and multiple-set programs, and they showed that untrained individuals respond well to either, but advanced individuals need multiple sets for higher rates of progression (38). There is great variability in selecting the number of sets per workout. Often training studies have incorporated 15 to 40 sets per workout (3-6 sets or one to two exercises per muscle group) for total body workouts (59). A meta-analysis showed that 4 to 8 sets per muscle group yielded the highest effects in trained individuals, whereas 4 sets per muscle group produced the highest effects in untrained individuals (56). Typically, 3 to 6 sets per exercise are common, but more or fewer can be used depending on the exercise and training goals. If a muscle group is trained once per week, then a high number of sets can be performed. However, if a muscle group is trained two to three times per week (within a total body or upper and lower body split workout), then fewer sets are performed per workout (35). The number of sets per workout depends on whether or not the tactical athlete is integrating resistance training with sprint, plyometric, agility, or possibly aerobic training.

Set Structures for Multiple-Set Programs

Set structuring determines the load patterning for multiple-set programs. The load and repetition number during each set can increase, decrease, or stay the same. Set structuring is exercise dependent, and various structures may be used within the same workout. There are three basic structures (as well as many integrated systems), and advantages and disadvantages exist for each. Because all are effective, the chosen structure may be up to the personal preference of the tactical athlete.

1. A constant load and repetition system uses a constant loading and repetition number across all sets. Most studies examining training in tactical athletes have used constant load and repetition systems because they work well within classic and undulating periodization models (33, 34, 37). A disadvantage is the lack of variety per workout

in loading and repetitions performed. However, that may be addressed by manipulating the loading and repetitions performed within a periodized scheme.

2. A second method is to use a light to heavy system. The weight increases each set while repetitions remain the same or decrease (i.e., ascending pyramid when repetitions are decreased). This offers the advantage of performing a warm-up progression before lifting the heaviest weight, especially for the first exercise in the workout. Ascending pyramids are commonly used for structural multijoint strength exercises that are performed for at least three sets. A disadvantage is that the heaviest set is performed last, and thus fatigue could be present during the heaviest set.

3. The third set structure is to work from heavy to light by decreasing the weight with each set and either maintaining or increasing the repetition number (i.e., descending pyramid when repetitions are increased). The advantage of this approach is that the heaviest set is performed first, when fatigue is minimal, which may be beneficial for the tactical athlete working out while on duty. However, the lifter may not properly be warmed up for the heaviest set, especially if it is the first exercise in the sequence and requires heavy loading. This system is effective when short rest intervals are used and weight needs to be reduced for subsequent sets.

All systems are effective for increasing strength, power, hypertrophy, and local muscular endurance (59) and can be adapted into resistance training programs for tactical athletes.

Rest Intervals

Length of rest intervals between sets and exercises depends on training intensity, goals, fitness level, and targeted energy system, and it is affected by the muscle groups trained, equipment available, and time needed to change weights and relocate to other equipment. Lifting performance becomes more difficult with short rest intervals. Fewer repetitions are performed with rest intervals <2 minutes compared with intervals >2 minutes (60-63, 80, 88, 89), and total volume for multiple sets of an exercise is higher with long versus short rest intervals (62, 84). A continuum exists where the fewest repetitions are performed with 30-second rest intervals and the largest numbers of repetitions are performed with 5-minute rest intervals (62), with a similar pattern of fatigue between single-joint and multijoint exercises (80). This is the case when exercises are performed in sequences that stress similar muscle groups (61). Recent studies have shown that factors such as gender, aerobic capacity, and muscular strength play key roles (60, 63). For example, women have been shown to maintain resistance exercise volume to a greater extent than men when short (1-minute) rest intervals are used (60, 63). In addition, men with greater strength may require more time to rest to maintain resistance exercise volume than men with lower levels of strength (60). Athletes with higher aerobic capacity ($\dot{V}O_2$max) tend to tolerate short rest intervals to a larger extent, especially during lower body resistance exercise, than athletes with lower $\dot{V}O_2$max values (63).

Strength and Power

Several studies showed greater strength increases with long versus short rest intervals between sets (e.g., 2 to 3 minutes versus ≤1 minute) (57, 70, 77), although some showed similar strength increases between 1- to 2-minute and 2.5- to 5-minute intervals (3, 89), and one showed similar strength increases when rest intervals were gradually reduced from 2 minutes (compared with a standard 2-minute interval) (84). Thus, a number of factors must be considered when selecting rest interval lengths. Training for maximal strength and power requires the tactical athlete to perform heavy, high-velocity sets with quality repetitions. This is best accomplished in a state with minimal fatigue. Thus, greater recovery between sets and exercises (especially to allow ample time for ATP-PCr resynthesis and removal of waste and metabolic products) is needed. For strength and power training, the NSCA recommends that tactical athletes rest at least 2 to 5 minutes for core exercises using heavier loads (81). Each exercise may be prescribed with a specific rest interval length and modified when necessary based on the goals of that exercise and its location within the training session.

Hypertrophy Training

Muscle hypertrophy training encompasses a wide range of rest interval lengths depending on the intensity and volume of the set and exercise. Long rest intervals benefit tactical athletes during heavy lifting to increase strength and power (77), which is part of the muscle hypertrophy continuum targeting mechano growth-inducing factors. In contrast, short rest intervals limit recovery between sets, thereby increasing muscle hypoxia and subsequent metabolic stress. Short rest intervals are characteristic of endurance training. For hypertrophy training, the NSCA recommends 30- to 90-second rest intervals (81).

Local Muscular Endurance Training

Local muscular endurance training is best accomplished when higher levels of fatigue are induced by the training stimulus. Thus, limiting recovery between sets is a common method of local muscular endurance training. In addition, local muscular endurance training is accomplished using high-repetition sets where additional recovery between sets may allow more repetitions to be performed. Thus, multiple strategies may be used for local muscular endurance training. The NSCA recommends ≤ 30 seconds of rest between sets for local muscular endurance training (81). When circuit training, it is recommended that rest intervals encompass the time needed to get to the next station, but the goal should be <30 seconds. Minimal rest is customary for these muscular endurance training protocols. Tactical athletes should be cognizant of the metabolic stress associated with continuous resistance training programs and modify rest intervals based on conditioning levels and rates of muscular endurance, strength, power, and hypertrophy progression (36).

Repetition Velocity

Repetition velocity depends on loading, fatigue, and training goals (35). Tactical athletes have the ability to control repetition velocity for a specific exercise up to a certain point; that is, they can choose to lift the weight at slow, moderate, or fast velocities (35). Beyond this load, maximal effort is needed during the lifting of maximal and near-maximal loads, yet the bar velocity observed is relatively slow based on the muscle concentric force–velocity relationship. These velocities are referred to as *unintentionally slow lifting velocities*. They occur during the lifting of heavy loads and are paramount to maximal strength training. For nonmaximal lifts, the intent to control velocity is critical. Self-selected slow, moderate, and fast velocities invoke velocity-specific adaptations to resistance training with some carryover effects (35). Intentionally super-slow-velocity repetitions (5- to 10-second concentric phase; 5- to 10-second eccentric phase) are used with submaximal weights to increase muscular time under tension. The goal of this approach is to increase fatigue and potentiate endurance and hypertrophy enhancement. Strength enhancement is secondary because muscle force produced, weight lifted, and repetitions performed per workload are lower compared with moderate and fast velocities (22). Slower rates of strength increase occur with intentionally slow velocities (49), and higher rates occur when the weight is moved rapidly (28).

Strength and Power Training

For strength and power training, the intent to move the weight as quickly as possible appears to be the critical element (9). Because force is equal to mass multiplied by acceleration, the force exerted by the tactical athlete is proportional to the acceleration of the resistance per given level of mass lifted. For strength training, slow (2- to 3-second concentric phase; 2- to 3-second eccentric phase with minimal time between phases) and moderate (1- to 2-second concentric phase; 1- to 2-second eccentric phase) velocities are recommended for untrained lifters. This is a starting level while the trainees are learning proper technique and building a strength base. However, moderate to fast velocities are recommended for intermediate and advanced lifters whose technique is proficient (35). Unintentionally slow velocities that accompany heavy weightlifting are recommended during strength training phases. For power training, fast velocities (≤1-second concentric phase; ≤1-second eccentric phase) are recommended for power-specific training (35). High movement velocity is critical to increasing rate of force development, and this occurs with light to moderate loading. Because power is the product of force and velocity, strength training is part of the power training continuum. Thus, velocity may be moderate to fast for strength training and unintentionally slow when maximal and near-maximal loads are lifted (35).

Hypertrophy Training

Hypertrophy training encompasses a spectrum of velocities depending on intensity and volume. Slow, moderate, and fast velocities are recommended, which must interact with loading and repetition number (35). Because hypertrophy training involves a mixture of strength, power, and endurance training, tactical athletes can effectively use slow, moderate, and fast velocities.

Local Muscular Endurance Training

A spectrum of lifting velocities is beneficial for local muscular endurance training. Lifting velocity appears to interact with volume load and intensity in a manner that can be congruent to maximizing each. A slow velocity increases muscle time under tension to augment duration, but a faster velocity may do the same because more repetitions can be performed to match the time (35). Thus, the interaction of several variables, including velocity, appears critical to maximizing muscle endurance, and slow, moderate, and fast velocities are recommended for local muscular endurance training (35). The critical component is prolonged set duration; it is recommended to use intentionally slow velocities for a moderate number of repetitions (i.e., 10-15) and moderate to fast velocities for high-repetition sets (i.e., 15-25 or more) (35).

Frequency

Frequency refers to the number of training sessions per week or the number of times muscle groups are trained per week. As with other variables, frequency depends on several factors, such as volume, intensity, exercise selection, level of conditioning, training status, recovery ability, nutritional intake, and training goals. Two to 3 days per week is an effective training frequency for untrained individuals (59, 81). A meta-analysis has shown that 3 days per week produces the highest effect size in untrained individuals and 2 days per week produces the highest effect size

in trained individuals (66). Increased training experience does not necessitate a change in frequency for training each muscle group but may require alterations in other acute variables such as exercise selection, volume, and intensity. Increasing the frequency may enable greater exercise selection and volume per muscle group per workout (35).

Frequency varies considerably for advanced training. Advanced strength athletes have benefitted from frequencies of 4 to 5 days per week (24), and some elite strength and power athletes train at higher frequencies (more than once per day) (59). Studies examining resistance training in tactical athletes have used frequencies of 2 to 4 days per week (20, 37, 69, 74), with most studies targeting 3 days per week (31, 33, 45, 46, 54, 69-73). Thus, this appears to be a recommended frequency, especially for total body workouts. The U.S. Army recommends alternating resistance training workouts with endurance training and mobility workouts every other day (86). This involves a resistance training frequency of 2 to 3 days per week depending on whether the focus of the training week is strength or endurance (86). Caution must be used when determining frequency during integrated training with sprint, plyometric, agility, and aerobic endurance training. Because tactical training involves several fitness components, frequency must be adapted to allow adequate recovery between workouts to avoid overtraining.

Circuit and Metabolic Training

Circuit training has been a staple of tactical strength and conditioning for many years. Circuit programs increase training efficiency, yield substantial metabolic and cardiovascular responses, and are an excellent modality to improve anaerobic capacity. Circuit programs have been examined in firefighters (1, 53) and military personnel (20, 45, 46, 90). For example, firefighters performing two circuits of 12 exercises for 12 repetitions (or more for bodyweight exercises) plus 3 minutes of treadmill running and stair-climbing yielded average HRs at ~86% of max HR during the second circuit and blood lactate levels of ~11.7 mmol/L (1). The continuity is a stimulus for increasing aerobic capacity. Often, circuits consist of 6 to 12 exercises at a low to moderate intensity for 10 to 15 repetitions with <15 seconds between exercises to primarily improve local muscular endurance (1, 53). Large muscle mass resistance and bodyweight exercises increase the metabolic response and difficulty of the circuit. Muscle strength and power can improve with circuit training when circuits are designed to target each fitness component. To achieve the goals of strength and power, the intensity needs to be higher, exercises should be sequenced to allow partial rest for major muscle groups between exercise performance, and the repetition number must be lower.

It has become popular to include other modalities of training (e.g., sprint, agility, tactical, aerobic, and plyometric drills) within metabolic circuits. Circuit progression can take place by increasing the load, repetitions, or duration of the drills or by reducing the total time needed to complete the entire circuit (e.g., timed circuits). **Timed circuits** can stress the combination of speed, quickness, and agility in addition to muscle strength and power endurance, but correct form must be enforced. The tactical athlete can perform the entire circuit, rest 1 to 2 minutes, and repeat the circuit for the desired number of sets. Circuits depend on equipment availability and space, and they can be varied by altering the exercise selection and number per circuit, loading, and volume.

Several popular metabolic training programs have evolved over the years. Metabolic training is an aggressive form of circuit training. Structural and compound (large muscle mass) bodyweight, resistance, aerobic, plyometric, sprint, or agility exercises are performed with minimal rest between exercises. The high continuity and large muscle mass involvement (along with the intensity interaction) provide a strong metabolic stimulus for cardiovascular and muscular endurance improvements and body-fat reductions (20, 53). Metabolic training has become popular among military personnel, athletes, and general fitness enthusiasts (83). Following is a sample metabolic circuit workout, designed to decrease body fat and increase muscle strength, power, muscle and cardiovascular endurance, mobility, and coordination:

1. Conventional barbell deadlift × 10 reps
2. Blast-off push-up × 12 reps
3. Sandbag reverse lunge × 10 reps (alternate sides)
4. Kettlebell swing × 15 reps
5. Burpee × 15 reps
6. Inverted row × 10 reps
7. Plank × 30 seconds
8. Jump rope × 100 reps

The circuit is performed continuously with minimal rest (depending on conditioning level) between exercises. The tactical athlete can rest 1 to 3 minutes between circuits and perform two to four circuits in total.

These workouts can be challenging, so a gradual progression is needed, perhaps starting with a couple of drills for moderate duration. Volume can increase and rest can decrease progressively over time as the trainee becomes more conditioned. Increasing the workload too quickly or assigning a novice, deconditioned person to an advanced, competitive program could result in a greater risk of overuse injuries. Thus, prudent exercise prescription should be implemented as well as proper recovery between workouts and adequate nutritional and fluid intake.

Importance of Progressive Overload, Specificity, and Variation

There are a multitude of ways to design effective programs for tactical athletes following the programming guidelines discussed in this chapter. Three critical components of all tactical training programs are progressive overload, specificity, and variation (35, 59). **Progressive overload** involves the program gradually becoming more difficult, such as by adding weight, increasing repetitions with the current workload or duration of an exercise, adding more complex or challenging exercises, decreasing rest intervals, or using more advanced training techniques. **Specificity** means training adaptations are specific to the imposed stimulus. Specificity is seen with muscle groups trained, ROM, energy system targeted, velocity, muscle actions, and contraction patterns. In addition, specificity is achieved through exercise selection. The inclusion of strength and power exercises plus functional tactical movements (e.g., rope climbing, drags, partner carries) increases the likelihood that fitness gains can transfer to the tactical athlete's occupational movements. **Variation** entails altering the training stimulus through training periodization.

Key Point

Three critical components of tactical training programs are progressive overload, specificity, and variation. A training program can be highly effective, provided all three components are included in the design.

Periodization is a logical method of planning training (i.e., manipulating program variables) in a sequential and integrative fashion in order to maximize training-induced physiological and performance outcomes (see chapter 10). Although programs can be varied in many ways, a few basic models of periodization have been studied most frequently. The **classic (linear) model of periodization** involves a gradual increase in intensity and reduction in volume with each phase usually to peak strength and power following a period of hypertrophy training (67, 68). **Block periodization** involves dividing the training stimulus into highly specialized mesocycles. Typically, three or four mesocycle blocks two to four weeks in length are used (25). The focus of blocks can vary but often targets specific training components. An **undulating (nonlinear) periodization** model varies intensity and volume within each 7- to 10-day cycle by rotating protocols to emphasize specific fitness components (65, 67, 68). For example, for structural exercises in the workout, heavy, moderate, and lighter resistances may be rotated over a week (Monday, Wednesday, Friday), using 3 to 5 repetitions (with loads ≤3RM-5RM), 8 to 10 repetitions (with loads ≤8RM-10RM), and 12 to 15 repetitions (with loads ≤12RM-15RM) in the rotation. A variation of this model is the weekly undulated periodized model, where intensity and volume vary weekly as opposed to daily. Another model emphasizes peaking for hypertrophy or muscular endurance and is known as **reverse linear periodization**. This model begins with training phases emphasizing moderate to high intensity and low training volume, and it progresses to lower intensity, higher volume training with each successive phase (68).

All periodization models are effective for increasing fitness and performance, and most studies show periodized training to be superior to nonperiodized training (65). Reverse linear periodization produces inferior strength increases but superior endurance increases compared with linear and undulating models (68). In contrast, the undulating model is more effective than the classic model for increasing strength (67). Most studies involving tactical athletes have examined the classic and undulating models in military personnel, who showed substantial fitness and performance improvements (37, 71-73). In firefighters, undulating periodization was shown to produce more comprehensive improvements in fitness compared with the classic model (54).

CONCLUSION

Tactical athletes require sufficient muscular strength, endurance, flexibility, hypertrophy, and power as well as cardiorespiratory endurance, speed, agility, and mobility. Resistance training is a critical modality in the training programs of tactical athletes. Proper prescription and manipulation of the acute program variables is the most effective way to improve performance and reduce the risk of injury in tactical athletes. Many programming strategies can be effective as long as progressive overload, specificity, and variation are included in each training cycle.

Key Terms

assistance exercises
basic strength exercises
block periodization
classic (linear) model of periodization
closed chain kinetic exercises
concentric muscle action
core exercises
corrective exercises
eccentric muscle action
exercise order
exercise selection
free weights
isometric muscle action
lower cross syndrome
machines
multijoint exercises
muscle group split routines
needs analysis

open chain kinetic exercises
periodization
progressive overload
resistance training
reverse linear periodization
single-joint exercises
specificity
strength implements
timed circuits
total body exercises
total body workouts
training volume
undulating (nonlinear) periodization
upper and lower body split workouts
upper cross syndrome
variation
volume load
weight training

Study Questions

1. Which of the following must be addressed before a resistance training program can be designed for a tactical athlete?

   a. workout structure

   b. exercise selection

   c. needs analysis

   d. training frequency

2. All of the following are examples of strength implements EXCEPT

   a. kegs

   b. sleds

   c. dumbbells

   d. ropes

3. When programming for a strength or power training cycle, what is the most appropriate exercise order?

   a. squat, plank, power clean, bench press

   b. power clean, squat, bench press, plank

   c. plank, power clean, bench press, squat

   d. bench press, squat, plank, power clean

4. During power training, what is the recommended percentage of 1RM when performing a single-effort power exercise?

   a. 50%-60%

   b. 60%-70%

   c. 70%-80%

   d. 80%-90%

Chapter 10

Periodization for Tactical Populations

G. Gregory Haff, PhD, CSCS,*D, FNSCA

One of the key concepts in the preparation of athletes is periodized training. These training plans are essential when attempting to optimize the performance of tactical athletes (5, 68). Although periodization is a widely accepted concept, there is a large degree of confusion in both the scientific (1, 60, 61) and practical literature (17, 44) when trying to determine what periodization is and how to employ it. At the center of this confusion is a misinterpretation of the classic periodization literature, the terminology adopted by some scientists and practitioners, and the modern trend of isolating training factors without considering how they are integrated within a training period or phase (i.e., **vertical integration**) or sequenced over time (i.e., **horizontal integration**) (27-29).

Critical evaluation of the classic literature reveals that a true periodization model should exhibit nonlinearity, sequential variation (i.e., horizontal integration), and integration within a time period (i.e., vertical integration) of all training activities in order to optimize performance at predetermined time points related to the operational plan (5, 33, 47, 54, 55). Attention to these tenets removes training linearity and monotony in order to maximize the tactical athlete's development. To accomplish these goals, consideration must also be given to the logical application of training stressors so as to minimize any interference by one training factor on another.

Many classic periodization theorists emphasize that the training process must contain logical and systematic sequential or phasic alterations in workload, training focus, and training tasks in order to ensure that appropriate adaptations are stimulated to create the desired performance outcomes (2, 3, 6, 7, 34, 48-50, 54-56). Scientific inquiry has supported these earlier observations by revealing that sequential modeling results in superior physiological and performance outcomes (36, 51, 81). It is clear that periodization models used by tactical athletes must be nonlinear, have integrated training factors, be sequenced over time, progress loads logically, avoid random or excessive variation, and target specific training outcomes as determined by the athlete's operational plan.

Although periodization is essential for performance optimization, it is not a rigid framework.

Rather, it should be seen as a methodology that is easily adaptable to the specific programming needs of the tactical athlete (68), and its tenets allow the TSAC Facilitator to carefully craft a training intervention that targets the specific goals of the tactical athlete.

In order to develop a periodized training plan for the tactical athlete, the TSAC Facilitator must understand several central concepts. Therefore, the aim of this chapter is to define periodization, discuss its goals, explain its general principles, present its hierarchical structure, introduce the concept of integration and sequencing of training, and discuss how to apply these principles to the preparation of the tactical athlete.

DEFINING PERIODIZATION

The scientific literature contains numerous definitions of **periodization** with varying levels of complexity (1, 5, 56, 59). For example, Nádori (54, 55) and Nádori and Granek (56) define periodization as the theoretical and methodological basis for training and planning, while Plisk and Stone (59) define it as the logical and phasic manipulation of training factors in order to optimize the training process. Ultimately, periodization can be defined as a logical method of planning training interventions (i.e., volume, intensity, training density, training frequency, training focus, tactical practice, technical skills acquisition, modalities of training) in a sequential and integrative fashion in order to maximize training-induced physiological and performance outcomes (27-29).

Key Point

Periodization is a logical method of planning training interventions in a sequential and integrative fashion in order to maximize training-induced physiological and performance outcomes.

From an applied perspective, periodization contains both aspects of planning and programming in order to logically and systematically implement training units to develop the attributes that are critical to the tactical athlete's performance. In a tactical environment, it may be better to consider the periodized training plan as an **operational plan** that targets specific physiological adaptations and performance outcomes that are in line with the tactical athlete's operational goals.

Key Point

> The periodization plan for tactical athletes should be considered in the context of an operational plan, in which mission or operational requirements serve as the foundation for the training program.

GOALS OF PERIODIZATION

The primary goal of any periodized training intervention is to provide an adequate training stimulus for the development of specific physiological attributes that optimize performance at specific time points (5). This goal must also be balanced with a secondary goal where overtraining potential, reduced training monotony and linearity, and long-term athlete development are managed through the manipulation of the training stressors contained in the operational plan. It is important to note that operational goals are different from the goals of periodization. For example, an operational goal for a police officer may be to concurrently develop strength and endurance in order to better prepare him to pursue and subdue a suspect, whereas the operational goals for a firefighter may focus on increasing strength so that she may be able to better move hoses or injured individuals. Conversely, the periodization goals focus more on how things are planned and programmed to achieve these operational goals.

Using periodization to address operational goals requires systematic variation of training interventions that capitalize on the logical manipulation of training factors, including training volume, intensity, density, and frequency (27-29). Additionally, variation should be considered in the context of the exercise selection, targeted training focus, and overall mode of training (27-29). Variation should not be limited to an individual training session but should be included in the period or phase of training contained within the operational plan. Although there are limitless training variations, they should not be excessive or randomly applied because this can result in a less optimal training stimulus and failure to achieve the prescribed training outcomes (71).

PRINCIPLES OF PERIODIZATION MODELS

The end product of the training process is the stimulation of some training or performance outcome. The ability of the training process to accomplish this goal is tightly linked to the external load and the internal load, or the tactical athlete's characteristics that dictate responsiveness to the training process (figure 10.1).

The external load is the application of the training stimulus, which is largely dictated by the periodization model prescribed for the athlete. This model dictates the organization of the training interventions, including the integration and sequencing of training factors, and the quality and quantity of the training interventions (38). The tactical athlete's characteristics, such as genetic predisposition, current training status, training history, health status, and chronological age, all affect the internal load that is experienced in response to this external loading. Therefore, the physiological adaptations and training outcomes are directly stimulated by the tactical athlete's internal load, which is created by the external load (training stimulus) and the tactical athlete's individual characteristics, or **adaptive potential**. The ability of the periodized training plan to induce the targeted training outcomes is therefore based on the ability of the model to create an external load that balances recovery and adaptation while capitalizing on the tactical athlete's ability to tolerate the prescribed training stimulus.

Regardless of the tactical athlete's characteristics, three mechanistic theories are generally associated with the ability of the periodized plan to stimulate the desired outcomes: general adaptation syndrome (25, 71), stimulus-fatigue-recovery-adaptation theory (71), and fitness–fatigue theory (12, 82).

General Adaptation Syndrome

A core concept underlying the application of periodized training is the **general adaptation syndrome (GAS)** (71, 82, 83). The GAS was first theorized by Hans Selye in 1956 (65) to explain how the body responds to physical and psychosocial stress (figure 10.2). The basic response to

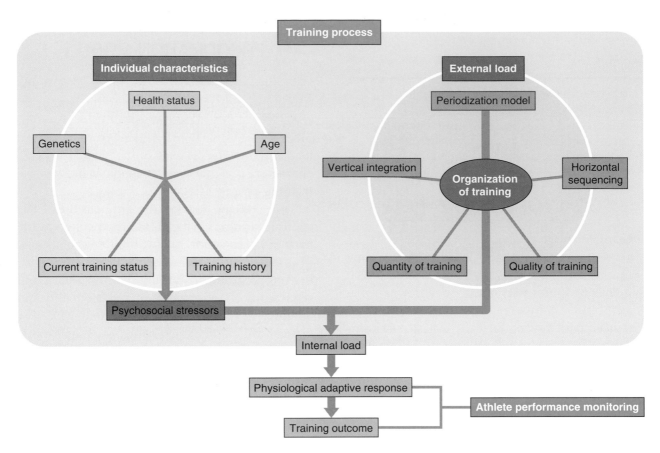

Figure 10.1   Training process and interaction of the internal and external loads.

Adapted from Impellizzeri, Rampinini, and Marcora (38).

stress appears to be similar regardless of how that stress is stimulated and may explain the tactical athlete's internal loading response to any applied external loading parameters associated with the training process (25, 71) or operational engagement.

The initial response to a training stimulus, or the alarm phase, is marked by a decreased performance capacity in response to accumulated fatigue, soreness, stiffness, and decreased energy reserves (71). During the alarm phase, the adaptive responses that occur in the resistance phase of the GAS are initiated. If the external load is structured appropriately, the primary adaptive responses occur during the resistance phase, and performance returns to baseline or elevates to a higher level (supercompensation). However, if the external load is excessive or illogically applied, performance will continue to decline as a result

of the athlete's inability to tolerate the training stressors, which would be indicative of an excessive internal load. If this situation occurs, there is a significantly higher potential for overtraining (19).

Even though the applied external load greatly influences the tactical athlete's internal loading, it is important to remember that all stressors are additive. Specifically, psychosocial stressors can significantly affect the tactical athlete's internal load (9, 43), resulting in an inability to recover from the external load and ultimately causing an overtraining response. This maladaptive response may even occur if the external load is well planned and appropriate for the tactical athlete (43). In some instances, excessive psychosocial stress can result in significant overtraining responses even when the external load is relatively low and seemingly adequate recovery is provided (20).

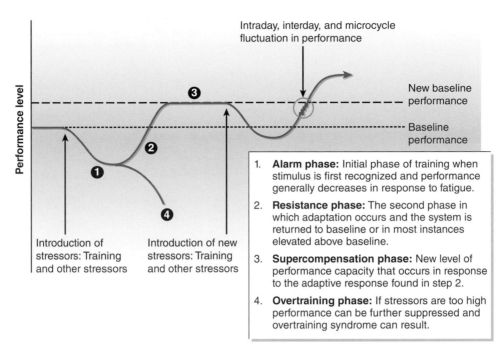

Figure 10.2 The general adaptive syndrome and its application to periodization.

Reprinted, by permission, from G.G. Haff and E.E. Haff, 2012, Training integration and periodization. In *NSCA's guide to program design*, edited by J. Hoffman (Champaign, IL: Human Kinetics), 215.

Stimulus-Fatigue-Recovery-Adaptation Theory

The **stimulus-fatigue-recovery-adaptation theory** (**SFRAT**) is an extension of the GAS theory that attempts to generalize the response to the external load (71). The initial response to an external load results in an accumulation of fatigue and a reduction in both **preparedness** and performance capacity. The magnitude of these reductions is largely predicated by the magnitude and duration of the external load applied by the periodized training plan (31). As recovery occurs, the accumulated fatigue dissipates and the individual's preparedness and performance capacity increase. Once the recovery adaptation response is complete, another external load must be introduced in order to stimulate continued adaptation. If a long duration of time exists between the completion of the recovery adaptation process and the introduction of a new external load, involution will occur, resulting in reduced preparedness and performance capacity (figure 10.3).

This response pattern to an external load occurs whenever a training exercise, unit, session, day, or cycle is engaged. The ability of the tactical athlete to recover is an integral part of this process, but complete recovery is not a prerequisite for undertaking another training bout or session (56). In fact, a better strategy for modulating fatigue, maximizing fitness, and inducing recovery is to use light and heavy days of training (10, 18). Accomplishing these goals is at the core of all sound periodized training programs where various training factors are manipulated in a logical and sequential fashion while considering how the training factors interact with one another. If the external loads are inappropriately prescribed, haphazardly applied, or not integrated correctly, the physiological adaptive responses necessary for performance gain will be greatly reduced as a result of a mismanagement of both fatigue and recovery.

Fitness–Fatigue Theory

The third mechanistic theory, the **fitness–fatigue theory**, attempts to explain the relationship between a training stimulus and the training aftereffects of **fatigue** and **fitness** (71, 82, 83). Every training activity, exercise, session, or cycle stimulates these two aftereffects, which are then

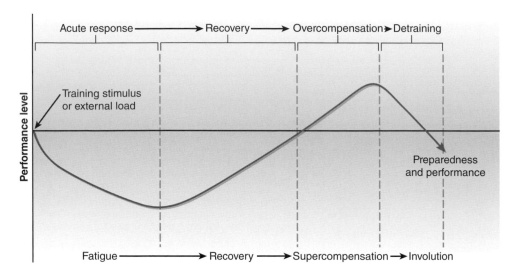

Figure 10.3 The stimulus-fatigue-recovery-adaptation theory.

Reprinted, by permission, from G.G. Haff and E.E. Haff, 2012, Training integration and periodization. In *NSCA's guide to program design*, edited by J. Hoffman (Champaign, IL: Human Kinetics), 216.

summated to determine the level of preparedness (12, 82). When training loads are the highest, the greatest increase in fitness occurs, along with the greatest increase in fatigue. When the fatigue and fitness aftereffects are then summated, preparedness and performance capacity are reduced in proportion to the magnitude of the external load (figure 10.4).

Because fatigue dissipates at a faster rate than fitness, overall preparedness and performance capacity increase (5, 71). The external load must be applied in a structured fashion to maximize fitness aftereffects while allowing fatigue to decrease in order to increase overall preparedness.

Figure 10.4 presents the classic fitness–fatigue relationship for one training factor. However, the fatigue–fitness paradigm should be viewed as a multifactorial response model; each training factor has its own fitness, fatigue, and preparedness aftereffects (figure 10.5)

The multifactorial fitness–fatigue relationship is a key concept in **sequential periodization models** (31) where aftereffects from one training period modulate the preparedness in subsequent periods depending on the organization of the periodized training plan. Central to the sequential model concept is the idea that the aftereffects of one period of training can raise the level of preparedness in subsequent training periods,

depending on which periodization model is followed (31, 36, 81). Additionally, because training aftereffects exhibit variable rates of decay, they may be maintained with minimal stimulus or periodic applications of the training factor (81).

When the GAS, SFART, and fitness–fatigue theory are examined collectively, it is clear that the ability to direct adaptive responses and elevate preparedness largely depends on the application of the external load and the ability to modulate the development of fitness and the reduction of cumulative fatigue (27-29, 59). The accomplishment of these goals is influenced by the ability to employ logical periodization models that integrate and sequence the external load in a way that manages the stimulated aftereffects (27).

STRUCTURAL COMPONENTS OF PERIODIZED TRAINING

Several planning levels create the backbone of the periodized training plan (table 10.1, page 188 and figure 10.6, page 189). Each level must be considered in the context of the tactical athlete's long-term and short-term performance goals. These goals are the foundation upon which the various training structures are interrelated and sequenced so that the tactical athlete develops the performance outcomes required by the individualized or team operational plan (31). Planning structures range from global or long-term structures, such as the multiyear or annual training plan, to individual training units within a training session (27-29, 31).

Eight interrelated planning levels (figure 10.7, page 190) can be created in the hierarchical structure of a periodized plan. These are the multiyear training plan, annual training plan, macrocycle, mesocycle, microcycle, training day, training session, and training unit.

Multiyear Training Plan

A key component of the long-term development of any tactical athlete is the multiyear training plan. This planning structure comprises several interlinked annual training plans that develop tactical

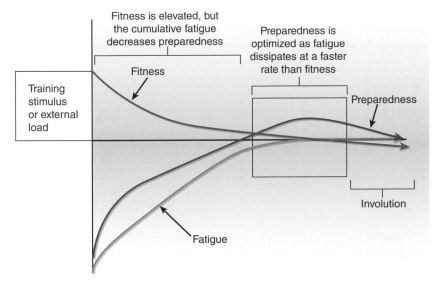

Figure 10.4   Fitness–fatigue paradigm.

Reprinted, by permission, from G.G. Haff and E.E. Haff, 2012, Training integration and periodization. In *NSCA's guide to program design*, edited by J. Hoffman (Champaign, IL: Human Kinetics), 219.

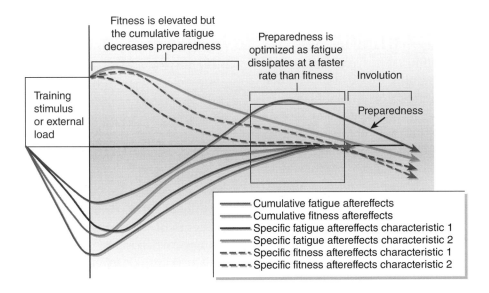

Figure 10.5   Modified fitness–fatigue paradigm depicting multiple training aftereffects.

Reprinted, by permission, from G.G. Haff and E.E. Haff, 2012, Training integration and periodization. In *NSCA's guide to program design*, edited by J. Hoffman (Champaign, IL: Human Kinetics), 219.

Table 10.1   Hierarchy of Training Structures in a Periodized Training Plan

Period	Duration	Description
Multiyear preparation	2-4 years	• Interlinked annual training plans • A 4-year plan is called a *quadrennial plan*
Annual training plan	1 year	• Overall training plan that contains macrocycles • Subdivided into preparation, competitive, and transition periods
Macrocycle	Several months to 1 year	• Sometimes referred to as an *annual plan* • Considered a season of training • Contains preparatory, competitive, and transition periods
Mesocycle	2-6 weeks	• Medium-sized training cycle consisting of microcycles linked together • Sometimes referred to as a *macrocycle* or *block of training*
Microcycle	Several days to 2 weeks	• Small-sized training cycle • Consists of multiple workouts designed in the context of its mesocycle
Training day	1 day	• Contains multiple training sessions that target individual training units • Designed in the context of its microcycle
Training session	Several hours	• Consists of several hours of training • If the workout has more than 30 min of rest between bouts of training, it would be considered to have multiple training sessions
Training unit	Minutes to hours	• Targeted training item • Could be a tactical drill or a conditioning activity

Reprinted, by permission, from G.G. Haff and E.E. Haff, 2012, Training integration and periodization. In *NSCA's guide to program design*, edited by J. Hoffman (Champaign, IL: Human Kinetics), 219.

athletes in accordance with their long-term goals (31). Because periodization is typically used with competitive athletes, the classic multiyear training plan has been associated with the Olympic cycle, linking four annual plans, or a quadrennial plan, to bridge between two successive Olympic Games. Recently, the use of quadrennial planning has expanded beyond the Olympic cycle and has been used in high school (42) and collegiate sport. Tactical athletes do not use the same organized structure for their training due to the irregular aspects of their job duties, operational plans, and training programs. Regardless, a key component of any multiyear training plan is its ability to sequence the athlete's training and performance goals in order to facilitate the physiological, psychological, and performance outcomes central to the tactical athlete's overall development (42). The benefit of the multiyear plan is that it establishes the goals of each annual training plan in a way that sets the long-term development path for the tactical athlete.

Annual Training Plan

The annual training plan, sometimes referred to as a *macrocycle* (13, 50), outlines all the training targets contained in one year of training (13, 57, 62) in accordance with the long-term development path established in the multiyear training plan. The structure of the annual training plan is largely dictated by important tactical engagements (5), the objectives of the multiyear plan (13, 42, 57), and the tactical athlete's level of development (5, 39, 40, 57).

Three annual training plan models are classically employed: the **monocycle** (one macrocycle), **bicycle** (two macrocycles), and **tricycle** (three macrocycles) (5). Additionally, at least 16 annual training plan variants can be employed when structuring an annual training plan (6). Because many tactical athletes don't have competitive seasons or deployment periods, it may be difficult to construct annual training plans for them. In these cases, the TSAC Facilitator can examine the annual calendar to determine when the most incidents of tactical operations may occur. For example, when in the calendar year are the most fires or criminal activity, and when are the least fires or criminal activity? The annual plan for a firefighter or police officer can then be constructed around the periods of increased risk. A similar approach can be taken when working with the military and ambulance services.

Macrocycle

The **macrocycle** has been referred to as a year of training (4, 5). This definition of a macrocycle was largely dictated by the fact that there was only one competitive period and thus only one macrocycle in the training year (figure 10.8) (13, 50, 70). This type of macrocycle is probably the most appropriate for the tactical athlete because the annual plan may be divided into periods of high and low risk of engagement.

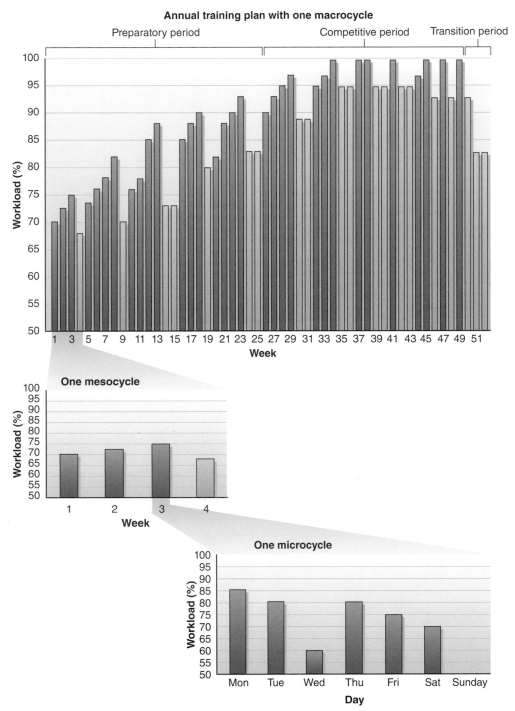

Figure 10.6 Breakdown of an annual training plan.

Reprinted, by permission, from G.G. Haff and E.E. Haff, 2012, Training integration and periodization. In *NSCA's guide to program design*, edited by J. Hoffman (Champaign, IL: Human Kinetics), 221.

An alternative planning approach is to break the annual training plan into multiple macrocycles to address the needs of the tactical athlete who has more tactical engagements during certain times of the year (figure 10.9) (27-29, 31). For example, there are more health emergencies during major holidays and other events, such as Thanksgiving, Christmas, Valentine's Day, Easter, and the Fourth of July. Therefore, the annual plan for emergency response personnel would be broken into three or four macrocycles, with the main periods of engagement centered on these holidays. In short, it is probably best to consider the tactical athlete's macrocycles in the context of periods of major tactical engagements, similar to a season in the sporting construct (31), because this allows the planning structure to prepare the tactical athlete for these periods of time (5).

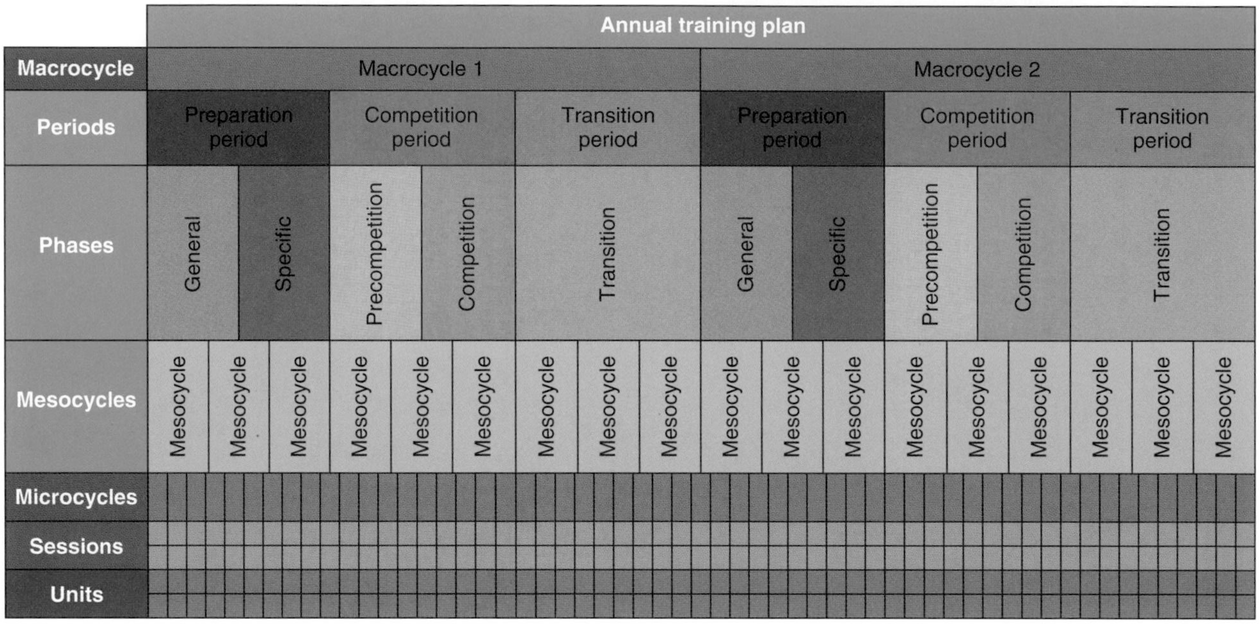

	Annual training plan																
Macrocycle	Macrocycle 1									Macrocycle 2								
Periods	Preparation period		Competition period			Transition period			Preparation period			Competition period			Transition period		
Phases	General	Specific	Precompetition		Competition	Transition			General	Specific		Precompetition		Competition	Transition		
Mesocycles	Mesocycle	Mesocycle	Mesocycle	Mesocycle	Mesocycle	Mesocycle	Mesocycle	Mesocycle	Mesocycle	Mesocycle	Mesocycle	Mesocycle	Mesocycle	Mesocycle	Mesocycle	Mesocycle	Mesocycle	Mesocycle
Microcycles																		
Sessions																		
Units																		

Figure 10.7   Hierarchical structure of a periodized training plan.

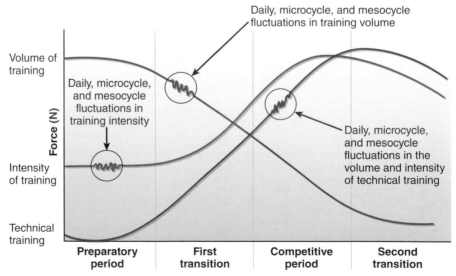

Figure 10.8   Classic annual training plan.

Reprinted, by permission, from G.G. Haff and E.E. Haff, 2012, Training integration and periodization. In *NSCA's guide to program design*, edited by J. Hoffman (Champaign, IL: Human Kinetics), 223.

Regardless of the number of macrocycles in the annual training plan, the load progression is from lower intensity, higher volume training toward higher intensity, lower volume training that is more technically oriented (32). This alteration in training volume, intensity, and technical development illustrates that the focus of training changes to meet the athlete's needs throughout the annual training plan. These changes in focus can also be seen in the main periods that structure the macrocycle: the preparatory period, competitive period, and transition period (5, 50, 62).

Preparatory Period

The **preparatory period** is the foundation of the macrocycle, where specific physiological, psychological, and technical skills are developed (5). This period might be the part of the annual plan where historically there have been the fewest tactical events. Depending upon the density of tactical events within the calendar year and the tactical athlete's individual needs, this period may last three to six months (5). People with shorter training histories tend to spend more time in the preparatory period, whereas those who are more experienced spend more time on tactical-specific training. Additionally, the overall amount of time dedicated to the preparatory period will be affected by the number of macrocycles, or periods of increased tactical engagements, contained in the annual training plan and by the time allocated for preparation in each macrocycle (5, 27-29). Preparatory activities designed to develop a training base are emphasized during the early part of the macrocycle, and tactical performance is emphasized during the latter part of the macrocycle.

From a structural standpoint, the preparatory period can be divided into the general preparation and specific preparation phases (31). The **general preparation phase** is the earliest portion of the preparatory period and targets the physical training base (5). This phase has a large training volume, lower intensity, and a multifaceted training approach in order to develop the general motor abilities and skills required by the tactical athlete (40, 50). It lasts longer for less developed tactical athletes, who require a much greater focus on developing a training base.

As tactical athletes progress through the preparatory period, they move from the general preparation phase to the **specific preparation phase**. This progression shifts from overall development toward more specific motor ability and technical development, focusing on attributes that are

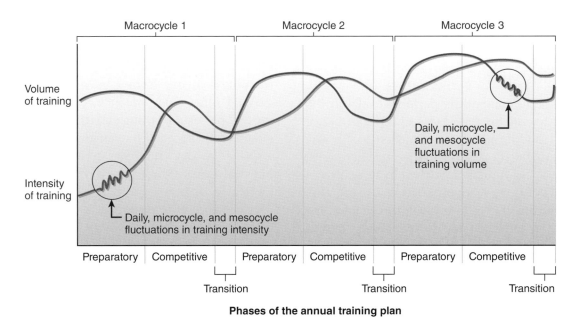

Phases of the annual training plan

Figure 10.9 Sample annual training plan with three macrocycles.

Reprinted, by permission, from G.G. Haff and E.E. Haff, 2012, Training integration and periodization. In *NSCA's guide to program design*, edited by J. Hoffman (Champaign, IL: Human Kinetics), 223.

directly related to the tactical activities required of the athlete (13). This phase combines higher training loads with periods of high intensity and targeted technical development. In sport situations, a central goal of this phase is to strengthen the sport-specific training base while assisting athletes in their transition into the competitive period of the macrocycle (13, 27-29, 31). For tactical athletes, this is a period in which training is more closely aligned with their tactical requirements. As such, the training practices in this period are specific to the needs of the individual tactical athlete or tactical operations team.

In the classic literature on periodization, the trend is to sequence the general and specific preparation phases (5). Another approach is to run these two phases concurrently and modulate the focus of each phase at any given time point (6, 31). This alternative approach of concurrently targeting general and specific preparation is based on the belief that the preparatory period should last only long enough to elevate training status and should not be determined by the constraints of an annual training plan that contains two or three macrocycles (6). This alternative may be ideally suited for tactical athletes, who rarely have defined tactical engagements and need to be at a higher level of preparedness more frequently during the calendar year. Concurrently training these targets can increase the tactical athlete's ability to undergo more frequent tactical engagements (39).

Competitive Period

The goal of the **competitive period** is to elevate the athlete's overall preparedness and performance at key competitions or engagements (5). For the tactical athlete, the competitive period aligns with the part of the annual plan when historically the most tactical engagements occur. During this part of the macrocycle, physiological adaptations and skills acquired during the preparatory period are maintained or slightly elevated in order to modulate performance capacity (56). The period is marked by an overall reduction in general physical conditioning units and an increase in specific training units that target precise technical and tactical elements related to the tactical athlete's engagements. Additionally, the period often contains activities such as skill-based conditioning

units, which continue to develop the technical and tactical skills necessary for success while maintaining overall fitness (27-31).

When compared with the preparatory period, the competitive period is marked by reduced training volume, increased training intensity, and increased emphasis on technical and tactical training units (31). Even though this general loading pattern is exhibited in this period, there will be fluctuations in training volume, intensity, density, and frequency to account for the schedule, travel, modulation of recovery, and potential density of tactical engagements (27-29). In order to better plan the competitive period and appropriately sequenced training, it is traditionally recommended to break the period into the **precompetitive phase** and **main competitive phase** (5, 27-30). For the tactical athlete, the precompetitive phase is the time period immediately before deployment, and the competitive phase is the deployment period itself. In other words, the precompetitive phase occurs before periods of time when historically there are more tactical events, and the competitive phase is when the increased density of tactical events occurs.

The main role of the precompetitive phase is to link the preparatory period and the main competitive phase of the competitive period (5, 31). During this crucial phase, the tactical athlete may undergo simulations of key elements associated with the operational plan. For example, a firefighter may practice key aspects related to rescuing someone from a burning car, whereas a SWAT officer may practice breaching a building and perform training activities that optimize strength and speed of movement. Consider these activities as dry runs that continue to develop physical fitness while practicing technical and tactical elements related to the engagements undertaken by the tactical athlete. Additionally, these activities allow the tactical commander to evaluate the inner workings of the team as well as determine the effectiveness of certain technical and tactical elements. These simulations or dry runs serve only as training tools and tests of operational readiness; they should not be considered as main objectives (31).

After performance is honed during the precompetitive phase, the main competitive phase should be initiated. The primary objective of this phase is to optimize overall preparedness and performance capacity for specific tactical operations or common tactical engagements contained in this portion of the annual training plan (27-29). The length of this phase is largely dictated by the deployment length or, for nondeployed tactical athletes, historical data on the typical lengths of the heightened occurrence of tactical events. A key element of this phase is a structured modulation of training workloads that are in balance with both the engagement and travel schedules (27-30). This is essential in order to maintain or elevate tactical fitness and skills that have been developed in the previous training periods.

One key consideration during this phase is that performance cannot be maintained at its maximum for the duration of the period. In fact, maximal performance can only last 7 to 14 days when an appropriate taper is employed. If a taper is too long, involution will occur because of a reduction in overall fitness that occurs in response to the reduced training volume and cumulative fatigue associated with competitive schedules and travel. Thus, tapers are not recommended because the tactical athlete likely needs to optimize performance over a period of time longer than two weeks. Instead, the main competitive period should be designed to maintain performance over longer amounts of time. The main competitive phase is probably the most difficult to structure because travel, known and unknown tactical demands, and ability to manage recovery and injuries all come into play.

Key Point

The tactical athlete's annual training plan should be designed around the historical periods of increased tactical engagements. For example, the time of year when there is the greatest risk of fires is the competitive period for the firefighter, and the period of least risk of fires is the preparatory period.

Transition Period

The **transition period** serves as the bridge between multiple macrocycles or annual training plans (5, 56, 62). This period is marked by large reductions in training volume and intensity and an emphasis on maintaining fitness levels (5, 56) and technical proficiency (56). It occurs during the time of year when the tactical athlete is given leave or is off duty. Depending on the location of the transition period within the overall macrocycle, it generally lasts two to four weeks (5, 15, 46). If the transition period lasts too long, fitness will greatly decrease, which can have ramifications for subsequent macrocycles. In some instances an extended transition period is warranted—when the competitive period, macrocycle, or annual plan is particularly stressful or the tactical athlete has an injury, the transition period can be extended to six weeks (5, 15, 46).

Complete or passive rest is usually avoided, but in certain instances a complete cessation of training may be warranted for some portion of the period (56). However, as mentioned, if the transition period is extended or complete rest occurs, the athlete's overall physical capacity will be markedly reduced (5), and the preparatory period of the next macrocycle must contain an increased emphasis on the general preparation phase in order to return fitness to the level obtained in the previous macrocycle (5). If the transition period is constructed and employed appropriately, this period will refresh the tactical athlete both physically and mentally (56) while allowing them to prepare for the training stress of the next macrocycle or annual training plan.

Mesocycle

The main building block of all macrocycles is the medium-sized planning unit known as the **mesocycle**. Sometimes a mesocycle is also referred to as a **block** of training (31) or **summated microcycle** (59, 71). The mesocycle lasts two to six weeks (39, 40, 46, 57, 71, 75, 82, 83), with four weeks being the most common duration (59, 79, 82, 83). Four weeks are typically used because asymptotic training effects begin to occur around this time, and the onset of involution begins to manifest as either a stagnation or decline in the physiological adaptive responses and performance gain (79). Manipulating various training units in the mesocycle in order to alter the training focus can offset the asymptotic effects so that continued adaptations and development can occur (27-29, 31, 32).

In the classic literature, there are 8 to 10 potential classifications (table 10.2) of mesocycles that can be created based on the target training goal (13, 35, 39, 50, 82). These blocks of training can then be sequenced and interlinked to create the training structure (31).

For example, starting in the general preparation phase, one might sequence the following classic blocks of training to create the macrocycle that ends with a competitive period:

Preparation → buildup → recovery → competition → competitive buildup

For the tactical athlete, mesocycles may start with a preparatory mesocycle and end with a mesocycle designed to stabilize the tactical athlete's engagement-specific fitness and tactical skills:

Preparation → buildup → recovery → buildup → stabilization → recovery

The idea behind sequencing mesocycle blocks of training is to develop training residuals and allow these residuals, or delayed training effects, to be superimposed across each block of training (39, 40, 71, 82, 83). In turn, this allows for the exploitation of the collective training residuals during the competitive period of the macrocycle (45, 71).

In order to simplify the sequencing process, proponents of block periodization (7, 39, 40, 77, 82) have divided the mesocycle classification system into three training blocks: the accumulation, transmutation, and realization blocks (table 10.3).

Accumulation

One of the foundational mesocycle blocks is the **accumulation** (39, 40) or **concentrated loading** block (59), where the athlete is exposed to substantial workloads that target a primary training factor such as muscular strength, anaerobic

Table 10.2 Traditional Mesocycle Classifications

Type	Average duration (weeks)	Characteristics
Basic sport specific	6	Elevates sport-specific fitness where performance in specific skills is targeted
Buildup	3	• General training and conditioning enhances foundational skills or fitness • May be used after a period of specific or high-load training
Competition	2-6	• Mesocycle that targets a competition during the mesocycle • Used in the competitive period of the annual training plan
Competitive buildup	3	• Increases training loads during a long competitive phase • Reestablishes foundational skills or fitness
General	Any duration	• Basic or general education and training that targets the development of basic fitness • Occurs in the preparatory period of the annual training plan
Immediate preparation	2	• Occurs prior to a competition • Targets peaking and restoration • May be considered a taper • May precede a testing period
Precompetition	6	• Maximizes preparedness and performance for a specific competition or series of competitions • Marked by sport-specific training • Designed to peak fitness, performance, and preparedness
Preparation	6	• Develops a base necessary for competitive performance • Training moves from extensive to intensive • Fitness is established and used to develop skills
Recovery	1-4	• Induces restoration • May follow a series of competitions • Prepares the individual for subsequent training
Stabilization	4	• Perfects technique and fitness base • Targets technical errors targeted as well as fitness deficits • Develops sport-specific fitness and skills base

Reprinted, by permission, from G.G. Haff and E.E. Haff, 2012, Training integration and periodization. In *NSCA's guide to program design*, edited by J. Hoffman (Champaign, IL: Human Kinetics), 229.

endurance, muscular power, aerobic endurance, technical or tactical ability, or some specified training factor (31). Regardless of the primary mesocycle target, this block of training typically lasts two to six weeks depending on the time necessary to acquire the target ability, the rate of involution, and the competitive schedule that the block is preparing the athlete for (27-29, 31).

From a structural standpoint, the stability of the residuals created by this block of training is proportional to the length of time used to develop the targeted factor (71, 82). Additionally, the longer the duration of this block, the longer the training residual will last, the greater the delayed training effect (i.e., time before adaptations are realized as performance gains) will be, and the greater the time course of involution associated with the residuals created in response to the mesocycle will be (39, 40, 59, 71).

As a whole, during accumulation mesocycles, the athlete is saturated with more intense training that is designed to elevate performance at a later date (27-29, 31). If planned appropriately, these blocks serve as the foundation for subsequent mesocycles.

Transmutation

After the completion of an accumulation block, a **transmutation block** (6, 39, 40, 82) or **phase potentiation mesocycle** (59, 71) is used. Transmutation blocks are periods of reduced loading and shifted training focus that capitalize on the residual training effects established from the accumulation block, thus leading the tactical athlete to better operational preparedness. This block can be two to six weeks long but rarely extends beyond four weeks (27-29). The length of the transmutation phase is based on the magnitude of the residuals established and the rate of involution of the residuals created in response to the accumulation block, the levels of fatigue generated, and the time course for the appearance of asymptotic training effects (29). If a longer accumulation block is used, the time course before involution of the established training residuals will be extended and a longer transmutation block can be employed. This longer transmutation block is necessary in order to dissipate fatigue and capitalize on the delayed training effects created by the training residuals. However, if this block is too long (>4 weeks in most cases), there is a greater potential for involution in which the training residuals are reduced prior to entering the realization block. If this scenario occurs, the tactical athlete's preparedness and performance will be compromised (27, 29, 31).

Realization

The next block in this structural plan is the **realization block**, which is employed before a specified or predetermined tactical operation or at the end of a series of mesocycles that are particularly taxing. Regardless of their application, these

Table 10.3   Simplified Sequential Mesocycle Structures

Phase	Alternative names	Duration	Methods	Characteristics
Accumulation	Concentrated loading	2-6 weeks	General physical development: endurance, muscular strength, and basic technique that underpin the needs of athlete-specific tactical scenarios	• Tends to have the longest training residuals • Creates the greatest amount of fatigue • Increases general fitness the most
Transmutation	Normal training	2-4 weeks	Engagement-specific abilities: anaerobic conditioning (mixed), muscular endurance, and targeted techno-tactical preparedness that directly translate to tactical scenarios	• Shortened training residuals • Elevations in preparedness • Fatigue can become an issue
Realization	Peaking or tapering	7-14 days	Engagement modeling: maximal speed work, active recovery, and optimization of techno-tactical scenarios that translate to tactical scenarios	• Reduced training loads • Elevation in preparedness • Recovery

Reprinted, by permission, from G.G. Haff and E.E. Haff, 2012, Training integration and periodization. In *NSCA's guide to program design*, edited by J. Hoffman (Champaign, IL: Human Kinetics), 230.

blocks are designed to optimize both prepared-ness and tactical performance capacity (8, 37, 41, 52, 53) while reducing accumulated fatigue. Conceptually, the realization block is similar to a taper and should only be used from the 7 to 14 days leading into a predetermined tactical opera-tion or as a linkage to another accumulation block of training (27-29, 31). Typically this block reduces training workload while maintaining both train-ing frequency and intensity (27) and increasing focus on tactical training. This structure helps dissipate accumulated fatigue while elevating preparedness and tactical performance capacity. The main concept underlying this block is that a convergence of the residual training effects is established in the accumulation and transmuta-tion blocks so that supercompensation occurs at the end of this block, when the primary tactical operation is scheduled (27-29, 31).

In a periodized training plan, these three sim-plified blocks serve as the foundation for creating a sequential training model. As interchangeable training structures, these basic structures can be employed in a repetitive fashion to direct the tactical athlete toward the engagement-specific performance goals of the operational plan (39, 40).

Regardless of the mesocycle classification, there are several methods for manipulating the train-ing load within a mesocycle. The most common method for modulating the workload is the 3:1 loading paradigm (3 microcycles of increasing workload followed by 1 microcycle of decreasing workload) (5, 22). Other loading structures can be created, such as 2:1, 2:2, 3:2, 4:1, and 4:2 (figure 10.10). The overall ratio of loading to recovery

across the mesocycle is dictated by the tactical athlete's level of development, ability to recover, and training objectives for the mesocycle.

Microcycle

Probably the most important and detailed training structure is the **microcycle**, which contains the daily training sessions (27, 31, 78). The typical length of a microcycle can range from 2 to 14 days, with the most common duration being 7 days (21, 22, 31, 78). Ultimately, a series of microcycles are linked in order to create the mesocycle, with each microcycle being constructed in accordance with the objectives of that mesocycle (31).

The various mesocycle structures in a peri-odized training plan make it obvious that not all microcycles contain the same content or training objectives (27). The periodization literature dem-onstrates that numerous microcycle structures can be used when developing a training plan (62, 78). These microcycles can be divided into four broad categories: developmental, preparation, competition, and restoration microcycles (78). Because so many microcycles are possible, it is difficult to give exact microcycle structures that can be used by all tactical athletes. However, it is widely accepted that the microcycle should contain heavy and light days so as to maximize both recovery and adaptation (27-29), be inte-grated so as to optimize adaptive potential, and be designed in accordance with the mesocycle objectives. Typically, microcycles are structured with both training and recovery sessions or days (5). Several variations of the microcycle can be

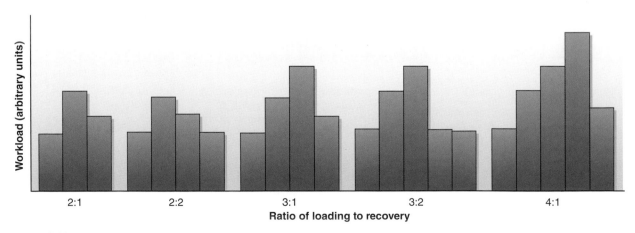

Figure 10.10 Sample mesocycle loading structures.

created, such as 2+2, 3+1, 5+1, or 5+1+1 (training session + recovery session) (table 10.4).

Training Day

A **training day** is structured in accordance with the goals established for the individual microcycle in which it is contained. Each training day targets specific goals and objectives by employing one or more interrelated training sessions. The density (number) of training sessions in the training day is often dictated by the tactical athlete's physical development, ability to handle training activities, time allocated for training, and goals of the training phase.

It is widely accepted that spacing multiple training sessions throughout the day results in significantly greater training adaptations (6, 34, 47-50, 56, 58, 59, 67, 72-76). Interspersing training sessions with periods of recovery throughout the training day increases work capacity while better managing fatigue (31).

Training Session

The workout, or **training session**, as it is more appropriately termed, is a structural unit in a periodized training plan. A session is a series of training units with <30 minutes of rest between units (39, 40, 82). Generally, each training day contains multiple training units designed to target specific outcomes in accordance with the overall structure of each cycle of the periodized training plan (40, 82).

Training Unit

The **training unit** is the smallest planning component of a periodized training program. It contains focused training activities that are used to create an individual training session (27-29). A training session may be composed of several training units, such as warm-up, plyometric, technical, strength, and flexibility units. The units in a training session are dictated by the targeted goals established for the session in accordance with the overall training plan.

SEQUENCING AND INTEGRATING TRAINING

A key aspect of periodization is sequencing and integrating training factors in order to direct training outcomes. Although this concept is not new (49), recent scientific evidence reveals the superiority of appropriately sequenced (51, 81) and integrated training programs (14, 24, 36) when compared with traditional training models.

From a sequential standpoint, it is important to remember that the training residuals created in one mesocycle will directly influence the training outcomes of subsequent mesocycles. If, for example, the targeted outcome of a series of mesocycles is the development of muscular power, a horizontally sequenced series of mesocycles might proceed as follows (81):

Strength endurance → strength → power

Table 10.4 Sample Microcycle Loading Structures

Loading structure	Session time	Day						
		Monday	Tuesday	Wednesday	Thursday	Friday	Saturday	Sunday
2+2	a.m.	Training		Training		Training		
	p.m.	Training		Training		Training		
3+1	a.m.	Training	Training	Training	Training	Training	Training	
	p.m.	Training		Training		Training		
5+1	a.m.	Training	Training	Training	Training	Training	Training	
	p.m.	Training	Training		Training	Training		
5+1+1	a.m.	Training	Training	Training	Training	Training	Training	Training
	p.m.	Training	Training		Training	Training		

Adapted, by permission, from T.O Bompa and G.G. Haff, 2009, *Periodization: Theory and methodology of training*, 5th ed. (Champaign, IL: Human Kinetics), 207, 208.

In this traditional example, the strength endurance phase develops the fitness foundation from which strength can then be maximized. After the athlete's maximal strength is increased, the ability to optimize power output with specific training interventions is maximized as a result of architectural changes and neuromuscular adaptations of the muscle (51, 81).

Though sequencing of training is a critical aspect of periodization, it is also important to consider how the individual training factors integrate. Appropriate integration of training factors allows for compatible factors (table 10.5) to be trained simultaneously without creating interference effects that mute or hinder the targeted performance gain (27-29). Vertical integration of training factors is important for tactical athletes, who may need to develop several training outcomes in preparation for their operational engagement.

When the training plan is appropriately integrated and sequenced, the ability to manage workloads and enhance tactical performance is maximized.

A lack of sequencing and integration is most noted in training programs that address or emphasize all training factors at the same time (27-29) without consideration for how these factors interrelate. This lack of sequencing and integration creates the **blender effect** (27): excessive accumulated fatigue that makes it impossible to optimize performance at appropriate times (26, 78), increases the risk of overtraining (69), and increases the potential for injury (23). These effects are even greater for tactical athletes than sport athletes because failure to be prepared for operational engagements can have worse outcomes (i.e., extreme bodily harm or death).

Conversely, in a well-crafted periodized training program, the ability to determine when

Table 10.5 Compatible Training Factors

Dominant (primary) training emphasis	Compatible training factors
Aerobic endurance	• Strength endurance training • Maximal strength training • Anaerobic endurance training • Technical and tactical training (if done first)
Anaerobic endurance	• Strength endurance training • Aerobic-anaerobic mixed endurance training • Power endurance training • Sprint and agility training • Explosive strength/power training • Muscular strength training • Technical and tactical training (if done first)
Sprint ability	• Maximal strength training • Plyometric training • Explosive strength/power training • Agility training • Technical and tactical training (if done first)
Maximal strength	• Sprint training • Agility training • Explosive strength/power training • Anaerobic endurance training • Technical and tactical training (if done first)
Explosive strength/power	• Sprint training • Agility training • Maximal strength training • Plyometric training • Technical and tactical training (if done first)
Technical training	Any emphasis as long as it is performed after the technical work
Tactical training	Any emphasis as long as it is performed after the tactical work

Reprinted, by permission, from G.G. Haff and E.E. Haff, 2012, Training integration and periodization. In *NSCA's guide to program design*, edited by J. Hoffman (Champaign, IL: Human Kinetics), 235.

optimal performance occurs is greatly increased, overtraining potential is reduced, and injury potential is markedly reduced (27-29). The periodized training plan is able to accomplish these goals thanks to the vertical integration and horizontal sequencing of training factors. Vertical integration involves looking at how the various training factors interact within a specific mesocycle block, whereas horizontal sequencing deals with how the factors are sequenced.

Figure 10.11 presents an example of how several training factors can be vertically integrated or prioritized in accordance with their mesocycle block. Additionally, it presents a horizontal sequential pattern in which the targeted factors vary in their emphasis in each mesocycle block. For example, in block 1, the main emphasis is endurance development, with strength being the secondary emphasis and technique being a tertiary emphasis. In mesocycle block 2, strength becomes the primary emphasis and endurance becomes secondary. After completing block 2, tactical training is the primary emphasis and tactical employment of techniques is the secondary emphasis. So for these three mesocycles, the targeted emphasis progresses from endurance to strength and ends with tactical performance. Conceptually, vertical integration is a modulation of emphasis within a block, while horizontal sequencing is the sequential prioritization of specific training factors over time.

The success of the periodized training plan is largely influenced by the ordering of successive mesocycles in relationship to the mechanical specificity (5, 59), metabolic specificity (59, 71), and time course for the involution of residual training factors (39, 40). Additionally, how the training factors are vertically integrated will influence the success of the sequential model. For example, if the targeted outcome is maximal strength, then including large volumes of endurance work can result in interference effects that mute the ability to develop strength (27).

APPLYING PERIODIZATION THEORY TO DEPLOYMENT-BASED TACTICAL ATHLETES

Applying periodization theory to deployment-based tactical athletes may seem daunting. However, this task can be made simpler by considering periodization in the context of a mission plan, operational plan, or tactical guide. Operational plans must be modifiable in order to meet the ever-changing environment, unit schedules, and mission status of the deployment-based tactical athlete while staying focused on the operational objectives or goals. Using periodization modeling for the tactical athlete is a sound idea and may help prevent injury, avoid overtraining, and maximize mission effectiveness. In fact, a major problem

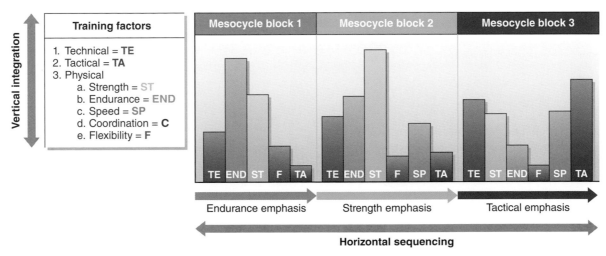

Figure 10.11   Vertical integration and horizontal sequencing.

with conventional preparation programs for tactical athletes is overtraining and injuries that are directly related to physical preparation (64). Sell (64) recently revealed that 48.5% of the injuries in a cohort of airborne soldiers occurred to the lower extremity (62.6% of all injuries) during physical preparation activities, which may be linked to overtraining. Further, Bullock (11) revealed that preventing overtraining during the preparation of the tactical athletes is a high priority because of its large impact on the tactical athlete's mission readiness.

Periodization modeling offers an excellent tool for addressing the issues brought to light by Sell (64) and Bullock (11). To address the mission readiness of the tactical athlete, Sell and colleagues (63) developed a periodized strength and conditioning model (table 10.6). Even though this was a relatively short intervention (eight weeks), the model had all the earmarks of a successful periodized training plan (vertical integration and horizontal sequencing) and revealed that periodized training can be used in the preparation of tactical athletes.

When considering periodization modeling for the tactical athlete, it is important to relate the classic periods of training with the traditional tactical mission (table 10.7). For example, the predeployment period should be considered as a preparation period in which the tactical athlete prepares for deployment.

The goal of the predeployment period is developing the physiological attributes necessary for tactical success, including strength, endurance, high-intensity endurance, power, speed, agility, and balance. Consider this early portion of the predeployment period as the general preparation phase when the foundation is developed with higher volumes and lower intensities of training. The later stages of the predeployment period would then bring in higher intensities of training and reorient focus toward tactical-specific training activities that better prepare the tactical athlete for deployment. Deployment should be considered as the competitive period and should contain both precompetitive and main competitive phases. The deployment period will most likely change the means, modes, or methods of

Table 10.6 Relating Sell's Training Model to Periodization Periods and Phases

Phase of preparation	Duration	Objectives	Periodization Period	Periodization Phase
Phase 1	2 weeks	General adaptation and introduce training activities	Preparation	General preparation
Phase 2	2 weeks	Gradually increase training volume	Preparation	General preparation
Phase 3	2 weeks	Increase intensity and decrease volume	Preparation	Specific preparation
Phase 4	2 weeks	Reduce volume before deployment	Preparation	Specific preparation

The model by Sell et al. (63) was designed to test a basic preparation model. More research is required to determine how this would be integrated into a large predeployment period.

Based on Sell et al. (63).

Table 10.7 Relating Periodization to Tactical Mission Terminology

Tactical mission Period	Tactical mission Phase	Periodization Period	Periodization Phase
Predeployment	General deployment preparation	Preparation	General preparation
	Specific deployment preparation		Specific preparation
Deployment	Initial deployment	Competition	Precompetition
	Main deployment		Main competition
Postdeployment	Transition	Transition	Transition

training based on the availability of equipment. However, even though these items may change, the targeted goals should remain constant. The challenge of the deployment period is adjusting the training stressors in accordance with the ever-changing tactical environment.

Key Point

> Periodized training programs for deployment-based tactical athletes can be based on macrocycles, which have predeployment, deployment, and postdeployment training periods. These are similar to the preparatory, competitive, and transition periods used to prepare sport athletes.

When developing an operational plan, the most important thing is to establish the training or outcome goals. These goals are based on the strengths and weaknesses of the tactical athlete as well as the operational constraints under which that tactical athlete will operate.

According to the literature, it appears that tactical athletes should not solely rely on long marching or distance running to develop their physical preparedness (11, 63). Instead, a more balanced training approach is warranted that includes muscular strength, speed, agility, power, and high-intensity exercise endurance. These elements need to be balanced with technical and tactical development. An additional item of concern is developing a lean mass reserve during the predeployment period (11).

A basic periodization model can be developed to address the phases of a mission (figure 10.12). In this generic model, the predeployment period focuses on improving strength, lean body mass reserve, high-intensity endurance capacity, speed, agility, and endurance capacity. During this period, tactical athletes will probably have numerous methods and modes of training at their disposal, including gym and field-based activities.

Once tactical athletes are deployed, the main goals are to manage operational fatigue, maintain strength levels, maintain or slow the decline in lean body mass associated with deployment, maintain high-intensity endurance capacity, maintain overall endurance, and maintain speed and agility. Because of the ever-changing environment during deployment, the program must offer flexibility in the modes and methods for targeting these training goals and often must rely on field-based training methods.

Upon return from deployment, tactical athletes undergo a transition phase. This is classified as the postdeployment period and is designed to transition the tactical athlete from deployment into the next predeployment training period. This period also allows tactical athletes to recover from deployment stressors, deal with any injuries or wounds suffered during deployment, begin low-level training to prepare for the next predeployment period, and determine what training factors must be addressed before the next deployment.

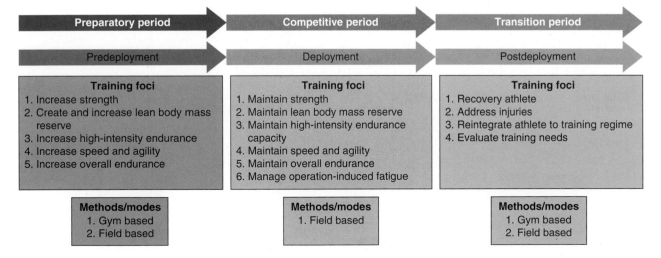

Figure 10.12 Generic periodization model with training foci for the tactical athlete.

Predeployment Period

The construction of the predeployment period should be individualized to the tactical athlete or unit. However, a sample mesocycle model is shown in figures 10.13 through 10.15, which depict a series of mesocycles that vertically integrate and horizontally sequence training factors that are of particular interest to the tactical athlete.

Figure 10.13 depicts the first mesocycle of a series that could be contained in a predeployment period. In block 1 of this series, the primary emphasis is hypertrophy with a secondary emphasis on aerobic-anaerobic endurance capacity. These targets may be addressed with hypertrophy training (high-volume resistance training with moderate loads) and *aerobic-anaerobic endurance training* (high-intensity interval training of varying distances and time lengths that develops both aerobic and anaerobic capacities). A microcycle is then structured that allows for better management of training stressors. It is important to consider tactical or technical training as part of the training plan to account for traditional training activities such as target practices. This first mesocycle block would generally last around four weeks.

After completing the first mesocycle block, the second block begins (figure 10.14). This block develops maximal strength as a primary target;

increasing lean body mass in the first block serves as a foundation from which strength can be enhanced (51, 81). This block also increases emphasis on power development and tactical training. Because large volumes of endurance work interfere with strength development, this training target is de-emphasized. As with the first mesocycle block, four weeks is the typical duration.

The final block of this example is presented in figure 10.15. In this mesocycle block, the emphasis shifts to strength and power development, tactical and technical work, and speed and agility. The idea is to enhance performance capacity for four weeks of training before deployment occurs. However, if the predeployment period is longer than 12 weeks, the sequence of mesocycle blocks could be repeated.

Deployment Period

The deployment period would be synonymous with the long competitive period typically seen in college and professional sport. Its objective is to maintain the training adaptations developed in the predeployment period (5). Typically, this is accomplished using a structured program that keeps intensity relatively high while modulating training frequency around major engagements. Because of the ever-changing tactical environment, this period is probably the hardest to

Predeployment mesocycle blocks		
Block type 1	**Block type 2**	**Block type 3**

	Block type 1	Block type 2	Block type 3
Primary	Hypertrophy	Maximal strength	Strength-power
Secondary	Aerobic-anaerobic endurance	Strength-power	Tactical-technical
Tertiary	Power-endurance	Tactical-technical	Speed/agility/plyometric
Quaternary	Tactical-technical	Speed/agility/plyometric	Aerobic-anaerobic endurance
Quinary	Speed/agility/plyometric	Aerobic-anaerobic endurance	Maximal strength

Block type 1 training factor breakdown							
	Monday	Tuesday	Wednesday	Thursday	Friday	Saturday	Sunday
Hypertrophy							
Aerobic-anaerobic endurance							Day of rest
Power-endurance							
Tactical-technical							
Speed/agility/plyometric							

Figure 10.13 Sample predeployment period mesocycle 1 with structures and targets.

construct a periodized plan for. Additionally, the modes and methods may not be set, and the availability of some training tools may be limited. As a rule of thumb, a strength program should have a minimum of two nonconsecutive days per week and one to two days per week of anaerobic-aerobic endurance training. However, if the tactical engagements require large amounts of aerobic or anaerobic intervals, this may be reduced because the tactical engagements may be adequate to maintain these characteristics. Finally, it is important to keep in mind the density of tactical engagements because they are physiologically and psychologically stressful. If there are many tactical engagements, then additional recovery may be warranted.

Predeployment mesocycle blocks

	Block type 1	Block type 2	Block type 3
Primary	Hypertrophy	Maximal strength	Strength-power
Secondary	Aerobic-anaerobic endurance	Strength-power	Tactical-technical
Tertiary	Power-endurance	Tactical-technical	Speed/agility/plyometric
Quaternary	Tactical-technical	Speed/agility/plyometric	Aerobic-anaerobic endurance
Quinary	Speed/agility/plyometric	Aerobic-anaerobic endurance	Maximal strength

Block type 2 training factor breakdown

	Monday	Tuesday	Wednesday	Thursday	Friday	Saturday	Sunday
Maximal strength							Day of rest
Strength-power							
Tactical-technical							
Speed/agility/plyometric							
Aerobic-anaerobic endurance							

Figure 10.14 Sample predeployment period mesocycle 2 with structures and targets.

Predeployment mesocycle blocks

	Block type 1	Block type 2	Block type 3
Primary	Hypertrophy	Maximal strength	Strength-power
Secondary	Aerobic-anaerobic endurance	Strength-power	Tactical-technical
Tertiary	Power-endurance	Tactical-technical	Speed/agility/plyometric
Quaternary	Tactical-technical	Speed/agility/plyometric	Aerobic-anaerobic endurance
Quinary	Speed/agility/plyometric	Aerobic-anaerobic endurance	Maximal strength

Block type 3 training factor breakdown

	Monday	Tuesday	Wednesday	Thursday	Friday	Saturday	Sunday
Strength-power							Day of rest
Tactical-technical							
Speed/agility/plyometric							
Aerobic-anaerobic endurance							
Maximal strength							

Figure 10.15 Sample predeployment period mesocycle 3 with structures and targets.

APPLYING PERIODIZATION THEORY TO NONDEPLOYED TACTICAL ATHLETES

When working with tactical athletes who are not deployment based, such as firefighters, police officers, and emergency response personnel, classic periodization modeling becomes more challenging. Two strategies can be used to create an annual training plan. The first strategy is to use statistical analyses to determine times in the calendar year when there is an increased occurrence of tactical events. If TSAC Facilitators are able to quantify these time points, they can follow the same principles for designing a periodized training program as when they work with deployment-based tactical athletes. For example, it is well documented that there is a 10% increase in the demand for emergency response services when the temperature becomes oppressively hot (16). Additionally, there is an additional increase in emergency response demand when extreme cold weather occurs (80). Because temperatures rise during the summer, these months could be classified as one of the main tactical demand periods (i.e., a competitive period). Conversely, when the temperature drops in the winter months, a second main tactical demand period could be determined. The TSAC Facilitator could create an annual plan that divides the calendar year into two macrocycles based on these two key periods (figure 10.16).

For example, in figure 10.16 the annual plan is based on spring, summer, fall, and winter. The preparatory periods are the spring and fall months, and the competitive periods are the summer and winter months. The TSAC Facilitator can then create training targets for each period of training.

Another strategy is to create blocks of training that cycle through accumulation, transmutation, and realization phases. For example, police officers may need to use this strategy, where general physical preparation activities (accumulation) are undertaken for the first microcycle each month, specific preparation activities (transmutation) are undertaken during the second and third microcycles, and peaking of performance (realization) occurs during the fourth microcycle each month (figure 10.17).

Spring	Summer	Fall	Winter

Macrocycle 1	Macrocycle 2

Preparatory period	Competitive period	Preparatory period	Competitive period
Training foci 1. Increase strength 2. Create and increase lean body mass reserve 3. Increase high-intensity endurance 4. Increase speed and agility 5. Increase overall endurance	**Training foci** 1. Maintain strength 2. Maintain lean body mass reserve 3. Maintain high-intensity endurance capacity 4. Maintain speed and agility 5. Maintain overall endurance	**Training foci** 1. Increase strength 2. Create and increase lean body mass reserve 3. Increase high-intensity endurance 4. Increase speed and agility 5. Increase overall endurance	**Training foci** 1. Maintain strength 2. Maintain lean body mass reserve 3. Maintain high-intensity endurance capacity 4. Maintain speed and agility 5. Maintain overall endurance

Figure 10.16 Sample annual training plan for an EMS provider.

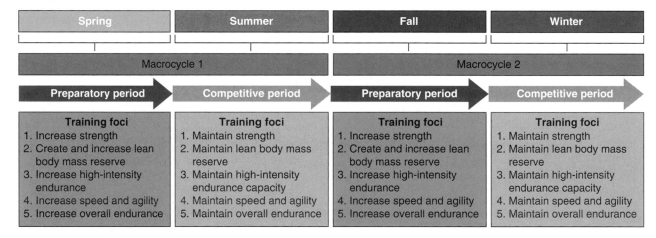

Figure 10.17 Sample block model of periodization for a police officer.

Regardless of the type of tactical athlete being trained, the TSAC Facilitator can manipulate the various periodization strategies to provide structured training that prepares the tactical athlete for operational engagements.

CONCLUSION

Periodization is a well-documented theoretical and practical paradigm typically associated with the preparation of athletes at various levels. When adapting periodization theory to the tactical environment, it is important to consider the paradigm as a form of operational planning. As such, periodization should be a central concept in the preparation of tactical athletes. Regardless of the environment, the application of periodization is based on a logical integrative sequencing of training factors in order to optimize performance, reduce overtraining potential, manage fatigue, and enhance recovery. Ultimately, periodized training models in the tactical environment can optimize operational effectiveness and maintenance of the tactical athlete's overall well-being.

Key Terms

accumulation block
adaptive potential
aerobic-anaerobic endurance training
competitive period
bicycle
blender effect
block
concentrated loading
fatigue
fitness
fitness–fatigue theory
general adaptation syndrome (GAS)
general preparation phase
horizontal integration
macrocycle
main competitive phase
mesocycle
microcycle
monocycle

operational plan
periodization
phase potentiation mesocycle
precompetitive phase
preparatory period
preparedness
realization block
sequential periodization models
specific preparation phase
stimulus-fatigue-recovery-adaptation theory (SFRAT)
summated microcycle
training day
training session
training unit
transition period
transmutation block
tricycle
vertical integration

Study Questions

1. What is the primary consideration when designing a periodization program for a tactical athlete?
   a. adaptive potential
   b. proper variation
   c. peaking season
   d. operational plan

2. What level of the periodization hierarchy structure consists of several hours of training?
   a. training day
   b. training session
   c. training unit
   d. microcycle

3. When designing a tactical athlete's program, which period of training will typically be planned for when fewer tactical events are predicted?
   a. preparatory
   b. precompetitive
   c. main competitive
   d. transition

4. During which block of training is workload decreased while frequency and intensity are maintained?
   a. accumulation
   b. concentrated loading
   c. transmutation
   d. realization

Chapter 11

Resistance Training Exercise Techniques

Jason Dudley, MS, CSCS,*D, TSAC-F*D

Brad Schoenfeld, PhD, CSCS, NSCA-CPT, FNSCA

After completing this chapter, you will be able to

- design a warm-up for a resistance training session; and
- describe proper exercise technique and instructional cues for resistance training exercises using free weights, machines, and alternative modes or equipment.

To perform a resistance training session with proper technique, the exerciser should perform a warm-up first. Proper technique, including body posture, stance, and breathing, is paramount when performing strength and conditioning exercises. If the tactical athlete is unable to initiate or maintain proper technique for a given exercise, an exercise **regression** should be selected. Tactical athletes within a group should each be given exercises that are appropriate for their individual fitness and ability levels, which will ensure they can safely and effectively complete the exercise. When necessary, exercises can be performed with alternative implements, provided that proper exercise technique can be maintained.

Key Point

Tactical athletes should only perform exercises they are able to successfully complete with the proper technique.

PERFORMING EXERCISES WITH ALTERNATIVE IMPLEMENTS

It may be necessary to perform the following exercises with alternative equipment when in the field or when the equipment described is not available. Choose alternative equipment that allows the tactical athlete to maintain the proper technique. For example, if no dumbbells are available for a farmer's walk, use an ammo can, a battering ram, or another piece of equipment that can be safely carried. The objective is to achieve the same training result intended while ensuring that the alternative equipment is not damaged.

Key Point

When traditional exercise equipment is not available, use alternative equipment that allows the tactical athlete to perform the exercise safely and effectively.

WARM-UP BEFORE RESISTANCE TRAINING

At the beginning of a resistance training session, a warm-up should be completed. The warm-up should include both general and specific components. The purpose of the general warm-up is to elevate the core temperature and increase blood flow, which in turn enhances the speed of nerve impulses, increases nutrient delivery to working muscles and removal of waste by-products, and facilitates oxygen release from hemoglobin and myoglobin (4). The general warm-up usually consists of 5 to 10 minutes of light cardiorespiratory activity at approximately 50% of maximal heart rate (MHR). The goal is to work up a light sweat, not to elicit cardiorespiratory adaptations.

The specific warm-up is designed to enhance neuromuscular efficiency for an exercise by rehearsing the movement before it is performed at a high intensity (4). This is believed to improve performance during training sets. The specific warm-up should involve movements as similar as possible to those that will be completed during the training session. Movements during the specific warm-up should be performed with light weight or body weight at a controlled speed. The movements will depend on the equipment and space available. Additionally, the selected movements should allow the tactical athlete to go through a full ROM and should increase body temperature and HR without undue fatigue.

GUIDELINES ON BODY STANCE AND ALIGNMENT, BREATHING, AND SPOTTING

Proper body stance and alignment, breathing, and spotting when necessary should be implemented in resistance exercises. Use the following guidelines with primary exercises as well as when using alternative equipment.

Body Stance and Alignment

Stability during lifting is essential to maximize force production and ensure safety. To achieve a stable base of support, exercises performed from a standing position should generally be executed with feet slightly wider than shoulder-width apart and feet remaining firmly in contact with the ground. The spine should remain as upright as possible with preservation of the natural curves

(3). Supine exercises should be carried out using five points of contact, where the head, shoulders, upper back, and buttocks are firmly situated on the bench and both feet are flat on the ground (1).

Breathing

Correct breathing technique facilitates exercise performance. As a general rule, lifters should exhale during the **sticking point** of an exercise (i.e., the most difficult portion of the concentric action) and inhale during the eccentric component. In certain cases, particularly structural exercises (movements that directly place load on the vertebrae) performed with heavy loads, it can be beneficial to use the **Valsalva maneuver** as a breathing strategy. The Valsalva maneuver involves expiring against a closed glottis, which increases torso stiffness and thus attenuates compressive forces on the vertebral discs (2).

Spotting

For certain exercises, a spotter can facilitate performance while ensuring lifter safety. The following are general guidelines for spotting (1):

- Exercises performed overhead and with the bar on the back or front of the shoulders should be carried out in a power rack with crossbars set to safely allow full ROM. Spotters should remain close enough to the lifter to be able to assist if needed.

- Barbell exercises performed over the face should be spotted with an **alternating grip** (one hand pronated, the other supinated) to provide maximal safety and leverage. Over-the-face dumbbell exercises should be spotted by grasping the lifter's arm as close to the wrist as possible. This helps prevent the elbows from collapsing during performance (which could lead to the weights falling on the face or torso).

- No spotting should be done for power exercises such as the snatch or clean. Rather, the lifter should be instructed to push away the bar or drop it and clear the area as quickly as possible.

Free Weight Exercises

Machine-Based Exercises

Bodyweight Exercises

Alternative Exercises

FREE WEIGHT EXERCISES

BARBELL DEADLIFT: PRIMARY EXERCISE

Starting Position

Stand with the feet about hip-width apart. Grasp a barbell with an overhand or alternating grip and the arms outside the knees. The barbell should be on the ground and touching the lower legs at midshin level. The knees, hips, and ankles should be flexed with the back in a neutral position at approximately a 45° angle to the ground.

Upward Movement

Extend the knees and then the hips, keeping the elbows extended and allowing the barbell to travel upward in close proximity to the legs. The back should remain in a neutral position throughout the exercise. Continue the upward movement until the knees and hips are extended with the barbell at midthigh level and the torso perpendicular to the ground.

Downward Movement

Flex the hips (sit backward), knees, and shoulders while keeping the elbows extended, allowing the barbell to travel downward in close proximity to the legs.

The back should remain in a neutral position throughout the exercise. Continue descending until the barbell is back in the starting position.

Common Errors

- Allowing the spine to round forward
- Fully extending the knees before starting to extend the hips
- Hyperextending the back at the top of the exercise

Major Muscles Involved

gluteus maximus, semimembranosus, semitendinosus, biceps femoris, vastus lateralis, vastus intermedius, vastus medialis, rectus femoris

Field Alternative

This exercise can be performed in the field with a weighted piece of equipment (e.g., artillery box or weighted rucksack) as long as the equipment can be lifted using safe and effective technique.

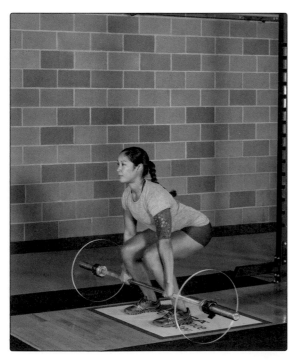

Starting position

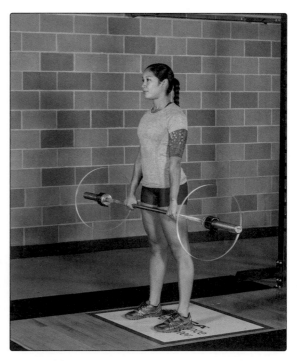

Top position

FREE WEIGHT EXERCISES

■ SUMO DEADLIFT

Starting Position

Stand with the feet wider than hip-width apart. Grasp a barbell with an overhand or alternating grip with the arms inside the knees. The barbell should be on the ground and touching the lower legs at mid shin level. The knees, hips, and ankles should be flexed with the back in a neutral position at approximately a 45° angle to the ground.

Upward Movement

Extend the knees and then the hips, keeping the elbows extended and allowing the barbell to travel upward in close proximity to the legs. The back should remain in a neutral position throughout the exercise. Continue the upward movement until the knees and hips are extended with the barbell at midthigh level and the torso perpendicular to the ground.

Downward Movement

Flex the hips (sit backward), knees, and shoulders while keeping the elbows extended, allowing the barbell to travel downward in close proximity to the legs.

The back should remain in a neutral position throughout the exercise. Continue descending until the barbell is in the starting position.

Common Errors

- Allowing the spine to flex or round forward
- Fully extending the knees before starting to extend the hips
- Hyperextending the back at the top of the exercise

Major Muscles Involved

gluteus maximus, semimembranosus, semitendinosus, biceps femoris, vastus lateralis, vastus intermedius, vastus medialis, rectus femoris

Field Alternative

This exercise can be performed in the field with a weighted piece of equipment (e.g., artillery box, weighted rucksack) as long as the equipment can be lifted using safe and effective technique.

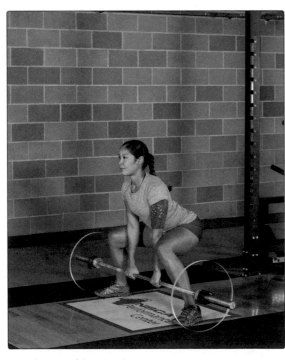

Starting position

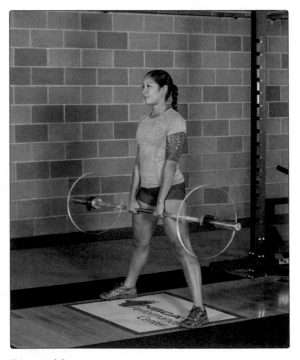

Top position

FREE WEIGHT EXERCISES

BARBELL ROMANIAN DEADLIFT: PRIMARY EXERCISE

Starting Position

Stand with the feet about hip-width apart. Grasp a barbell with an overhand grip with the barbell resting across the front of the thighs. The knees should be slightly flexed and the back in a neutral position.

Downward Movement

Flex the hips (sit backward) and the shoulders while keeping the elbows extended, allowing the barbell to travel downward in close proximity to the legs. The back should remain in a neutral position throughout the exercise. Continue descending as far as the flexibility of the hamstrings will allow and proper posture can be maintained.

Upward Movement

Extend the hips to bring the pelvis forward toward the bar. Continue ascending until the starting position is achieved while maintaining a slightly flexed knee.

Common Errors

- Allowing the shoulders and back to round forward
- Allowing the knees to fully extend and lock out
- Hyperextending the lower back at the top of the movement
- Allowing the barbell to travel forward away from the legs

Major Muscles Involved

gluteus maximus, semimembranosus, semitendinosus, biceps femoris, erector spinae

Field Alternative

Perform using a weighted rucksack or other equipment.

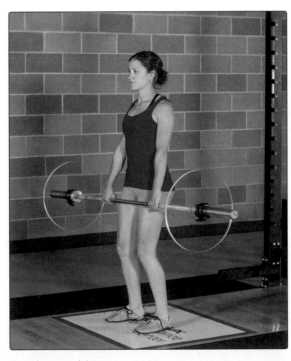

Starting position

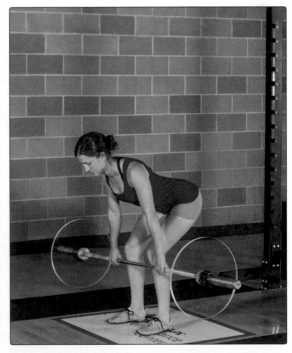

Bottom position

FREE WEIGHT EXERCISES

DUMBBELL ROMANIAN DEADLIFT: BARBELL ROMANIAN DEADLIFT REGRESSION

Starting Position

Stand with the feet about hip-width apart. Grasp a dumbbell in each hand with an overhand grip with the dumbbells resting across the front of the thighs. The knees should be slightly flexed and the back in a neutral position.

Downward Movement

Flex the hips (sit backward) and the shoulders while keeping the elbows extended, allowing the dumbbells to travel downward in close proximity to the legs. The back should remain in a neutral position throughout the exercise. Continue descending as far as the flexibility of the hamstrings will allow and proper posture can be maintained.

Upward Movement

Extend the hips to bring the pelvis forward toward the dumbbells. Continue ascending until the starting position is achieved while maintaining a slightly flexed knee.

Common Errors

- Allowing the shoulders and back to round forward
- Allowing the knees to fully extend and lock out
- Hyperextending the lower back at the top of the repetition
- Allowing the dumbbells to travel forward away from the legs

Major Muscles Involved

gluteus maximus, semimembranosus, semitendinosus, biceps femoris, erector spinae

Field Alternative

Perform using an ammo can or other equipment in each hand.

Regression

This exercise can be performed using body weight to accommodate all ability levels.

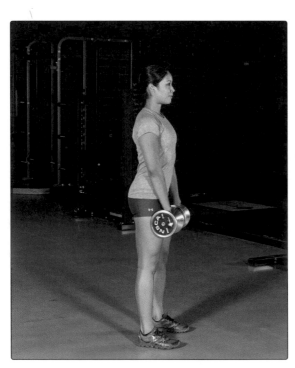

Starting position

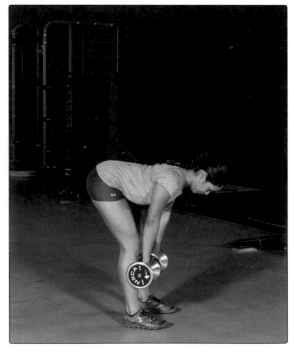

Bottom position

FREE WEIGHT EXERCISES

SINGLE-ARM, SINGLE-LEG ROMANIAN DEADLIFT: PRIMARY EXERCISE

Starting Position

Stand with the feet about hip-width apart. Grasp a dumbbell in one hand with an overhand grip with the dumbbell resting across the front of the thigh. The knees should be slightly flexed and the back in a neutral position.

Downward Movement

This exercise can be performed two ways. One variation is to hold the dumbbell in the hand opposite the supporting leg (the leg staying on the ground). The second variation is to hold the dumbbell in the hand on the same side as the supporting leg. Flex the hip of the supporting leg while keeping the opposite leg extended at the knee and the hip, allowing the foot to come off the ground. The arm holding the dumbbell will remain extended at the elbow while the shoulder flexes, allowing the dumbbell to move downward. Keep the hip and knee extended so the leg that comes off the ground remains in line with the torso. The back should remain in a neutral position throughout the exercise. Continue descending until the torso and leg are parallel to the ground or as far as the flexibility of the hamstrings will allow and proper posture can be maintained.

Upward Movement

Extend the hip of the supporting leg to bring the opposite leg forward. Continue ascending until the starting position is achieved while maintaining a slightly flexed knee.

Common Errors

- Allowing the shoulders and back to round forward
- Allowing the knee of the supporting leg to fully extend and lock out
- Allowing the pelvis to tilt to either side during the movement

Major Muscles Involved

gluteus maximus, semimembranosus, semitendinosus, biceps femoris, erector spinae

Field Alternative

Perform using an ammo can, water jug, or other equipment.

Regression

This exercise can be performed using body weight to accommodate all ability levels.

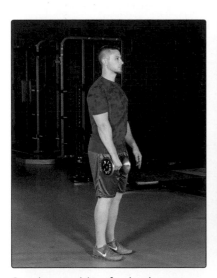

Starting position for both movements

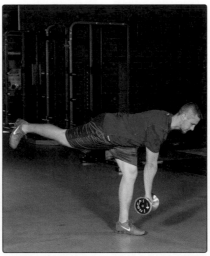
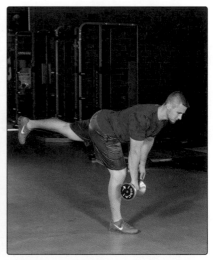

Bottom position for each movement: Dumbbell in hand on the side opposite the support leg and dumbbell in hand on the same side as the support leg

FREE WEIGHT EXERCISES

DOUBLE-ARM, SINGLE-LEG ROMANIAN DEADLIFT: PRIMARY EXERCISE

Starting Position

Stand with the feet about hip-width apart. Grasp a dumbbell in each hand with an overhand grip with the dumbbells resting across the front of the thighs. The knees should be slightly flexed and the back in a neutral position.

Downward Movement

Flex the hip of the supporting leg (the leg that will remain on the ground) while keeping the opposite leg extended at the knee and the hip, allowing the foot to come off the ground. The arms holding the dumbbells will remain extended at the elbow while the shoulders flex, allowing the dumbbells to move downward. The back should remain in a neutral position throughout the exercise. Continue descending until the torso and rear leg are parallel to the ground or as far as the flexibility of the hamstrings will allow with proper posture being maintained.

Upward Movement

Extend the hip of the supporting leg to bring the opposite leg forward. Continue ascending until the starting position is achieved while maintaining a slightly flexed knee.

Common Errors

- Allowing the shoulders and back to round forward
- Allowing the knee of the supporting leg to fully extend and lock out
- Allowing the pelvis to tilt to either side during the movement

Major Muscles Involved

gluteus maximus, semimembranosus, semitendinosus, biceps femoris, erector spinae

Field Alternative

Perform using ammo cans, water jug, or other equipment.

Regression

This exercise can be performed using body weight to accommodate all ability levels.

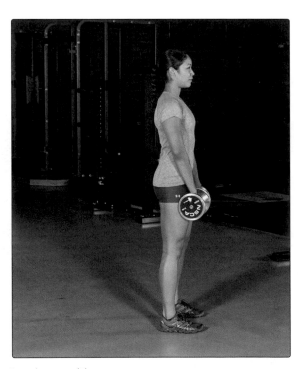

Starting position

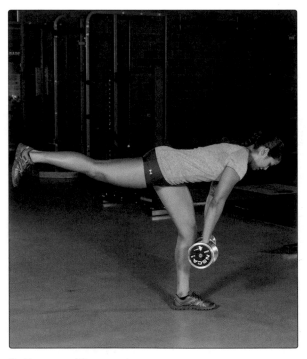

Bottom position

FREE WEIGHT EXERCISES

FRONT SQUAT: PRIMARY EXERCISE

Starting Position

Place a barbell across the front of the shoulders, with the elbows and shoulders flexed and wrists extended. In this position, the upper arms should be approximately parallel to the ground with the fingers supporting the bar and elbows pointing straight ahead. The feet should be shoulder-width or slightly wider than shoulder-width apart with a *neutral back position.* As an alternative, the lifter can cross the arms, placing each hand over the barbell on the opposite shoulder. This can be especially useful if the lifter has any trouble with wrist mobility.

Downward Movement

Simultaneously flex the hips (sit backward) and knees to descend in a controlled manner. The knees should stay positioned over the feet. The torso should remain erect throughout the movement, and the head should maintain a neutral position with the eyes focused either straight ahead or slightly upward. Continue the downward movement until the thighs are parallel to the ground or as far as quality technique can be maintained.

Upward Movement

While keeping the feet flat on the ground, simultaneously extend the knees and hips to return to the starting position.

Spotter

The preferred spotting method is with two spotters: The spotters stand at opposite ends of the bar and hold the hands 2 to 3 inches (5-8 cm) below the ends of the bar, thumbs overlapping. If only one spotter is used, the spotter should be positioned directly behind the lifter with the arms underneath the upper arms of the lifter and the hands near the lifter's torso just below the lifter's elbows. The spotter mimics the motion of the lifter throughout the exercise, staying a few inches (about 5 cm) away from the lifter. If help is required, the spotter immediately places the hands on the lifter's torso and begins lifting by extending the hips and knees.

Common Errors

- Allowing the shoulders and back to round forward
- Allowing the knees to move toward each other and lose alignment over the feet
- Allowing the elbows to point downward so that the upper arms do not maintain a position that is parallel to the ground

Major Muscles Involved

gluteus maximus, semimembranosus, semitendinosus, biceps femoris, vastus lateralis, vastus intermedius, vastus medialis, rectus femoris

Field Alternative

The Zercher squat can be performed in the field with heavy equipment when a squat rack in not available.

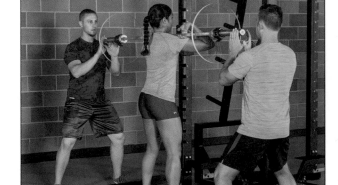

Starting position with two spotters

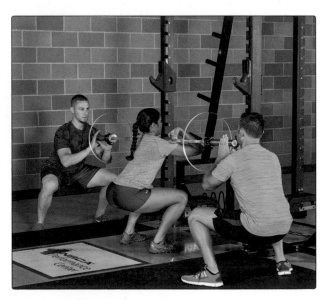

Bottom position with two spotters

ZERCHER SQUAT: FIELD ALTERNATIVE FOR FRONT SQUAT

Starting Position

Place a piece of equipment across the *antecubital area* (crease of the elbows), with the elbows and shoulders flexed. In this position, the forearms should be approximately parallel to the upper torso. The feet should be shoulder-width or slightly wider than shoulder-width apart with a neutral back position.

Downward Movement

Simultaneously flex the hips (sit backward) and knees to descend in a controlled manner. The knees should stay positioned over the feet. The torso should remain erect throughout the movement, and the head should maintain a neutral position with the eyes focused either straight ahead or slightly upward. Continue the downward movement until the thighs are parallel to the ground or as far as quality technique can be maintained.

Upward Movement

While keeping the feet flat on the ground, simultaneously extend the knees and hips to return to the starting position.

Common Errors

- Allowing the shoulders and back to round forward
- Allowing the knees to move toward each other and lose alignment over the feet

Major Muscles Involved

gluteus maximus, semimembranosus, semitendinosus, biceps femoris, vastus lateralis, vastus intermedius, vastus medialis, rectus femoris

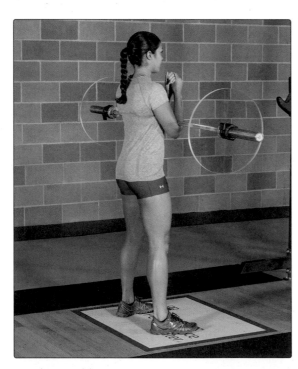

Starting position

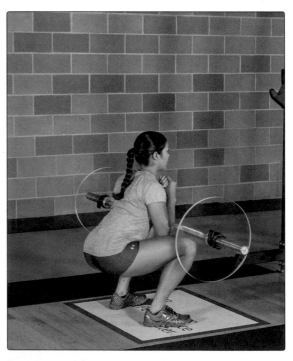

Bottom position

FREE WEIGHT EXERCISES

DUMBBELL GOBLET SQUAT: FRONT SQUAT REGRESSION

If the exerciser has never performed a front squat or is unable to perform a front squat properly, or the appropriate equipment is not available to perform a barbell front squat, a dumbbell (or other implement) goblet squat can be performed as a substitute.

Starting Position

Position the dumbbell (or other implement) vertically next to the sternum, just underneath the chin, holding the dumbbell on each side with the palms facing in and the forearms against the side of the dumbbell as much as possible. The upper arms and elbows should be in contact with the torso. The feet should be shoulder-width or slightly wider than shoulder-width apart.

Downward Movement

Simultaneously flex the hips (sit backward) and knees to descend in a controlled manner. The knees should stay aligned over the feet. The torso should remain erect throughout the movement, and the head should maintain a neutral position with the eyes focused either straight ahead or slightly upward. Continue the downward movement until the thighs are parallel to the ground or as far as quality technique can be maintained.

Upward Movement

While keeping the feet flat on the ground, simultaneously extend the knees and hips to return to the starting position.

Common Errors

- Allowing the shoulders and back to round forward
- Allowing the knees to move toward each other and lose alignment over the feet
- Allowing the implement to move forward or away from the torso

Major Muscles Involved

gluteus maximus, semimembranosus, semitendinosus, biceps femoris, vastus lateralis, vastus intermedius, vastus medialis, rectus femoris

Field Alternative

The goblet squat can be performed with any piece of weighted equipment.

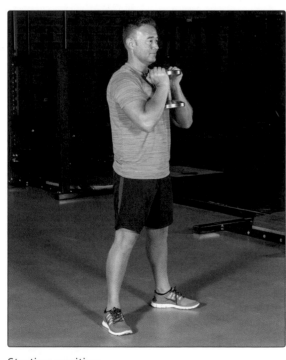

Starting position

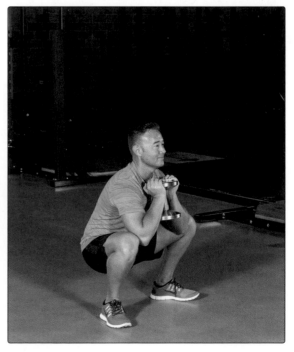

Bottom position

FREE WEIGHT EXERCISES

■ DOUBLE-ARM DUMBBELL WALKING LUNGE: PRIMARY EXERCISE

Starting Position

Grasp a dumbbell in each hand in a standing position, arms hanging down at the sides of the body. Maintain a neutral back position.

Downward Movement

Take a step forward with one leg and leave the other leg in place. Descend by flexing the knee and hip of the front leg while simultaneously flexing the knee of the back leg. Continue descending until the knee of the trail leg is about an inch (2.5 cm) off the ground, or as low as possible, maintaining good form. The torso should remain erect throughout the movement, and the head should maintain a neutral position with the eyes focused either straight ahead or slightly upward. At the bottom position, the knee of the trail leg, the hips, and the shoulders should all be aligned vertically. The knee of the front leg should be aligned with the front foot.

Upward Movement

Simultaneously extend the knee and hip of the front leg while bringing the trail leg forward until it is alongside the front leg. Repeat this process with the other leg forward to complete a full repetition.

Common Errors

- Allowing the shoulders and back to round forward
- Allowing the forward knee to move inward and lose alignment over the front foot
- Taking too long of a stride to begin the movement, so the knee of the trail leg does not stay aligned under the hips and shoulders

Major Muscles Involved

gluteus maximus, semimembranosus, semitendinosus, biceps femoris, vastus lateralis, vastus intermedius, vastus medialis, rectus femoris, iliopsoas

Field Alternative

Pushing a sled or vehicle can be used as a field alternative. Ammo cans, water jugs, or any other piece of equipment can also be held in each hand to perform this exercise in the field.

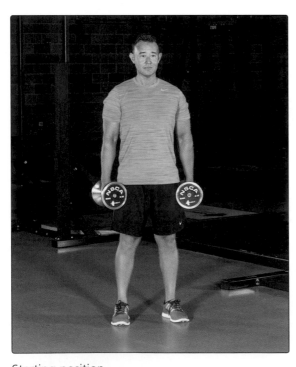

Starting position

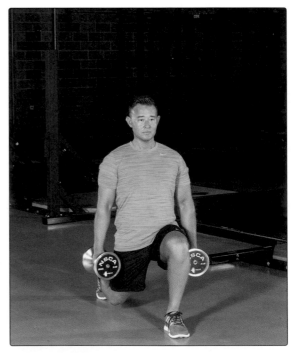

Bottom position

FREE WEIGHT EXERCISES

DUMBBELL STEP-UP: DOUBLE-ARM WALKING LUNGE REGRESSION

If the exerciser has never performed a walking lunge or is unable to perform a walking lunge properly, a dumbbell (or other implement) step-up can be performed instead.

Starting Position

Grasp a dumbbell in each hand in a standing position facing a box (or a solid step). The box or step height should be set so when the lifter places a foot on the box, the knee is at the same height or lower than the hip. This exercise can be performed with body weight or lower steps to accommodate all fitness levels.

Upward Movement

Flex the knee and hip of one leg to place the foot flat on the box. Then extend the knee and hip of the front leg, keeping the trail leg relatively extended to ensure the front leg does the majority of the work. The torso should remain erect throughout the movement, and the head should maintain a neutral position with the eyes focused either straight ahead or slightly upward. Continue extending the front leg to bring the trail leg forward until it is alongside the front leg on the box.

Downward Movement

Step backward from the box with the trail leg while controlling the descent with the front leg, which is still on the box. Continue descending until the foot of the trail leg reaches the ground. Return to the starting position by removing the front leg from the box and returning it to the ground. The torso should remain erect and the knee of the front leg should be aligned with the foot throughout the movement. Repeat this process with the other leg on the box to complete a full repetition.

Common Errors

- Allowing the shoulders and back to round forward
- Allowing the front knee (of the foot that is on the box) to move inward and lose alignment over the front foot
- Pushing off with the back leg to assist the upward movement

Major Muscles Involved

gluteus maximus, semimembranosus, semitendinosus, biceps femoris, vastus lateralis, vastus intermedius, vastus medialis, rectus femoris

Field Alternative

Pushing a sled or vehicle can be used as a field alternative. Ammo cans, water jugs or any other piece of equipment can also be held in each hand to perform this exercise in the field.

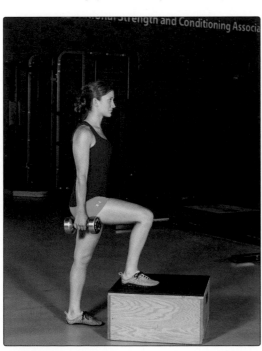

Starting position

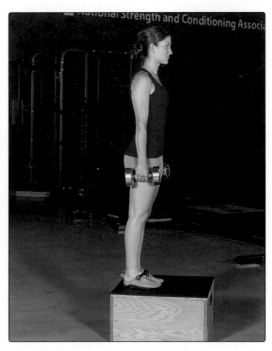

Top position

FREE WEIGHT EXERCISES

SINGLE-ARM DUMBBELL OVERHEAD WALKING LUNGE: PRIMARY EXERCISE

Starting Position

In a standing position with a neutral back position, grasp a dumbbell in one hand and press the dumbbell directly overhead.

Downward Movement

Take a step forward with one leg while leaving the other leg in place. Descend by flexing the knee and hip of the front leg and flexing the knee of the trail leg so it lowers toward the ground. Continue descending until the knee of the trail leg is about an inch (2.5 cm) off the ground, or as low as possible, maintaining good form. The torso should remain erect throughout the movement and the dumbbell held overhead with the elbow fully extended. The head should maintain a neutral position with the eyes focused either straight ahead or slightly upward. At the bottom position, the knee of the trail leg, the hips, the shoulders, and the dumbbell should all be aligned vertically. The knee on the front leg should be aligned with the front foot.

Upward Movement

Simultaneously extend the knee and hip of the front leg while bringing the trail leg forward until it is alongside the front leg. Repeat this process with the other leg to complete a full repetition. Complete an equal number of repetitions with the dumbbell in each hand.

Common Errors

- Allowing the shoulders and back to round forward
- Allowing the front knee to move inward and lose alignment over the front foot
- Taking too long of a stride to begin the movement, so the knee of the trail leg does not stay aligned under the hips and shoulders

Major Muscles Involved

gluteus maximus, semimembranosus, semitendinosus, biceps femoris, vastus lateralis, vastus intermedius, vastus medialis, rectus femoris, iliopsoas, anterior and medial deltoids, triceps brachii

Field Alternative

Perform with a sandbag or other implement instead of the dumbbell.

Regression

The exercise can be modified to accommodate all ability levels by removing the implement from the hand, reducing the ROM during the downward phase of the movement, or both.

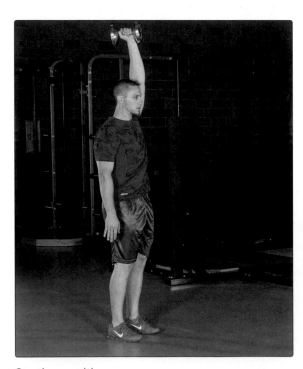

Starting position

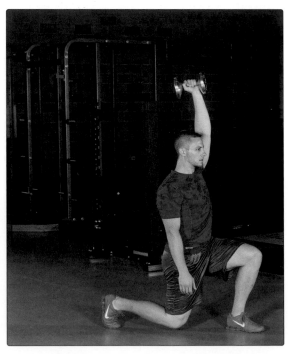

Bottom position

FREE WEIGHT EXERCISES

DUMBBELL REVERSE LUNGE: PRIMARY EXERCISE

Starting Position

Grasp a dumbbell in each hand in a standing position with a neutral back position.

Downward Movement

Take a step backward with one leg while leaving the other leg in place. Descend by flexing the knee of the trail leg while simultaneously flexing the knee and hip of the front leg. Continue descending until the knee of the trail leg is about an inch (2.5 cm) off the ground, or as low as possible, maintaining good form. The torso should remain erect throughout the movement, and the head should maintain a neutral position with the eyes focused either straight ahead or slightly upward. At the bottom position, the knee of the trail leg, the hips, and the shoulders should all be aligned vertically. The knee of the front leg should be aligned with the front foot.

Upward Movement

Simultaneously extend the knee and hip of the front leg while bringing the trail leg forward until it is alongside the front leg. Repeat this process with the other leg to complete a full repetition.

Common Errors

- Allowing the shoulders and back to round forward
- Allowing the front knee to move inward and lose alignment over the front foot
- Taking too long of a stride backward to begin the movement so that the knee of the trail leg does not stay aligned under the hips and shoulders

Major Muscles Involved

gluteus maximus, semimembranosus, semitendinosus, biceps femoris, vastus lateralis, vastus intermedius, vastus medialis, rectus femoris

Field Alternative

Hold equipment or another implement across the front of the torso with both arms instead of dumbbells.

Regression

The exercise can be modified to accommodate all ability levels by removing the dumbbells from the hands, reducing the ROM during the downward phase of the movement, or both.

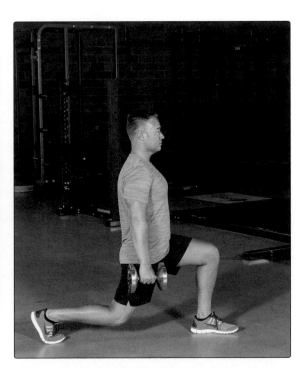

Starting position

Bottom position: Step backward with one leg

FREE WEIGHT EXERCISES

DUMBBELL FARMER'S WALK: PRIMARY EXERCISE

Starting Position

Grasp a dumbbell in each hand in a standing position with a neutral back position.

Movement

This exercise is completed by performing a walking motion while carrying a dumbbell or other training implement in each hand. The torso should remain upright with the eyes focused forward or slightly upward and elbows extended throughout the exercise. This exercise can be performed for a prescribed number of steps, time, or distance.

Common Errors

- Allowing the shoulders and back to round forward
- Allowing the dumbbells or training implements to fall to the ground upon completion of the set
- Using too much weight, so the lifter is unable to maintain quality posture
- Flexing the elbows during the movement

Major Muscles Involved

forearm flexors, trapezius, and middle deltoids

Field Alternative

Replace the dumbbells with heavy rucksacks or other pieces of equipment.

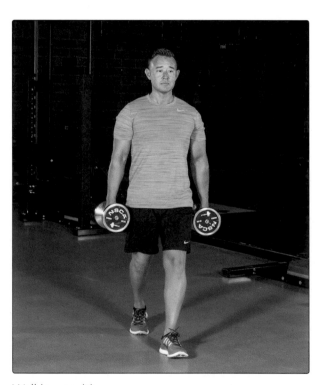

Walking position

FREE WEIGHT EXERCISES

DOUBLE-ARM ARNOLD PRESS: PRIMARY EXERCISE

Starting Position

Stand with the feet hip-width or slightly wider than hip-width apart. The knees and hips should be slightly flexed and remain in this position throughout the movement. Grasp two dumbbells, flex at the elbows, and internally rotate the forearms to bring the dumbbells to a position where they are directly under the chin, with the palms facing each other and the head of the dumbbells touching the sternum.

Upward Movement

Simultaneously extend the elbows while abducting and flexing the shoulders and externally rotating the forearms until the dumbbells are overhead with the palms facing forward and the elbows fully extended.

Downward Movement

Flex the elbows while adducting and extending the shoulders and rotating the hands so the dumbbells descend inward. Continue until the starting position is achieved.

Common Errors

- Using the lower body to generate momentum to propel the dumbbells upward
- Not fully extending the elbows at the top of each repetition
- Not bringing the dumbbells back underneath the chin at the bottom of each repetition

Major Muscles Involved

anterior and medial deltoids, triceps brachii

Field Alternative

This exercise can be performed by holding a sandbag or other implement in each hand.

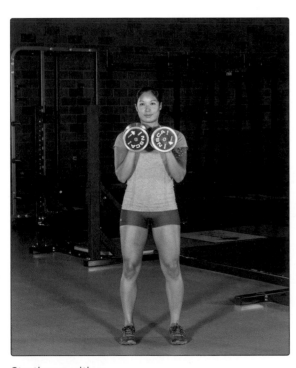

Starting position

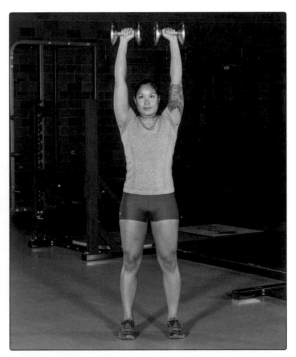

Top position

FREE WEIGHT EXERCISES

SINGLE-ARM ARNOLD PRESS FROM SPLIT STANCE: PRIMARY EXERCISE

Starting Position

Stand with the feet staggered with both feet flat on the ground. Place the front foot ahead of the hips and the back foot behind the hips. The more narrowly aligned the feet are, the more this will challenge the lifter's balance. The knees should be slightly flexed and remain in this position throughout the movement. Hold a dumbbell in the hand of the arm on the same side as the trail leg, with the dumbbell directly under the chin and the palm facing inward. The head of the dumbbell should lightly touch the sternum. The arm that does not have a dumbbell should remain relaxed at the lifter's side.

Upward Movement

Simultaneously extend the elbow while abducting and flexing the shoulder and externally rotating the forearm until the dumbbell is overhead with the palm facing forward and the elbow fully extended.

Downward Movement

Flex the elbow while adducting and extending the shoulder and rotating the hand so the dumbbell descends inward. Continue until the starting position is achieved. When the desired number of repetitions is reached, repeat on the opposite side.

Common Errors

- Placing the opposite hand on the hip to assist with balance
- Not allowing the elbow to fully extend and the shoulder to fully flex at the top of each repetition
- Not bringing the dumbbell back underneath the chin at the bottom of each repetition

Major Muscles Involved

anterior and medial deltoids, triceps brachii

Field Alternative

This exercise can be performed using a sandbag, other implement, or other piece of equipment.

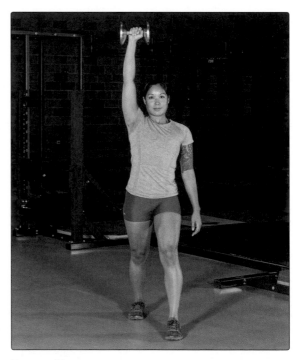

Starting position   Top position

FREE WEIGHT EXERCISES

BARBELL MILITARY PRESS: PRIMARY EXERCISE

Starting Position

Place a barbell across the front of the shoulders. The elbows should be flexed and directly underneath the bar with the palms facing forward. The feet should be shoulder-width or slightly wider than shoulder-width apart with the knees slightly flexed.

Upward Movement

Simultaneously extend the elbows and flex the shoulders to press the barbell upward. Continue the movement until the elbows are fully extended with the barbell pressed directly overhead.

Downward Movement

Flex the elbows while extending the shoulders so that the bar travels downward. Continue until the barbell returns to the starting position. The lower body and torso should remain in the starting position throughout the movement.

Spotter

A spotter is needed, but one is not shown in the photos. If the lifter performs the exercise in a seated position (such as in a shoulder press bench), the spotter should stand directly behind the lifter with the hands just outside the hands of the lifter a few inches (about 5 cm) below the bar. If the lifter performs the exercise in a standing position, the spotter may not be able to spot the bar due to height differences, especially toward the end of the upward movement and the beginning of the downward movement. Thus, it may be necessary to stand on an elevated stable surface to assist the lifter at the top of the exercise.

Common Errors

- Performing the exercise with the barbell moving behind the head
- Using the lower body to generate momentum to drive the barbell upward
- Hyperextending the lower back during the exercise

Major Muscles Involved

anterior and medial deltoids, triceps brachii

Field Alternative

This exercise can be performed with any implement or piece of equipment that can be pressed overhead safely.

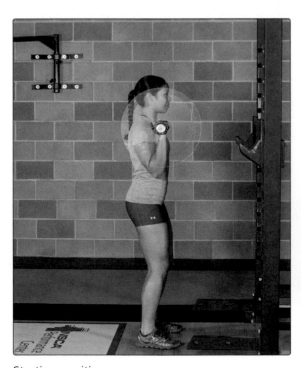

Starting position

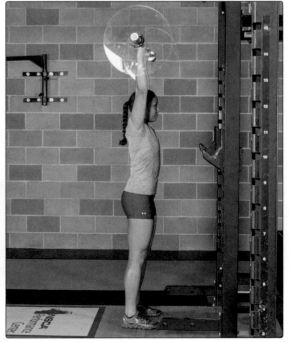

Top position

FREE WEIGHT EXERCISES

BARBELL PUSH PRESS: PRIMARY EXERCISE

Starting Position

Place a barbell across the front of the shoulders. The elbows should be flexed and directly underneath the bar with the palms facing forward. The feet should be shoulder-width or slightly wider than shoulder-width apart with the knees slightly flexed.

First Downward Movement

Flex the knees and hips. Continue descending until the hips are approximately 6 inches (15 cm) below the starting position.

Upward Movement

Simultaneously extend the elbows and flex the shoulders to press the barbell upward while quickly extending the knees and hips and plantar flexing the ankles. Continue the upward movement until the elbows are fully extended and the barbell is pressed directly overhead in a standing position with the knees slightly flexed. This movement is performed quickly to generate momentum to drive the barbell vertically.

Second Downward Movement

Flex the elbows while extending the shoulders so that the bar travels downward. Continue until the barbell returns to the starting position.

Common Errors

- Performing the exercise with the barbell moving behind the head
- Performing a second downward movement (the same as the first downward movement) while the barbell is traveling vertically
- Hyperextending the lower back during the exercise

Major Muscles Involved

gluteus maximus, semimembranosus, semitendinosus, biceps femoris, vastus lateralis, vastus intermedius, vastus medialis, rectus femoris, soleus, gastrocnemius, deltoids, trapezius, triceps brachii

Field Alternative

This exercise can be performed with any implement or piece of equipment that can be pressed overhead safely.

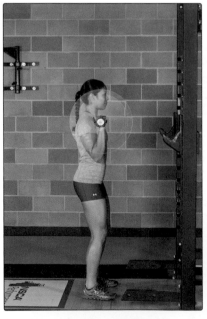
Starting position

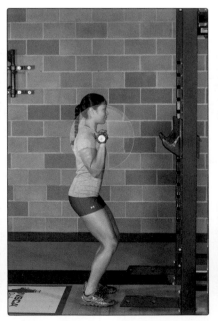
Dip

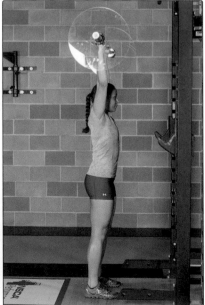
Press

FREE WEIGHT EXERCISES

ALTERNATE-ARM DUMBBELL BENCH PRESS: PRIMARY EXERCISE

Starting Position

Lie supine on a bench with a dumbbell in each hand. Flex the shoulders and extend the elbows so the arms are perpendicular to the ground. The head, shoulders, and buttocks should be in contact with the bench with both feet flat on the ground. These five points of contact should be maintained throughout the exercise.

Downward Movement

Flex the elbow and extend the shoulder of one arm so that the arm achieves a 45° angle from the torso. The other arm should remain motionless during this motion. Continue the downward movement until the bottom of the dumbbell is in line with the top of the chest.

Upward Movement

Simultaneously extend the elbow and flex the shoulder of the lifting arm. Continue this movement until the dumbbell returns to the starting position. Repeat this process with the other arm to complete a full repetition.

Spotter

The spotter should be at the head of the bench with the hands around, but not touching, the lifter's wrist. If spotting is necessary, the spotter should grasp the lifter's wrist, not lift up on the lifter's upper arm or elbow.

Common Errors

- Failing to keep the uninvolved arm motionless while the other arm is moving
- Arching the low back so the buttocks come off the bench
- Lifting the head off the bench

Major Muscles Involved

pectoralis major, anterior deltoids, triceps brachii

Field Alternative

Use the alternate-arm medicine ball (or other implement) push-up when dumbbells are not available. For this exercise, the lifter places one hand on the medicine ball while in a push-up position and then completes a push-up. The hand that is elevated should be changed with each repetition to mimic the alternation of the dumbbell bench press.

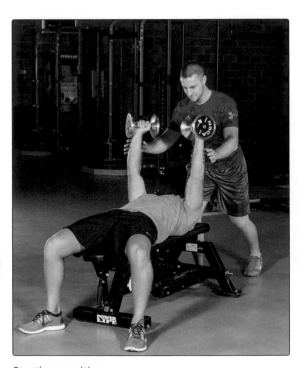

Starting position

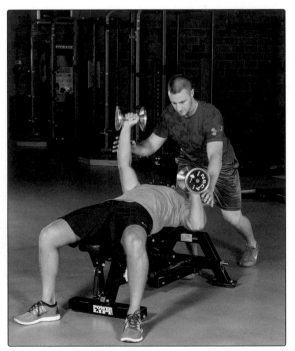

Bottom position

FREE WEIGHT EXERCISES

BENT-OVER BARBELL ROW: PRIMARY EXERCISE

Starting Position

Stand with the feet hip-width or slightly wider than hip-width apart with the knees and hips flexed and the torso approximately parallel to the ground. The arms should be perpendicular to the ground with the hands grasping a barbell with an overhand grip. The barbell should be directly in front of the shins. The position of the legs and torso should be maintained throughout the movement.

Upward Movement

Flex the elbows and extend the shoulders to pull the barbell toward the lower chest. Continue this movement until the barbell touches the sternum. The position of the legs and torso should not change, and only the arms should move.

Downward Movement

Extend the elbows and flex the shoulders to lower the barbell toward the ground. Continue this movement until the starting position is achieved.

Common Errors

- Using the legs or torso to generate momentum to lift the barbell toward the sternum
- Allowing the torso to flex and extend during the movement

Major Muscles Involved

latissimus dorsi, rhomboid minor and major

Field Alternative

This exercise can be performed with any equipment that can be lifted safely, such as a weighted rucksack or ammo can.

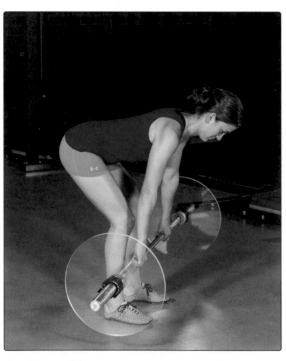

Starting position

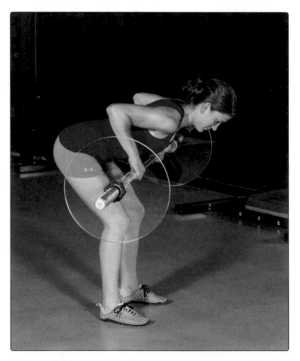

Top position

FREE WEIGHT EXERCISES

SINGLE-ARM BENT-OVER DUMBBELL ROW: PRIMARY EXERCISE

Starting Position

Stand with the feet hip-width or slightly wider than hip-width apart, with the knees and hips flexed and the torso at a 45° angle from the ground. The arms should be perpendicular to the ground, with one hand grasping a dumbbell with a neutral grip. The dumbbell should be between the feet, in line with the arches. The position of the legs and torso should be maintained throughout the movement.

Upward Movement

Flex the elbow and extend the shoulder of the arm holding the dumbbell to pull the dumbbell toward the lower chest. As the dumbbell is pulled upward, the hand should rotate, allowing the palm to face inward. Continue this movement until the dumbbell touches the side of the torso with the palm facing inward. The position of the legs, torso, and other arm should not change throughout the movement, and only the arm holding the dumbbell should move.

Downward Movement

Extend the elbow and flex the shoulder of the arm holding the dumbbell to lower the dumbbell toward the ground. Continue this movement until the starting position is achieved. At the end of the set, repeat the movement with the opposite arm.

Common Errors

- Using the legs or torso to generate momentum to lift the dumbbell upward
- Allowing the torso to rotate, flex, or extend during the movement

Major Muscles Involved

latissimus dorsi, teres major, middle trapezius, rhomboids, posterior deltoids

Field Alternative

This exercise can be performed with any equipment that can be lifted safely, such as a weighted ammo can.

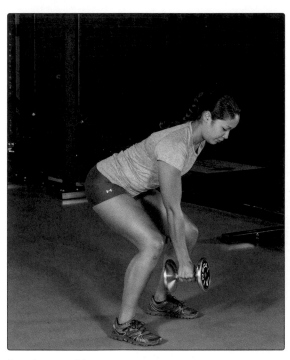

Starting position

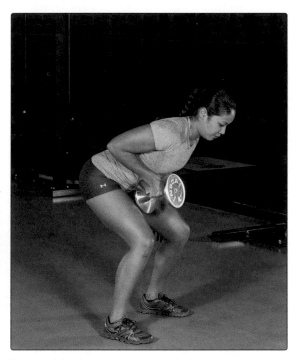

Top position

MACHINE-BASED EXERCISES

WIDE-GRIP PULLDOWN: WIDE-GRIP PULL-UP REGRESSION

Starting Position

From a seated position, grasp the bar of a pulldown machine slightly wider than shoulder-width with palms facing forward. The torso should remain upright with a slight lean backward to allow the bar to pass in front of the face and with the elbows fully extended. The eyes should be focused forward or slightly upward.

Downward Movement

Simultaneously flex both elbows and adduct the shoulders to pull the bar toward the upper chest. The torso should remain upright with a slight lean backward throughout the movement. Continue the downward movement until the bar crosses below the chin.

Upward Movement

Extend the elbows and abduct the shoulders, allowing the bar to rise. Continue the upward movement until the starting position is achieved.

Common Errors

- Rocking the torso backward to generate momentum to bring the bar downward
- Not allowing the elbows to fully extend at the end of each repetition
- Not bringing the bar low enough to cross below the chin

Major Muscles Involved

latissimus dorsi, teres major, middle trapezius, rhomboids, posterior deltoids

Field Alternative

Perform an assisted pull-up from an object that is strong enough to support the body weight.

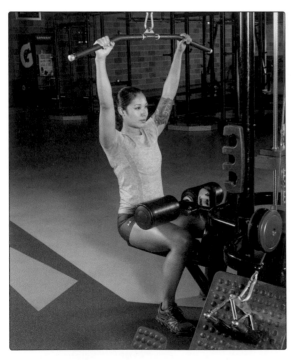

Starting position

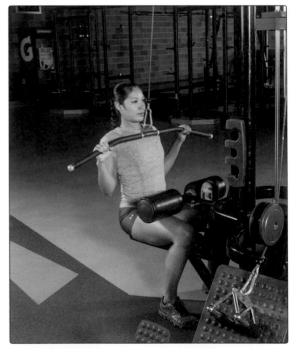

Bottom position

MACHINE-BASED EXERCISES

CLOSE-GRIP PULLDOWN: CLOSE-GRIP PULL-UP REGRESSION

Starting Position

From a seated position, grasp the bar of a pulldown machine several inches (about 5 cm) apart with palms facing toward one another. The torso should remain upright with a slight backward lean and the elbows fully extended. The eyes should be focused forward or slightly upward.

Downward Movement

Simultaneously flex the elbows and extend the shoulders to pull the bar toward the upper chest. The torso should remain erect with a slight backward lean throughout the movement. Continue the downward movement until the bar crosses below the chin.

Upward Movement

Extend the elbows and flex the shoulders to allow the bar to rise. Continue the upward movement until the starting position is achieved.

Common Errors

- Rocking the torso backward to generate momentum to bring the bar downward
- Not allowing the elbows to fully extend at the end of each repetition
- Not bringing the bar low enough to cross below the chin

Major Muscles Involved

latissimus dorsi, teres major, middle trapezius, rhomboids, posterior deltoids

Field Alternative

Perform an assisted close-grip pull-up from an object that is strong enough to support the body weight.

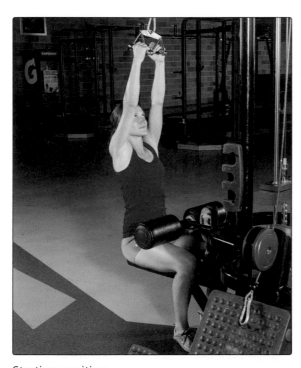

Starting position

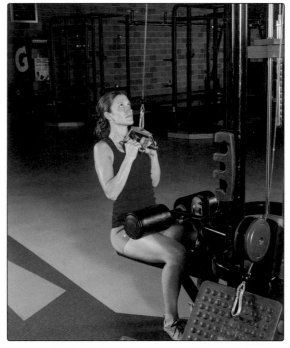

Bottom position

MACHINE-BASED EXERCISES

REVERSE-GRIP PULLDOWN: REVERSE-GRIP PULL-UP REGRESSION

Starting Position

From a seated position, grasp the bar of a pulldown machine slightly wider than shoulder-width with the palms facing the body. The torso should remain upright with a slight backward lean and with the elbows fully extended. The eyes should be focused forward or slightly upward.

Downward Movement

Simultaneously flex the elbows and extend the shoulders to pull the bar toward the upper chest. The torso should remain erect with a slight backward lean throughout the movement. Continue the downward movement until the bar crosses below the chin.

Upward Movement

Extend the elbows and flex the shoulders to allow the bar to rise. Continue the upward movement until the starting position is achieved.

Common Errors

- Rocking the torso backward to generate momentum to bring the bar downward
- Not allowing the elbows to fully extend at the end of each repetition
- Not bringing the bar low enough to cross below the chin

Major Muscles Involved

latissimus dorsi, teres major, middle trapezius, rhomboids, posterior deltoids

Field Alternative

Perform an assisted pull-up from an object that is strong enough to support the body weight.

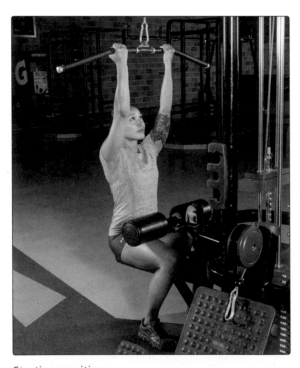

Starting position

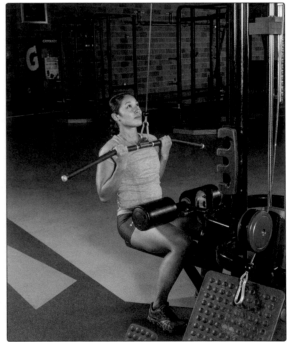

Bottom position

MACHINE-BASED EXERCISES

SINGLE-ARM PULLDOWN: PRIMARY EXERCISE

Starting Position

From a seated position, grasp a single-hand attachment of a pulldown machine with the palm facing forward. The torso should remain upright with the elbow of the lifting arm fully extended. The arm that is not holding the handle should remain relaxed at the side of the body. The eyes should be focused forward or slightly upward.

Downward Movement

Simultaneously flex the elbow, extend the shoulder, and rotate the hand so that the palm faces inward to pull the handle toward the upper chest. The torso should remain perpendicular to the ground throughout the movement. Continue the downward movement until the bottom of the handle is in line with the top of the shoulder.

Upward Movement

To allow the handle to rise, extend the elbow and flex the shoulder while simultaneously rotating the palm to face forward. Continue the upward movement until the starting position is achieved.

Common Errors

- Rocking the torso backward to generate momentum to bring the handle downward
- Not allowing the elbow of the lifting arm to fully extend at the end of each repetition
- Not bringing the handle low enough to complete the repetition

Major Muscles Involved

latissimus dorsi, teres major, middle trapezius, rhomboids, posterior deltoids

Field Alternative

Rope climbing is a useful field alternative.

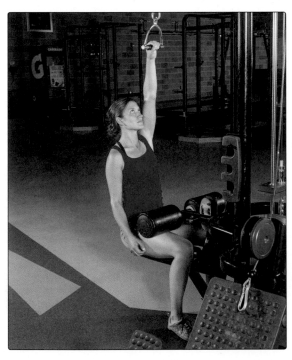

Starting position

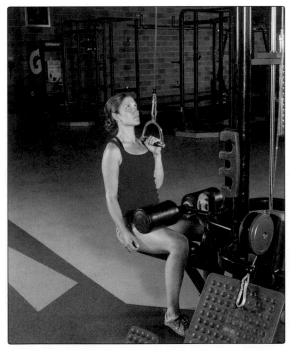

Bottom position

MACHINE-BASED EXERCISES

SINGLE-ARM CABLE ROW FROM SQUAT STANCE: PRIMARY EXERCISE

Starting Position

Stand with the feet shoulder-width or slightly wider than shoulder-width apart, keeping the knees and hips flexed approximately 90° so the upper leg is close to parallel to the ground. The torso should be perpendicular to the ground, slightly more than arm's length from a cable machine. One arm should be relaxed at the lifter's side, with the other arm in front of the lifter. The shoulder should be flexed, allowing the entire arm to achieve a parallel position to the ground. The hand of the arm that is out front should be holding a single-handle attachment that is attached to the cable column, with the palm facing downward and the elbow fully extended.

Backward Movement

Simultaneously flex the elbow and extend the shoulder of the arm holding the handle to pull the handle toward the lower chest. As the hand approaches the chest, it should rotate so that it faces inward. Continue this movement until the handle of the cable column is in line with the torso.

Forward Movement

Extend the elbow, flex the shoulder, and rotate the palm downward so that the arm moves forward.

Continue this movement until the starting position is achieved. At the end of the set, repeat the movement with the opposite arm.

Common Errors

- Rotating the torso to generate momentum during the movement
- Failing to control the movement during the forward motion
- Allowing the torso to flex and extend during the movement

Major Muscles Involved

latissimus dorsi, teres major, middle trapezius, rhomboids, posterior deltoids

Field Alternative

This exercise can be performed with a resistance band or by tying a rope to a weighted implement and performing a rope row.

Regression

Perform the same exercise while seated on a bench.

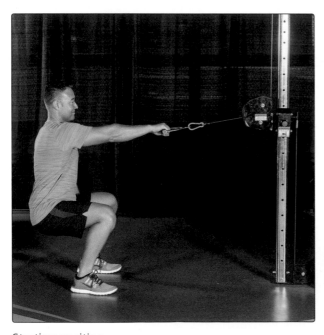

Starting position

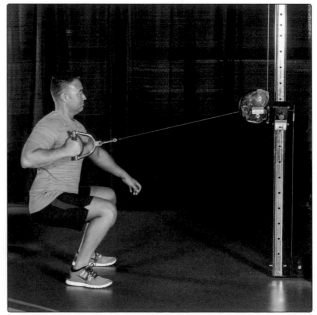

Backward position

MACHINE-BASED EXERCISES

SEATED MACHINE ROW: PRIMARY EXERCISE

Starting Position

Sit upright in a seated row machine slightly farther than arm's length away from the cable column. The hips and knees should be flexed, with the feet placed flat on the foot pedals. Grasp the handle attached to the cable on the cable column with a neutral grip. (The type of grip may change based on the type of attachment or handle of the machine.)

Backward Movement

Simultaneously flex the elbows and extend the shoulders to pull the handle toward the sternum. Continue this movement until the handle touches the sternum. The position of the torso and the lower body should remain constant during this movement.

Forward Movement

Extend the elbows and flex the shoulders to allow the handle to travel away from the torso.

Continue this movement until the starting position is achieved.

Common Errors

- Extending the knees to generate momentum
- Using the torso to generate momentum to pull the handle on the cable column
- Allowing the torso to flex and extend during the movement

Major Muscles Involved

latissimus dorsi, teres major, middle trapezius, rhomboids, posterior deltoids

Field Alternative

This exercise can be performed by sitting down and pulling a rope, hose, or cable (tied to a piece of equipment) inward.

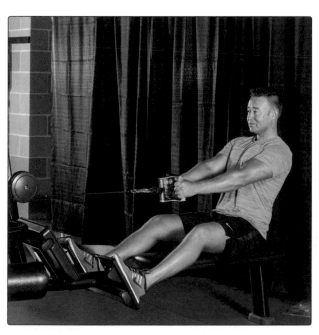

Starting position

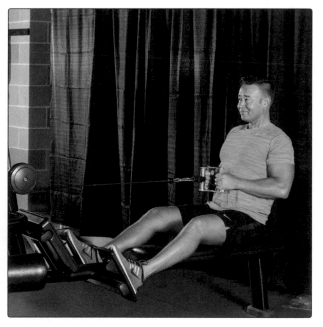

Backward position

BODYWEIGHT EXERCISES

BACK EXTENSION: PRIMARY EXERCISE

Starting Position

Place both feet in a back extension or glute-ham machine, with the knees slightly flexed and the hips supported by the machine pads. The body should be aligned from the heels to the shoulders, either parallel to the ground or at a 45° angle from the ground, depending on the machine. The knees should remain slightly flexed throughout the exercise.

Downward Movement

Allow the hips to flex so the shoulders lower. The torso should remain extended throughout the exercise with the back in a neutral position. Continue descending until the torso is perpendicular to the ground, or as low as possible, maintaining proper form.

Upward Movement

Extend the hips so that the shoulders rise upward while keeping the knees slightly flexed. Continue until the starting position is achieved.

Common Errors

- Allowing the shoulders and back to round forward
- Hyperextending the lower back at the top of the movement
- Locking out the knees

Major Muscles Involved

erector spinae, gluteus maximus, semimembranosus, semitendinosus, biceps femoris

Field Alternative

Perform with body weight or perform a weighted good morning.

Regression

Increase the angle of the machine so the body is closer to perpendicular to the ground.

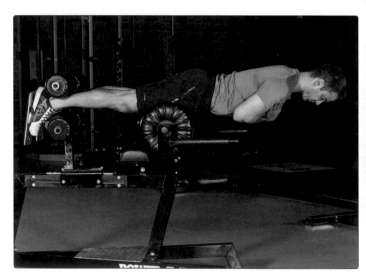

Starting position

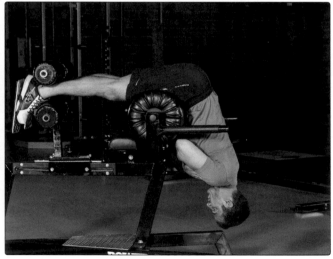

Bottom position

BODYWEIGHT EXERCISES

WIDE-GRIP PULL-UP: PRIMARY EXERCISE

Starting Position

Grasp a pull-up bar slightly wider than shoulder-width apart with palms facing forward. Hang from the bar with the elbows fully extended. The eyes should be focused forward or slightly upward.

Upward Movement

Simultaneously flex the elbows while adducting the shoulders so the body rises. The entire body should remain perpendicular to the ground throughout the movement. Continue the upward movement until the chin crosses above the pull-up bar.

Downward Movement

Extend the elbows and abduct the shoulders so that the body lowers. Continue the downward movement until the starting position is achieved.

Common Errors

- Using the lower body to generate momentum to propel the body upward
- Not allowing the elbows to fully extend at the end of each repetition
- Not raising the body enough to allow the chin to cross above the bar

Major Muscles Involved

latissimus dorsi, teres major, middle trapezius, rhomboids, posterior deltoids

Field Alternative

This exercise can be performed by hanging from any structure that is strong enough to support the body weight.

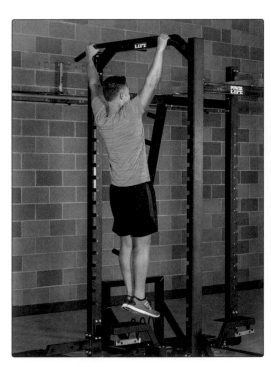

Starting position

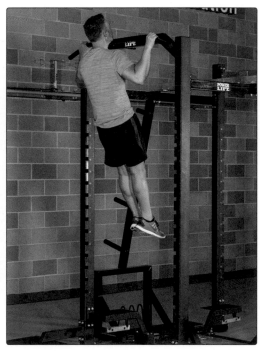

Top position

BODYWEIGHT EXERCISES

CLOSE-GRIP PULL-UP: PRIMARY EXERCISE

Starting Position

Grasp a pull-up bar with the palms facing each other. Hang from the bar with both arms fully extended. The eyes should be focused forward or slightly upward.

Upward Movement

Simultaneously flex the elbows and extend the shoulders so the body rises. The entire body should remain perpendicular to the ground throughout the movement. Continue the upward movement until the chin crosses above the pull-up bar.

Downward Movement

Extend the elbows and flex the shoulders to lower the body. Continue the downward movement until the starting position is achieved.

Common Errors

- Using the lower body to generate momentum to propel the body upward
- Not allowing the elbow to fully extend at the end of each repetition
- Not raising the body enough to allow the chin to cross above the bar

Major Muscles Involved

latissimus dorsi, teres major, middle trapezius, rhomboids, posterior deltoids

Field Alternative

This exercise can be performed by hanging from any structure that is strong enough to support the body weight.

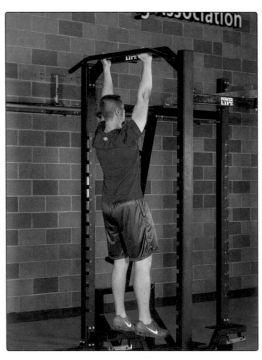

Starting position

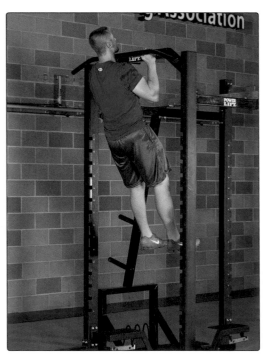

Top position

BODYWEIGHT EXERCISES

REVERSE-GRIP PULL-UP: PRIMARY EXERCISE

Starting Position

Grasp a pull-up bar at a shoulder-width distance with the palms facing the body. Hang from the bar with the elbows fully extended. The eyes should be focused forward or slightly upward.

Upward Movement

Simultaneously flex the elbows and extend the shoulders so the body rises. The entire body should remain perpendicular to the ground throughout the movement. Continue the upward movement until the chin crosses above the pull-up bar.

Downward Movement

Extend the elbows and flex the shoulders so that the body lowers. Continue the downward movement until the starting position is achieved.

Common Errors

- Using the lower body to generate momentum to propel the body upward
- Not allowing the elbows to fully extend at the end of each repetition
- Not raising the body enough to allow the chin to cross above the bar

Major Muscles Involved

latissimus dorsi, teres major, middle trapezius, rhomboids, posterior deltoids

Field Alternative

This exercise can be performed by hanging from any structure that is strong enough to support the body weight.

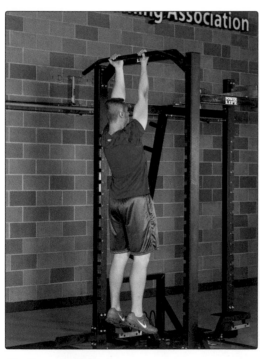

Starting position

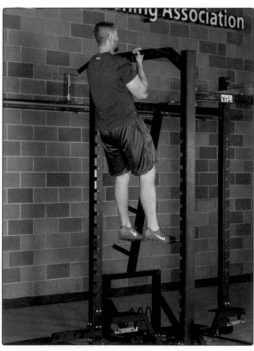

Top position

BODYWEIGHT EXERCISES

PUSH-UP: PRIMARY EXERCISE

Starting Position

Lie prone on the ground with the toes extended so the bottoms of the toes are flat on the ground. Place the hands slightly wider than shoulder-width apart, in line with the shoulders. The hands should be flat on the ground in a position that allows the upper arm to achieve a 45° angle from the torso.

Upward Movement

Simultaneously extend the elbows and flex and adduct the shoulders. The toes should stay flat on the ground, and the torso and legs should remain in line throughout the movement. Continue the upward movement until the elbows are fully extended.

Downward Movement

Flex the elbows and extend and abduct the shoulders. The torso and legs should remain in line, and the toes should remain flat on the ground. Continue the downward movement until the torso is a few inches (about 5 cm) from the ground.

Common Errors

- Failing to maintain alignment from the shoulders to the heels
- Failing to fully extend the elbows at the top of the movement

Major Muscles Involved

pectoralis major, anterior deltoids, triceps brachii

Regression

Elevate the hands on a box or other implement, leave the knees on the ground during the exercise, or do both.

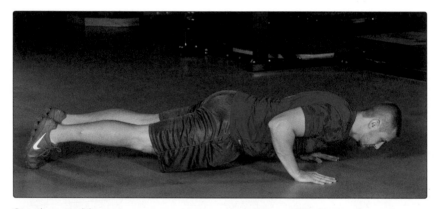

Starting position

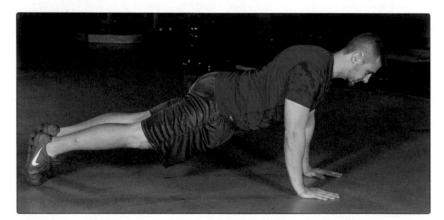

Upward movement

BODYWEIGHT EXERCISES

SINGLE-LEG PUSH-UP: PRIMARY EXERCISE

Starting Position

Lie prone on the ground with the toes of one foot extended and flat on the ground. Place the hands slightly wider than shoulder-width apart and in line with the shoulders. The opposite leg should be elevated off the ground a few inches (several centimeters) by slightly extending the hip. The elevated leg will remain in this position throughout the movement. The hands should be flat on the ground in a position that allows the upper arms to achieve 45° angles from the torso.

Upward Movement

Simultaneously extend the elbows and flex and adduct the shoulders. The toes of the foot on the ground should stay flat on the ground, and the torso and legs should remain in line throughout the movement. Continue the upward movement until the elbows are fully extended.

Downward Movement

Flex the elbows and extend and abduct the shoulders. The torso and legs should remain in line, and the toes of the foot on the ground should remain flat on the ground. Continue the downward movement until the torso is a few inches (about 5 cm) from the ground. Switch the starting position of the feet by placing the lifted foot on the ground and then lifting the foot that was on the ground, and then repeat to complete one repetition.

Common Errors

- Failing to maintain alignment from the shoulders to the heels
- Failing to fully extend the elbows at the top of the movement
- Allowing the pelvis to lose a parallel position with the ground

Major Muscles Involved

pectoralis major, anterior deltoids, triceps brachii

Regression

Elevate the hands on a box or other implement.

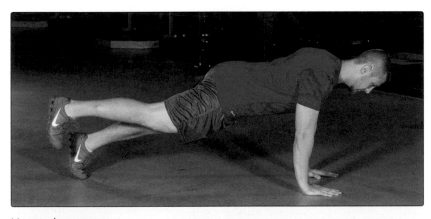

Upward movement

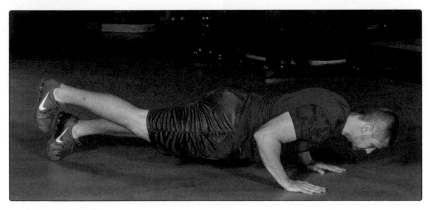

Bottom position

BODYWEIGHT EXERCISES

INVERTED ROW: PRIMARY EXERCISE

Starting Position

Stand with the feet flat on the ground and the hands holding handles attached to straps or another implement that allows the torso to achieve an angle of less than 90° from the ground. The shoulders should be flexed with the arms perpendicular to the body. The torso should be inclined backward at an angle that is appropriate for the lifter; the lower the angle of the torso from the ground, the greater the difficulty of the movement. The greatest difficulty will be achieved by elevating the feet slightly so the entire body is parallel to the ground.

Upward Movement

Flex the elbows and extend the shoulders to pull the torso toward the strap handles. Continue this movement until the handles are in line with the front of the chest. The body should remain in line from the heels to the shoulders throughout the movement, and only the arms should move.

Downward Movement

Extend the elbows and flex the shoulders to lower the body. Continue this movement until the starting position is achieved.

Common Errors

- Allowing the hips to flex or extend during the movement
- Failing to control the downward motion of the movement
- Flexing or extending the neck during the movement
- Failing to fully extend the elbows at the bottom of the movement

Major Muscles Involved

latissimus dorsi, teres major, middle trapezius, rhomboids, posterior deltoids

Field Alternative

This exercise can be performed with any piece of equipment that can be grasped and will support the body weight.

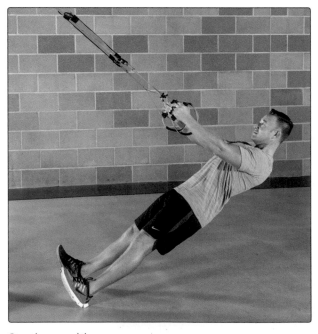

Starting position

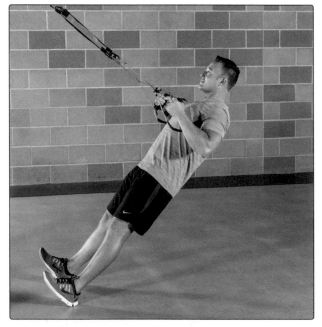

Top position

ALTERNATIVE EXERCISES

KETTLEBELL SWING: PRIMARY EXERCISE

Starting Position

Stand with the feet approximately hip-width apart. Grasp a kettlebell with both hands and an overhand grip with the arms inside the knees. The kettlebell should be at approximately knee height between the legs. The knees and hips should be flexed with the back in a neutral position at approximately a 45° angle to the ground and the feet flat on the ground.

Upward Movement

Extend the hips and knees, keeping the elbows extended and allowing the shoulders to passively flex so that the kettlebell travels up in front of the body. The back should remain in a neutral position throughout the exercise. Continue the upward movement until the knees and hips are extended with the kettlebell at chest level, with the elbows extended and the torso perpendicular to the ground.

Downward Movement

Flex the hips (sit backward) and knees and extend the shoulders while keeping the elbows extended, allowing the kettlebell to travel downward between the legs. The back should remain in a neutral position throughout the exercise. Continue descending until the kettlebell has traveled between the legs and is slightly behind the hips.

Common Errors

- Allowing the spine to flex round forward
- Using the upper body rather than the hips to create momentum
- Hyperextending the back at the top of the exercise

Major Muscles Involved

gluteus maximus, semimembranosus, semitendinosus, biceps femoris, vastus lateralis, vastus intermedius, vastus medialis, rectus femoris

Field Alternative

This exercise can be performed in the field with a weighted piece of equipment (e.g., an ammo can) as long as the equipment can be lifted using safe and effective technique.

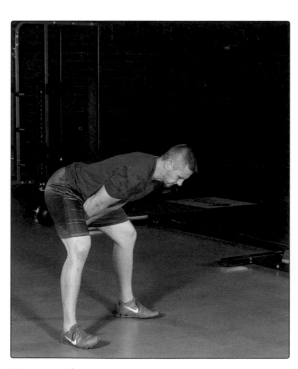

Downward movement

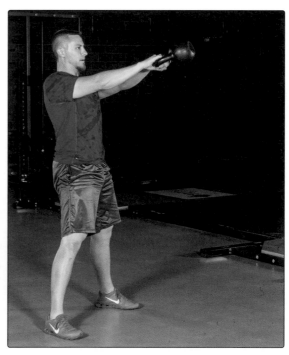

Top position

ALTERNATIVE EXERCISES

SINGLE-ARM KETTLEBELL SWING: PRIMARY EXERCISE

Starting Position

Stand with the feet approximately hip-width apart. Grasp a kettlebell with an overhand grip with one hand and the arm inside the knees. The kettlebell should be at approximately knee height between the legs. The opposite arm (without the kettlebell) should remain at the lifter's side out of the path of the kettlebell. The knees and hips should be flexed with the back in a neutral position at approximately a 45° angle to the ground and the feet flat on the ground.

Upward Movement

Extend the hips and knees, keeping the elbow extended and allowing the shoulder to passively flex so that the kettlebell travels in front of the body. The back should remain in a neutral position throughout the exercise. Continue the upward movement until the knees and hips are extended with the kettlebell at chest level, with the elbow extended and the torso perpendicular to the ground.

Downward Movement

Flex the hips (sit backward) and knees and extend the shoulder while keeping the elbow extended, allowing the kettlebell to travel downward between the legs. The back should remain in a neutral position throughout the exercise. Continue descending until the kettlebell has traveled between the legs and is slightly behind the hips.

Common Errors

- Allowing the spine to flex round forward
- Using the upper body rather than the hips to create momentum for the lift
- Hyperextending the back at the top of the exercise

Major Muscles Involved

gluteus maximus, semimembranosus, semitendinosus, biceps femoris, vastus lateralis, vastus intermedius, vastus medialis, rectus femoris

Field Alternative

This exercise can be performed in the field with a weighted piece of equipment (e.g., an ammo can) as long as the equipment can be lifted using safe and effective technique.

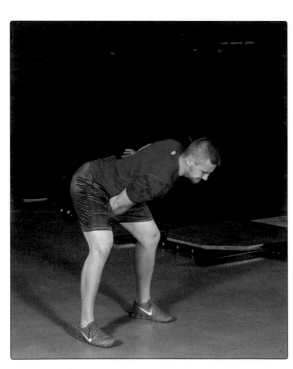

Downward movement

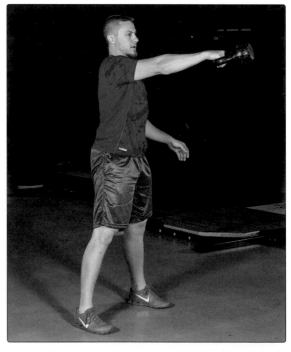

Top position

ALTERNATIVE EXERCISES

SUSPENSION SQUAT: FRONT SQUAT REGRESSION

Starting Position

Grasp the handles (one in each hand) of the extended suspension strap with a closed, neutral grip and stand approximately arm's length away with the upper arms next to the torso and the elbows flexed to approximately 90°. The feet should be shoulder-width or slightly wider than shoulder-width apart with a neutral back position.

Downward Movement

Simultaneously flex the hips (sit backward) and knees to descend in a controlled manner. The knees should stay positioned over the feet with the feet flat on the ground. The torso should remain erect throughout the movement, and the head should maintain a neutral position with the eyes focused either straight ahead or slightly upward. Continue the downward movement until the thighs are parallel to the ground or as far as quality technique can be maintained. Throughout the movement, maintain a hold on the suspension strap; the shoulders will flex and the elbows will extend as the body descends.

Upward Movement

Simultaneously extend the knees and hips to return to the starting position. Keep the knees positioned over the feet with the feet flat on the ground. Use the suspension strap as needed to provide assistance during the upward movement by pulling on the strap handles while extending the shoulder and flexing the elbows.

Common Errors

- Leaning too far backward during the downward phase of the movement
- Allowing the knees to move toward each other and lose alignment over the feet
- Allowing the heels to come off the ground during the exercise

Major Muscles Involved

gluteus maximus, semimembranosus, semitendinosus, biceps femoris, vastus lateralis, vastus intermedius, vastus medialis, rectus femoris

Field Alternative

This exercise can be performed in the field by holding onto the bumper of a vehicle or any other surface that will safely support the body weight.

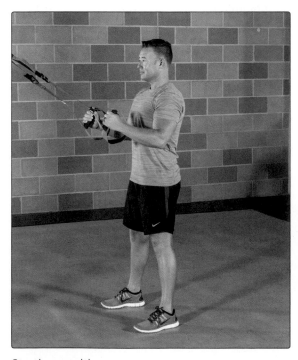

Starting position

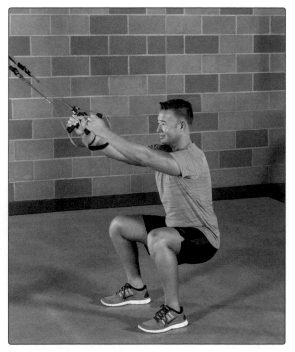

Bottom position

ALTERNATIVE EXERCISES

SUSPENSION PISTOL SQUAT: PRIMARY EXERCISE

Starting Position

Grasp the handles (one in each hand) of the extended suspension strap with a closed, neutral grip and stand approximately arm's length away with the upper arms next to the torso and the elbows flexed to approximately 90°. The foot of one leg (support leg) should remain in contact with the ground throughout the movement. The other leg should be flexed at the hip with the knee extended so the foot is off the ground and the leg is in front of the body.

Downward Movement

Flex the hip (sit backward) and knee of the support leg to descend in a controlled manner. The knee should stay positioned over the foot, and the foot should remain flat on the ground. The torso should remain erect throughout the movement, and the head should maintain a neutral position with the eyes focused either straight ahead or slightly upward. Continue the downward movement until the thigh of the support leg is parallel to the ground or as far as quality technique can be maintained. Throughout the movement, maintain a hold on the suspension strap; the shoulders will flex and the elbows will extend as the body descends.

Upward Movement

Simultaneously extend the knee and hip of the support leg to return to the starting position. Keep the knee of the support leg positioned over the foot, and keep the foot flat on the ground. Use the suspension strap as needed to provide assistance during the upward movement by pulling on the strap handles while extending the shoulder and flexing the elbows. At the end of the set, switch the support leg and the leg in front, and then repeat the movement.

Common Errors

- Leaning too far backward during the downward phase of the movement
- Allowing the knee of the support leg to lose alignment over the foot
- Allowing the heel of the support leg to come off the ground during the exercise

Major Muscles Involved

gluteus maximus, semimembranosus, semitendinosus, biceps femoris, vastus lateralis, vastus intermedius, vastus medialis, rectus femoris

Field Alternative

This exercise can be performed in the field by holding onto the bumper of a vehicle or any other surface that will safely support the body weight.

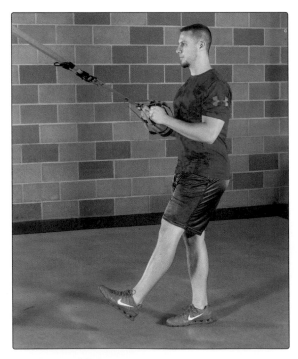

Starting position

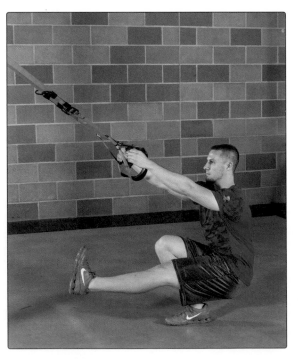

Bottom position

ALTERNATIVE EXERCISES

SUSPENSION SPLIT SQUAT: PRIMARY EXERCISE

Starting Position

Stand with one foot flat on the ground in front of the body (support leg), with the hip and knee slightly flexed. The foot of the opposite leg (trail leg) should be placed in the handle of the suspension strap behind the body, with the hip extended and the knee flexed. The torso should be in an upright position perpendicular to the ground.

Downward Movement

Simultaneously flex the hip and knee of the support leg and extend the hip and flex the knee of the trail leg to descend in a controlled manner. The knee of the support leg should stay aligned with the foot, and the foot should stay flat on the ground. The torso should remain erect throughout the movement, and the head should maintain a neutral position with the eyes focused either straight ahead or slightly upward. Continue the downward movement until the thigh of the support leg is parallel to the ground or as far as quality technique can be maintained.

Upward Movement

Simultaneously extend the knee and hip of the support leg to return to the starting position. Keep the knee of the support leg positioned over the foot, and keep the foot flat on the ground. The trail leg in the suspension strap should be used only for support and should not be used to assist the upward movement. At the end of the set, switch the support leg and the trail leg, and then repeat the movement.

Common Errors

- Leaning forward during the downward phase of the movement
- Allowing the knee of the support leg to lose alignment over the foot
- Using the trail leg to push during the upward phase of the movement

Major Muscles Involved

gluteus maximus, semimembranosus, semitendinosus, biceps femoris, vastus lateralis, vastus intermedius, vastus medialis, rectus femoris

Field Alternative

This exercise can be performed in the field by holding onto the bumper of a vehicle or any other surface that will safely support the body weight.

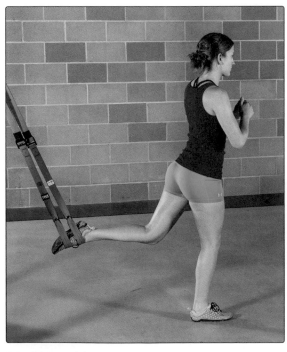

Starting position

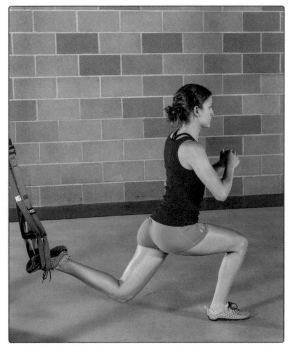

Bottom position

ALTERNATIVE EXERCISES

▌ MEDICINE BALL SQUAT TO PRESS: PRIMARY EXERCISE

Starting Position

Pick up a medicine ball and hold it directly in front of the chest with the elbows flexed. Place one hand on each side of the medicine ball with the base of each palm slightly underneath the medicine ball. The feet should be shoulder-width or slightly wider than shoulder-width apart.

Downward Movement

Flex the hips (sit backward) and knees. The knees should stay aligned over the feet, and the feet should stay flat on the ground. Continue descending until the thighs achieve a position parallel to the ground or as far as quality technique can be maintained. The medicine ball should remain directly in front of the chest during the downward movement.

Upward Movement

Simultaneously extend the knees and hips while flexing the shoulders and extending the elbows to push the medicine ball upward, allowing it to leave the hands. This movement should be done as quickly as possible while maintaining proper technique.

Continue pushing the medicine ball up until the elbows and knees are fully extended. Allow the medicine ball to fall to the ground before beginning the next repetition.

Common Errors

- Allowing the shoulders and back to round forward or hyperextend
- Allowing the knees to move toward each other and losing alignment over the feet

Major Muscles Involved

gluteus maximus, semimembranosus, semitendinosus, biceps femoris, vastus lateralis, vastus intermedius, vastus medialis, rectus femoris, soleus, gastrocnemius, deltoids, trapezius, triceps brachii

Field Alternative

This exercise can be performed with a sandbag or any implement that can be thrown into the air safely without damaging the surface on which it will land.

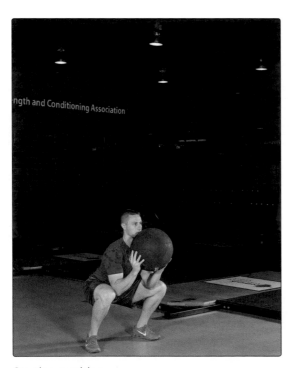

Starting position

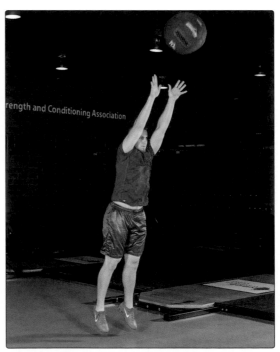

Top position

ALTERNATIVE EXERCISES

KETTLEBELL HALF GET-UP: PRIMARY EXERCISE

Starting Position

Lie on the ground in a supine position with a kettlebell in the left hand. The left arm should be flexed at the shoulder and extended at the elbow to hold the kettlebell over the chest. The right arm should be flat on the ground at approximately a 45° angle to the torso. The left knee and hip should be flexed so the left foot is flat on the ground. The right leg should be extended at the hip and knee so it is flat on the ground.

Upward Movement

While keeping the eyes focused on the kettlebell, begin the exercise by pushing up against the kettlebell. To do so, simultaneously push into the ground with the left foot to rotate the hips and torso so that the body is balanced on the right forearm and right hip. Continue to press up against the kettlebell and transition from the right forearm to the right hand. With the left foot still flat on the ground, continue extending the left hip until the left knee is flexed approximately 90°. The top position is with the arms in a straight line nearly perpendicular to the ground and the kettlebell directly above the shoulders, elbows, and right hand.

Downward Movement

Begin the downward movement by flexing the hips and shoulder to lower the torso toward the ground. Continue the downward movement until the starting position is achieved. At the end of the set, repeat the movement with the opposite arm.

Common Errors

- Allowing the arm holding the kettlebell to lose perpendicular alignment with the ground
- Allowing the arm holding the kettlebell to lose alignment with the torso
- Allowing the legs to come off the ground during the upward movement

Major Muscles

gluteus maximus, semimembranosus, semitendinosus, biceps femoris, vastus lateralis, vastus intermedius, vastus medialis, rectus femoris, anterior deltoid, pectoralis major, triceps brachii, rectus abdominis

Field Alternatives

This exercise can be performed with any piece of equipment that can be safely held in the hand during the movement (e.g., an unloaded weapon, axe, or shovel).

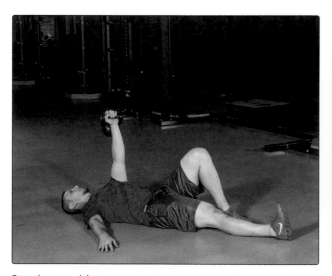

Starting position

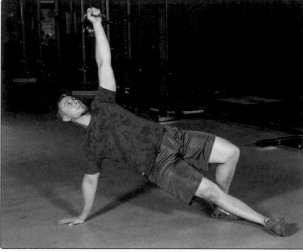

Top position

■ BOTTOMS-UP KETTLEBELL PRESS

Starting Position

Stand with the feet about shoulder-width apart. The knees should be slightly flexed and remain in this position throughout the movement. Hold a kettlebell in the hand of one arm, with the other arm relaxed at the side of the torso. The kettlebell should be gripped with the weighted portion (the bell of the kettlebell) above the hand and the handle (a tight grip must be maintained throughout the movement to keep the kettlebell in this upright position) and the hand directly under the chin and the palm facing inward.

Upward Movement

Simultaneously extend the elbow while abducting and flexing the shoulder and externally rotating the forearm until the dumbbell is overhead with the palm facing forward and the elbow fully extended. Continue the upward movement until the elbow is fully extended with the palm facing forward.

Downward Movement

Flex the elbow while adducting and extending the shoulder and rotating the hand so the kettlebell descends inward. Continue until the starting position is achieved. After performing the desired number of repetitions, repeat on the opposite side.

Common Errors

- Placing the opposite hand on the hip to assist with balance
- Not allowing the elbow to fully extend and the shoulder to fully flex at the top of each repetition
- Not bringing the kettlebell back underneath the chin at the bottom of each repetition

Major Muscles Involved

anterior and medial deltoids, triceps brachii

Field Alternative

This exercise can be performed using a sandbag, other implement, or other piece of equipment.

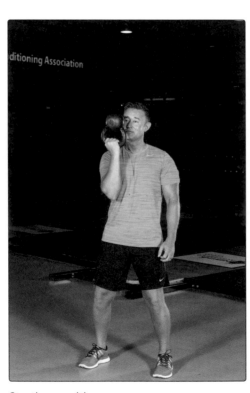

Starting position

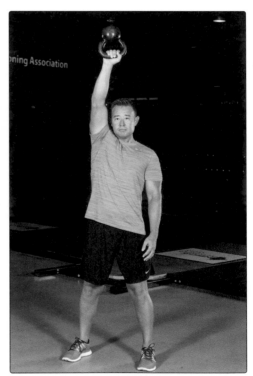

Top position

ALTERNATIVE EXERCISES

MEDICINE BALL SLAM: PRIMARY EXERCISE

Starting Position

Stand with the feet slightly wider than hip-width apart while holding a medicine ball overhead. The shoulders should be flexed and the elbows should be slightly flexed. This exercise should be performed on a surface that will not be damaged by the medicine ball and that will not damage the medicine ball. A medicine ball that does not bounce is recommended for safety reasons.

Downward Movement

Simultaneously flex the hips and knees while extending the shoulders to bring the medicine ball in front of the body toward the ground. The torso should remain upright throughout the movement with the eyes focused forward. When the upper arms are a few inches (about 5 cm) from the torso, extend the elbows to continue the path of the medicine ball toward the ground. As the elbows approach full extension, throw the medicine ball toward the ground.

Upward Movement

Pick up the medicine ball and return to the starting position.

Common Errors

- Allowing the torso to lose a perpendicular position with the ground
- Not allowing the hips to flex during the downward movement
- Not allowing the knees to flex during the downward movement

Major Muscles Involved

latissimus dorsi, deltoids, triceps brachii, rectus abdominis

Field Alternative

This exercise can be performed with a sandbag or any other implement that will not be damaged during the exercise or cause damage to the surface on which it will land.

Regression

This exercise can be performed at a very controlled speed in order to accommodate all ability levels.

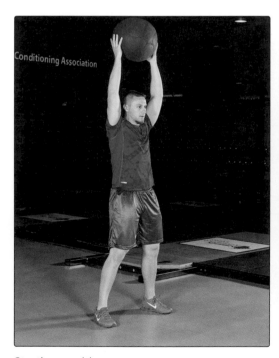

Starting position

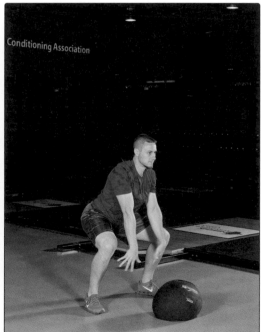

Bottom position

ALTERNATIVE EXERCISES

MEDICINE BALL CHEST PASS FROM SPLIT STANCE: PRIMARY EXERCISE

Starting Position

Facing an open area or wall that can withstand the impact of the medicine ball, assume a staggered stance with the front foot forward of the hips and the trail foot behind the hips. Hold a medicine ball slightly lower than chest level, with the elbows flexed and one hand on each side of the medicine ball. The shoulders should be extended so the forearms are parallel to the ground. Both knees should be slightly flexed.

Forward Movement

Push off the trail leg by extending the knee and the hip to propel the body forward. Simultaneously extend the elbows and flex the shoulders to push the medicine ball forward. Continue this movement until the trail foot begins to leave the ground, coming forward. At this point the elbows should be extended and the shoulders flexed so the arms are parallel to the ground. This momentum will allow the medicine ball to continue forward after leaving the hands.

Recovery Phase

As soon as the medicine ball leaves the hands, the trail leg will continue to come forward by flexing the hip and the knee until it crosses the opposite leg (which started in front and remains on the ground throughout the movement). At this point, place the foot on the ground and continue to flex the knee and the hip to soften the landing. Recover the medicine ball and repeat with the opposite foot starting forward to complete one repetition.

Common Errors

- Starting the exercise with the forearms perpendicular to the ground
- Letting the trail leg return to the ground before the medicine ball is released
- Failing to push with the trail leg while simultaneously pushing forward with the arms
- Rotating the torso to push primarily with one arm

Major Muscles Involved

pectoralis major, anterior deltoids, triceps brachii

Field Alternative

This exercise can be completed with a sandbag or any other implement that can be thrown safely.

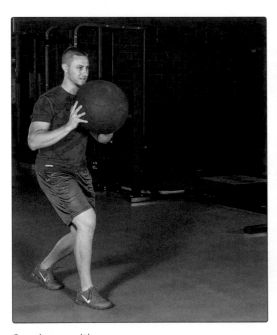

Starting position

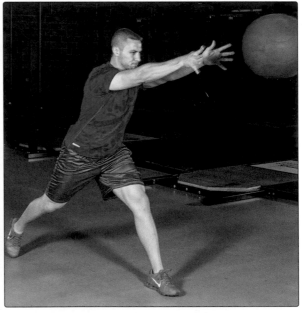

Release position

ALTERNATIVE EXERCISES

SUSPENSION PUSH-UP: PUSH-UP PROGRESSION

Starting Position

Lie prone on the ground with the feet hooked in the handles of a suspension strap, approximately 1 foot (30 cm) off the ground. Place the hands slightly wider than shoulder-width apart, in line with the shoulders. The hands should be flat on the ground in a position that allows the upper arm to achieve a 45° angle from the torso.

Upward Movement

Simultaneously extend the elbows and flex and adduct the shoulders. The feet should stay together while hooked in the suspension straps, with the torso and legs in line throughout the movement. Continue the upward movement until the elbows are fully extended.

Downward Movement

Flex the elbows and extend and abduct the shoulders. The torso and legs should remain in line, and the feet should remain hooked in the suspension strap. Continue the downward movement until the torso is a few inches (about 5 cm) from the ground.

Common Errors

- Failing to maintain alignment from the shoulders to the heels
- Failing to fully extend the elbows at the top of the movement
- Allowing the feet to separate or sway side to side during the movement

Major Muscles Involved

pectoralis major, anterior deltoids, triceps brachii

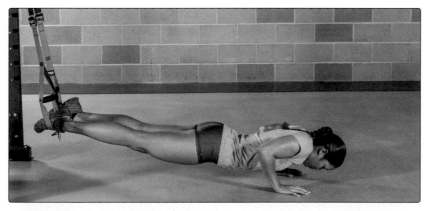

Starting position

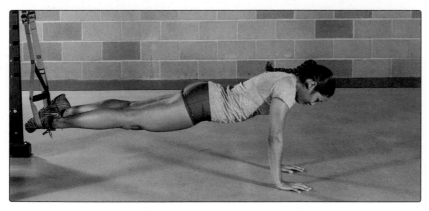

Upward movement

ALTERNATIVE EXERCISES

SINGLE-ARM SUSPENSION ROW: INVERTED ROW PROGRESSION

Starting Position

Stand with the feet flat on the ground and one hand holding a handle (or both handles, depending on the design) of a suspension strap that allows the torso to achieve an angle of less than 90° from the ground. The arm that is not holding the suspension handle should be held at the lifter's side. The shoulder of the arm holding the strap should be flexed with the arm perpendicular to the body. The torso should be inclined backward at an angle that is appropriate for the lifter; the lower the angle of the torso from the ground, the greater the difficulty of the movement. The greatest difficulty will be achieved by elevating the feet slightly so the entire body is parallel to the ground.

Upward Movement

Flex the elbow and extend the shoulder to pull the torso toward the strap handle. Continue this movement until the handle is in line with the front of the chest. The body should remain in line from the heels to the shoulders throughout the movement, and the torso should not rotate during any portion of the movement.

Downward Movement

Extend the elbow and flex the shoulder to lower the body. Continue this movement until the starting position is achieved. At the end of the set, repeat the movement with the opposite arm.

Common Errors

- Allowing the hips to flex or extend during the movement
- Allowing the torso to rotate during the movement
- Flexing or extending the neck during the movement

Major Muscles Involved

latissimus dorsi, teres major, middle trapezius, rhomboids, posterior deltoids

Field Alternative

This exercise can be performed with any piece of equipment that can be grasped and will support the body weight.

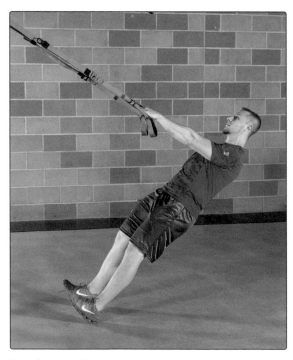

Starting position

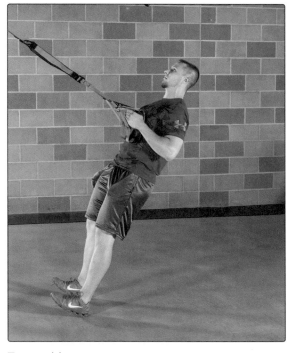

Top position

CONCLUSION

During any training session, regardless of the setting, it is imperative to use proper technique during each repetition of each exercise to reduce injury risk and to achieve the desired training result. If a tactical athlete is unable to perform the proper technique for an exercise, use a regression exercise to allow the athlete to perform the exercise successfully and work toward the training objective. In a field setting or an environ-ment where traditional training equipment is not available, use alternative training implements to perform alternative exercises.

Key Point

Regardless of the training environment and equipment, tactical athletes should use proper technique for each repetition of each exercise to ensure their health is maintained and performance improved.

Key Terms

alternating grip
antecubital area
inguinal fold
neutral back position

regression
sticking point
structural exercise
Valsalva maneuver

Study Questions

1. Spotting should be used for safety purposes during all of the following exercises EXCEPT

   a. power snatch

   b. back squat

   c. dumbbell shoulder press

   d. bench press

2. Which of the following is a common error of the barbell deadlift exercise?

   a. extending the knees and hips until the torso is perpendicular to the ground

   b. fully extending the knees before starting to extend the hips

   c. keeping the barbell in close proximity to the legs

   d. maintaining a neutral back position throughout the exercise

3. Which of the following is an exercise regression for an athlete who is unable to properly perform the front squat?

   a. Zercher squat

   b. goblet squat

   c. back squat

   d. single-leg squat

4. Which of following exercises specifically targets the gluteus maximus, semitendinosus, semimembranosus, biceps femoris, and erector spinae muscles?

   a. step-up

   b. push press

   c. front squat

   d. Romanian deadlift

Chapter 12

Flexibility and Mobility Exercise Techniques and Programming

Mark Stephenson, MS, ATC, CSCS,*D, TSAC-F

Daniel J. Dodd, PhD, CSCS

After completing this chapter, you will be able to

- describe various types of flexibility exercises and myofascial release (MR) techniques;
- describe proper technique and instructional cues for flexibility and mobility exercises; and
- design flexibility and mobility programs based on the training status, goals, and occupational demands of tactical athletes.

Increasing the performance of tactical athletes often involves a focus on the development of muscular strength, muscular endurance, muscular power, and cardiorespiratory efficiency. Although these areas are crucial for tactical athletes, mobility and flexibility are equally significant. Mobility and flexibility programs contribute to the development of the aforementioned fitness components, but more importantly, they enhance the ability of tactical athletes to perform occupational duties. In addition, including a well-designed mobility and flexibility program in a strength and conditioning intervention can help tactical athletes recover so they can repeat their duties over time.

The demands placed on tactical athletes vary significantly, and the athlete's ability to perform optimally depends on a multitude of factors, such as age, training and injury history, years of service, and job requirements. Regardless, the ability to move efficiently and effortlessly remains vital for all tactical athletes. This chapter addresses the importance of both mobility and flexibility for the tactical athlete's performance. Mobility and flexibility are essential for not only the efficiency but also the coordination of movement (21), and prescribing individualized, job-specific mobility and flexibility exercises will enhance tactical athletes' ability to meet their occupational demands while minimizing functional limitations (39). The purpose of this chapter is to explore mobility and flexibility, including the various types of each modality; identify appropriate exercises and technique; and discuss program design for the tactical athlete.

COMPARISON OF MOBILITY AND FLEXIBILITY

For the purposes of this chapter, **mobility** refers to the coordination and efficiency of movement throughout joint **range of motion (ROM)**. For example, in the forward lunge, the exerciser takes an exaggerated step forward with one leg to a position where there is a 90° knee angle in both legs. Mobility often involves movements using multiple joints and relies on the activation and coordination of neuromuscular action along

with joint stability to perform a controlled movement. **Flexibility** refers to the ability of muscles and tendons to go through the full ROM about a joint. For instance, when an exerciser sits with the legs extended and bends forward as far as possible, the ability to reach the toes indicates the level of flexibility at the hip joint and lumbar spine. Flexibility differs from mobility in that it typically focuses on one joint and measures the capacity to move throughout the joint ROM. Mobility, on the other hand, is concerned with how well a person can perform movements without having to compromise or make an adjustment to complete the movement. Both mobility and flexibility are key components for the optimal function of the kinetic chain during dynamic movements (53).

The daily demands of tactical athletes such as firefighters, police officers, and military personnel are ever evolving and thus may result in alterations to the athlete's physical structure, particularly over time. To sustain functional performance and maintain health and physical fitness, it is essential to regularly assess and address flexibility and mobility, just as one should for muscular strength, power, and cardiorespiratory endurance (26).

Mobility

The coordination and efficiency of movement are vital to tactical athletes, who may find themselves undertaking tasks such as squatting, kneeling, or crawling for prolonged durations, sometimes while under load (equipment). By maintaining appropriate mobility, tactical athletes improve their ability to successfully complete tasks. In addition, these athletes often perform unilateral and bilateral movements, and they need to maintain mobility and prevent imbalances or alignment issues from decreasing their motor coordination and movement efficiency. A lack of mobility is closely associated with faulty alignment and restricted movement due to tight muscles, or the inability of weaker muscles to move a body part through its ROM (35).

Aging is one factor that may lead to reduced mobility. Tactical athletes encompass a wide range of ages and experience, the youngest being

18 years of age and the oldest beyond 50 years, each with varied years of service and job-specific demands. The ability to perform at a necessary level becomes extremely important as one ages. With age, fibrous connective tissue gradually replaces degenerating muscle tissue, a process known as **fibrosis** (3, 15). This new fibrous tissue is not as pliable as the original tissue, therefore increasing joint stiffness and limiting flexibility. A gradual decline in flexibility as a result of muscle and connective tissue degradation can affect the health and performance of a tactical athlete. For example, a significant decrease in flexibility is often accompanied by a decrease in joint mobility, and as result, it can decrease performance and increase injury risk. The tactical athlete must be able to move efficiently with coordinated movement in many positions and environments, and improving and maintaining mobility is an issue of safety and effectiveness on the job.

Tactical athletes may also find themselves in a static position (e.g., sitting) during nontraining hours, which has been shown to lead to adaptive shortening, a tightness resulting from muscles remaining in a shortened position (35). Thus, the need for a structured program becomes even more critical.

Key Point

> Flexibility and joint mobility provide the foundation for movement and are key to developing strength, speed, agility, power, and endurance. The tactical athlete needs flexibility to generate movement and mobility to perform well with negligible limitations.

Factors Affecting Mobility and Flexibility

The ability to develop and sustain mobility and flexibility can be directly affected by **physiological factors** (e.g., age, gender, physical activity level, body composition) and **kinesiological factors** (e.g., origin and insertions of muscle and tendons, joint structure and integrity, muscle CSA). These distinct factors affect mobility and flexibility in varying ways. Although some of these factors cannot be altered with training, others, such as physical activity and body composition, can be manipulated to develop the necessary mobility and flexibility for tactical occupations (3, 15).

Physiological Factors

The age, gender, range of physical activity, and body composition of an individual can all affect mobility and flexibility. As people age, there appears to be a common decline in not only function but flexibility, and the level of decline is associated with both the development of limiting conditions and a reduction in physical activity (2). Conditions such as **sarcopenia** (loss of muscle tissue), fibrosis (increased muscle stiffness), and **arthritis** (joint pain and stiffness) have been shown to decrease flexibility with age. Additionally, physical inactivity and disuse also lead to a loss of joint mobility and flexibility (29). In contrast, increased amounts of exercise, particularly resistance training, have been shown to decrease the impact of the aforementioned conditions (19, 34), helping to maintain joint and tissue integrity and thus maintain movement capabilities.

Body composition, specifically the distribution of body fat and muscle mass, also influences mobility and flexibility. The size of a body segment may prevent or greatly reduce ROM around or about the joint (15), particularly if neighboring tissue or body segments (whether due to high levels of subcutaneous fat or muscle mass) hinder the movement. This may limit the ability to perform certain movements; however, it does not necessarily indicate a lack of flexibility in the muscles or joints (29).

Kinesiological Factors

Muscles, tendons, ligaments, and bones are all involved in movement and ROM. The primary function of muscle and connective tissue is to produce movement through contraction and the development of tension. When muscles contract, tension develops, which is then transmitted to bones by the attaching tendons, and subsequently movement occurs (2). The interaction of muscle, tendon, and bone along with the support of adjoining connective tissue and the individual joint capsule is where flexibility is needed to promote movement throughout the body. Each of these elements is integral in not only allowing muscle shortening but also muscle lengthening, and it is within these elements that a direct physiological relationship to levels of mobility and flexibility occurs (2).

Myofibrils are elements of muscles that contract, relax, and elongate. They are composed of functional units called *sarcomeres*, which contain myosin and actin filaments, along with a connecting filament called *titin* (2). Myosin and actin are adjoining contractile elements of muscle, and they are directly responsible for the shortening of and development of tension within the muscle. When muscles are stretched, the myosin and actin filaments begin to separate and the titin filaments begin to lengthen. As stretching continues, titin filaments lengthen further until reaching a resting tension, at which point resistance to the stretch occurs. If stretching continues, the integrity of the sarcomere may be compromised or injured. Research has shown that a sarcomere can stretch to 150% of its resting length before injury occurs (62).

Both neurophysiological and mechanical factors are thought to be responsible for the acute response to the stretching of muscles. When changes in muscle length occur, neural receptors detect the extent of change and initiate a response to prevent **overstretching** and injury. To prevent injury, skeletal muscles contain two types of nerve fiber receptors that monitor when muscle lengthening is occurring: **Golgi tendon organs (GTOs)** and **muscle spindles**. GTOs detect levels of muscle tension, particularly during muscle contraction, and are activated during excessive stretching. Muscle spindles primarily respond to dynamic (length and speed of stretch) and tonic (length of stretch) response (2). Muscle spindles are also responsible for initiating the **stretch reflex**, a neuromuscular response to sudden increases in muscle length resulting in a subsequent shortening contraction of the muscle to prevent further elongation. However, the influence of the stretch reflex can be somewhat negated through **reciprocal inhibition**. When a muscle (agonist) contracts to cause movement, typically an opposing muscle (antagonist) relaxes to allow contraction to take place. It is this neural response that can allow a muscle to become more flexible. When stretching a muscle (or muscle group), the active contraction of the opposing muscle allows the stretched

muscle to relax and inhibits the stretch reflex, so the muscle further lengthens. The goal of flexibility training is to minimize the reflex activity of a muscle, reducing resistance to the stretch and therefore increasing joint ROM (38). Understanding these concepts is helpful for choosing stretching exercises to make the greatest impact on a person's flexibility.

Other kinesiological factors, such as the origin and insertion points of muscle and tendons, joint structure and integrity, and muscle CSA, all differ among individuals, leading to various levels of flexibility as well as responses to mobility and flexibility training. The point of origin and insertion of a tendon to a bone could largely affect the ROM about a joint. ROM could depend upon limb lengths and the relationship of muscle to bone, as well as the corresponding joint structures and the supporting connective tissue.

The structure of a joint often dictates the ROM that occurs at a particular segment of the body. Joint structure pertains to the overall dynamics of a joint, including joint capsule, ligaments, tendons, and muscle spanning the joint, as well as joint geometry (29). For example, hip and shoulder joints provide greater ROM in multiple directions compared with more fixed joints, such as the elbow, knee, ankle, and wrist, which are limited by their anatomical structure and have less ROM and less directional movement.

In addition, the surrounding and supporting connective tissue is an important component of flexibility. Connective tissue affects mobility by determining the ROM of the joint. In particular, two types of connective tissue contribute to flexibility: collagen and elastic tissue. Because connective tissue is made up of varying amounts of **collagen** and **elastin** (i.e., elastic tissue), it has a major effect on both mobility and flexibility (15). Tissue that contains collagen, such as ligaments and tendons, is rigid and restricts ROM, whereas elastic tissue allows greater ROM. Connective tissue such as fascia is composed primarily of elastic tissue (15). This is particularly important in designing flexibility programs because incorrect stretching may result in excessive stretching of the joint. Joint integrity is based predominantly on the stiffness and stability of the joint and can be explained by the amount of stiffness of the joint capsule and ligaments (47% of total joint stiffness), muscle fascia (41%), tendons (10%), and skin (2%) (33).

The joint capsule, ligaments, and tendons account for the majority of joint stiffness; however, they contain lower levels of elastic tissue than muscle fascia, the key to improving flexibility. The more elastic the muscle fascia, the greater the flexibility can be obtained and the less resistance to joint elongation. On the other hand, lack of elasticity in the capsule, ligament, and tendons may create instability in the joint if they are over-stretched (2). The less stable and less stiff a joint becomes, the more flexibility it has; however, the more stable the joint becomes, the less flexible the surrounding muscles and connective tissue are (35). This is the primary reason why mobility and flexibility programs should be based on individual needs and undergo regular assessment.

Key Point

Ideal levels of flexibility and mobility require a balance between joint stiffness and joint instability, and they are largely affected by genetic makeup as well as controllable factors such as physical activity, body composition, and recovery. Achieving optimal flexibility and mobility depends on how well these factors are taken into consideration.

TYPES OF FLEXIBILITY AND MOBILITY EXERCISES

There are many forms of mobility and flexibility, and each plays a distinct role in the development and sustainment of optimal performance and health. Stretching the muscles, tendons, and connective tissue is common among athletes of all kinds (9, 17, 26). The four main types of stretching are static, ballistic, dynamic, and proprioceptive neuromuscular facilitation (PNF). All four types have been shown to improve ROM within the muscle (25); however, certain types may be more beneficial depending on the circumstances, goal, or needs of the individual (40).

Static Stretching

Static stretching involves a slow stretch of the muscle to its end ROM with a static hold for up to 90 seconds. Historically, it has been the most common type of flexibility exercise, especially during warm-ups (5, 15, 54, 55). It requires little energy, and the slow, controlled movement allows the stretch to be performed easily and safely (54). The two types of static stretching are static passive and static active.

1. *Static passive*: The more common of the two, it involves slowly bringing the muscle to its furthest end ROM and holding it for 15 to 90 seconds without further movement.

2. *Static active*: Involves contracting the opposing muscle group to bring the muscle to its furthest end point and then holding the limb in position for 15 to 90 seconds.

Static stretching has been widely regarded as an effective method of increasing flexibility and mobility (54). It is also thought to decrease the risk of injury, although there is no conclusive evidence to support this (7, 12, 20, 32, 46, 66). There is some controversy regarding the effects of static stretching before exercise (53). Studies have suggested that static stretching may actually decrease maximal force production, jump height, and sprint speed, as well as increase reaction time and impair proprioceptive balance (46, 48, 67). This effect has been referred to as **stretch-induced strength loss**, and it has been linked to a loss of neural activation in the stretched muscle, an important mechanism for strength, power, and speed output (40). Rubini et al. (48) also showed significant reductions in strength due to preexercise static stretching, and they concluded that for people whose jobs require strength and power, static stretching prior to activity may compromise the ability to perform with optimal strength and power. The long-term effects of static stretching on performance, however, are unknown (7).

Proprioceptive Neuromuscular Facilitation (PNF) Stretching

Proprioceptive neuromuscular facilitation (PNF) uses muscle contractions and relaxation to increase ROM. Usually done with the assistance of a partner, PNF involves both passive movement and active muscle contractions (3, 15). The voluntary action of the agonist muscle causes neural activation, thereby causing reciprocal inhibition of the antagonist muscle group and allowing greater ROM (20). It is commonly believed that

PNF stretching is the most effective technique to increase flexibility (11, 18, 30, 44, 51, 58, 61); however, there is inconsistent evidence to support this (14, 16). There are three types of PNF techniques: hold-relax (8, 10, 11, 51, 58), contract-relax (8, 11), and hold-relax with agonist contraction (10, 42). Performing the hold-relax coupled with an agonist contraction is more effective for increasing flexibility than using the hold-relax or contract-relax techniques independently (25).

Hold-Relax

The muscle is passively stretched by the partner to the point of discomfort and held for 10 seconds. At this point, the exerciser performs an isometric contraction while the partner resists for 6 seconds before relaxing the stretched muscle. Then the muscle is passively stretched further, to the new point of discomfort, and held for 30 seconds. Repeat three to four times.

Contract-Relax

The muscle is passively stretched to the point of discomfort and held for 10 seconds. The exerciser then performs a concentric contraction of the stretched leg while the partner resists through the full ROM and then relaxes. Then the muscle is passively stretched further, to the new point of discomfort, and held for 30 seconds. Repeat three to four times.

Hold-Relax With Agonist Contraction

As in the hold-relax technique, the muscle is passively stretched to the point of discomfort and held for 10 seconds before performing an isometric contraction while the partner resists for approximately 6 seconds. The exerciser relaxes before contracting the agonist muscle group while the partner passively stretches it further, to the new point of discomfort, and holds for 30 seconds. Repeat three to four times.

Dynamic and Ballistic Stretching

Dynamic stretching uses controlled movements to help activate the muscles and tendons prior to activity. It typically involves activity-specific movements and forcefully controlled movements within an active range of motion in which an individual should function for a given sport (3,

12, 15). Dynamic stretching has been shown to negate any stretch-induced strength loss (28, 31) and to improve sprinting, jumping, and generating peak force (46). This is perhaps due to the neuromuscular preparation and activation of the musculotendinous junctions (60).

Ballistic stretching involves forceful movements such as bouncing, swinging, or jerking using one's own body weight to produce the force, and the end point is not held. This style of stretching generally exceeds the end ROM, may produce more pain and microtears to the muscle fibers, and usually triggers the stretch reflex, which does not allow the muscle to relax, a key component of increasing flexibility. Ballistic stretching involves similar movements as static passive stretching, but in a fast bobbing or jerking motion (14). Historically, it has been commonly used as a warm-up before activities involving high-acceleration sprints or jerky movements, such as in track, dance, or gymnastics (3, 5, 12, 15). However, because it may result in connective tissue trauma, local muscular soreness, and heightened injury risk, it is not recommended for tactical athletes. Though tactical athletes work in environments that require periods of acceleration and explosive power, such as law enforcement personnel sprinting after a suspect or military personnel moving between positions, the potentially negative outcomes of ballistic stretching may compromise job performance (14, 59).

Key Point

> A dynamic warm-up is a general warm-up (5-10 minutes of aerobic activity) combined with a dynamic flexibility routine. It is commonly used with athletic populations before practice and games to elicit physiological and sport-specific responses in preparation for the activity.

Myofascial Release (MR): Massage and Foam Rolling

Myofascia or fascia is the connective tissue that covers the muscles. It can be restricted by injury, disease, inactivity, or inflammation, and as a result it loses elasticity and begins to bind together, causing **fibrous adhesions** (36). These adhesions may not only become painful but also decrease ROM, muscle length, strength, endurance, motor coordination, and soft tissue extensibility (6, 13, 56). Fascia has an important link to mobility and flexibility due to its elastic qualities, providing the greatest potential for stretch (15).

Myofascial release (MR) is a manual therapy developed by Barnes (6) to help relieve and reduce adhesions within the fascia. It involves massage or trigger-point therapy in which a health care provider, such as an athletic trainer, physical therapist, or a licensed massage therapist, provides manual pressure to the affected area (22). Physiotherapists spend approximately 45% of their time providing massage therapy to aid recovery and improve sport performance (22). Massage therapy is often an underrated and underutilized therapeutic procedure that improves circulation, promotes muscle relaxation, loosens scar tissue, stretches tight muscles and fascia, and relieves muscle spasms (35). It has also been shown to help HR and DBP recover to preexercise levels after high-intensity exercise (4) and to reduce exercise-induced fatigue (42, 44). This is particularly important for tactical athletes who experience episodes of high cardiovascular demand, such as firefighters, where the risk of a cardiac event is significant. Massage therapy may not always be practical because it requires a third-party therapist. However, **self-myofascial release (SMR)**, which uses foam rollers or dense implements such as baseballs or golf balls, can be performed by an individual without the assistance of others. It is becoming a more common practice and may provide a suitable alternative to massage therapy.

Implements such as foam rollers allow the user to manipulate the soft tissue by applying the sustained pressure needed to help release fascial adhesions. Individuals are able to use their own body weight in varying positions to isolate soft tissue areas and apply pressure to those areas in a manner similar to massage therapy (27). This pressure helps soften and lengthen the fascia. The generation of friction between the fascia and the implement (foam roller) warms the fascia, helping it take on a fluid form (known as the *thixotropic property* of fascia); breaks down scar tissue and adhesions between the skin, muscle, and bone; and restores soft tissue extensibility (52). There is limited peer-reviewed research on SMR for improving mobility and flexibility; however, MacDonald et al. (36) showed that as little as 2 minutes of slow, undulating rolling on a high-pressure foam roller enhanced quadriceps ROM to levels similar to those resulting from static stretching. The foam rolling had no effect on force output, an argument commonly used against static stretching (36). The research on SMR and performance enhancement is also minimal (23, 65), but there have been studies supporting the use of SMR to enhance mood and reduce exercise-induced fatigue (27, 39, 63, 64). Healey et al. (27) showed postexercise fatigue to be significantly less after foam rolling and suggested that the reduced fatigue might allow participants to extend their acute workout time and volume and possibly enhance long-term performance.

EXERCISE TECHNIQUE AND CUEING GUIDELINES

The following section contains exercise technique and cueing guidelines for the primary types of stretching:

- Static stretching exercises
- PNF stretching exercises
- Dynamic stretching exercises, including mobility exercises (mobility hurdles and a medicine ball circuit), yoga, and other dynamic stretches
- MR exercises, with instructions for foam rolling

As with any exercises—whether resistance exercises, aerobic training, or stretching—care must be taken by the TSAC Facilitator to ensure that the given exercises are implemented at the appropriate time (given the targeted training goals) and with the optimal technique. Failure to do so may not only increase risk of injury but also inhibit the likelihood of optimizing training goals. A TSAC Facilitator cannot assume that tactical athletes are aware of the correct stretching techniques or aware of bad habits they are unintentionally using in their training. An understanding of optimal stretching technique is a critical component of any training program.

The advantage of static stretching lies primarily in the ability to hold a stretch for a prolonged time, decreasing passive resistance to the stretch (40). The elastic properties of muscle allow a stretched muscle to return to its original length once the stretch has ceased; however, if a stretch is held for a prolonged time (i.e., 15-90 seconds), muscle compliance increases (1), thus increasing the time the muscle takes to return to its original length. If continued, over time it may lead to changes in the viscoelastic properties of muscle and explain gains in ROM (13).

An optimal static stretching prescription of intensity, frequency, and duration to decrease passive resistance has been indeterminate. Intensity is the subjective assessment of discomfort by the exerciser and largely depends on individual pain tolerance (40). Given the differences in individual pain tolerance, length of stretch-hold time appears to be a more suitable prescription item. Research has shown that a static stretching frequency and duration of two to five sets of 15- to 90-second stretches decreases resistance to stretch and increases acute levels of flexibility (37, 38, 41, 49). Based on these recommendations, four to five sets of 30- to 60-second stretches are suggested to decrease resistance and improve flexibility (24, 40). Note, however, that if both agonist and antagonist muscles of the major segments of the body are stretched using these guidelines, it may take 40 to 60 minutes to complete the exercises (40), certainly a major consideration in terms of goals, objectives, and priorities in program design.

QUADRICEPS

STANDING QUADRICEPS STRETCH

In a standing position, bring one foot toward the hips and grasp the ankle. Pull the ankle toward the buttocks and gently push the hip forward. Hold for 30 to 60 seconds per leg, and repeat four to five times.

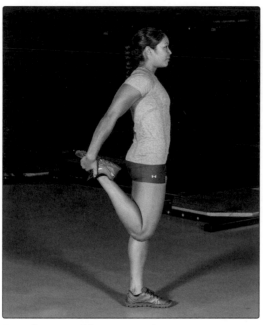

Standing quadriceps stretch

LYING QUADRICEPS STRETCH

Lying on one side, flex the knee, bring one foot toward the hips, and grasp the ankle. Pull the ankle slightly toward the buttocks and gently push the hip forward. Hold for 30 to 60 seconds per leg, and repeat four to five times.

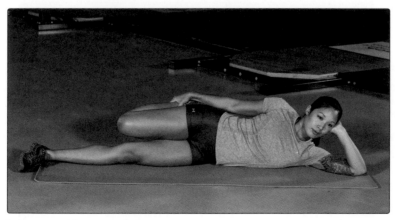

Lying quadriceps stretch

HAMSTRINGS

STANDING HAMSTRING STRETCH

In a standing position, step forward with one foot, keeping the back leg straight and the front leg slightly bent. Point the toes on the front foot back toward the shin and bend forward (keeping the spine neutral) until a stretch is felt in the back of the front leg. Progress to a slightly straighter front leg if an increase in stretch is required. Hold for 30 to 60 seconds per leg, and repeat four to five times.

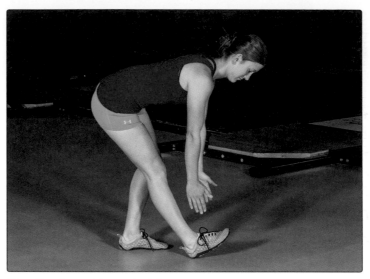

Standing hamstrings stretch

SEATED HAMSTRING STRETCH

In a seated position, keeping one leg straight and one knee flexed (foot of the flexed leg positioned on the inner thigh of the straight leg), slowly bend forward along the line of the extended leg until the point of discomfort is met, and hold for 30 to 60 seconds. Repeat four to five times per leg.

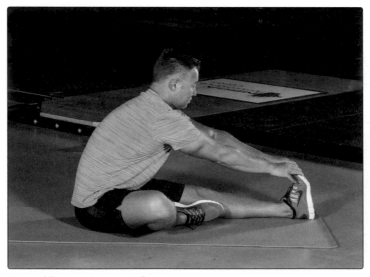

Seated hamstring stretch

ADDUCTORS (GROIN)

SEATED ADDUCTOR STRETCH

In a seated position, bring the soles of the feet together in front of the body. Place a hand on the inner surface of the lower leg and rest the forearm across the inner surface of knee of each leg; gently push down until the point of discomfort is met. Hold for 30 to 60 seconds, and repeat four to five times.

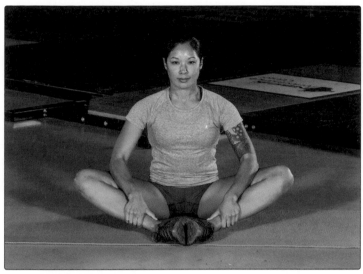

Seated adductor stretch

LATERAL ADDUCTOR STRETCH

In a wide stance with the feet pointing forward, bend one knee and slowly lower the body to the same side while keeping the opposite leg straight until the point of discomfort is met. Hold for 30 to 60 seconds, and repeat four to five times per leg.

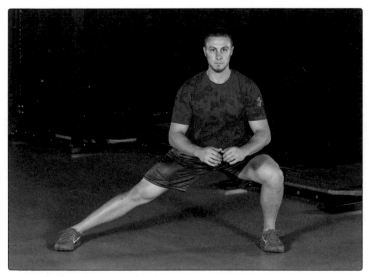

Lateral adductor stretch

CALF

GASTROCNEMIUS AND SOLEUS STRETCH

In a staggered stance with one foot forward (knee bent) and the other foot back (leg straight), lean forward while maintaining a flat rear foot until the point of discomfort is met in the rear lower leg. Hold this position for 30 to 60 seconds per leg, and repeat four to five times.

Additional progression: Repeat the movement, but instead of maintaining a straight rear leg, bend the back knee and lower the body toward the ground while keeping the back foot flat against the ground.

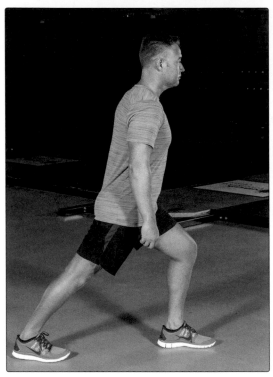 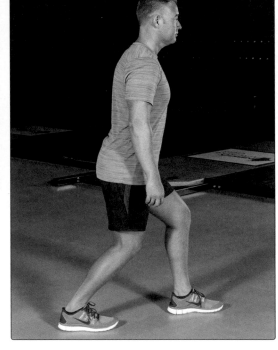

Gastrocnemius and soleus stretch

HIP AND LOW BACK

PRETZEL STRETCH

In a supine lying position, bend the right knee so that the right foot is flat on the floor. Cross the left leg over the right so that the left ankle rests on the lower third of the right thigh. Use the hands to grab the left knee and pull it gently toward the opposite shoulder until the point of discomfort is met in the hips and buttocks. Hold for 30 to 60 seconds per leg, and repeat four to five times.

Adjustment: If unable to raise the leg toward the chest, perform this stretch in a seated position, as shown in the second photo.

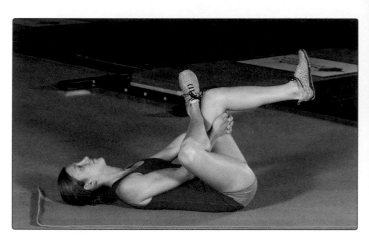
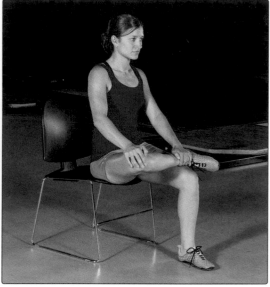

Pretzel stretch

FORWARD LUNGE

From a standing position, take an extended step forward and lower the body toward the ground until the back knee is resting on the ground and the front leg achieves a 90° angle. While maintaining an upright torso, gradually move the hips forward until slight discomfort is felt in the anterior hip of the rear leg. Hold for 30 to 60 seconds per leg, and repeat four to five times.

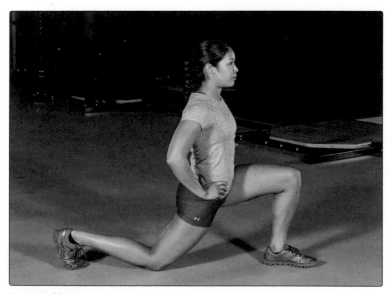

Forward lunge

HIP AND LOW BACK

KNEE TO CHEST

From a supine lying position with one leg extended and the other knee flexed, grasp the flexed leg with both hands just below the knee, pulling the knee toward the chest until the point of discomfort is met. Hold for 30 to 60 seconds per leg, and repeat four to five times.

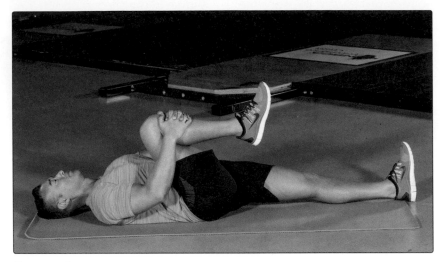

Knee to chest

NECK

LATERAL NECK FLEXION

From a seated or standing position, laterally flex the head to one side until the point of discomfort is felt on the opposing side. Hold for 30 to 60 seconds each side, and repeat four to five times.

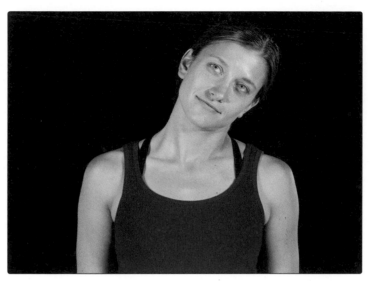

Lateral neck flexion

LATERAL NECK ROTATION

From a seated or standing position, laterally rotate the head to one side as if looking over the shoulder until the point of discomfort is felt on the opposing side. Hold for 30 to 60 seconds each side, and repeat four to five times.

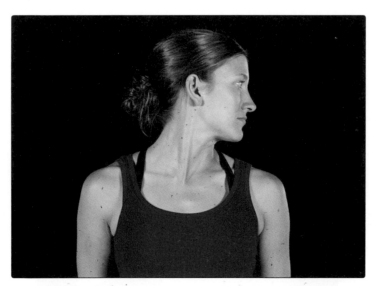

Lateral neck rotation

SHOULDERS AND CHEST

ANTERIOR SHOULDER AND CHEST STRETCH

From a standing position with arms fully extended behind the body, clasp the hands and gently move them upward while pushing the chest forward. Hold for 30 to 60 seconds, and repeat four to five times.

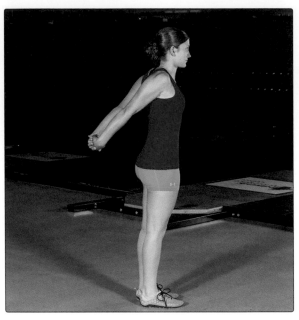

Anterior shoulder and chest stretch

CROSS-ARM STRETCH

From a seated or standing position, extend one arm across the body, keeping the shoulder depressed. Using the other arm, gently pull the extended arm until the point of discomfort is felt in the extended arm. Hold for 30 to 60 seconds per arm, and repeat four to five times.

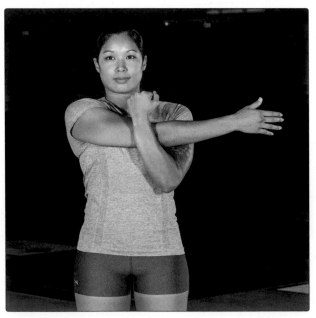

Cross-arm stretch

TORSO

SIDE BEND

From a standing position with arms fully extended overhead, clasp the hands and laterally flex to one side. Hold for 30 to 60 seconds per side, and repeat four to five times.

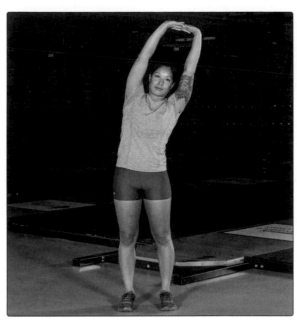

Side bend

PROPRIOCEPTIVE NEUROMUSCULAR FACILITATION (PNF) STRETCHING EXERCISES

Before undergoing any PNF routine, it is imperative that the person being stretched and the assisting partner both understand the proper technique. Both people should have thorough knowledge of the correct exercises to use, the appropriate placement of supporting hands or equipment, the amount of stretch to be performed (to the point of discomfort, not pain), and the degree of resistance being applied. Failure to do so may result in injury to the stretched person. As discussed earlier, three major techniques can be used in PNF stretching: hold-relax, contract-relax, and hold-relax with agonist contraction. Descriptions of these techniques and examples of exercises, including correction positioning, are outlined in this section.

HOLD-RELAX

Perform a passive stretch of the muscle to the point of mild discomfort and hold for 10 seconds. Apply an isometric hold against the PNF partner for 6 seconds before a short relaxation of the stretched muscle. Finally, perform a second passive stretch to the point of discomfort for 30 seconds.

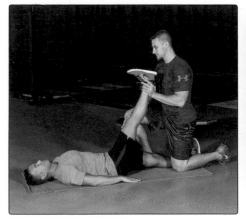 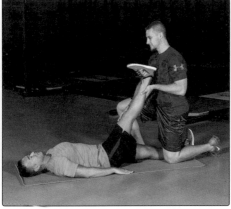 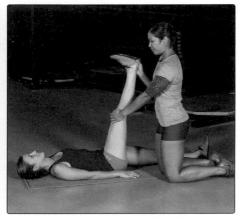

Passive stretch   Isometric resist   Passive restretch

CONTRACT-RELAX

Passively stretch the muscle to the point of mild discomfort and hold for 10 seconds. Perform a concentric muscle action of the stretched muscle through full ROM while the partner provides gentle resistance. Temporarily relax before a passive stretch is applied for 30 seconds to the point of mild discomfort.

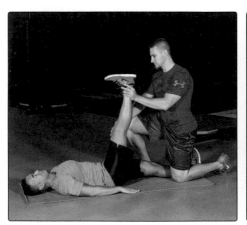 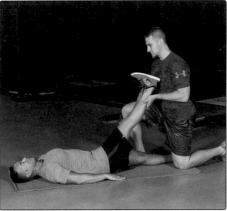 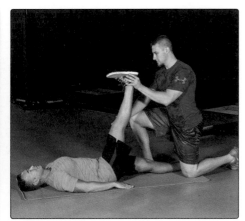

Passive stretch   Concentric contraction with resist   Passive restretch

HOLD-RELAX WITH AGONIST CONTRACTION

Perform a passive stretch of the muscle to the point of mild discomfort and hold for 10 seconds. Apply an isometric hold against the PNF partner for 6 seconds before a short relaxation of the stretched muscle. Finally, apply a concentric muscle action of the muscle (agonist) opposing the stretched muscle while a passive stretch is performed for 30 seconds.

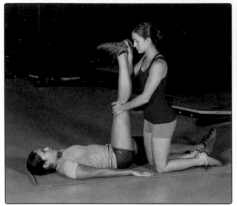

Passive stretch

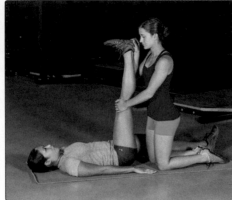

Isometric resist

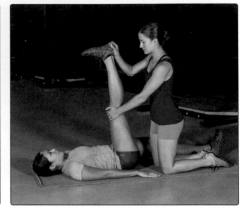

Agonist contraction

HAMSTRING STRETCH

Lie in a supine position with extended legs and hands by the sides (palms down). One leg will be passively raised to the point of discomfort. The assisting partner straddles the grounded leg and places one hand on the foot and the other on the thigh (just above the knee) on the stretched leg. Photos of hamstring PNF stretches using the three techniques were shown previously.

CALF STRETCH

Start in a seated position with the legs extended straight out. The partner can be positioned at the feet or raise the extended leg onto his shoulder.

The partner's hands are placed on the upper third of the feet.

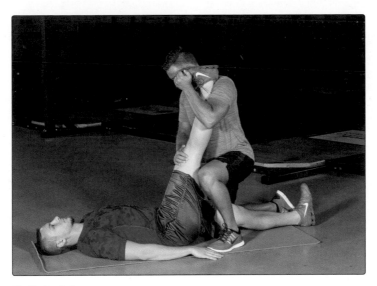

Calf stretch

GROIN STRETCH

Sit with both knees flexed and the soles of the feet together (butterfly position). The partner can be kneeling and positioned behind the exerciser.

The partner places one hand on the inner portion of each knee.

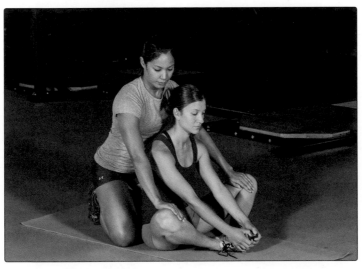

Groin stretch

QUADRICEPS AND HIP FLEXOR STRETCH

Lie in a prone position with both legs extended. The partner is positioned between the thighs of the exerciser and places one hand on the lower third of the stretched thigh.

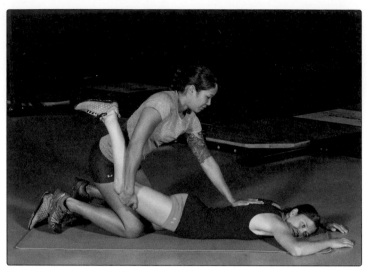

Quadriceps and hip flexor stretch

CHEST STRETCH

Sit or kneel with both arms abducted and hands interlocking behind the head. The partner stands behind the exerciser with one hand just above each elbow.

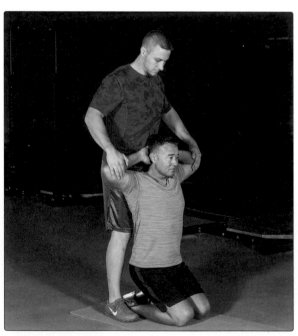

Chest stretch

SHOULDER STRETCH

Sit or kneel with both arms extended behind the body. The partner stands behind the exerciser with one hand grasping each wrist.

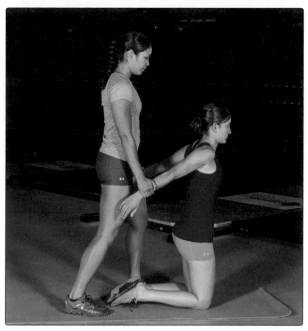

Shoulder stretch

Dynamic stretching should include exercises with movement patterns similar to job tasks. Body segments move through patterns intended to stretch the desired body part or muscle group. The goal of dynamic stretching is to elongate the muscle through a desired movement while maintaining blood flow, increasing body temperature, and promoting neuromuscular activation, all of which develop and maintain flexibility for the desired skill. Because this style of stretching focuses on sport-specific or occupation-specific movement patterns, it is an appropriate flexibility choice to prepare the individual for the upcoming physical activity.

Mobility exercises can be included in a warm-up to prepare for the upcoming session. Movements should progress from low to high intensity through full ROM. They can also be performed during the main workout session to address any deficiencies or maintain mobility for optimal performance during the session.

Yoga is a blend of static and dynamic movements that improve both flexibility and mobility. It is an ancient practice that brings the mind and body together, and it incorporates a variety of poses that both stretch and strengthen the muscles and tendons (47). Each pose incorporates a focus on breathing and requires the exerciser to pay attention to the body's alignment during the stretch. Yoga also includes static postures held for an extended time (i.e., 15-90 seconds). It gently lengthens the muscles, increases ROM, and relieves muscle tension and soreness (32).

The exercises in this section are just a few that can be used for dynamic flexibility. Other exercises may be added to the warm-up to gradually progress intensity and incorporate movements similar to those in the workout ahead.

MOBILITY HURDLES

Mobility hurdles can be used to train mobility and flexibility. For many of the following exercises, line up four to six mobility hurdles and place them at intervals of 2 feet (61 cm). Alternate the heights of each hurdle, beginning with low (stepping over) and then high (stepping under). Do not let the knee go to the side when stepping over. In most cases, set low hurdles at midthigh height and high hurdles at waist height.

FORWARD OVER AND UNDER

Standing in front of the low hurdle, raise one knee as high as possible. Step over the hurdle so the lead heel moves directly over the hurdle and lands flat on the ground. Bring the trail leg over the hurdle to return to a standing position. In one motion, squat to a height lower than the hurdle, step forward with the lead leg through the hurdle, and move the body under the hurdle so the trail leg returns to the start position. Continue through the hurdle series using the same lead leg. Change the lead leg and repeat the hurdle series. Repeat the hurdle series one to two times per leg.

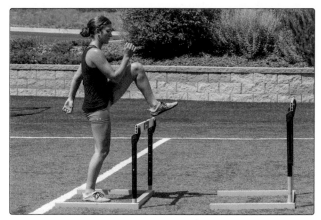

Stepping over the hurdle

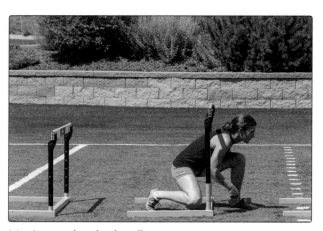

Moving under the hurdle

BACKWARD OVER AND UNDER

Standing with the back to the low hurdle, raise one knee as high as possible. Lean slightly forward and reach back over the hurdle so the lead heel moves directly over the hurdle and lands flat on the ground. Bring the trail leg over the hurdle to return to a standing position. In one motion, squat to a height lower than the hurdle, step back with the lead leg through the hurdle (unlike what is shown in the photo; the other leg should have been used), and move the body under the hurdle so the trail leg returns to the start position. Continue through the hurdle series using the same lead leg. Change the lead leg and repeat the hurdle series. Repeat the hurdle series one to two times per leg.

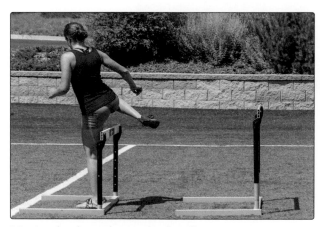

Moving backward over the hurdle

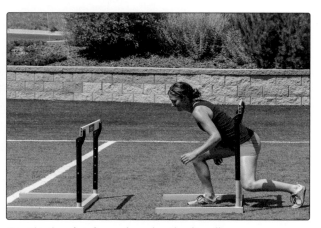

Continuing backward under the hurdle

MOBILITY HURDLES

LATERAL OVER AND UNDER

Standing to the side of the low hurdle, raise the knee of the lead leg (the leg next to the low hurdle) as high as possible. In one motion, abduct the lead leg and step over the hurdle. Raise the knee of the trail leg, adduct the leg, and bring it over the hurdle to return to a standing position. From this position, descend into a squat where the thighs are parallel to the hurdle or lower. Take a lateral step with the lead leg to reach through the high hurdle to the other side and then move the body under the hurdle to return to the starting position. Continue through the hurdle series using the same lead leg. Change the lead leg and repeat the hurdle series. Repeat the hurdle series one to two times per leg.

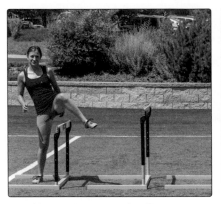

Lead leg going over the first hurdle

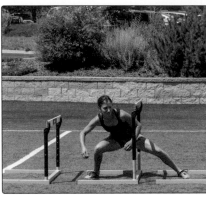

Lead leg going under the second hurdle

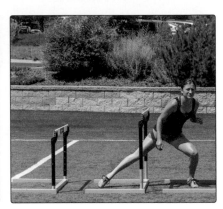

Trail leg going under the second hurdle

HIGH STEP

Line up four to six mobility arches and place them 1 foot (30 cm) apart or end to end. Set the hurdle to just below groin height. Begin by moving forward, stepping over the hurdle, and swinging the knee outward. The trail leg follows through, swinging the knee outward around the hurdle to return to a standing position. After completing the series moving forward, repeat it while moving backward, with the lead leg stepping back over the hurdle. The trail leg swings outside the hurdle and returns to a standing position.

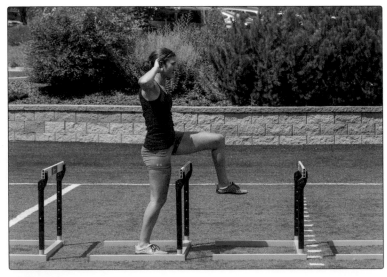

High step

MEDICINE BALL CIRCUIT

The following exercises can be used in a medicine ball circuit. All movements begin from an athletic position (see the photos) where the exerciser is in a half-squat position with the feet hip-width apart, shoulders back, and spine neutral. Be sure to follow the medicine ball with the head throughout the entire movement. Though these exercises are shown using a medicine ball, it is possible to use a dumbbell, kettlebell, or resistance band instead.

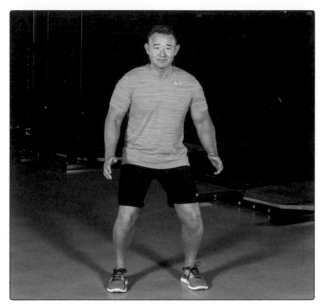

Athletic position: front view

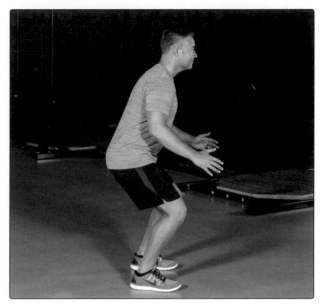

Athletic position: side view

ROCKY TWIST

Extend the arms holding a medicine ball at chest level. Rotate the arms to one side of the body, following the medicine ball with the head. Unlock the hips so they rotate with the arms. The back foot should also rotate toward the medicine ball. Repeat 5 to 10 times per side.

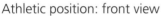

Starting position

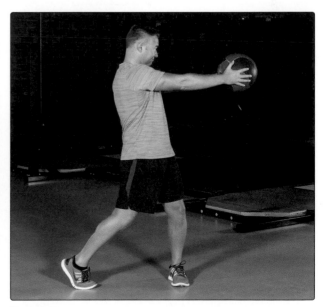

Rotation

MEDICINE BALL CIRCUIT

DIAGONAL CHOP TO HIP

Extend the arms holding a medicine ball over one shoulder. Swing the extended arms downward diagonally toward the opposite hip. Return to the starting position. Repeat 5 to 10 times per side.

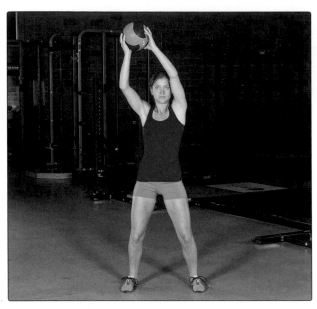

Starting position

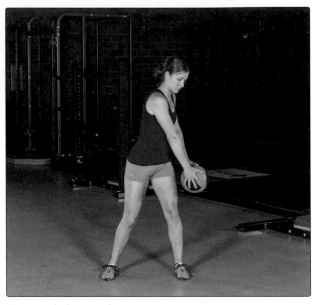

Diagonal chop to hip

DIAGONAL CHOP TO KNEE

Extend the arms holding a medicine ball over one shoulder. Begin by swinging the extended arms downward diagonally toward the opposite knee. Return to the starting position. Repeat the movement 5 to 10 times per side.

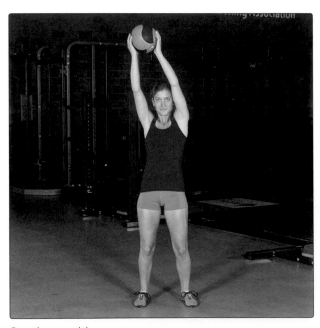

Starting position

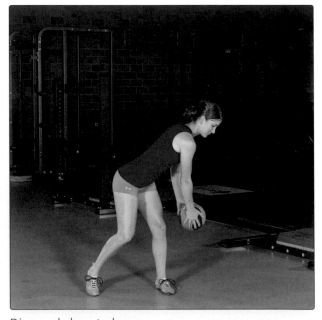

Diagonal chop to knee

MEDICINE BALL CIRCUIT

▌ DIAGONAL CHOP TO ANKLE

Extend the arms holding a medicine ball over one shoulder. Swing the extended arms downward diagonally toward the opposite ankle. Return to the starting position. Repeat the movement 5 to 10 times per side.

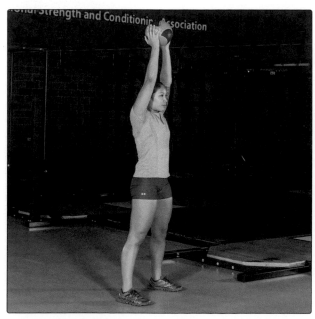

Starting position

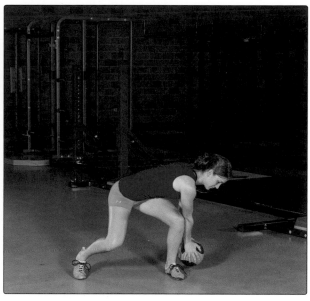

Diagonal chop to ankle

▌ WOOD CHOP

Extend the arms holding a medicine ball overhead. Swing the medicine ball with the extended arms downward through the legs. Be sure to squat during the downward motion and bend slightly forward to allow the medicine ball to pass through the legs. Maintain a neutral spine throughout the movement to avoid any rounding of the back.

Starting position

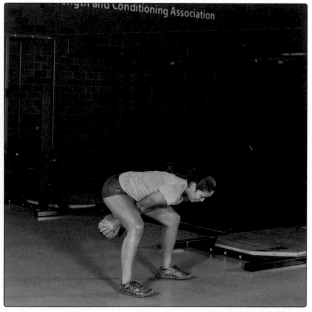

Downward swing

HIGH LUNGE

Step back with one leg and place the ball of the back foot flat on the floor. The front knee should be bent to about 90° with the front foot remaining flat on the ground. Lean forward, bringing the torso toward the front thigh. Hold for 30 to 60 seconds. Return to the starting position and repeat with the opposite leg. Repeat three to four times.

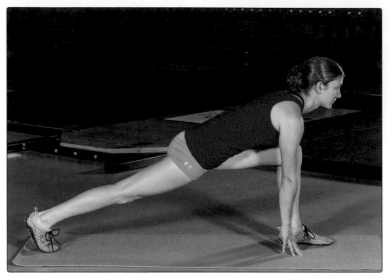

High lunge

LOW LUNGE

Step back with one leg to an extended lunge position and place the instep of the back foot on the floor. The front knee should be bent and should remain behind the line of the front toes. Drop the back knee to the floor, stretching the groin and thigh of the back leg and reaching up with both arms to elongate the torso. Hold for 30 to 60 seconds. Return to the starting position and repeat with the opposite leg. Repeat three to four times.

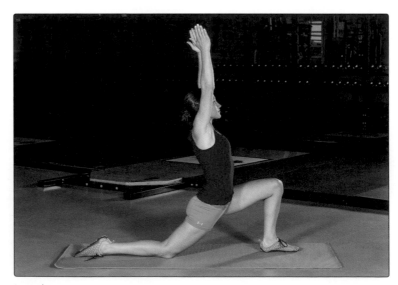

Low lunge

WARRIOR I

Step back with one leg and place the heel of the back foot on the floor with the toes pointed out at 45 degrees. The front knee should be slightly bent with the foot flat on the floor and the toes pointed forward. Reach up with both arms, elongating the torso. Hold for 30 to 60 seconds. Return to the starting position and repeat with the opposite leg. Repeat three to four times.

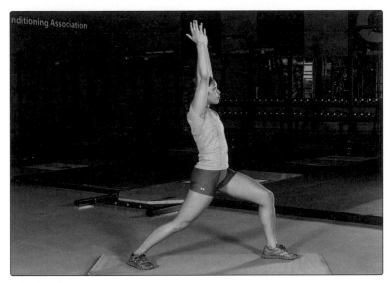

Warrior I

EXTENDED SIDE ANGLE

Get into a lunged position with the heel of the back foot on the floor. Rotate the torso to face perpendicular to the front leg. Rotate the back foot so that the toes face outward the same direction as the torso. The front knee should be bent to about 90° with the foot flat on the floor and the toes pointed forward. Reach up toward the head with the arm closest to the back leg, leaning the torso toward the front thigh. Reach down with the opposite arm, grasping the foot of the front leg. Hold for 30 to 60 seconds. Return to the starting position and repeat with the opposite leg. Repeat three to four times.

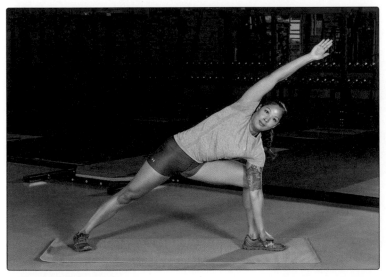

Extended side angle

DEAD PIGEON

Lie on the floor in a supine position and bring both knees toward the chest. Cross one ankle over the thigh of the opposite leg. Grasp the knee of the leg with the ankle crossed over it with both hands and pull the knee gently toward the chest. Hold for 30 to 60 seconds. Repeat with both legs three to four times.

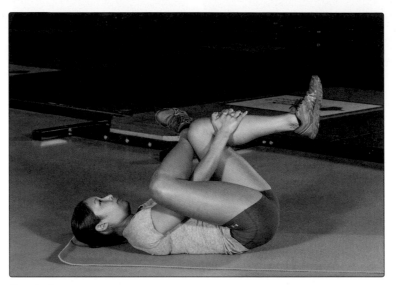

Dead pigeon

MODIFIED PIGEON

Begin in a quadruped position on both hands and knees. Bring one leg forward with the knee bent and place the outside of the knee on the floor with the foot behind the hand on the opposite side of the body. Bring the opposite leg straight back with the knee on the floor behind. Lean the torso forward gently and hold for 30 to 60 seconds. Repeat with both legs three to four times.

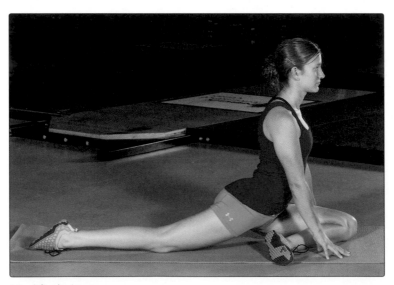

Modified pigeon

LOW BACK SERIES

Lie supine on the floor, arms abducted and extended, hips and knees at 90°, holding the feet off the ground. Slowly lower the bent knees to one side toward the floor, raise them back to the starting position, and repeat to the other side. Repeat 5 to 10 times per side.

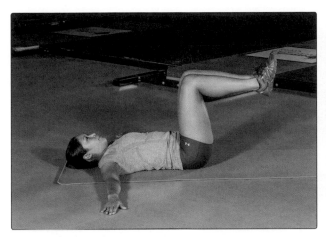

Low back: bent knee

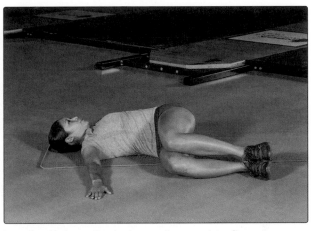

Low back: bent knee, knees lowered to floor

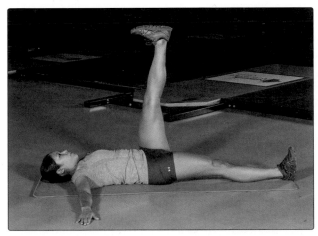

Low back: single leg

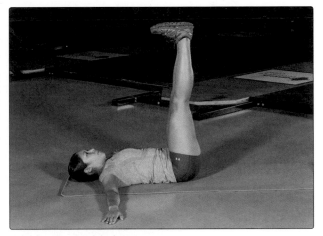

Low back: double leg

PRONE SPINAL TWIST

Lie prone on the floor, with arms abducted and extended to the sides, pressed firmly to the floor. Raise a heel toward the opposing hand by extend-ing and rotating at the hips. Return to the starting position. Alternate legs and repeat 5 to 10 times per side.

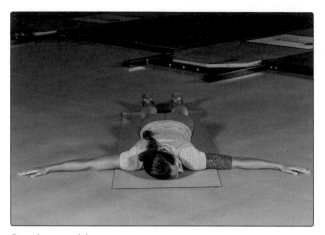

Starting position

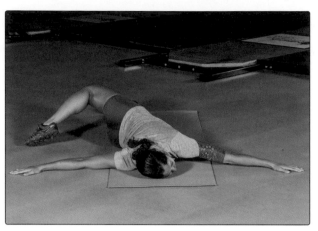

Stretched position: heel raised, hip rotated and extended

FORWARD LUNGE

Standing straight, take a large step forward with one leg to create a 90° angle of flexion in both knees. Keep the lower leg from touching the ground. Return to the starting position and alter-nate lead legs. Repeat 5 to 10 steps with both legs.

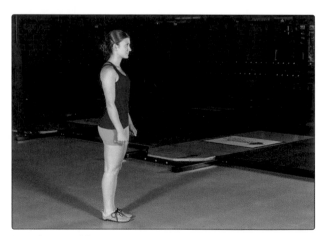

Starting position

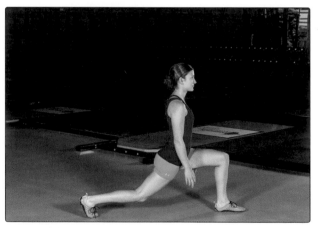

Forward lunge

LUNGE PROGRESSION

Lunge into an elbow-to-instep position and then move to a knee extension position: Repeat the forward lunge and then flex forward at the hips to bring the forearm of the same side as the lead leg toward the ground. After reaching the end point of the forward stretch, slowly shift the body weight backward and extend the lead leg into a hamstring stretch.

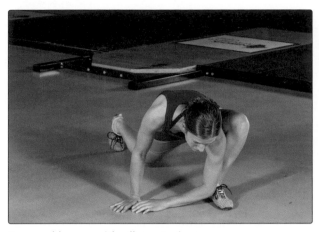

Forward lunge with elbow to instep

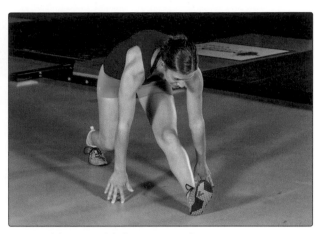

Forward lunge with knee extension

BACKWARD LUNGE WITH A TWIST

Standing straight, take a large step backward with one leg to create a 90° angle of flexion in both knees. Keep the lower leg from touching the ground. Twist the torso to the same side as the lead leg and back to the lunge position. Return to the start position and alternate legs. Repeat 5 to 10 steps with both legs.

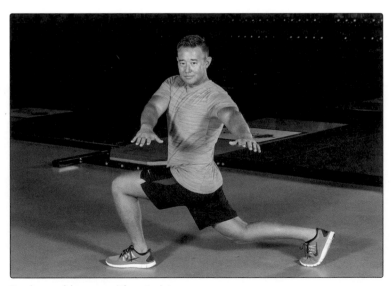

Backward lunge with a twist

SIDE LUNGE

From a standing position, step out to the right and shift the body weight over the right leg, squatting to a 90° angle while maintaining a neutral spine and keeping the left leg straight and both feet flat on the ground. It is important to sit back, keeping the weight on the heels and keeping the knees from reaching over the toes. Return to the starting position and repeat 5 to 10 steps with both legs.

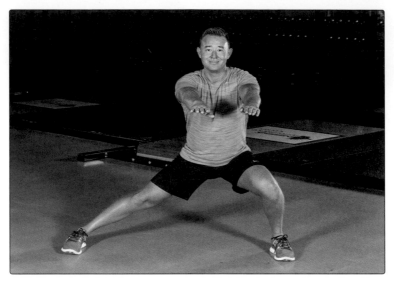

Side lunge

SUMO STRETCH

Stand with the feet slightly wider than shoulder-width apart. Move into a deep squat, keeping the hips back and weight over the heels of the feet while maintaining a neutral spine. Grab the toes and slowly extend the knees to the point of mild discomfort while keeping a neutral spine. Return to the starting position and repeat 5 to 10 times, aiming for a slightly deeper squat and slightly straighter legs in extension.

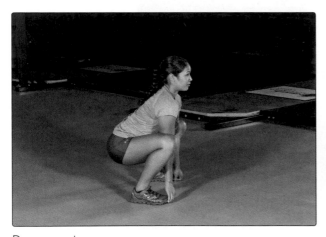

Deep squat

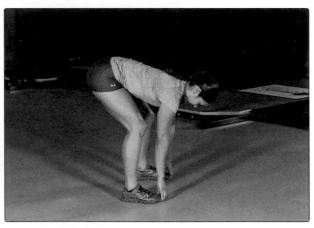

Knees somewhat extended

LEG CRADLE

In a standing position, lift one knee as high as possible and turn it outward. With one hand, grasp the knee, and with the other, grasp the ankle. Pull the lower leg up toward the chest and then release to the starting position. Alternate legs and repeat 5 to 10 times. The leg cradle can be performed in one spot or walking forward.

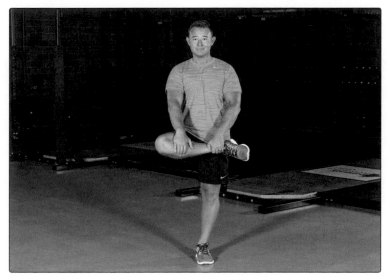

Leg cradle

INVERTED HAMSTRING STRETCH

In a standing position, while balancing on one foot and keeping both legs straight, bend forward at the waist so that the upper body (with neutral spine) and nonbalancing leg are parallel to the ground. Return to the starting position and alternate legs. Repeat 5 to 10 times.

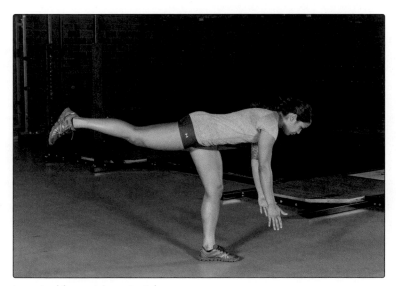

Inverted hamstring stretch

HAND WALK (INCHWORM)

From a standing position with knees slightly flexed, bend forward at the waist and place both hands on the floor. While keeping the legs as straight as possible, gradually walk the hands out to a push-up position. From this position, gradually walk the feet toward the hands with small steps, keeping the legs as straight as possible (minimal bend in the knees).

Variation: After the initial walk to the push-up position, return to the starting position with the hands returning to the feet rather than the feet to the hands. A push-up can also be added at the midway point to increase the difficulty of the shoulder stability in conjunction with the hand walk.

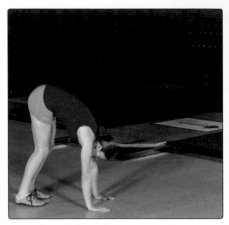

Hips flexed, hands on ground

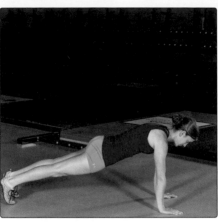

Push-up position

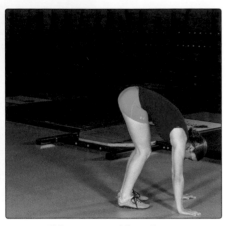

Feet walking toward hands

T PUSH-UP

Starting in a push-up position with hands directly under the shoulders, take one hand off the ground and rotate the torso 180° until the extended arm is pointing straight up in the air. Return to the starting position and change arms. Repeat 5 to 10 times per arm.

Variation: Include a push-up between alternating arms.

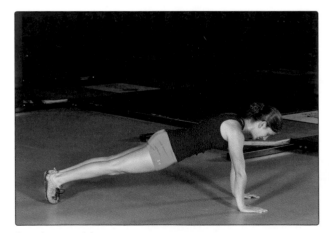

Starting position

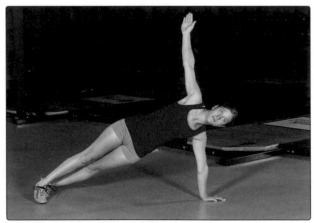

Torso rotated 180°

SMR devices such as foam rollers are becoming popular, not only because of their health benefits (4, 43, 45) but also because they are relatively inexpensive, light and compact, and portable. Foam rollers come in a variety of shapes and sizes; however, a denser foam roller provides significantly more pressure on the soft tissue (12). This should be considered when selecting an implement. Other considerations for using foam rollers include the following:

- Avoid rolling over joints or areas where there is little soft tissue.
- Position the roller directly over or under the area of focus.

- Begin by applying gentle pressure above or below the target area, rolling back and forth, slowly working through the middle of the selected area toward the end point before returning to start position.
- Roll each area for 15 to 30 seconds. In extremely sensitive areas, stop at the point of sensitivity and apply gradual pressure for 30 to 60 seconds before continuing.
- Focus on areas with restrictions in ROM or muscles with soreness or tightness.

Beginners may want to take a day off between sessions until the fascial adhesions become softer or more tolerable.

GLUTEAL AREA

Sit on the floor with the knees bent or legs straight. Place a foam roller under one side of the buttocks. Begin by rolling back and forth across the area, starting in a small area and widening as tolerated.

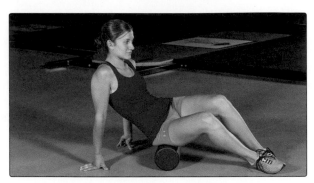

Gluteal foam roller exercise

HAMSTRINGS

Sit with the legs straight out in front of the body, and place a foam roller under the posterior thigh of one leg. Begin by rolling back and forth, using small motions, migrating from the bottom of the buttocks to just above the back of the knee.

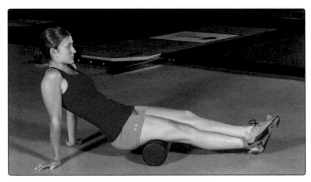

Posterior thigh (hamstring) foam roller exercise

QUADRICEPS

Lie facedown and place a foam roller under one thigh, just below the hip. Begin by rolling back and forth along the thigh, working small areas, migrating from just below the hip to just above the knee.

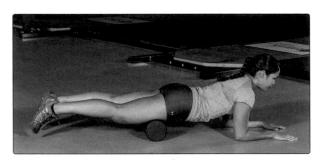

Anterior thigh (quadriceps) foam roller exercise

HIP FLEXORS

Lie facedown and place a foam roller under the pelvis, just below the hip but above the thigh. Begin by rolling back and forth, working small areas, just at the fold of the hip.

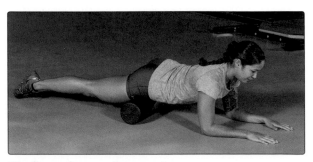

Hip flexor foam roller exercise

HIP ADDUCTORS (GROIN)

Lie facedown and place a foam roller under the inner thigh of one leg, just below the groin. Begin by rolling back and forth, working small areas, migrating from just below the groin to just above the knee.

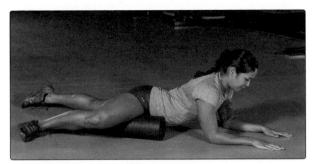

Hip adductor foam roller exercise

IT BAND

Lie on one side of the body. Place a foam roller under the outer thigh of bottom leg, just below the hip. The top leg can either be stacked on top of the other leg or shifted to the front to assist with balance. Begin by rolling back and forth, working small areas, migrating from just below the hip to just above the knee.

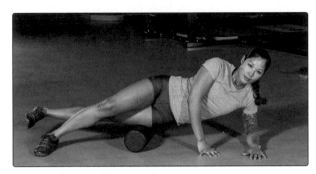

IT band foam roller exercise

CALVES

Sit with the legs straight out in front of the body, and place a foam roller under the calf of one leg. Begin by rolling back and forth, using small motions, migrating from just below the knee to just above the ankle.

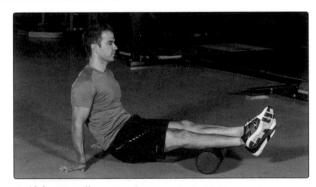

Calf foam roller exercise

UPPER BACK

Lie in a supine position. Place a foam roller under the scapulae, perpendicular to the spine. With knees bent and feet flat on floor, raise the buttocks off the floor by extending the hips. Roll back and forth from the top of the shoulder blades to the thoracic region of the back.

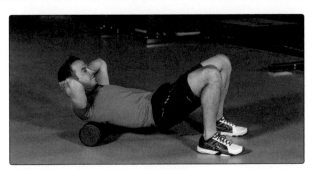

Upper back foam roller exercise

LATISSIMUS DORSI

Lie on one side of the body with the bottom arm extended and a foam roller under the axillary region (armpit). Roll back and forth from the axillary region to just above the waist.

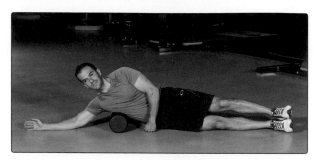

Latissimus dorsi foam roller exercise

PROGRAM DESIGN

The scope of mobility and flexibility has been heavily detailed throughout this chapter, along with substantial options for integrating exercises into a tactical training program and daily life. However, certain considerations need to be addressed in order to provide a safe and beneficial program.

Training Status and Goals

No single mobility and flexibility program is effective for everyone. The prescription of any mobility and flexibility program must focus on the needs of the individual and the goal of maintaining or improving functioning for health or for performance in a tactical environment (40). Before adding mobility and flexibility exercises to a program, the TSAC Facilitator must become familiar with the types of flexibility and mobility exercises discussed throughout this chapter. Failure to do so may put a tactical athlete at risk for injury or may compromise the athlete's other training.

The extent to which flexibility and mobility exercises are implemented into a training program depends on the status and goals of the tactical athlete, number of training sessions, available resources, and time available to complete the exercises. Many people fail to include flexibility or mobility exercises in a regularly scheduled session or weekly program because they do not prioritize mobility and flexibility. However, flexibility and mobility should be addressed the same as other fitness components such as muscular strength or power. If incorporated correctly, these exercises not only improve flexibility and mobility but also improve preparedness for other task-specific variables, such as field and job-specific duties (40). To design an appropriate flexibility and mobility program, it is important to establish the most suitable position for the previously discussed styles of flexibility and mobility training.

The intended purpose of stretching before and during an event or training session is to ensure that the person has sufficient ROM to perform optimally and to decrease any muscle stiffness (or increase muscle compliance) to theoretically decrease the risk of injury (40). The purpose of stretching after an event or training session (including periods between sessions) is to maintain or improve flexibility and mobility.

TSAC Facilitators should consider the most suitable styles of mobility and flexibility training for tactical athletes when establishing training goals and programs. Though static and PNF stretching benefit flexibility, they may not benefit muscular force and power output, and thus they primarily should be performed in the cool-down or between sessions as a way to focus on maintaining flexibility levels (if optimal) and address any identified limitations. Ballistic stretching has also been shown to increase flexibility; however, due to its harsh nature and possible increase in injury risk, it has fallen out of favor (59) and may not be suitable for tactical athletes.

Dynamic stretching is the more suitable presession and in-session activity because it imitates occupation-specific movements, thus preparing the tactical athlete for the intended workout or actions. It also has the advantage of developing mobility without compromising the integrity of the session (i.e., decrease in HR, body temperature, circulation, and force and power output common with static stretching). Finally, the inclusion of MR through massage therapy or SMR using foam rollers can decrease fatigue and improve recovery, in addition to improving pain management and mood state, and as such it can be used during the session, immediately after the session, or between sessions.

Demands Specific to Tactical Populations

Mobility and flexibility training should not just be part of the warm-up or cool-down. It is a workout in its own right and should be just as much of a priority as strength training for tactical athletes (21). Achieving whole-body mobility requires a structured program. As always, the TSAC Facilitator must be aware of time, equipment, and personnel constraints. For example, PNF stretching may be more advantageous than static stretching for increasing flexibility, but it requires a substantial amount of time per stretch as well as an assisting partner. Static stretching, on the other hand, still increases flexibility but is much simpler and takes less time. In addition, the tactical athlete's environment may or may not be conducive to massage therapy or SMR (e.g., lack of time, limited access to equipment or personnel).

Tactical athletes can use many methods to achieve flexibility and mobility when under time constraints. For example, a typical workout may begin with a dynamic warm-up (light aerobic exercise and dynamic stretches) for 10 to 15 minutes, followed by the focus of the day (e.g., strength, speed, agility, cardio). In addition, mobility exercises such as SMR or corrective exercises for identified areas of concern can be performed in the main body of the program as isolated exercises between major movements, during recovery between sets of major movements, or at the end of the workout as a complement to the session. Include any static or PNF stretches targeting flexibility as part of the cool-down. Each workout

session should be followed by a recovery session that includes flexibility or mobility exercises (e.g., yoga, static stretching, PNF); four to five sets of 60-second bilateral static stretches of target muscle groups are the most suitable frequency and duration to decrease passive resistance and increase flexibility (40).

The style of mobility or flexibility work must be chosen carefully to prepare the tactical athlete for a specific exercise session. In addition, it must consider future exercise sessions and work schedules. As with other program design considerations (e.g., training for muscular strength, power, endurance, or cardiorespiratory gains), the TSAC Facilitator should complete a needs analysis to structure a program accordingly. A primary risk factor for injury in tactical athletes is overuse of training errors (40). By planning a schedule for work, rest, and training, the facilitator can identify the frequency, intensity, volume, and modality for recovery, maintenance or improvement of flexibility and mobility, and, most importantly, optimal performance. Tactical athletes are not always able to warm up before an occupational demand arises, such as an alarm callout for firefighters, a response to fire for military personnel, or a forced entry for law enforcement. Flexibility and mobility are essential for tactical athletes so that they can respond optimally, lower the possible risk for injury, and recover quickly.

Key Point

A tactical conditioning program must address all key fitness components; however, the attention paid to each component depends on the needs analysis. Factors may include current physical readiness; physical demands of work and life; time, equipment, and personnel available; and individual health and performance goals.

Following are guidelines to increase and maintain flexibility and mobility (29):

1. Perform a general warm-up before stretching to increase body temperature and blood flow to the working muscles.

2. Include all major muscle groups, particularly common areas such as the low back, hips, quadriceps, hamstrings, and calves.

3. Follow a logical anatomical order, such as starting with the lower legs and moving to the upper extremities or vice versa, to allow exercises to stretch similar muscles. Stretch through various planes of movement to improve ROM at each joint.

4. Complete at least two to five repetitions per exercise, and hold the stretch for 15 to 90 seconds as long as it feels comfortable. Stretches should never be taken to the point of pain; they should only cause mild discomfort.

5. Breathe slowly and rhythmically while holding a stretch to assist in releasing muscle tension and avoid the Valsalva maneuver and subsequent increase in blood pressure.

6. Perform a dynamic warm-up before any moderate to vigorous physical activity, include mobility exercises within or at the end of the workout to maintain or improve any areas of concern, and finish with static stretching during the cool-down to focus on overall flexibility improvement.

CONCLUSION

This chapter has discussed mobility and flexibility for tactical athletes. Mobility and flexibility exercises are one component of a health and fitness program; however, due to their direct link to the ability to move, they may have implications for other program components. The ever-changing theater of operations for tactical athletes highlights the importance of flexibility and mobility. Whether a firefighter, police officer, first responder, or soldier, all tactical athletes need to be supple and flexible to perform their required tasks. As with any program, individualization is crucial. To prescribe an efficient, effective routine, the TSAC Facilitator must consider the status of and the demands placed on the tactical athlete, individual and program goals and objectives, and physiological and kinesiological factors that affect flexibility and mobility.

Key Terms

arthritis
ballistic stretching
collagen
dynamic stretching
elastin
fibrosis
fibrous adhesions
flexibility
Golgi tendon organ (GTO)
kinesiological factors
mobility
muscle spindles
myofascia

myofascial release (MR)
overstretching
physiological factors
proprioceptive neuromuscular facilitation (PNF)
range of motion (ROM)
reciprocal inhibition
sarcopenia
self-myofascial release (SMR)
static stretching
stretch-induced strength loss
stretch reflex

Study Questions

1. Which of the following is a kinesiological factor that affects mobility and flexibility?

   a. age
   b. muscle origin and insertion
   c. physical activity level
   d. body composition

2. Which of the following structures is responsible for initiating the stretch reflex?

   a. muscle spindle
   b. Golgi tendon organ
   c. myosin and actin
   d. collagen and elastin

3. Which of the following stretching techniques involves controlled activity-specific movements that extend the muscles to exceed end ROM?

   a. static

   b. PNF

   c. dynamic

   d. ballistic

4. Which of the following guidelines applies to using a foam roller?

   a. Roll each area for 5 to 10 seconds.

   b. Go around any extremely sensitive areas.

   c. Position the roller 4 in. (10.2 cm) away from the area of focus.

   d. Avoid rolling over joints or areas where there is little soft tissue.

Chapter 13

Plyometric, Speed, and Agility Exercise Techniques and Programming

Mike Barnes, MEd, CSCS, NSCA-CPT

Jay Dawes, PhD, CSCS,*D, NSCA-CPT,*D, FNSCA

After completing this chapter, you will be able to

- describe the plyometric, speed, and agility training needs for tactical populations;
- describe optimal types of plyometric, speed, and agility training exercises and drills;
- design a warm-up protocol for a plyometric, speed, and agility training session;
- describe proper exercise technique and instructional cuing for plyometric, speed, and agility exercises; and
- design plyometric, speed, and agility training programs based on the training status, goals, and occupational demands of tactical athletes.

actical athletes are often required to perform physically demanding tasks as part of their occupational duties. Depending on the situation, these tasks may range from routine to potentially life threatening. Regardless, each situation requires varying degrees of physical abilities. Based on the physiological demands and stresses of their jobs, it is evident that tactical athletes may be required to perform feats of significant power and strength. For example, a law enforcement officer requires a high degree of neuromuscular control to maintain speed and balance while navigating uneven terrain and wearing a utility belt with various tools, and a military soldier navigating urban warfare needs a high degree of strength and effective use of the nervous system to execute the task safely.

This chapter discusses the fundamentals of plyometric, speed, and agility training. By incorporating these conditioning methods into a comprehensive strength and conditioning program, tactical athletes will better be able to accomplish the physical functions of their occupations.

PLYOMETRIC TRAINING

Power is frequently defined as the ability of the body to do work, or the rate at which work is performed (31). However, in terms of performance, power may best be defined as the optimal expression of force and velocity to perform a given task. One method of developing power is plyometric training. Plyometric drills consist of hopping, jumping, and bounding movements that rely heavily on the series elastic components (SECs) of the muscles and tendons, as well as the **stretch–shortening cycle (SSC)**, to improve reactive strength (23, 26).

This section provides examples of plyometric drills. Additionally, guidelines for teaching and cuing drill techniques will be emphasized to assist the TSAC Facilitator in refining movement quality. Finally, program design recommendations—including progressions based on training status, goals, and demands specific to tactical populations—will be addressed.

Plyometric drills consist of three major phases. The first is the eccentric, or loading, phase. During this stage of the movement, rapid loading of the agonist muscle groups occurs. As a result,

the SECs within the muscles and tendons store elastic energy. This rapid eccentric muscle action also activates the muscle spindles, which prevent overstretching of the agonist muscle by causing muscular contraction. The eccentric loading of the musculotendinous tissues is then immediately followed by the **amortization phase**. This phase occurs between the end of eccentric muscle action and the initiation of concentric muscle action (figure 13.1) (40). During this transitional phase, the Type Ia afferent motor neurons are stimulated and synapse with the alpha motor neurons in the spinal cord. When this occurs, the alpha motor neurons transmit signals to the agonist muscle groups to initiate a more powerful contraction during the final stage of the drill, or the concentric phase. However, if the amortization phase is too long, the majority of energy stored in the SEC dissipates as heat (40).

Need for Power Within Tactical Populations

For tactical athletes, the ability to produce force rapidly is critical to success in many situations. Due to the physiological demands and stresses of their jobs, tactical athletes may be required to perform feats of power and strength similar to those performed by competitive sport athletes. For example, to be effective, tactical athletes must be able to sprint to an objective to avoid gunfire or when in pursuit of an assailant; lift, carry, push, or drag an object or a victim to safety; jump and vault over barriers and obstacles of varying sizes; climb stairs; and perform hand-to-hand combat (14, 39, 47).

Several studies have identified the importance of anaerobic power for people who work in physically demanding occupations (38, 46, 48). For example, Sell (45) found a strong relationship between time to completion on simulated firefighting task scenarios (SFTS) and vertical jump height. The study discovered that firefighters with a vertical jump height of at least 17 inches (43 cm) were more likely to achieve passing scores on the SFTS. Similarly, Michaelides et al. (35) found significant correlations between vertical jump and a simulated rescue using a mannequin. Research conducted by Dawes et al. (14) found a significant relationship between direct and indirect measures

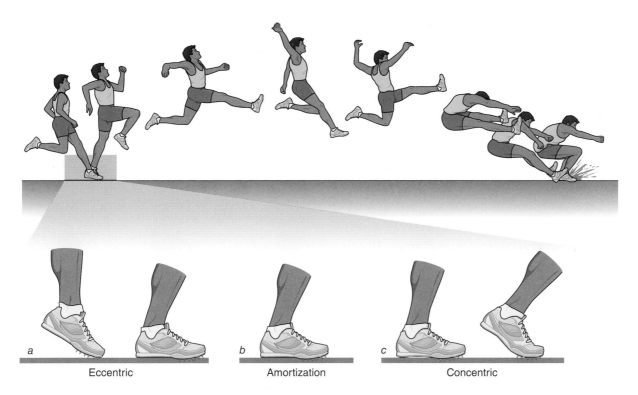

a	b	c
Eccentric	Amortization	Concentric

Figure 13.1   The long jump and SSC. *(a)* The eccentric phase begins at touchdown and continues until the movement ends. *(b)* The amortization phase is the transition from eccentric to concentric phases; it is quick and without movement. *(c)* The concentric phase follows the amortization phase and comprises the entire push-off time, until the athlete's foot leaves the surface.

Reprinted, by permission, from NSCA, 2016, Program design and technique for plyometric training, D.H. Potach and D.A. Chu. In *Essentials of strength training and conditioning*, 4th ed. (Champaign, IL: Human Kinetics), 474.

of power and **speed** over 5, 10, and 20 m among members of a part-time SWAT team. Furthermore, Rhea, Alvar, and Gray (41) discovered a significant relationship between time to completion of a series of simulated firefighting tasks and sustained anaerobic power as measured by 400 m run time.

Improving absolute power among tactical athletes should have a direct impact on occupational performance, especially during tasks that require sprinting, jumping, vaulting, lifting, dragging, and carrying. Because improving absolute power should improve the amount of force the tactical athlete is able to exert at foot strike (13), training for power may also contribute to sustained power.

In addition, although there is a paucity of research on the topic, upper body **plyometrics** that use body weight and other forms of light external resistance (e.g., medicine balls, sandbags) may also be useful for developing power in this population. The SAID (specific adaptation to imposed demands) principle, sometimes used interchangeably with *specificity principle*, refers to the adaptation that is made to a specific demand or stimulus (6, 39, 51). For example, rotational throws and tosses may aid the development of power in the transverse plane, which may directly relate to specific tactical tasks such as breaching, throwing, striking, and using force. For these reasons, developing power should be a primary consideration when designing a comprehensive training program for the tactical athlete, and plyometrics should be considered for developing this attribute.

Types of Plyometric Drills

Plyometric drills are typically classified by their degree of intensity (2, 3, 40). The intensity of a plyometric drill can vary drastically based on several factors, such as the height and distance traveled, the complexity of the drill, the speed at which the drill is performed, the loading parameters selected (e.g., bodyweight versus weighted jumps), and the rate of the SSC (i.e., the transition time between eccentric and concentric muscle actions and the amplitude of the movements performed). These factors may be influenced by the displacement of the center of mass, horizontal speed, body mass, individual effort, and reactive strength.

Warm-Up

Warm-ups have two components: the general warm-up and the specific warm-up. The general warm-up increases blood flow, HR, respiration rate, deep muscle temperature, and perspiration; decreases viscosity of joint fluids (30); and improves joint ROM. This phase lasts 5 to 10 minutes and incorporates low-intensity continuous movements such as jogging or stationary cycling. As the general warm-up proceeds, so does the corresponding intensity of the drill; however, this should produce little to no fatigue.

The second phase is the specific warm-up. This phase incorporates movements that are more dynamic, require higher power outputs over larger ROMs, and are similar to the actions observed in operations or the training to follow. It is recommended to first use general movement patterns before performing more specific movements. When training plyometrics, include both a general and specific warm-up before skills and drills (40).

The incorporation of dynamic flexibility movements into the specific warm-up is advised if strength and power capabilities are required for the activity. Note that warming up and stretching are not the same thing; stretching is designed to cause chronic adaptations in muscle tissue extensibility and joint ROM, whereas the purpose of a warm-up is to progressively increase muscle temperature, breathing rate, perspiration rate, and HR in preparation for more vigorous activity. Additionally, static stretching prior to activity may quell neural activity and compromise power output (30, 36). Therefore, for chronic adaptations in muscle tissue extensibility and joint ROM, postactivity static stretching is advised (19). This suggests that if improvement in mobility for immediate use is required, then a dynamic warm-up is recommended. However, if the individual has limitations in muscle or joint ROM, then postactivity static stretching to enhance ROM is advised (19). The TSAC Facilitator should make an educated decision on which warm-up activities are most appropriate for the training activity and the tactical athlete. Training segments specifically focusing on flexibility can be added to further increase joint ROM.

Dynamic flexibility movements often are multiplanar, are held briefly, address opposing muscle groups, and replicate movements similar to the upcoming activity or training. Depending on the activity or the training that follows, some warm-up activities, including flexibility, may be more appropriate than others. For specific warm-up guidelines, refer to chapter 12.

LANDING DRILLS

Tactical personnel should be taught, and must demonstrate, appropriate landing technique before progressing to plyometric drills.

■ DROP SQUAT

Purpose

To teach proper landing mechanics

Start

Stand in a tall, upright position with the arms hanging at the sides of the body, the hips and knees extended, and the feet slightly narrower than hip-width apart.

Action

Raise the heels by plantar flexing the ankles. Jump the feet outward so they are approximately shoulder-width apart, with the toes pointed slightly outward and the knees lined up with the second toe on the same-side foot.

Finish

Land in the universal athletic position, with the chest up, the shoulder blades retracted and slightly depressed, and a slight bend in the ankles, knees, and hips.

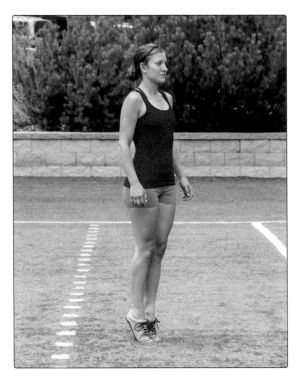 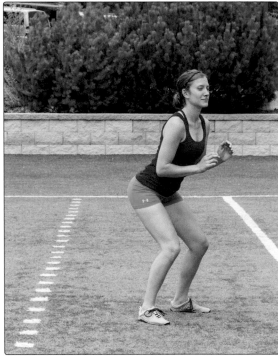

LANDING DRILLS

DROP LUNGE

Purpose

To teach proper landing mechanics, develop eccentric strength, and emphasize appropriate arm action for improved **change-of-direction speed**

Start

Stand in a tall, upright position with the arms hanging at the sides of the body, the hips and knees extended, and the feet slightly narrower than hip-width apart.

Action

Raise the heels by plantar flexing the ankles. Then jump the feet outward so they are approximately shoulder-width apart, with the toes pointed slightly outward and the knees lined up with the second toe on the same-side foot.

Finish

Quickly split the feet and land in a lunge position.

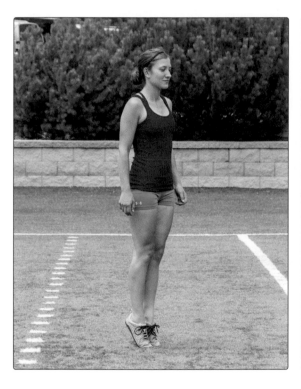
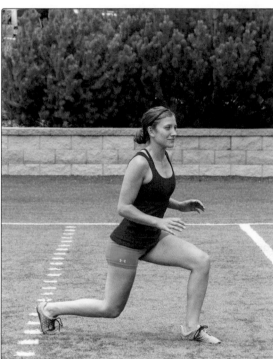

LANDING DRILLS

DROP FREEZE

Purpose
To teach proper landing mechanics and develop eccentric strength

Start
Stand on top of a 12- to 24-inch (30-61 cm) plyometric box.

Action
Step forward off the box.

Finish
Both feet should contact the ground simultaneously. Land in the universal athletic position, with the chest up, the shoulder blades retracted and slightly depressed, and a slight bend in the ankles, knees, and hips.

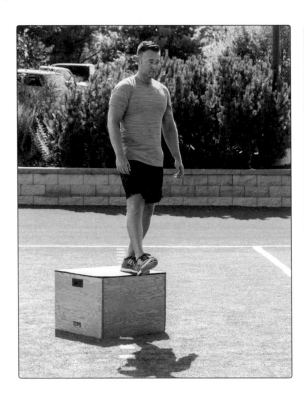
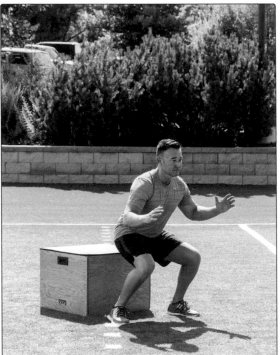

LANDING DRILLS

DROP PUSH-UP

Purpose
To develop eccentric strength in the upper body

Start
Start in a push-up position with the arms extended and hands placed slightly wider than shoulder-width apart on a set of 4- to 6-inch (10-15 cm) steps or risers.

Action
Simultaneously shift the hands inward so they are approximately shoulder-width apart and land with both hand in full contact with the ground. Upon landing, allow the wrists, elbows, and shoulders to flex slightly in order to absorb the landing. The trunk should remain rigid upon landing, and the legs should remain straight.

Finish
Return to the starting position and repeat for the desired number of repetitions.

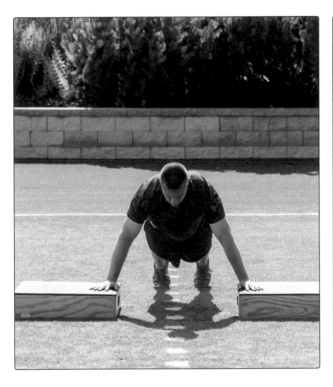 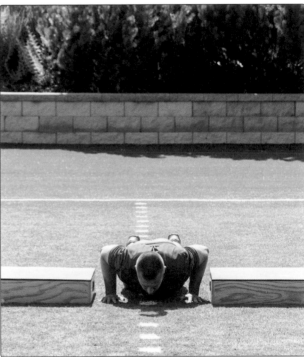

LOW INTENSITY

When performing plyometric drills, maintaining proper technique is critical. The TSAC Facilitator should monitor fatigue during every drill and repetition. Particular attention should be given to body alignment and fatigue that may increase risk of injury. The following section describes a variety of lower body plyometric drills.

DOUBLE-LEG JUMP

Purpose

To develop explosive plantar flexion at the ankles, improve utilization of the SSC, and teach proper landing mechanics

Start

Stand in the universal athletic position with the feet approximately hip-width apart and the arms bent at a 90° angle at the elbows.

Action

Rapidly swing the arms backward while maintaining a 90° bend at the elbows. At the same time, quickly flex the ankles, knees, and hips. Jump upward, with primary motion occurring at the ankle joint (similar to jumping rope).

Finish

Land in the starting position. Immediately repeat this action for the desired number of repetitions.

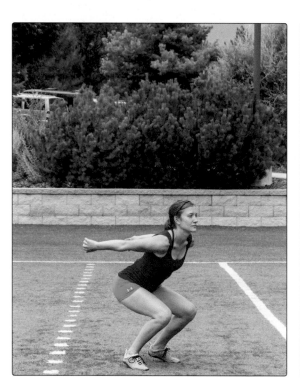
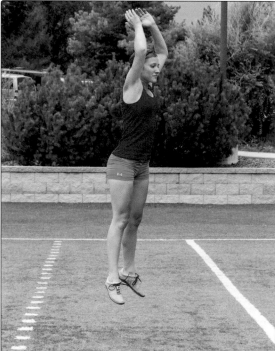

LOW INTENSITY

SKIP

Purpose

To develop rhythm and tempo, as well as improve triple extension of the drive leg and triple flexion of the front leg

Start

Begin by lifting one leg to approximately 90° of hip and knee flexion. Simultaneously lift the opposite arm.

Action

Extend the ankle, knee, and hip of the stance leg to skip forward, with the front leg still flexed 90° at the hip and knee. The arms should remain bent at 90°, and the arms and legs should act in a recipro-cal manner (i.e., when the left leg is forward, the left arm swings forward) to counterbalance the rotational forces of the lower body.

Finish

Return the flexed leg to the ground. Immediately repeat the skip with the opposite leg.

Note: This drill can also be performed backward as well as laterally. Additionally, the intensity can be increased by performing the drill over a longer distance or attempting to cover a greater distance without increasing the number of repetitions.

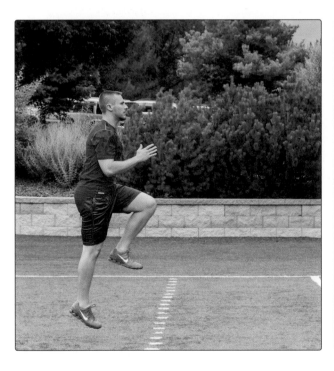
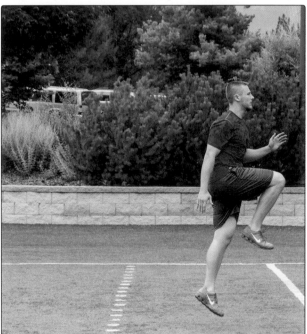

LOW INTENSITY

SQUAT JUMP

Purpose

To develop lower body power from a stationary start

Start

Stand in the universal athletic position with the hands on the hips.

Action

Squat until the tops of the thighs are parallel to the ground, count to 2, and then jump vertically as high as possible while keeping the hands on the hips.

Finish

Land in the starting position. Repeat for the desired number of repetitions.

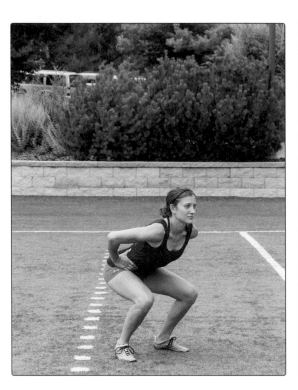
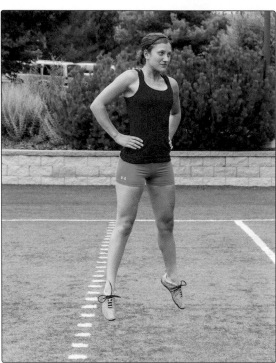

LOW INTENSITY

COUNTERMOVEMENT JUMP

Purpose

To develop lower body power via rapid prestretching action (i.e., countermovement)

Start

Stand in the universal athletic position with the hands on the hips.

Action

Rapidly squat to approximately 110° to 120° of knee flexion, and then immediately jump upward as high as possible while keeping the hands on the hips.

Finish

Land in the starting position. Repeat for the desired number of repetitions.

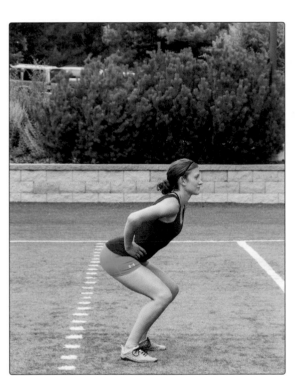 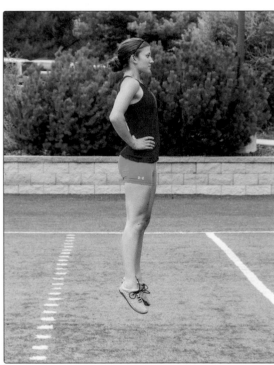

LOW TO MODERATE INTENSITY

The following drills are classified as low to moderate intensity. The low-intensity drills should be mastered before progressing to the following drills.

TUCK JUMP

Purpose

To develop lower body power and improve dynamic hip mobility

Start

Stand in the universal athletic position.

Action

Perform a countermovement jump while pulling the knees to the chest. Quickly touch the knees with both hands at the peak height of the jump.

Finish

Land in the starting position. Repeat for the desired number of repetitions.

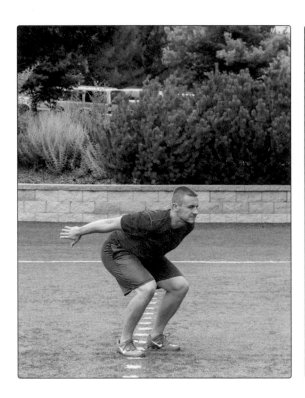
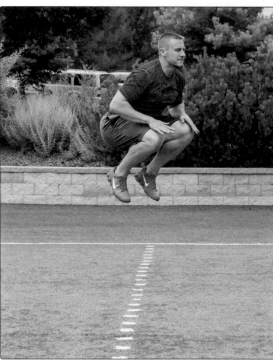

LOW TO MODERATE INTENSITY

CONE AND BARRIER JUMP

Purpose

To develop lower body power

Start

Stand in the universal athletic position with the feet approximately shoulder-width apart.

Action

Perform a countermovement and then jump over a cone or barrier.

Finish

Land in the starting position. Repeat for the desired number of repetitions.

Note: The height of the cones or barriers can increase as the tactical athlete becomes more proficient at this drill. The height can also be used to adjust the intensity (i.e., lower cones or barriers = lower intensity, taller cones or barriers = higher intensity).

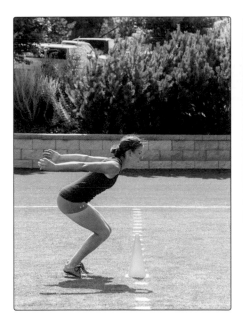 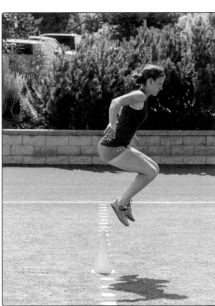 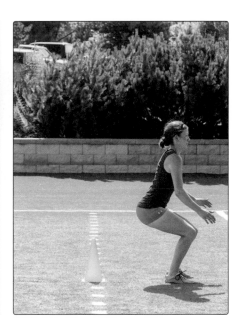

LOW TO MODERATE INTENSITY

BOX JUMP

Purpose

To develop lower body power

Start

Stand in the universal athletic position with the feet approximately hip-width apart facing a box.

Action

Perform a countermovement with arm swing (as previously described), and then rapidly extend the ankles, knees, and hips.

Finish

Flex the hips, knees, and ankles and land in the universal athletic position on top of the box. Step down from the box. Repeat for the desired number of repetitions.

Note: Do not jump off the top of the box; this increases the force one must absorb upon landing.

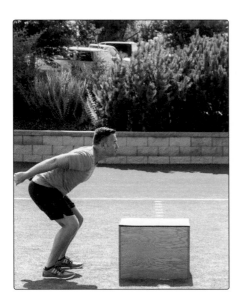 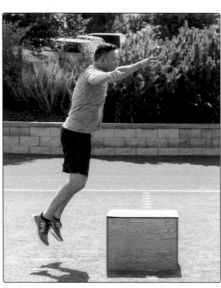 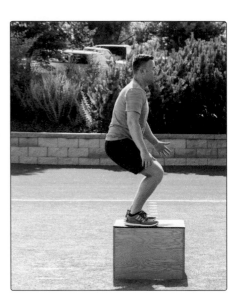

LOW TO MODERATE INTENSITY

BOX PUSH-OFF

Purpose

To develop lower body power off a single leg

Start

Stand behind a 12- to 24-inch (30-61 cm) plyometric box. Place one foot on top of the box.

Action

Explode upward by pushing off the lead foot and rapidly extending the hip, knee, and ankles. The arms should simultaneously swing upward to help generate greater total body power.

Finish

Land in the starting position, with the same foot on top of the box. Upon landing, the foot should be in full contact with the box. Repeat for the desired number of repetitions and then switch legs.

Note: Make certain the center of mass remains over the box throughout the drill. The intensity of this drill may be increased by performing the movement in an alternating fashion (i.e., the right leg starts on top of the box, and then the legs switch at the apex of the jump and the left foot lands on the box) while attempting to minimize the time between jumps. This drill can also be performed laterally off a single leg or in an alternating fashion (i.e., step-box-change). As tactical athletes transition over the box, they will shift their body mass from one side of the box to the other.

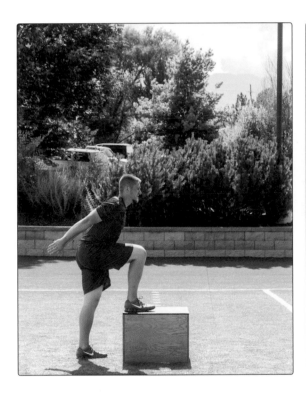
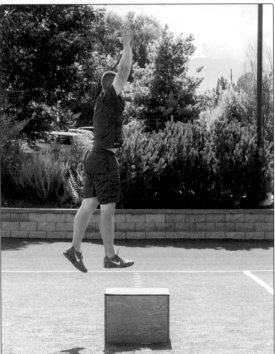

SPLIT SQUAT JUMP

Purpose

To develop lower body power off a single leg

Start

Start in a lunge position with one leg positioned forward (hip and knee flexed approximately 90°) and the other behind the midline of the body.

Action

Explosively jump as high as possible while simultaneously swinging the arms upward. At the peak of the jump, the legs should be fully extended and parallel to one another.

Finish

Land in the starting position with the same leg forward. Repeat for the desired number of repetitions and then switch legs.

Note: The intensity of this drill may be increased by performing the movement in an alternating fashion (i.e., right leg forward and then switch at the apex of the jump to land with the left leg forward) while attempting to minimize the time between jumps.

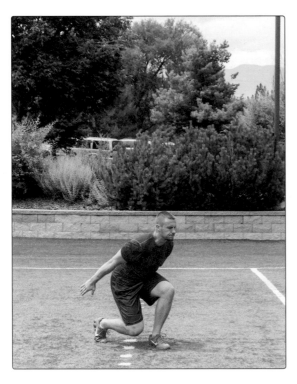
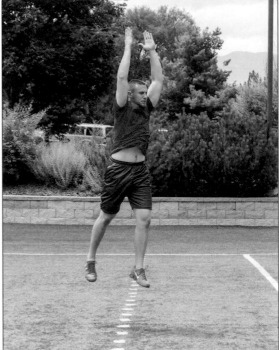

MODERATE TO HIGH INTENSITY

The following drills are classified as moderate to high intensity. The low- and moderate-intensity drills should be mastered before progressing to the following drills.

BROAD JUMP

Purpose

To develop vertical and horizontal lower body power

Start

Stand in the universal athletic position with the feet approximately shoulder-width apart.

Action

Perform a countermovement arm swing while simultaneously flexing the hips, knees, and ankles.

Jump horizontally as far as possible, using both arms to assist.

Finish

Land in the starting position, allow a few seconds to recover, and then repeat for the desired number of repetitions.

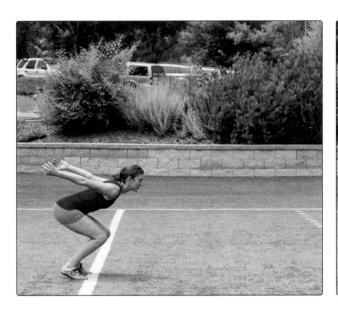
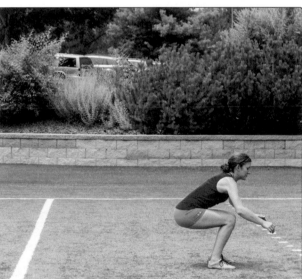

MODERATE TO HIGH INTENSITY

TRIPLE JUMP

Purpose

To develop vertical and horizontal lower body power

Start

Stand in the universal athletic position with the feet approximately shoulder-width apart.

Action

Bound forward on a single leg. Upon landing, immediately bound forward off the opposite leg.

Upon landing from the second bound, perform a broad jump and stick the landing.

Finish

Once the three jumps have been completed, walk back to the starting line. Repeat for the desired number of sets.

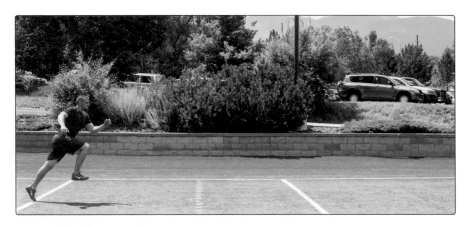

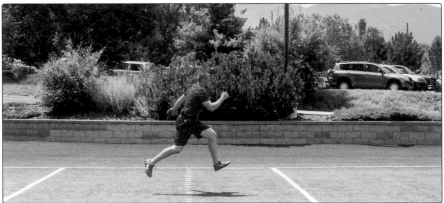

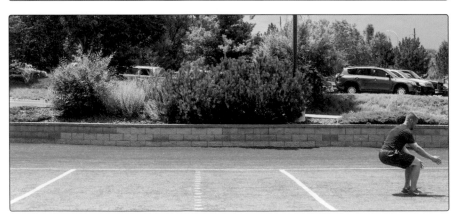

MODERATE TO HIGH INTENSITY

LATERAL CONE OR BARRIER JUMP

Purpose

To develop lower body power in multiple directions

Start

Stand in the universal athletic position with the feet approximately shoulder-width apart.

Action

Perform a countermovement by rapidly flexing the ankles, knees, and hips and jumping with both legs laterally over a cone or barrier.

Finish

Land in the starting position on the opposite side of the cone or barrier. Immediately repeat the jump to the starting side.

Note: Intensity of the lateral barrier jump can be increased from medium to high by progressively increasing the height of the barrier or by performing hops with one leg only.

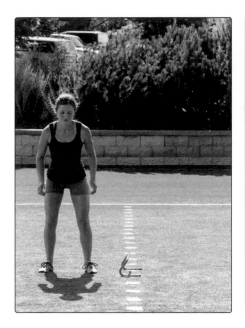 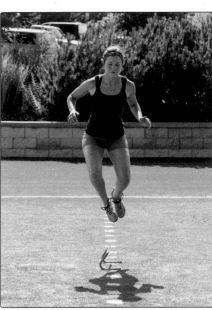 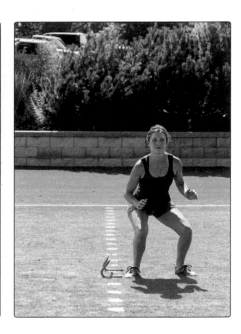

SINGLE-LEG HOP

Purpose

To develop lower body power off a single leg

Start

Stand on a single leg.

Action

While standing on a single leg, perform a counter-movement with arm swing and then jump vertically as high as possible.

Finish

Land in the starting position, and after balance on the stance leg has been achieved, repeat the action.

Note: Intensity of this drill can be increased by performing this action horizontally or by adding cones or barriers to clear.

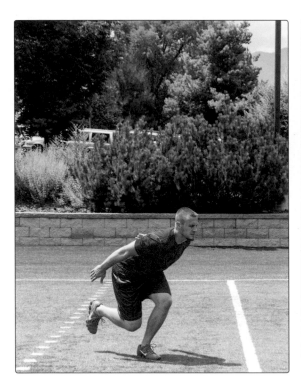 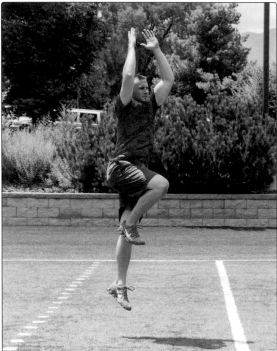

MODERATE TO HIGH INTENSITY

▌ BOUNDS

Purpose
To develop explosive horizontal and vertical power

Start
Jog at a comfortable pace.

Action
Explosively extend the front leg. During push-off, bring the opposite leg forward by flexing the hip until the thigh is approximately parallel to the ground and the knee is bent 90°. During this flight phase of the drill, reach forward with the arm opposite the front leg (i.e., if the left leg is forward, the right arm will be forward). Attempt to cover as great a distance as possible during each stride.

Finish
Land on the leg that extended, and immediately repeat the sequence with the other leg. Continue bounding for the desired distance.

Note: A bound is simply an exaggerated version of a normal running gait. To increase the intensity of this drill, perform a double-arm swing (both arms moving in the same direction at the same time) rather than a single-arm swing.

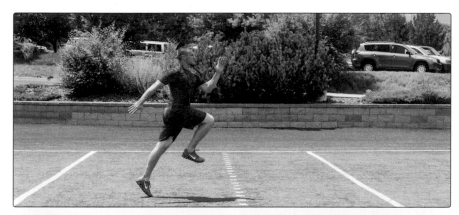

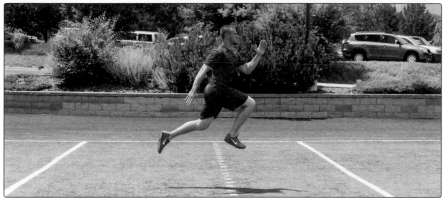

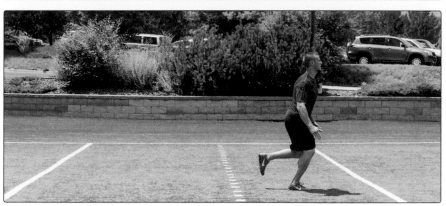

DEPTH JUMP

Purpose

To develop lower body power using high eccentric loading to create more powerful concentric muscle action upon takeoff

Start

Stand in the universal athletic position on the edge of a plyometric box with the toes near the edge of the box.

Action

Step straight out off the box. Upon landing, immediately jump as high as possible. Immediately upon landing, try to minimize ground contact time and jump as high as possible as quickly as possible.

Finish

Land in the universal athletic position, step back onto the box, and repeat for the desired number of repetitions.

Note: Intensity may be increased by raising the height of the box. Begin with a height of 12 inches (30 cm). This drill may also be performed by stepping off the box and jumping laterally or by jumping for maximal horizontal distance rather than maximal vertical height. Tactical athletes may also perform this drill by jumping up to another box.

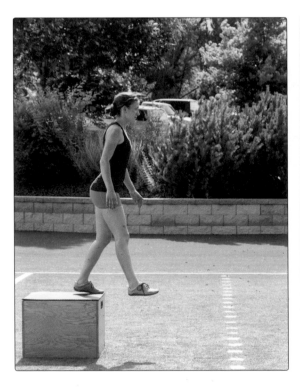
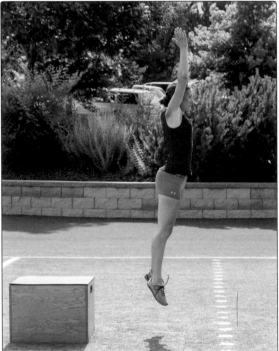

LOW INTENSITY

This section features several upper body and total body plyometric drills. Some of the drills use an implement such as a medicine ball. Some are multiplanar and emphasize total body rotational development. These may be of particular value to the tactical athlete when training to improve performance in use-of-force situations where the upper body or whole body is emphasized. Low-intensity upper body plyometrics can be used to improve SSC function of the upper body.

MEDICINE BALL CHEST PASS

Purpose

To improve upper body power

Start

Hold a medicine ball and stand in the universal athletic position with feet shoulder-width apart facing a wall or partner approximately 10 feet (3 m) away.

Action

Raise the medicine ball to chest level with the elbows flexed. Perform a rapid countermovement by cocking the arms (i.e., moving the arms slightly backward before the actual throw, similar to passing a basketball). Using both arms, throw the ball to the wall or partner by extending the elbows and wrists.

Finish

When the wall or partner returns the ball, catch it, return to the starting position, and immediately repeat the movement.

Note: Intensity may be increased by using a heavier medicine ball.

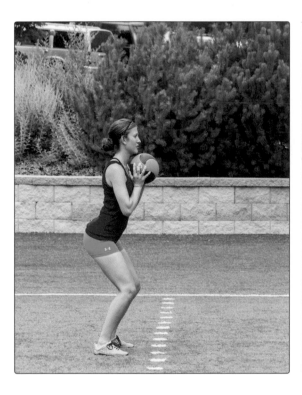
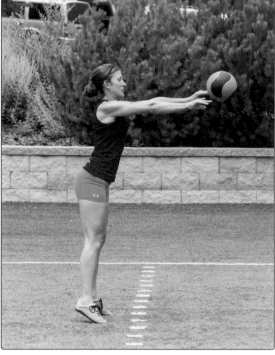

MODERATE INTENSITY

The following drills are classified as moderate intensity. The low-intensity drills should be mastered before progressing to the following drills.

BACKWARD OVERHEAD MEDICINE BALL (BOMB) TOSS

Purpose

To develop total body power and emphasize triple extension of the ankle, knees, and hips

Start

Stand in the universal athletic position with the feet approximately shoulder-width apart, holding a medicine ball in the front of the body.

Action

Perform a countermovement by rapidly squatting to approximately 110° to 120° and swinging the medicine ball back and downward between the legs. Immediately perform a vertical jump while explosively throwing the medicine ball overhead and backward.

Finish

Land in the universal athletic position, retrieve the ball, and repeat for the desired number of repetitions.

Note: Intensity may be increased by using a heavier medicine ball.

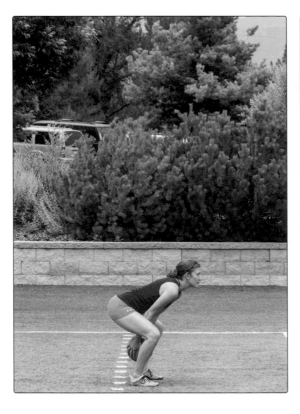 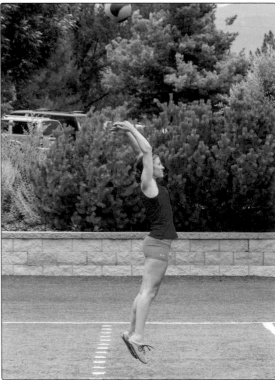

MODERATE INTENSITY

ROTATIONAL TOSS

Purpose

To improve rotational power

Start

While holding a medicine ball in front of the body with both hands between chest and navel height, stand in the universal athletic position with feet shoulder-width apart and lateral to a wall or partner approximately 10 feet (3 m) away.

Action

Quickly rotate and bring the ball to the hip farthest away from the partner or wall. Rapidly rotate the torso toward the partner or wall while keeping the arms straight, and toss the ball to the wall or partner.

Finish

Repeat for the desired number of repetitions, and then repeat on the opposite side.

Note: Intensity may be increased by using a heavier medicine ball.

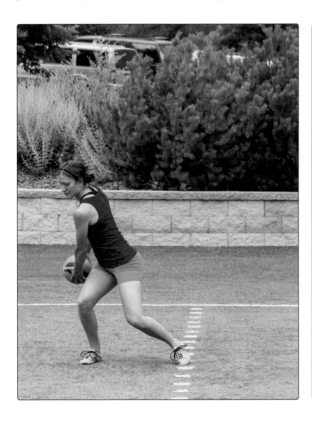

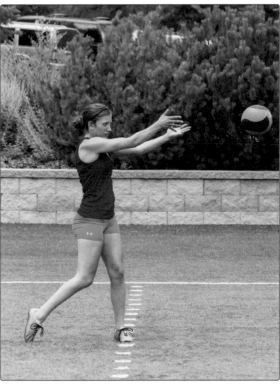

MODERATE TO HIGH INTENSITY

The following drills are classified as moderate to high intensity. The low- and moderate-intensity drills should be mastered before progressing to the following drills.

POWER DROP

Purpose

To develop explosive upper body power

Start

The tactical athlete lies supine on the ground with the elbows extended and both shoulders at approximately 90° of flexion; the head should be near the base of the box. The partner should be on the box, holding the medicine ball above the tactical athlete's arms.

Action

When the partner drops the ball, the tactical athlete catches it with both hands and throws it back to the partner.

Finish

The partner catches the ball and then repeats for the desired number of repetitions.

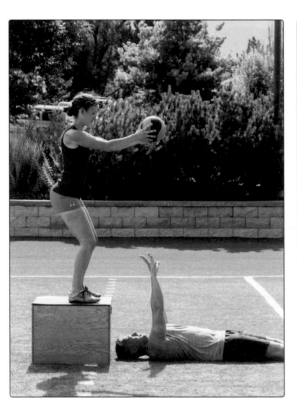 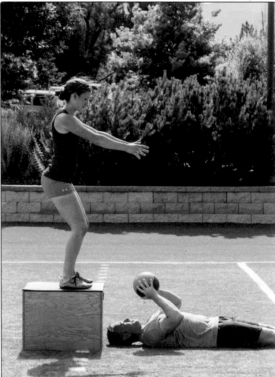

MODERATE TO HIGH INTENSITY

CLAP PUSH-UP

Purpose
To develop upper body power

Start
Start in a push-up position.

Action
Perform a countermovement by allowing the elbows to flex and the shoulders to extend. Once the upper arms are approximately parallel to the ground, explosively push off the ground and clap the hands.

Finish
Allow the elbows to flex when the hands return to the floor. Return to the starting position and then repeat for the desired number of repetitions.

Note: The torso should remain rigid throughout this drill.

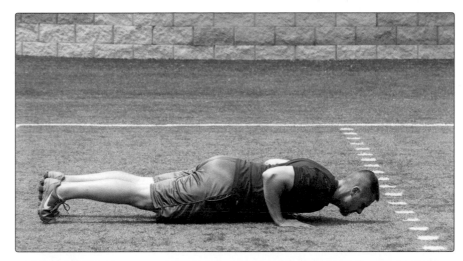

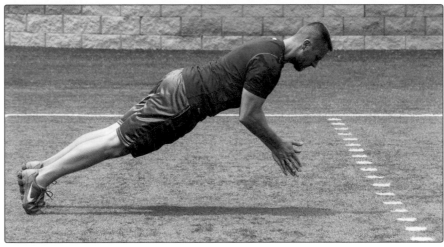

MODERATE TO HIGH INTENSITY

DEPTH PUSH-UP

Purpose

To develop explosive upper body power

Start

Start in a push-up position, with the hands on a medicine ball and elbows extended.

Action

Quickly remove the hands from the medicine ball slightly wider than shoulder-width apart and drop down. Contact the ground with the hands slightly wider than shoulder-width apart and elbows slightly flexed. Allow the chest to touch the medicine ball by letting the elbows flex. Then immediately and explosively push up by fully extending the elbows and wrists.

Finish

Return to the starting position.

Note: When the upper body is at maximal height during the upward movement, the hands should be higher than the medicine ball.

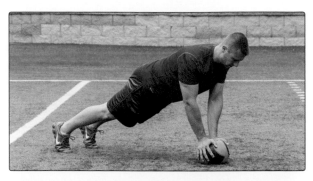

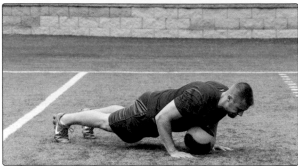

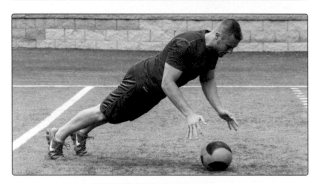

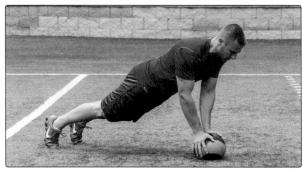

MODERATE TO HIGH INTENSITY

OVERHEAD FORWARD THROW

Purpose

To improve upper body power

Start

Hold a medicine ball and stand in the universal athletic position with the feet shoulder-width apart while facing a wall or partner approximately 10 feet (3 m) away.

Action

Keep the arms straight and lift the medicine ball overhead. Simultaneously step forward with one foot and use both arms to throw the ball forward.

Finish

Repeat the action leading with the opposite foot.

Note: Intensity may be increased by increasing the weight of the medicine ball.

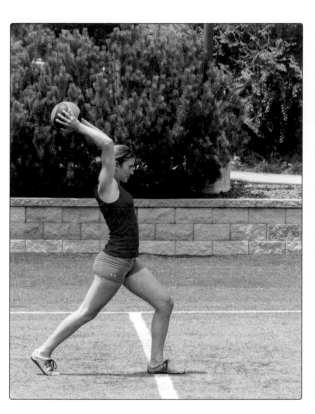
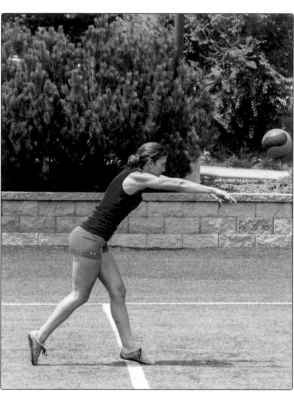

SCOOP TOSS

Start

Stand in the universal athletic position with the feet approximately shoulder-width apart, holding a medicine ball.

Action

Perform a countermovement by rapidly squatting to approximately 110° to 120° and swinging the medicine ball back and downward between the legs. Immediately perform a vertical jump, and while keeping the arms straight, explosively throw the medicine ball forward as far as possible.

Finish

Land in the universal athletic position, retrieve the ball, and repeat for the desired number of repetitions.

Note: Intensity may be increased by using a heavier medicine ball.

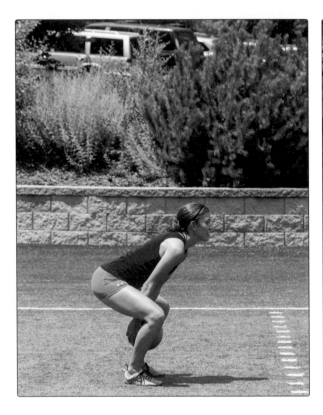
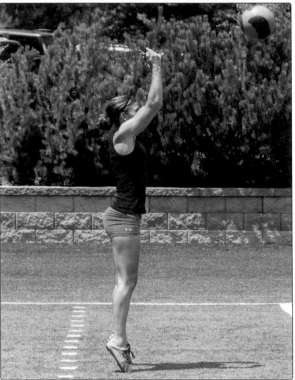

Program Design Recommendations

Before implementing plyometric training in the training program of a tactical athlete, there are several factors to consider. Addressing these factors will help maximize safety and ensure that the tactical athlete is physically prepared to engage in this form of training. Use the following program design recommendations when designing a plyometric training program.

General Considerations

Before implementing a plyometric training program, there are several factors to consider. These include training age and experience, body weight, injury history and status, strength requirements, proper technique, landing mechanics, attire, training surface and equipment, fatigue, and resistance.

Training Age and Experience   Due to the intensity of some plyometric drills and the potential risk of injury, it is imperative that a tactical athlete have a solid foundation of muscular strength. Moreover, a tactical athlete with a low skill level may require additional training at lower intensities and progressively higher volumes to improve technical proficiency before advancing to more complex drills. High-intensity plyometrics should be used with caution for middle-aged or older adults, who may be more prone to injury (1, 40).

Body Weight   Drills may need to be modified in order to reduce the amount of stress on the musculoskeletal system for larger individuals (>220 lb or 100 kg). This is due to the greater amount of force people of this size must absorb upon landing, as well as the high demands placed on the SSC, in relation to their body mass (2, 40). However, as long as the tactical athlete has an adequate amount of strength to accommodate these forces, there is likely no need to make significant adaptations to the training program. A more prudent strategy is to adjust intensity and volume based on recovery from training and the ability to maintain proper form and technique when performing these drills.

Injury History and Status   Areas of injury associated with lower body plyometrics typically include the feet, ankles, knees, hips, and lower back. For upper body plyometric drills, the fingers, wrists, elbows, and shoulders may be particularly vulnerable, especially if the tactical athlete has a preexisting injury. For this reason, a comprehensive physical evaluation should be performed before initiating plyometric training to determine whether a person can safely engage in this form of training.

Strength Requirements   For high-intensity lower body plyometric drills (e.g., bound, depth jump), it is recommended that a tactical athlete be able to back squat a minimum of one-and-a-half times their body weight before performing these drills (2, 40). This helps ensure that tactical athletes have the strength necessary to control the body when exposed to the high eccentric forces experienced when landing. An alternative to this recommendation is to perform five squats in 5 seconds or less with 60% of the tactical athlete's total body weight (40, 50). For example, a tactical athlete weighing 200 pounds (91 kg) should be able to squat 120 pounds (54 kg) five times in 5 seconds or less. However, these recommendations may be overly conservative when tactical athletes will be performing low- to moderate-level plyometrics. If tactical athletes are able to land properly with good form and technique, they should be able to safely perform the majority of the low- to moderate-level plyometric drills (34).

Proper Technique   When performing plyometric drills, proper form and technique must be maintained at all times. If a tactical athlete is allowed to perform a drill incorrectly, it may not only interfere with motor program development but may also increase injury risk. Tactical athletes who are unable to perform a drill correctly should be assessed to determine if additional strength training is required before performing plyometric work.

Landing Mechanics   As mentioned previously, plyometric drills can be intense due to the high eccentric loads that must be absorbed upon landing from a jump. Consequently, if the landing mechanics are improper, the tactical athlete will not be able to use the SSC to create a more powerful concentric action upon takeoff and may be more likely to experience an injury due to poor posture upon landing. Additionally, many times tactical athletes must absorb high eccentric loads during occupational tasks, such as when climbing over a fence or stepping off a truck in full kit. If tactical athletes have not developed sufficient eccentric strength and cannot support their body weight as well as body armor and equipment, they may be more likely to become injured when they experience high eccentric loads. For these reasons, the landing mechanics should be taught before incorporating plyometrics into a training program.

Attire When performing plyometric drills, athletic attire that allows unrestricted movement should be worn. In most cases, performing these drills in uniform or tactical gear would be contraindicated because movement may be impaired, increasing injury risk. For instance, if an officer were to wear a full tactical kit weighing 40 to 70 pounds (18-32 kg), the stress on the musculoskeletal system when performing these drills would be significantly higher than when wearing normal exercise attire. Additionally, the gear may shift during movement, leading to acute and sudden displacement of the tactical athlete's center of mass, which may alter body mechanics and technique. This sudden change may occur too rapidly for the individual to adjust to, which may lead to injury. As an advanced progression, it may be more prudent to use weighted exercise vests; they are typically designed to hang closer to the body than many tactical vests. Proper footwear that provides good foot and ankle support, such as a pair of cross-training shoes, is also recommended to increase safety when performing lower body plyometric drills. Running shoes may not be appropriate because they typically have a narrow sole and offer poor ankle support (2, 40).

Training Surface and Equipment Plyometric drills should always be performed on a nonslip, shock-absorbing surface, such as a grass or turf field, suspended wood flooring, or rubberized gym flooring (2, 40). Any boxes used for box and depth jumps should also have a nonslip surface on the top to reduce the risk of slipping and falling (40).

Fatigue To maximize the safety and effectiveness of plyometric drills, they should be performed early in a training session (i.e., before aerobic and resistance training) to ensure adequate recovery, maximum effort during each repetition, and reduced injury risks (40). Furthermore, plyometric drills should not be used as a form of metabolic conditioning. The main intent of these drills is to develop power. As fatigue ensues, an individual will be unable to perform these drills at maximal effort and may find it more challenging to maintain proper technique. This may not only lead to subpar performance gains but also injury.

Key Point

> The TSAC Facilitator must consider the health and training status as well as overall readiness of the tactical athlete when selecting plyometric drills for a training session.

Weight Selection for Medicine Ball Drills Currently, there are no standard recommendations for the training loads one should use when performing medicine ball throws and tosses. However, as with many implements used during plyometric exercise, a medicine ball that allows for correct form during a drill is a prudent starting point when determining an appropriate training load (10). In all cases, the load should be dictated by the desired movement speed and the ability to perform the drill with proper form.

Key Program Design Variables

When designing a plyometric training program, the four key variables to consider are frequency, intensity, volume, and rest (FIVR). By considering these factors, an individualized plyometric training program can be developed to meet the specific needs and demands of a tactical athlete.

Frequency The frequency of training for a plyometric program that emphasizes a particular body region (e.g., upper body, lower body, torso) may be performed as many as three days per week. Ultimately the frequency of plyometric training depends on the types and intensities of the drills selected, the volume of work performed, other physical and tactical skills sessions, travel, and ability to recover from training. For example, given the same volume, if a tactical athlete performs low-intensity drills in the plyometric training sessions, then two days of plyometric training may be better tolerated and easier to recover from than performing two days of moderate- to high-intensity plyometrics. Additionally, up to four sessions may be performed in a week if the upper and lower body plyometrics alternate between training sessions (e.g., lower body plyometrics on Monday and Thursday, upper body plyometrics on Tuesday and Friday). A minimum of 48 hours, depending on the intensity of the given training session (e.g., low or high intensity), should be allotted between plyometric training sessions that stress the same muscles or muscle groups to allow recovery from the previous sessions (26, 39).

Intensity   The intensity (e.g., one or two hands or feet) of a plyometric drill depends on the rate of stretch in the SSC (2). This rate of stretch depends on several variables, such as elevation and displacement of center of gravity, movement velocity or speed, body mass, use of a single leg versus both legs, and relative strength levels (3). Drill intensity should ultimately be based on the tactical athlete's current training status and experience, strength and technique level, physiological age, injury profile, and specific needs and goals. Table 13.1 displays a framework for plyometric drill progressions, with drills ranging from low to high intensities. TSAC Facilitators can use this table to decide which drills are most appropriate for their tactical athletes and how to increase the intensity of a plyometric training session as these individuals progress.

Volume   Training volume of plyometric drills is measured by foot or hand contacts or by distance traveled (3, 34). For example, if a tactical athlete performed four sets of 10 squat jumps, the total volume of training would be 40 contacts. If a tactical athlete performed a bounding drill over 120 m (131 yd), the total volume of training would be 120 m (131 yd). Table 13.2 provides guidelines for training volume based on training experience and time of year. Unlike a sport athlete with a set competitive season, a tactical athlete can be called upon at any time to perform. However, it is still prudent to use a periodized training model when incorporating plyometric drills into the training program to allow for the reduction of fatigue and overtraining effects. Periodization of plyometric training may be based on a personal fitness test, a deployment, other tactical training commitments (e.g., a block of defensive tactics training, rucking), travel commitments, or other fitness goals the tactical athlete may have outside of the occupation (e.g., 10K run, powerlifting competition).

Table 13.1 Plyometric Drill Progressions Based on Intensity

Intensity level	Classification	Description	Examples
Low intensity	Jumps in place	These drills involve vertical jumps performed while remaining in the same place or over a barrier. These drills should be performed for a single response (performed once, with a brief rest between reps).	• Squat jump • Tuck jump • Split squat jump • Countermovement jump • Cone and barrier jump* • Box jump*
	Standing jumps	These drills involve maximal jumps that emphasize horizontal displacement. These drills should be performed for a single response.	• Broad jump • Triple jump • Lateral jump • Cone and barrier jump* • Box jump*
	Multiple jumps and hops	These drills involve repeated jumps or hops.	• Double-leg hop • Single-leg hop • Lateral hop
	Bounds	These drills involve alternate landings from one foot to another, primarily aimed at achieving maximal horizontal distance.	• Double leg • Single leg
High intensity	Shock	These drills call for high-intensity nervous system activity and place a great deal of stress on the musculoskeletal system.	• Depth jump (vertical) • Depth jump (horizontal)

*May be used in multiple categories with slightly different training emphasis.

Adapted from Potach and Chu (40).

Table 13.2   Guidelines for Plyometric Training Volume

	Beginner	Intermediate	Advanced	Intensity
Off-season	60-100 foot contacts	100-150	120-200	Low to moderate
Preseason	100-150	150-300	150-450	Moderate to high
In-season	Dependent on other training commitments	Dependent on other training commitments	Dependent on other training commitments	Low to moderate

Based on Allerheiligen and Rogers (3).

Rest   *Rest* can be defined as the amount of time between repetitions, sets, or training sessions. Rest interval lengths for plyometric drills are load and goal specific. Longer rest periods for sufficient recovery between sets are required between drills of higher intensity in comparison to those of lower intensity. High-intensity plyometric drills (e.g., depth jumps) require adequate rest between sets to mitigate fatigue. Although plyometric drills are commonly conducted with little to no rest, this method of training is contraindicated because it does not allow for full recovery of the ATP-PCr energy system. It may accelerate fatigue, compromise power production, and increase the risk for injury.

SPEED TRAINING

Speed is the time required to cover a given distance and encompasses the skills and abilities needed to achieve high movement velocities (16). For the purpose of this text, speed will be explained in terms of linear running. Note that, in this chapter, plyometric, speed, and agility training are performed with an emphasis on neuromuscular and anaerobic capabilities.

Speed is an essential element for the tactical athlete when performing most critical job tasks. Whether running to seek cover from gunfire, running on uneven surfaces, rescuing a victim from a burning building, or chasing a fleeing assailant, speed matters. This section discusses running technique and form, and it features several drills for improving speed. An endless number of tactical situations could require running speed. The key for the tactical athlete is to be prepared for the various physical requirements that may arise.

Need for Speed Training in Tactical Populations

Many complicated movements take place in a short period of time during running. The ability of the nervous system to link the actions of the muscles in the most appropriate sequence will determine the ability to run fast and with control. In other words, all other physical capabilities being equal, the limiting factor in speed production is technique (13). Technique is important for performance, and it is also important for the prevention of injuries (4). Poor running technique can place too much strain on the lower leg, hamstrings, and groin and lead to injuries in those areas, to name a few. Therefore, a significant portion of training should use drills that are designed to develop an ideal running technique (4).

Running Technique

Linear running velocity is often divided into two phases: support and flight (16). The support phase is when one foot is in contact with the ground, and the flight phase is when the body is unsupported by the ground. A more detailed analysis of these phases of running follows.

Support Phase

The support phase starts when the lead foot makes contact with the ground, and it ends when the foot breaks contact. The lead foot should land on the ground slightly ahead of the body's center of gravity (16). Overstriding, or placing the foot farther than necessary in front of the center of mass, results in unnecessary braking forces that will slow the tactical athlete down and decrease running efficiency. The foot should be driven down by the hip extensors, and the hamstrings and gluteal muscles should perform the majority of the work during hip extension. The quadriceps are the primary movers and activate at ground contact in order to keep the knee from flexing excessively (11). At foot strike, the ankle should be dorsiflexed, with the big toe extended to help maximize elastic force production (11). The outside of the forefoot should contact the ground (11).

The tactical athlete should think about pulling herself over the foot and should continue exerting force until the center of gravity passes over and in front of the foot. When the toes leave the ground, the support phase ends.

Flight Phase

The flight phase starts when the aforementioned foot leaves the ground and lasts until it makes contact with the ground again (16). As the tactical athlete enters the flight phase and the foot leaves the ground, the ankle should immediately be dorsiflexed, with the big toe pulled up (11, 16). As the foot leaves the ground, the tactical athlete should flex the knee and bring the heel up to the hip as quickly as possible. This movement allows the tactical athlete to swing the recovery leg faster by shortening the lever and bringing the mass of the leg and thigh closer to the hip's axis of rotation. Knee flexion and hip flexion are executed by the hamstrings and knee flexors, respectively. As the heel reaches the hip, the leg should swing forward. The tactical athlete should aim to step over the opposite knee with the ankle to keep the lever shorter for a longer period of time. As the tactical athlete steps over the opposite knee, the knee extends and leg unfolds. The hip and knee extension is due to a transfer of momentum, not an active quadriceps contraction. As the leg unfolds, the tactical athlete aims to drive it down via hip extension, thus returning to the support phase (16). The swinging of the leg is where many hamstring injuries occur (12). As the leg swings forward, the hamstrings activate to keep the leg from unfolding too much (i.e., to keep the knee from hyperextending). Chumanov, Heiderscheit, and Thelen (12) found that the force the hamstrings exert during the unfolding increases as speed increases. This reinforces the need for tactical athletes to have well-conditioned hamstrings.

Additional Technique Considerations

While running, the head should remain in natural alignment with the spine. The shoulders and trunk should remain steady. Excessive twisting or rotating should be avoided. The exact angle of the body will depend upon **acceleration**, but at maximum speed it should be near vertical. The muscles of the face, neck, shoulders, arms, and hands should be relaxed. Tension in these areas may slow down limb speed and shorten ROM (11).

Arm action during maximum-velocity running is crucial. The swinging of the arms balances the forces created by the legs and initiates the actions of the legs (11). According to Bodyen (7), the total power output during sprinting can be no more than the latitude allowed by the weakest link. In other words, a weak and ineffective arm swing may limit maximum running speed. Therefore, the action of the arms during running is important to achieving and improving maximum velocity.

The elbow angle should range from 60° when the arm is in the front of the body to 140° when the arm is behind the body. The emphasis should be on driving the arm backward as opposed to forward. If the arm is driven back with enough force, it will be pushed forward due to the stretch reflex at the shoulder (11). Once the movement is automatic, the tactical athlete does not have to think about pushing the arm forward. The following guidelines will help tactical athletes achieve proper arm action.

- The arms should not cross the midline of the body. This causes the body to rotate, interfering with maximal speed.

- If the arm is driven backward properly, the elbow will extend to 140° on its own.

- The hand should travel from the height of the face or shoulder to the hip.

Finally, a major consideration for running within tactical populations is the change in technique that occurs due to PPE, utility belts, equipment, weapons, and so on. With the addition of this gear and equipment, certain movement constraints may not allow the tactical athlete to execute flawless running technique. The athlete must adapt to the gear and environmental conditions.

Warm-Up

A warm-up (general and specific) similar to that described previously for plyometric drills is recommended before speed drills. A further description of stretching approaches can be found in chapter 12.

Drills described in this section are designed to break linear running motion into parts to make mastery of these motions easier. The drills should be taught in the following order to ensure a part-to-whole approach is followed:

1. Arm swing drills
2. Ankling drills
3. High-knee drills
4. Butt kick drills
5. A-drills
6. B-drills
7. Fast-leg drills
8. Stride-length drills

Numerous starting positions can be incorporated in tactical-specific speed drills. The following positions are not a complete list but rather options to consider when performing acceleration drills.

- Prone
- Supine
- Crawling
- Seated
- Kneeling
- Two-point
- Three-point
- Four-point

ARM SWING DRILLS

Arm swing drills teach the correct arm action during maximum-velocity running. This section starts with simple arm swing drills and moves to more complex ones. Tactical athletes should not progress to more advanced drills until they have mastered the basic drills.

ARM SWING DRILL—SEATED

Purpose

To teach correct arm swing mechanics

Start

Sit down and extend the legs in front of the body. The torso should be tall, with the shoulders back. The right elbow should begin at approximately 60° and should be near the body with the hand located between the shoulder and the eyes. The left arm should be positioned behind the body so that the left hand is next to the left hip, and the elbows should be at approximately 90° angles.

Action

While seated, drive the right arm backward aggressively so that the right hand ends up next to the right hip. At the same time, drive the left arm forward so that the left hand ends up between the left shoulder and eye. Maintain a 90° elbow position throughout the duration of the movement, understanding that flexion and extension of the elbow will occur throughout the movement. Repeat until the desired time has elapsed.

Finish

The drill is completed when the desired time has elapsed.

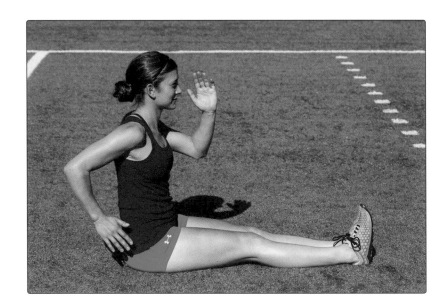

ARM SWING DRILLS

ARM SWING DRILL—STANDING

Purpose

To teach correct arm swing mechanics while standing

Start

Stand tall with the shoulders back. Keep the hands loose and flex both elbows. The right elbow should begin at approximately 60° and should be near the body, with the hand located between the shoulder and the eyes. The left arm should be positioned behind the body at approximately 140° so that the left hand is next to the left hip.

Action

While standing, drive the right arm backward aggressively so that the right hand ends up next to the right hip. At the same time, drive the left arm forward so that the left hand ends up between the left shoulder and eye. Maintain a 90° elbow position throughout the duration of the movement, understanding that flexion and extension of the elbow will occur throughout the action. Repeat until the desired time has elapsed.

Finish

The drill is completed when the desired time has elapsed.

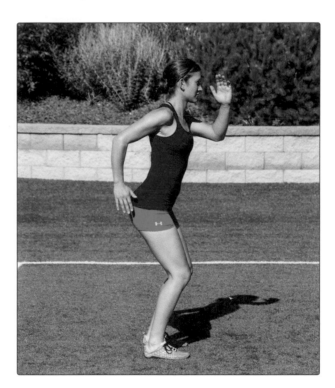

ARM SWING DRILLS

ARM SWING DRILL—WALKING

Purpose

To teach correct arm swing mechanics while moving

Start

Stand tall with the shoulders back. Keep the hands loose and flex both elbows. The right elbow should begin at approximately 60° and near the body, with the hand located between the shoulder and the eyes. The left arm should be positioned behind the body so that the left hand is next to the left hip. Maintain a 90° elbow position throughout the duration of the movement, understanding that flexion and extension of the elbow will occur throughout action.

Action

While walking forward for 10 to 20 yards (or meters), focus on driving the right arm backward aggressively so that the right hand ends up next to the right hip. At the same time, drive the left arm forward so that the left hand ends up between the left shoulder and eye. Try to swing the arms faster than the feet move.

Finish

The drill is completed when the desired distance has been covered.

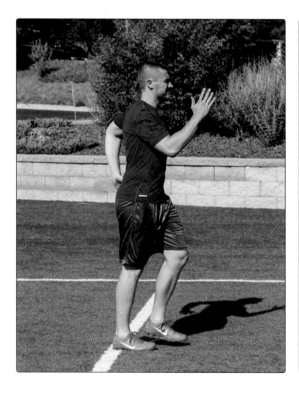 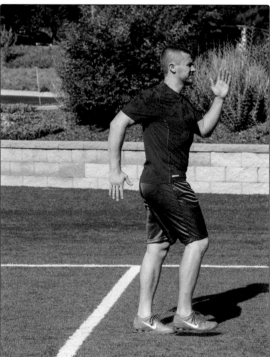

ARM SWING DRILLS

ARM SWING DRILL—JOGGING

Purpose

To teach correct arm swing mechanics while moving

Start

Stand tall with the shoulders back. Flex both elbows and make loose fists with both hands. The right elbow should begin at approximately 60° and near the body with the hand located between the shoulder and the eyes. The left arm should be positioned behind the body at approximately 140° so that the left hand is next to the left hip. Maintain a 90° elbow position, understanding that flexion and extension of the elbow will occur throughout the action.

Action

While jogging forward for 10 to 20 yards (or meters), focus on driving the right arm backward aggressively so that the right hand ends up next to the right hip. At the same time, drive the left arm forward so that the left hand ends up between the left shoulder and eye. Try to swing the arms faster than the feet move.

Finish

The drill is completed when the desired distance has been covered.

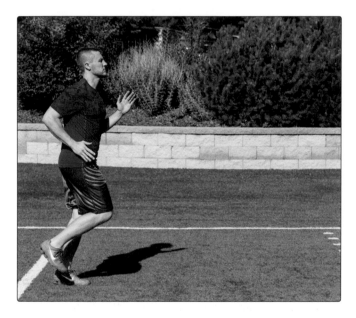
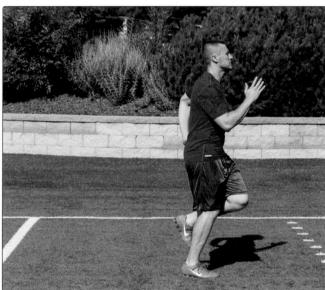

ANKLING DRILLS

Ankling drills teach the tactical athlete how to lift the feet off the ground during maximum-velocity running. These drills are designed to emphasize ankle plantar flexion and dorsiflexion. For sprint work, the dorsiflexed position should be empha- sized throughout the entire movement, with the exception of the explosive plantar flexion necessary to propel the body forward immediately after the foot strike.

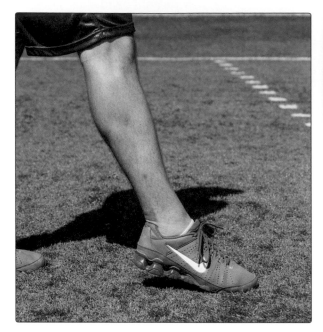

Plantar flexion

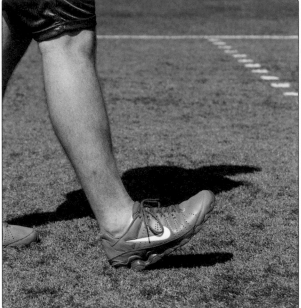

Dorsiflexion

ANKLING DRILLS

ANKLING DRILL

Purpose

To teach dorsiflexion of the ankle and proper sprint mechanics

Start

Stand tall with the shoulders back.

Action

Keeping the legs straight, alternately flex and extend the ankles to move forward with very short steps. Emphasize brief, explosive contact with the ball of the foot with each step while the legs remain straight. As each leg moves forward, the ankle should be dorsiflexed. Repeat these quick steps for the desired distance. Maintain a 90° elbow position, understanding that flexion and extension of the elbow will occur throughout the action.

Finish

The drill is completed when the desired distance has been covered.

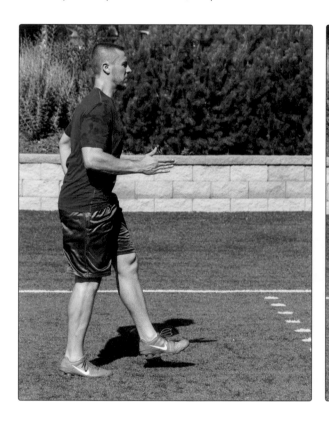
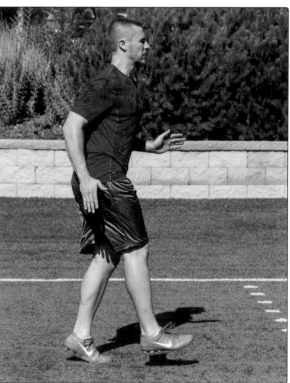

HIGH-KNEE DRILLS

High-knee drills teach the tactical athlete to lift the knees during maximum-velocity running. This technique is important to master because it results in a more powerful leg drive by using the gluteus maximus to help power the motion. High-knee drills start with a walking motion, focusing on one side at a time. Eventually, both sides are alternated, and then skipping is added to increase complexity. At first, these drills are performed without any emphasis on the arm motion. As the tactical athlete becomes more proficient, the arm motion can be added. High-knee drills are performed for 10 to 20 yards (or meters). The emphasis should be on quality of movement as opposed to speed.

■ HIGH-KNEE DRILL—WALKING, ONE SIDE

Purpose

To teach the high-knee motion while focusing on one side of the body at a time

Start

Stand tall with the shoulders back.

Action

Maintaining a tall posture, lift the right knee as high as possible. As the right knee is lifted, the right ankle should be dorsiflexed. Maintaining ankle dorsiflexion, lower the right foot to the ground and take a normal step forward with the left leg. The arms should move at the same rate as the leg, with minimal to no pausing of arm action between cycles. Repeat the drill with the right side for the desired distance, and then switch sides.

Finish

The drill is completed when the desired distance has been covered with both sides of the body.

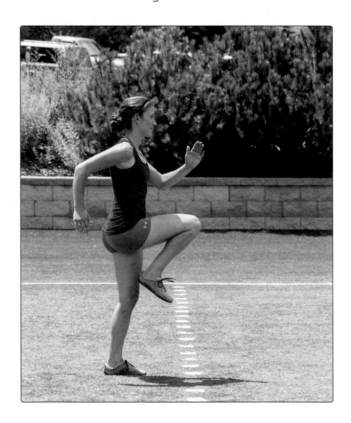

HIGH-KNEE DRILLS

HIGH-KNEE DRILL—WALKING, ALTERNATE SIDES

Purpose

To teach the high-knee motion while alternating both sides of the body

Start

Stand tall with the shoulders back.

Action

Perform the high-knee walking motion with the right leg with the ankle dorsiflexed. As the right foot lands on the ground, perform the high-knee walking motion with the left leg. The arms should move at the same rate as the leg, with minimal to no pausing of arm action between cycles. Continue alternating for the desired distance.

Finish

The drill is completed when the desired distance has been covered.

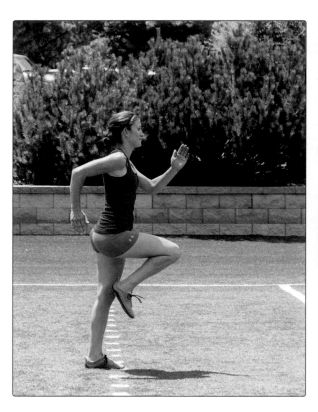 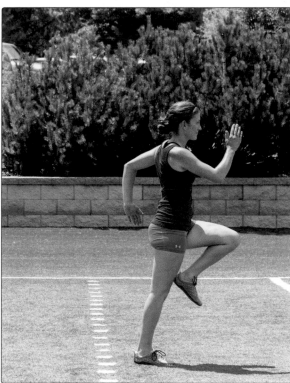

HIGH-KNEE DRILLS

HIGH-KNEE DRILL—SKIPPING, ONE SIDE

Purpose

To teach the high-knee motion in an explosive manner while focusing on one side of the body

Start

Stand tall with the shoulders back.

Action

Maintaining a tall posture, perform a forward skip with the left leg. As the left leg is extended, the right knee should be lifted high with the right ankle dorsiflexed. Maintain ankle dorsiflexion as the right foot lands on the ground. Take a normal step forward with the left leg and repeat the skip and high-knee motion of the right leg. The arms should move at the same rate as the leg, with minimal to no pausing of arm action between cycles. Repeat the skips for the desired distance and then switch sides.

Finish

The drill is completed when the desired distance has been covered with both legs.

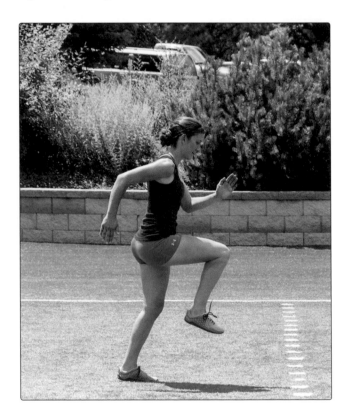

HIGH-KNEE DRILLS

HIGH-KNEE DRILL—SKIPPING, ALTERNATE SIDES

Purpose

To teach the high-knee motion in an explosive manner while alternating both sides of the body

Start

Stand tall with the shoulders back.

Action

Perform a skipping motion with the left leg to drive the high-knee motion of the right leg. As the right foot lands on the ground, perform the skipping motion with the right leg to drive the high-knee motion of the left leg. Repeat the alternated skips for the desired distance.

Finish

The drill is completed when the desired distance has been covered.

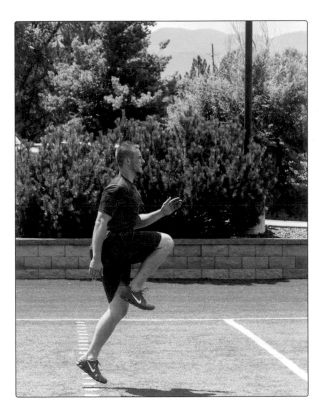
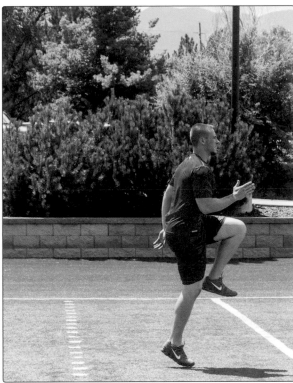

BUTT KICK DRILLS

BUTT KICKS

Purpose

To reinforce ankle dorsiflexion and to teach bringing the foot to the hip after push-off

Start

Stand tall with the feet directly below the hips.

Action

Lift the right foot off the ground, dorsiflexing the ankle it as it leaves the ground. Immediately bring the heel of the right foot to the buttocks, flexing the right hip somewhat so the knee does not point straight to the ground. The heel should align vertically with the hip. The arms should move at the same rate as the leg, with minimal to no pausing of arm action between cycles. As the right foot lands on the ground, repeat this drill with the left side. Continue alternating until 10 to 20 yards (or meters) have been covered. Note that this is a technique drill, not a speed drill.

Finish

The drill is completed when the desired distance has been covered.

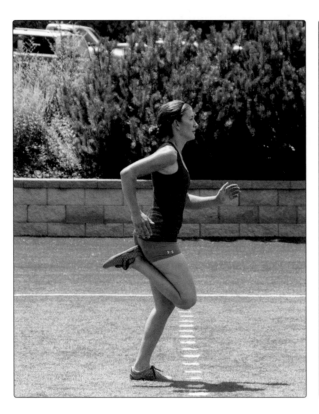 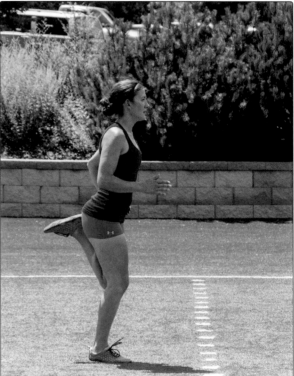

A-DRILLS

A-drills bring together ankling, high-knee drills, butt kicks, and arm swing drills. They are performed faster and more explosively than the basic drills and are meant to reinforce a tall posture, ankling, bringing the heel to the hip, high knees, ankle dorsiflexion, and driving the foot toward the ground. Like the high-knee drills, A-drills start with a walking motion, focusing on one side at a time. Eventually, both sides are alternated, and then skipping is added to make the movements more complex. At first, these drills are performed without any emphasis on the arm motion. As the tactical athlete becomes more proficient, the arm motion can be added. A-drills are performed for 10 to 20 yards (or meters). As with most technique drills, the emphasis should be on quality of movement as opposed to speed.

A-DRILL—WALKING, ONE SIDE

Purpose

To begin teaching the sprinting motion by focusing on one side of the body at a time

Start

Stand tall with the feet directly beneath the hips.

Action

Lift the right heel to the buttocks with the ankle dorsiflexed. When the heel reaches the buttocks, lift the right knee. As the knee is lifted, the foot will separate from the buttocks. The knee should be lifted high enough so that the right foot steps over the left knee. The ankle must remain dorsiflexed as this occurs. Using the hip, drive the leg into the ground slightly in front of the body's center of gravity. Use a pawing motion to pull the body's center of gravity over the foot. Take a normal step forward with the left leg. Repeat until the desired distance is covered. The arms should move at the same rate as the leg, with minimal to no pausing of arm action between cycles.

Finish

The drill is completed when the desired distance has been covered with both sides of the body.

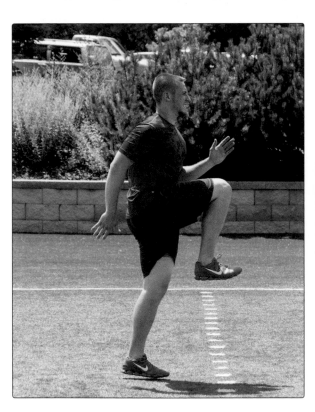
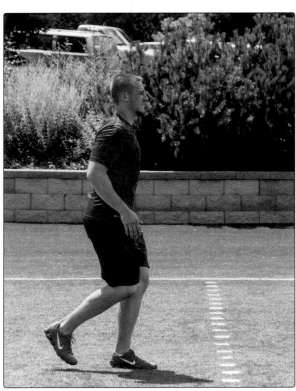

A-DRILLS

A-DRILL—WALKING, ALTERNATING SIDES

Purpose

To begin teaching the sprinting motion by focusing on alternating both sides of the body

Start

Stand tall with the feet directly beneath the hips.

Action

Perform the walking A-drill with the right side. As the body is pulled over the foot, lift the left heel to the buttocks and perform the walking A-drill with the left leg. Continue alternating legs until the desired distance has been covered.

Finish

The drill is completed when the desired distance has been covered.

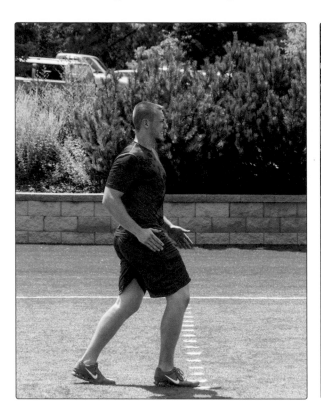
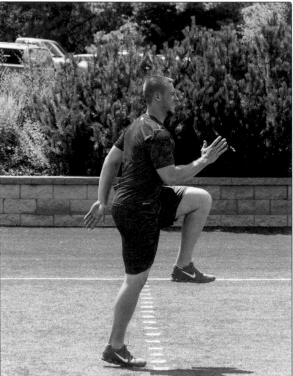

A-DRILLS

A-DRILL—SKIPPING, ONE SIDE

Purpose

To teach the sprinting motion in an explosive manner while focusing on one side of the body

Start

Stand tall with the feet directly beneath the hips.

Action

Maintaining a tall posture, perform a skip with the left leg. As the skip is performed, the right ankle should be dorsiflexed and the heel should be brought to the buttocks. The right knee should then be raised and the foot should be aggressively driven into the ground in a pawing motion. Step forward with the left leg. Repeat until the desired distance has been covered and then switch sides. The arms should move at the same rate as the leg, with minimal to no pausing of arm action between cycles.

Finish

The drill is completed when the desired distance has been covered with both sides of the body.

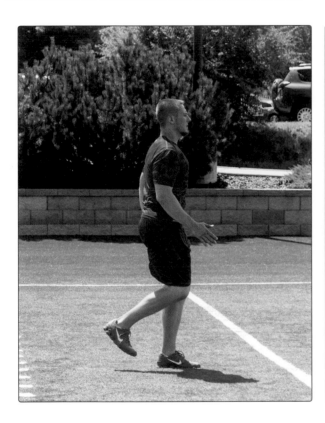 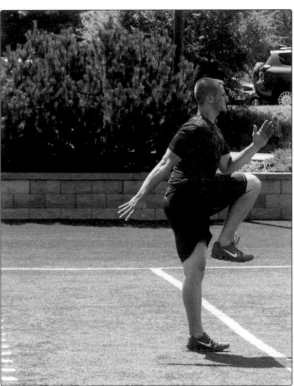

A-DRILLS

A-DRILL—SKIPPING, ALTERNATE SIDES

Purpose

To teach the sprinting motion in an explosive manner while focusing on alternating both sides of the body

Start

Stand tall with the feet positioned directly under the hips.

Action

Maintaining a tall posture, perform a skip with the left leg. As the skip is performed, the right ankle should be dorsiflexed and the heel should be brought to the buttocks. The right knee should then be raised and the foot should be aggressively driven into the ground in a pawing motion. As the right foot makes contact with the ground, immediately perform a skip with the right leg and bring the left heel to the buttocks with the ankle dorsiflexed. Strive to get off the ground as quickly as possible with each skip. Repeat until the desired distance has been covered. The arms should move at the same rate as the leg, with minimal to no pausing of arm action between cycles.

Finish

The drill is completed when the desired distance has been covered.

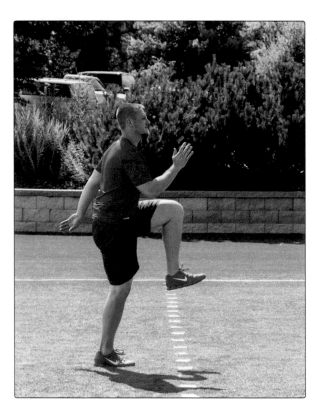
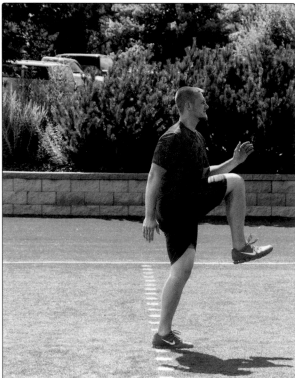

B-DRILLS

B-DRILL—SKIPPING, ONE SIDE

Purpose

To teach the active landing in an explosive manner, focusing on one side of the body

Start

Stand tall with the feet directly under the hips.

Action

Maintaining a tall posture, perform a skip with the left leg. As the skip is performed, the right ankle should be dorsiflexed and the heel should be brought to the buttocks. Raise the right knee and then allow it to extend as the foot travels out and away from the body. Remember to keep the ankle dorsiflexed throughout. The knee exten-sion should happen as a result of the hip flexion. It should not be forced or exaggerated. From the hip, aggressively drive the straight leg into the ground just in front of the body's center of gravity. Use a pawing motion to pull the body's center of gravity over the foot. Take a normal step forward with the left leg. Repeat until the desired distance is covered, and then switch sides. The arms should move at the same rate as the leg, with minimal to no pausing of arm action between cycles.

Finish

The drill is completed when the desired distance has been covered with both sides of the body.

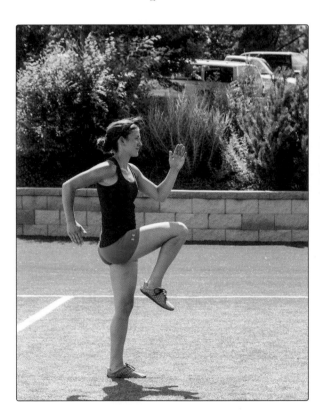 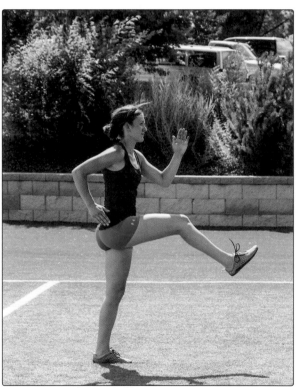

B-DRILLS

B-DRILL—SKIPPING, ALTERNATE SIDES

Purpose

To teach the active landing in an explosive manner, focusing on alternating both sides of the body

Start

Stand tall with the feet directly beneath the hips.

Action

The mechanics of skipping involve a step-hop pattern alternating from side to side. Bring the right heel to the buttocks with the ankle dorsiflexed. When the heel reaches the buttocks, lift the right knee. As the knee is lifted, the foot will separate from the buttocks. The knee should be lifted high enough so that the right foot steps over the left knee. Allow the right knee to extend so that the foot travels out in front of the body. Let this movement occur naturally as a result of the hip flexion. Do not force or exaggerate it. The right ankle must remain dorsiflexed as it moves in front of the body. Using the hip, drive the leg downward just in front of the body's center of gravity. Use a pawing motion to pull the body's center of gravity over the foot. Continue forward using a step-hop pattern, alternating sides. Continue this action for the desired distance. The arms should move at the same rate as the leg, with minimal to no pausing of arm action between cycles.

Finish

The drill is completed when the desired distance has been covered with both sides of the body.

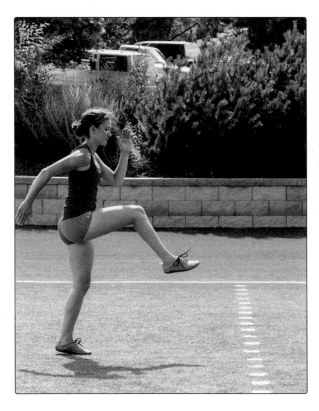
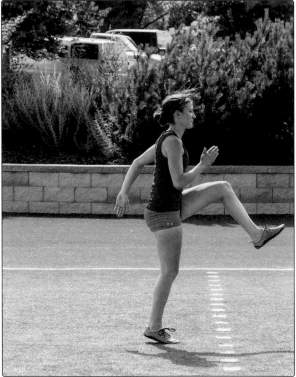

FAST-LEG DRILLS

Fast-leg drills are advanced drills that combine the qualities of a number of the drills described previously. Fast-leg drills should only be performed after the tactical athlete has mastered the more basic drills.

FAST-LEG DRILL

Purpose

To improve stride frequency

Start

Stand tall with the feet positioned approximately hip-width apart.

Action

Perform a fast ankling motion with straight legs, dorsiflexing each ankle as it leaves the ground. On every third step, perform a fast-leg motion by bringing the heel to the buttocks, cycling the leg forward (stepping over the opposite leg), lifting the knee, and allowing the foot to separate from the buttocks. Using the hip, drive the foot toward the ground in a pawing motion to pull the body's center of gravity over the foot. The ankle should remain dorsiflexed throughout. This fast-leg motion should take place as quickly as possible. Immediately take a normal step with the other foot. Perform the drill for 10 to 20 yards (or meters). A variation of this drill is to take every left (or right) stride as a fast leg. The arms should move at the same rate as the leg, with minimal to no pausing of arm action between cycles.

Finish

The drill is completed when the desired distance has been covered.

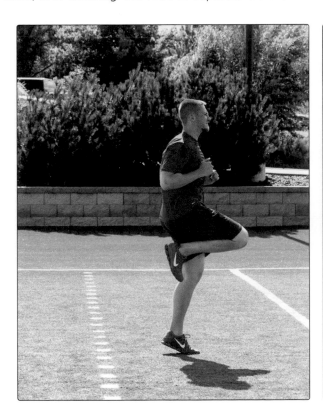
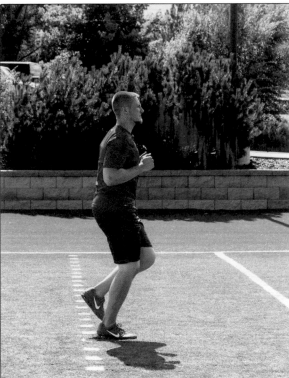

ACCELERATION DRILLS

Accelerating includes starting drills from a stationary or moving start and increasing velocity. Acceleration drills range from simple to occupation specific (e.g., running for cover, chasing an assailant, rushing up a hill):

1. Standing
2. Crouching
3. Lying
4. Changing directions
5. Occupation specific

STANDING START

Purpose

To teach the arm action that accompanies the start of a sprint and to develop acceleration

Start

The nonpower foot begins two foot-lengths behind the start line. The power foot begins three foot-lengths behind the start line. The feet are less than shoulder-width apart, and there is a slight bend in the ankles, knees, and hips. The head and spine should be kept neutral. Keep the weight on the balls of the feet.

Action

Begin acceleration by falling forward and then stepping with the power foot to break the fall. As the power foot steps forward, drive the arm on the same side of the body backward. Run the prescribed distance.

Finish

The drill is completed when the desired distance has been covered.

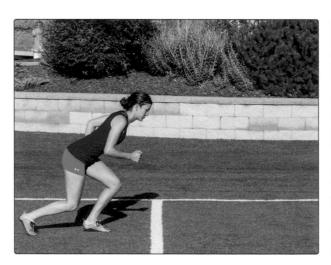
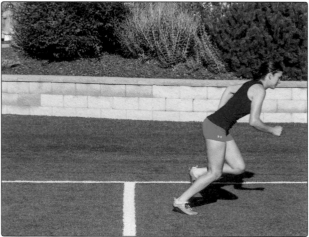

ACCELERATION DRILLS

CROUCH START

Purpose
To develop acceleration from a crouched position

Start
Assume a staggered stance with one foot two foot-lengths behind the start line. The other foot is three foot-lengths behind the start line.

Action
On command, sprint forward and cover the desired distance. As the lead foot steps forward, drive the arm on the same side of the body backward.

Finish
The drill is completed when the desired distance has been covered.

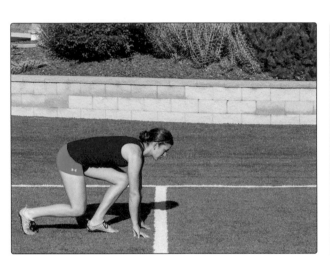
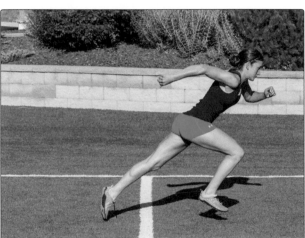

PUSH-UP START

Purpose
To make the starting motion more difficult by standing up before accelerating (similar to taking cover or performing a 3- to 5-second rush)

Start
Behind the start line, assume the starting position for push-ups.

Action
On command, stand up and sprint forward, covering the desired distance.

Finish
The drill is completed when the desired distance has been covered.

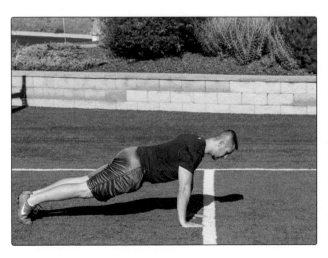
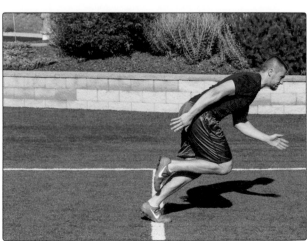

ACCELERATION DRILLS

PRONE START

Purpose

To make the starting motion more difficult by getting off the ground before accelerating

Start

Behind the start line, lie facedown in a push-up position.

Action

On command, stand up and sprint forward, covering the desired distance.

Finish

The drill is completed when the desired distance has been covered.

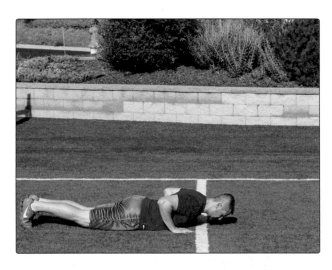 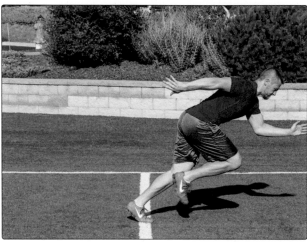

STANDING, BACK-TO-COURSE START

Purpose

To make the starting motion more difficult by changing direction before accelerating

Start

Stand with the back to the course.

Action

On command, turn around and sprint forward, covering the desired distance.

Finish

The drill is completed when the desired distance has been covered.

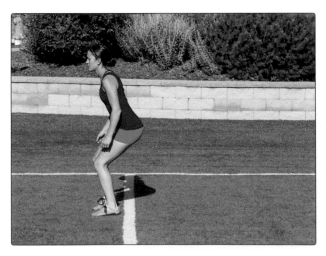 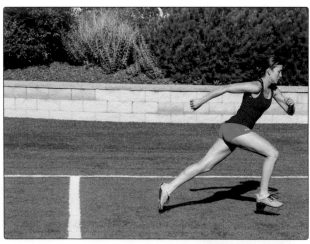

ACCELERATION DRILLS

BROAD JUMP + START

Purpose
To make the starting motion more complex and more sport specific by combining motions

Start
Stand tall with the feet directly under the hips and the hands at the sides of the body.

Action
Execute a standing broad jump. Upon landing, immediately sprint forward and cover the desired distance.

Finish
The drill is completed when the desired distance has been covered.

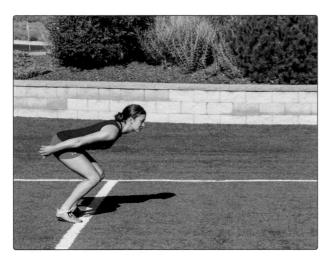
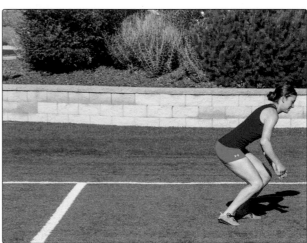

VERTICAL JUMP + START

Purpose
To make the starting motion more complex and more sport specific by combining motions

Start
Assume an athletic position with a slight bend in the ankle, knees, and hips; chest up; and shoulders back.

Action
Execute a vertical jump. Upon landing, immediately sprint forward and cover the desired distance.

Finish
The drill is completed when the desired distance has been covered.

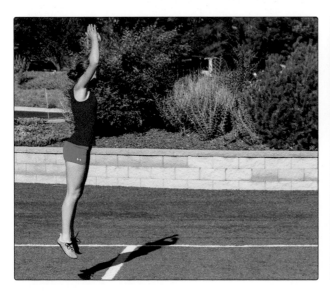
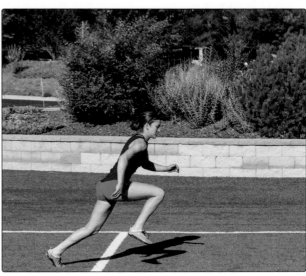

ACCELERATION DRILLS

MEDICINE BALL TOSS + START

Purpose

To make the starting motion more complex and more sport specific by combining motions

Start

Stand tall with the feet directly beneath the hips and the hands at the sides of the body.

Action

Execute a forward or backward medicine ball toss. Upon releasing the ball, sprint forward the desired distance.

Finish

The drill is completed when the desired distance has been covered.

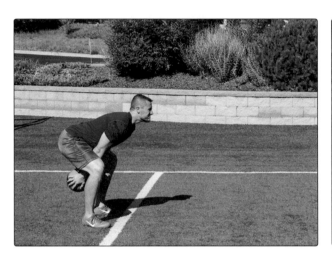
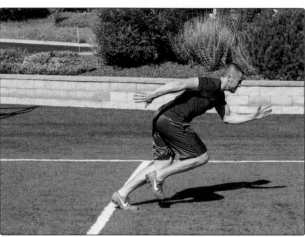

Program Design Recommendations

The following section discusses several program design variables. Manipulating these variables is the responsibility of the TSAC Facilitator. Care should be taken when designing programs to ensure optimal training adaptations.

Training Goals

The goal of linear, maximum-velocity running is to optimize stride length, maximize stride frequency, and minimize braking forces (20). Training for linear speed has three objectives (21, 32):

1. Minimize braking forces at ground contact. This is accomplished by planting the foot slightly in front of the center of mass and maximizing the velocity of the leg and foot at ground contact.

2. Emphasize brief ground-support times as a means of achieving rapid stride rate. This is achieved by high rates of force development.

3. Emphasize functional ability of the hamstrings. Because they simultaneously perform eccentric and concentric contractions at the hip and knee while running, the knee flexors are under extreme stress and subject to injury. Thus, tactical athletes require eccentric knee flexor strength (20).

Demands Specific to the Tactical Population

Specific speed drills for the tactical athlete will reflect loads, intensities, operational equipment, and environmental situations that are observed in the field of operation. Tactical personnel perform in a multitude of conditions with a variety of operational equipment and load requirements. The salient point is to train under field conditions while using the required clothing, equipment, and gear. Additionally, environmental conditions, such as temperature, humidity, time of day, altitude, surface (e.g., sand, mud, snow, water), and terrain, should be replicated to prepare for occupational conditions. The TSAC Facilitator should progress, load, assess, and monitor the tactical athlete to ensure optimal training adaptations are achieved while overloading the athlete in simulated conditions. The specific loading parameters should be predicated on technique mastery and the facilitator's discretion.

Additionally, although some linear speed training is warranted for all tactical athletes, the amount of speed training performed should be based on the occupational demands of the individual. For instance, firefighters perform many activities that are highly physically demanding, but it is their ability to sustain high power outputs that may be most important, such as when climbing stairs. Therefore, based on the terrain that firefighters must maneuver through (e.g., uneven ground, slick surfaces), maximal sprinting may put the firefighter in grave danger on the job. However, this does not mean that it cannot be used as a form of training; metabolic adaptations to sprint training may allow firefighters to work at a higher percentage of their overall aerobic capacity while fighting a fire. For law enforcement officers and military personnel, more sprint work may be warranted because they are more likely to be in a situation where a maximal sprint is imperative to safety and performance (e.g., taking cover from gunfire, chasing a fleeing assailant) (14).

In general, sprint training should be performed a minimum of twice per week; however, the volume is based on the tactical athletes' goals and how well they are able to recover between training sessions. Some individuals may benefit from shorter, more frequent bouts of speed training versus one concentrated session. For example, incorporating 5 to 10 sprints may improve or maintain this physical attribute. Furthermore, for drills that emphasize maximal speed or speed technique, the drill should last no more than approximately 10 seconds in order to focus on the development of the ATP-PCr energy system. This also requires longer rest periods between each sprint (e.g., 1:12 to 1:20 work:rest ratio). If performing speed work on the same day as other forms of training, it is best to perform speed training first, when the neurological system is less fatigued. If speed endurance is the goal, longer

sprints (>10 seconds) may be warranted. In this case, it may be best to perform these sprints after a traditional resistance training session or on a separate day to minimize the interference effect these types of training regimes may have on one another (27). As a guideline, maximal or near-maximal speed training should not exceed a total volume of approximately 600 yards (or meters) per session.

Key Point

Specific speed drills for the tactical athlete will reflect loads, intensities, operational equipment, and environmental situations that are observed in the field of operation.

AGILITY TRAINING

Agility is the interaction of perceptual motor abilities and physical abilities, or "the skills and abilities needed to change direction, velocity, or mode in response to a stimulus" (16). Historically there has been little to no difference between agility and change-of-direction training. However, current research suggests that agility is not only the ability to change direction but also the ability to change direction in response to a stimulus (i.e., auditory, kinesthetic, or visual cue) (1, 26, 46). Strength and conditioning practitioners most often use predetermined movement patterns to improve agility performance. However, when implementing an agility training program for tactical athletes, the specific tactical environment the athlete is required to perform in should be a consideration. Similar to most sporting situations, some tactical maneuvers are preplanned, but others require tactical athletes to respond to the opposition and their own team members, and some are a combination of the two. As a result, the TSAC Facilitator should implement change-of-direction speed drills to develop the appropriate physical qualities and movement patterns, as well as context-specific drills that require reaction to stimulus and decision-making requirements (perceptual-cognitive ability), to best address agility performance.

Following are seven primary abilities that contribute to agility.

1. Dynamic flexibility—the ROM around a joint while moving. Adequate dynamic flexibility allows the tactical athlete to place the body in optimal positions to move rapidly.

2. Multilimb coordination—the ability to coordinate the movement of multiple limbs simultaneously (22).

3. Power—the time rate of doing work, where work is the product of force exerted on an object and the distance the object moves in the direction in which the force is exerted (33).

4. Dynamic balance—the ability to maintain total body balance while moving (11).

5. Acceleration—change in velocity per unit of time (33).

6. Stopping ability—the ability to brake or decelerate (11)

7. Strength—the ability to exert force (33).

This is by no means an exhaustive list but rather a starting point to understand the underlying tenets of agility as a trainable skill.

Types of Agility Drills and Progression

Agility drills can be performed with a wide variety of patterns and tools, such as cones, hurdles, and ladders. Furthermore, the drills can be progressed from **closed drills** (performed in a known environment) to **open drills** (require the tactical athlete to respond to an auditory, visual, or kinesthetic stimulus or cue) or **semi-open drills** (a combination of closed and open drills).

This chapter features a wide variety of agility patterns and drills. However, although the

patterns of these drills may differ, there are some fundamental movement skills that are necessary to execute each drill effectively. Most agility drills can be classified as **serial tasks**, or the combination of two or more discrete tasks. A **discrete task** is an activity or movement with a clear beginning and ending. Several discrete patterns can be combined to create serial agility tasks (43). Each of these discrete tasks should be mastered before performing the agility patterns featured later in this chapter. Mastering these foundational movements will help develop the requisite movement skills for performing more complex agility movements. Table 13.3 presents the phases of learning to provide a framework for the TSAC Facilitator to determine the tactical athlete's level of understanding in regard to the movement skills required to execute an agility task.

When developing an agility program, it is prudent to use a mastery-based approach, in which each tactical athlete demonstrates competency in each of the discrete agility techniques featured in the following section. Furthermore, by establishing a movement curriculum or checklist for each of these drills, the TSAC Facilitator can better assess the tactical athlete's proficiency and ability to progress to higher intensity and complexity. A sample movement curriculum for the 90° agility turn is provided in table 13.4.

Warm-Up

Before agility drills, perform a warm-up (general and specific) similar to that described previously for plyometric drills. A further description of stretching approaches can be found in chapter 12.

Table 13.3 Phases of Learning

Phase of learning	Phase description
Early learning	Many errors, rigid, timid, inconsistent, stiff, inefficient, indecisive, inaccurate
Relatively proficient	Fewer errors, more adaptable, more confident, more consistent, more relaxed, more efficient, more decisive, accurate
Proficient	Few errors, adaptable, confident, consistent, automatic, efficient, certain, fluid, accurate

Adapted from Schmidt and Wrisberg (44).

Table 13.4 Checklist for 90° Agility Turn

Area of focus	Target mechanics
Foot position	Rapid, small steps Some lateral displacement Full contact of sole of foot while slowing Feet remain low to the ground
Leg position	Knees bent
Trunk position or posture	Neutral spine Shoulders square to the target Hips low to the ground
Arm position	Elbows close to the sides but not touching Elbows bent approximately 90° Short, rapid movements

Adapted from Jeffreys (29).

The fundamental agility skills are discrete tasks that should be mastered and performed correctly before the athlete performs the more complex agility patterns.

Fundamental Agility Skills

Agility Patterns

FUNDAMENTAL AGILITY SKILLS

◼ AGILITY TECHNIQUE: ACCELERATION

Purpose

To develop linear acceleration ability

Start

There are a number of starting positions to choose from. The key point is to start from a stationary position.

Action

Lower the center of mass by bending at the knees and hips. The spine remains neutral, and the torso angles forward. The knee and hip of the lead leg are flexed when the foot is not in contact with the ground. The support leg extends at the hip, knee, and ankle. Action at the arms and legs occurs on the sagittal plane.

Finish

The drill is completed when the desired distance is covered.

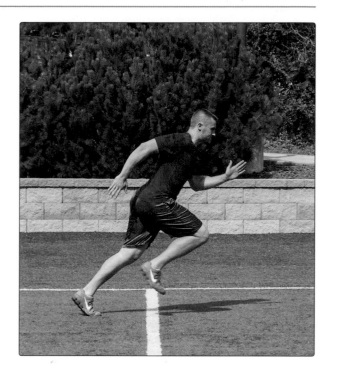

◼ AGILITY TECHNIQUE: DECELERATION

Purpose .

To develop the ability to come to a complete stop efficiently and quickly

Start

Start at running velocity that can be used to execute **deceleration** with desirable biomechanics.

Action

Lower the center of mass by bending at the knees and hips, placing the feet in front of the center of mass. This action accentuates eccentric contraction of the extensors of the hip, knee, and ankle. The spine remains neutral and the head remains up. The knee and hip of the lead leg are flexed, and the foot is in contact with the ground. Action at the arms and legs occurs on the sagittal plane.

Finish

The drill is completed when the desired number of repetitions have been achieved.

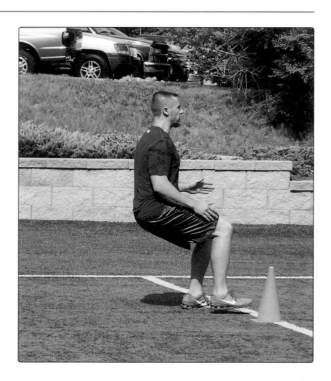

FUNDAMENTAL AGILITY SKILLS

■ AGILITY TECHNIQUE: BACKPEDAL

Purpose

To develop the ability to backpedal efficiently and quickly

Start

Start with the back to the direction of movement. Keep both the knees and hips flexed to the degree where there is no need to lower the center of mass before initiating the action.

Action

Keeping the center of gravity low and the shoulders over the base of support, alternate the feet and move backward. The lower body movement is from flexion and extension at the hips, knees, and ankles.

Finish

The drill is completed when the desired number of repetitions have been achieved over the desired distance.

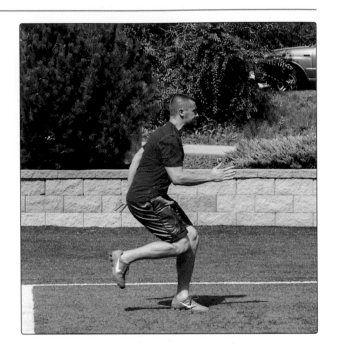

■ AGILITY TECHNIQUE: ROUNDING CONE

Purpose

To develop the ability to decelerate, turn efficiently, and accelerate

Start

Start by running toward a single cone that serves as the position to turn.

Action

Begin deceleration by lowering the center of mass (bending at the knees and hips and placing the feet in front of the center of mass). This action accentuates eccentric contraction of the extensors of the hip, knee, and ankle. The spine remains neutral and the head remains up. Use short, abbreviated steps. The knee and hip of the lead leg are flexed, and the foot is in contact with the ground. Lower the shoulder closest to the cone, and turn the head toward the intended direction. Use short steps to keep close to the cone while turning. The spine remains neutral while the torso angles forward. The knee and hip of the lead leg are flexed when the foot is not in contact with the ground. The support leg extends at the hip, knee, and ankle. Action at the arms and legs occurs on the sagittal plane.

Finish

The drill is completed when the desired number of repetitions have been achieved.

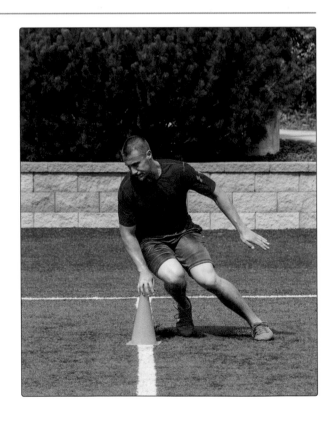

FUNDAMENTAL AGILITY SKILLS

AGILITY TECHNIQUE: SHUFFLE/CUTTING

Purpose

To develop the ability to move efficiently laterally

Start

Start in the universal athletic position. Face 90° from the direction of movement.

Action

Initiate the movement by stepping with the lead foot laterally in the desired direction. The support leg extends at the hip, knee, and ankle, pushing the body laterally. Keep the knees and hips bent and the center of mass low. Do not cross the feet. The spine remains neutral and the head remains up. The arms are at the sides with the elbows bent.

Finish

The drill is completed when the desired number of repetitions have been achieved over the desired distance.

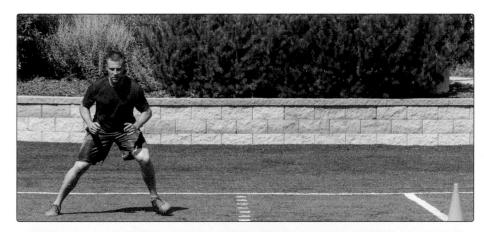

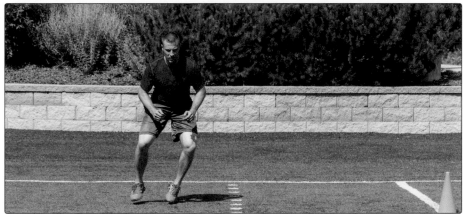

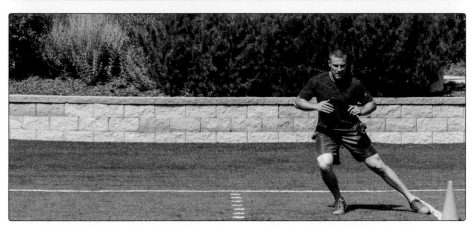

FUNDAMENTAL AGILITY SKILLS

AGILITY TECHNIQUE: OPEN STEP

Purpose

To develop the ability to transition from a backpedal to forward running

Start

Start by backpedaling in the desired direction.

Action

Initiate the open step by simultaneously turning the head, shoulders, and hips 180° in the intended direction. The hip of the lead leg externally rotates, pointing the foot and knee in the intended direction. Once the foot of the lead leg contacts the ground, the trail leg is lifted and the torso finishes turning in the intended direction. Keep the knees and hips bent and the center of mass low. The spine remains neutral and the head remains up.

Finish

The drill is completed when the desired number of repetitions have been achieved over the desired distance.

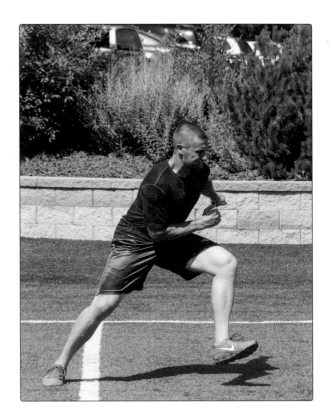

FUNDAMENTAL AGILITY SKILLS

AGILITY TECHNIQUE: CROSSOVER STEP

Purpose

To develop the ability to move efficiently laterally using a crossover step

Start

Start in the universal athletic position. Face 90° from the direction of movement.

Action

Initiate the movement by stepping across the body with the trail leg. The support leg extends at the hip, knee, and ankle, pushing the body laterally. Keep the knees and hips bent and the center of mass low. The spine remains neutral and the head remains up. The arms are at the sides with the elbows bent, alternating action with the legs. The initial step is required to turn the body 90° to face the desired direction. Once the body is turned in the desired direction, the knee and hip of the lead leg are flexed when the foot is not in contact with the ground. The support leg extends at the hip, knee, and ankle. Action at the arms and legs occurs on the sagittal plane.

Finish

The drill is completed when the desired number of repetitions have been achieved over the desired distance.

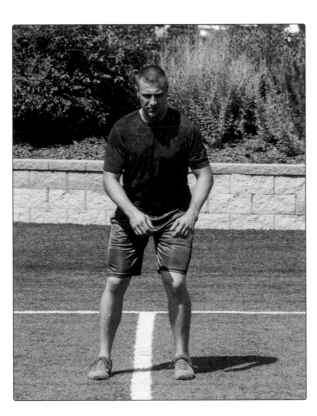 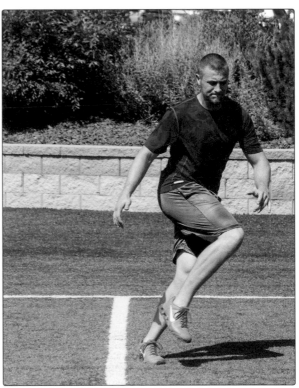

AGILITY PATTERNS

This section introduces several agility patterns that can be used when developing an agility program. However, a wide range of agility patterns and configurations can be used to make agility drills. Therefore, when performing any agility patterns, the basic mechanics previously discussed should be used to traverse the distance. It is the manner in which the drill is performed that has the biggest impact on performance.

CONE WEAVE

Purpose

To develop controlled running at maximal or near-maximal running speed

Objectives

- Incorporate decision making.
- Control unnecessary body movements.

Action

Use a rolling start (i.e., a slow to moderate jog). Run to the first cone, aiming to be at a maximal, controlled speed when reaching the first cone. Keep the corners tight when passing the cones. Keep the elbows relatively close to the sides of the body.

To Increase Complexity or Difficulty

- Stagger the distance of the cones.
- Stagger the width of the cones.
- The TSAC Facilitator can direct the tactical athlete in which direction to run (left or right) at the end of the drill.
- Use two identical patterns of cones so tactical athletes can race each other through the drill.

Work Interval

Varies depending on the distance of the cones and the ability of the tactical athlete but should be between 8 and 12 seconds.

Rest Interval

Once the drill has been mastered, the rest interval can be reduced to 2:1 rest-to-work interval.

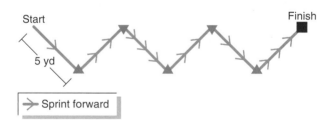

Setup for the cone weave drill

AGILITY PATTERNS

10 OUT, 5 BACK

Purpose

To develop acceleration and stopping ability

Objectives

- Simulate forward and backward movement patterns.
- Incorporate decision making.
- Reduce unnecessary body movements.

Action

Start on a yard line or at a cone and sprint forward 10 yards (or meters), backpedal 5, sprint forward 10, backpedal 5 again, and finish with a sprint forward to complete the drill. Use a forceful high-knee lift when initially accelerating. Accelerate with 100% effort, and optimize the forward lean. Minimize braking distance by quickly dropping the center of gravity, and use short, abbreviated steps to minimize the stopping distance.

To Increase Complexity or Difficulty

- Have the tactical athlete continue running at the end of the drill and perform an occupation-specific task (e.g., push, pull, drag, carry).
- Use two identical patterns of cones so tactical athletes can race each other through the drill.

Work Interval

Varies depending on the distance of the cones and the ability of the tactical athlete but should be between 8 and 12 seconds.

Rest Interval

Once the drill has been mastered, the rest interval can be reduced to a 2:1 rest-to-work interval.

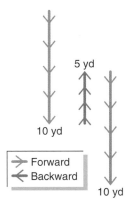

Setup for the 10 out, 5 back drill

AGILITY PATTERNS

5-10-15

Purpose

To develop acceleration, stopping ability, and body control

Objectives

- Simulate forward and backward movement patterns.
- Incorporate decision making.
- Reduce unnecessary body movements.

Action

Straddle a yard line or a cone and make a crossover step, moving forward 5 yards (or meters). Turn 180° and sprint 10 yards. Drop the inside shoulder and reach toward the ground with the same hand. Then turn 180° and finish the drill with a 15-yard sprint to finish. Use a forceful high-knee lift when initially accelerating. Accelerate with 100% effort, and optimize the forward lean. Minimize braking distance by quickly dropping the center of gravity, and use short, abbreviated steps to minimize the stopping distance.

To Increase Complexity or Difficulty

The TSAC Facilitator can indicate which direction the tactical athlete should start.

Work Interval

Varies depending on the distance of the cones and the ability of the tactical athlete but should be between 8 and 12 seconds.

Rest Interval

Once the drill has been mastered, the rest interval can be reduced to a 2:1 rest-to-work interval.

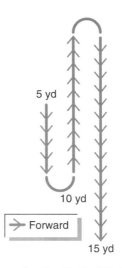

5 yd

10 yd

Forward

15 yd

Setup for the 5-10-15 drill

AGILITY PATTERNS

SIDE SHUFFLE

Purpose

To develop lateral acceleration, lateral stopping ability, and body control

Objectives

- Simulate movement patterns often seen while adjusting to external stimulus.
- Reduce unnecessary body movements.

Action

Begin in the universal athletic position. Side shuffle through the cone pattern. Do not cross the feet during the drill. Maintain an athletic position with a low center of gravity and ankles, knees, and hips flexed while shuffling. Accelerate with 100% effort. Lower the center of gravity further when transitioning from the shuffle to the forward sprint. Emphasize a forward lean when accelerating toward the last cone of the drill. Complete the initial series of cones and sprint toward the last cone in the drill.

To Increase Complexity or Difficulty

- The TSAC Facilitator can toss a ball to the tactical athlete while the athlete is shuffling.
- Backpedal instead of sprinting forward after completing the shuffle.
- Complete the drill by facing the opposite direction.
- Place the last cone of the drill farther away to increase the sprinting distance.
- Set up an identical series of cones so tactical athletes can race against each other.

Work Interval

Varies depending on the distance of the cones and the ability of the tactical athlete but should be between 8 and 12 seconds.

Rest Interval

Once the drill has been mastered, the rest interval can be reduced to a 2:1 rest-to-work interval.

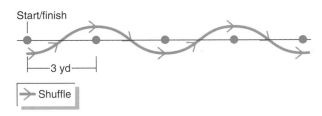

Setup for the side shuffle drill

AGILITY PATTERNS

FIGURE EIGHT

Purpose

To develop lateral acceleration, lateral stopping ability, and body control

Objectives

- Reduce unnecessary body movements.
- Train coordination of eye, hand, and foot.

Action

Place two cones 6 to 12 yards (or meters) apart. Run or shuffle in a figure-eight pattern around the cones, as shown in the diagram. Lower the center of gravity while moving through cones. Do not cross the feet while performing the drill. Drop the inside shoulder and extend the inside arm while turning. Emphasize a high-knee lift while accelerating off the turns. Move the feet as quickly as possible while shuffling.

To Increase Complexity or Difficulty

- The TSAC Facilitator can toss a ball back and forth with the tactical athlete while shuffling.

- Perform an operational-specific task during or at the end of the drill.
- Spread the cones farther apart to emphasize stopping mechanics while running.
- Time the drill for completed cycles through the pattern.
- Toss a ball for completed catches if shuffling, which will dictate the completion of the drill.

Work Interval

- Varies depending on the distance of the cones and the ability of the tactical athlete but should be between 8 and 12 seconds.
- If the drill is done with shuffling, toss a ball for completed catches to dictate the completion of the drill.

Rest Interval

Once mastery of the drill has been reached, the rest interval can be reduced to a 2:1 rest-to-work interval.

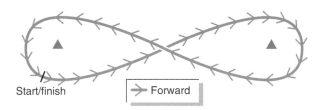

Setup for the figure-eight drill

AGILITY PATTERNS

V-PATTERN

Purpose

To develop acceleration, stopping ability, and body control

Objectives

- Reduce unnecessary body movements.
- Train coordination of eye, hand, and foot.

Action

Place two cones 10 to 15 yards (or meters) away from a third cone, as depicted in the diagram. Run in a straight line between the cones in the pattern illustrated. Lower the center of gravity while running around the cones. Do not cross the feet while performing the drill. Drop the inside shoulder and extend the inside arm while turning. Emphasize a high-knee lift while accelerating off the turns.

To Increase Complexity or Difficulty

- The TSAC Facilitator can serve as a starting cone and roll a medicine ball to the tactical athlete after he has finished turning around the other cones (the ball should be handed back to the TSAC Facilitator at the end of the pattern). The athlete's hands should be in a ready position to catch the ball when turning through the cones.
- Increasing the distance between cones can emphasize the acceleration and stopping mechanics.

Work Interval

- Varies depending on the distance of the cones and the ability of the tactical athlete but should be between 8 and 12 seconds.
- Time the drill for completed cycles through the pattern, or complete a prescribed number of repetitions.

Rest Interval

Once the drill has been mastered, the rest interval can be reduced to a 2:1 rest-to-work interval.

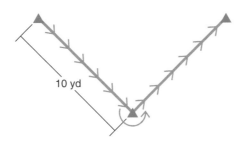

10 yd

Setup for the V-pattern drill

AGILITY PATTERNS

W-PATTERN

Purpose

To develop acceleration and stopping ability

Objectives

- Simulate movement patterns when transitioning from forward to backward.
- Reduce unnecessary body movements.

Action

Place five cones 5 to 10 yards (or meters) apart in a *W* pattern. Run forward and backward in the pattern illustrated. When changing direction, lower the center of gravity while moving through the pattern. Do not cross the feet while performing the drill. Emphasize a high-knee lift while transitioning directions. Transition from backpedaling to forward sprinting by slightly opening the hips, using full foot contact on the ground.

To Increase Complexity or Difficulty

The TSAC Facilitator can roll or throw a ball to the tactical athlete while the tactical athlete transitions from the backward to forward direction. The ball is tossed back to the TSAC Facilitator in each backward-to-forward direction change.

Increasing the distance from 5 to 10 yards (or meters) can increase the difficulty of the drill by emphasizing acceleration and stopping mechanics.

Work Interval

Varies depending on the distance of the cones and the ability of the tactical athlete but should be between 8 and 12 seconds.

Rest Interval

Once the drill has been mastered, the rest interval can be reduced to a 2:1 rest-to-work interval.

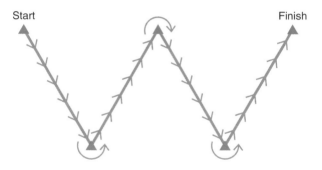

Setup for the W-pattern drill

AGILITY PATTERNS

T-DRILL

Purpose
To develop acceleration and deceleration mechanics

Objectives
Develop an effective change of direction.

Action
Set cones in a *T* pattern as shown in the figure. Sprint forward 10 yards (or meters), touch the center cone with the right hand, and then shuffle to the left. Touch the far cone with the left hand and shuffle right 10 yards (or meters). Touch the cone with the right hand. Shuffle back to the center and touch the cone with the left hand. Then backpedal to the starting cone.

To Increase Complexity or Difficulty
- The cones can be farther apart to increase the work interval.
- Two identical sets of cones can allow tactical athletes to compete against each other.

Work Interval
Varies depending on the distance of the cones and the ability of the tactical athlete but should be between 8 and 12 seconds.

Rest Interval
Once the drill has been mastered, the rest interval can be reduced to a 2:1 rest-to-work interval.

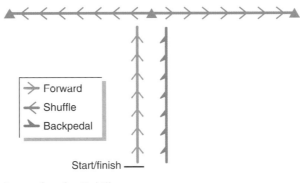

Setup for the T-drill

Program Design Recommendations

Many agility patterns are specific to operational practices. The TSAC Facilitator should be able to identify body mechanics and their associated criteria that allow for optimal movement. Jeffreys (29) identifies a three-step, target-based approach to developing agility that can easily be adapted to tactical situations:

1. **Identify and develop target movement patterns:** This step simply identifies, develops, and masters target movement patterns. For example, a 3- to 5-second rush to gain cover would require an acceleration pattern when running from one point to another in a straight line.

2. **Identify and develop key movement combinations:** This step combines two or more skills and becomes more task specific. For example, stand from a prone position, lift a fire hose, and run to another location.

3. **Identify key stimuli and subsequent reactions:** This step incorporates external stimuli and requires the tactical athlete to react or make a decision based on the situation. For instance, a law enforcement officer may have to run to a position, stop, and take a shot at more than one target. Determining which target to shoot first depends on the situation.

Agility biomechanics can be broken down into subcategories: foot position, leg position, trunk or posture, and arm position. For each of these subcategories, the TSAC Facilitator can establish criteria that reflect optimal location to execute the movement. Table 13.4 earlier in the chapter offers a movement checklist for the 90° agility turn. This same format can be used for any agility movement and is extremely useful for assessing movement technique.

Before implementing agility training in the training program of a tactical athlete, there are several factors to consider. Addressing these areas will help maximize safety and ensure that the person is physically prepared to engage in this form of training. The following considerations and guidelines are presented to help the TSAC Facilitator when designing an agility training program.

Training Status

Training status refers to a person's physical capacity to perform the agility movements outlined in this chapter. This is influenced by several factors, including heredity, injury status, nutritional status, training, and adaptive capabilities (49).

Key Point

> Training status is influenced by several factors, including heredity, injury status, nutritional status, training, and adaptive capabilities.

Training Age and Experience   Due to the intensity of some agility drills and the potential risk of injury, an individual must have a solid foundation of muscular strength, mobility, and speed before engaging in this form of training. Moreover, people with low motor abilities may require additional training at lower intensities to develop sufficient change-of-direction ability and perceptual-cognitive ability (e.g., pattern recognition) to improve their technical proficiency before advancing to more complex drills (16). High-intensity agility training should also be used with caution for middle-aged or older adults, who may be more prone to injury because of the aging process.

Body Weight and Body Composition   Excess body fat impairs the ability to execute agility movements at a high level. Because body fat does not actively contribute to force production, excessive levels may significantly impair movement ability

and increase overall movement time. Poor body composition may negatively affect several areas of performance for the tactical athlete, such as crawling (e.g., low and high crawling; functioning in crawl spaces, tunnels, vents, and shafts) and climbing (e.g., fences, walls, elevator shafts, multiple flights of stairs, ladders, fire escapes, ropes, poles, trees) to accomplish an objective or gain a tactical position (14, 35).

History of Injury   Agility training can be intense due to the nature of foot-strike impacts, demands placed on the neural system, and high-velocity muscle contractions. Areas of potential injury associated with the lower body in tactical populations usually include the ankles, knees, hips, and lower back (8, 24, 25). TSAC Facilitators should be aware of injury trends in the specific tactical athletes with whom they are working. The importance of progressing slowly and objectively monitoring the tactical athlete cannot be overstated.

Strength Requirements   There is no minimum strength requirement to perform agility training. The tactical athlete should have the ability to execute fundamental drills and move through key biomechanical positions with acceptable competency. To maximize their speed and agility potential, tactical athletes need to develop strength and power characteristics across the force–velocity spectrum (40).

Proper Technique   Proper agility technique cannot be overstated. The tactical athlete must be skilled in the fundamentals of starting, accelerating and decelerating, and other agility movements. To cover distance most effectively, it is desirable to be proficient at all phases (11).

General Considerations

In addition to training status, the TSAC Facilitator needs to take into account general considerations when designing an agility training program. These include attire, tactical gear, shoes and socks, training surface and equipment, and fatigue.

Attire   When learning agility mechanics, attire needs to be comfortable—not binding, not excessively loose or overly tight, and so on. The focus should be on mechanics and the associated effort for proper execution. A wide range of clothing is available for a variety of body sizes and shapes. Attire should be well fitting, breathable, and low in friction. Synthetic materials may offer some advantages depending on conditions. Unlike cotton, many synthetic materials do not hold sweat and actually wick moisture away from the skin. This may be advantageous in hot or humid environments when attempting to avoid excessive core temperature elevation (9).

Tactical Gear   Despite the effectiveness of the drills discussed throughout this chapter in promoting power, speed, and agility, when tactical personnel are wearing PPE, equipment, or other occupational attire, their ability to complete such drills and execute activities that require power, speed, and agility (as well as other fitness attributes) may be compromised (15, 18). Furthermore, the increased weight of PPE and carried equipment may increase fatigue, placing a great cardiorespiratory and thermoregulatory demand on the individual (5, 17, 18), and restrictive clothing and the presence of equipment (e.g., duty belt with weapons or tools) may alter gait, overall body mechanics, and movement patterns (37, 38). These factors may increase the rate of fatigue, falls, and injury. Consequently, if the TSAC Facilitator is inclined to have the tactical athlete train while wearing PPE, then the PPE should be introduced gradually and in a progressive manner; the individual should be acclimated to the training conditions and have demonstrated sufficient competency in the execution of the power, speed, and agility drills while not wearing PPE; and the rationale for doing so should be sound, all in a similar manner to training athletes wearing equipment during the preseason (9).

Shoes and Socks   Properly fitting shoes and socks can enhance performance and reduce the potential for injury (42). It is wise to buy one pair of shoes that can be worn for both speed and agility training. Obviously an athletic shoe that fits properly is important. There are many categories of athletic shoes, including distance running, biking, aerobic or group drills, walking, various cleats, court shoes, and cross-trainers. Buying athletic shoes at a specialty store with an educated staff will most likely be worth the time, money, and effort. When trying on the shoes, it is important to wear the type of athletic socks that will be worn during training. The shoes should be immediately comfortable after putting them on and require no breaking in. Feet tend to swell and get bigger at the end of the day, so it is recommended to try on shoes later in the day for the best fit.

Training Surface and Equipment

It is the responsibility of the TSAC Facilitator to inspect the training surface and equipment before training and to ensure the safety of the tactical athletes during training. To this end, the training surface should not be soft, wet, or slippery. The surface should be clear of any obstructions, and the training space should have a buffer area surrounding it that accounts for decelerations and outside interference (e.g., dogs, Frisbees, errant game balls, playground equipment, sidewalks, athletic gear, trees, drainage, parking lots).

Well-maintained natural grass offers training advantages such as shock-absorbing properties, and natural grass is often the medium in field operations (16, 28). Regardless, the surface should be free of any articles or objects that may interfere with safety and secure foot contact.

Fatigue   The accumulation of fatigue when training agility can be a rate-limiting factor. The TSAC Facilitator needs to recognize immediate and chronic accumulation of fatigue and its implications for speed training. In an effort to mitigate fatigue, particular attention needs to be paid to additional training (e.g., strength training, conditioning, speed training) that contributes to chronic fatigue and rest interval length that contributes to immediate or acute fatigue.

Ideally, the tactical athlete should be rested, fueled, hydrated, and motivated for training. Understanding that often the training state of the tactical athlete is less than optimal, the TSAC Facilitator needs to be particularly attentive to poor training technique. In other words, training for speed in a state that compromises quality training is most often counterproductive.

A well-planned agility program is coordinated with other training methods and cycle volume and intensities in an effort to optimize training adaptations. Ideally, fatigue is balanced and managed with the interaction of the individual's fitness capabilities and levels (7, 37).

Program Design Components

As with most types of strength training and conditioning, the program design for agility training should take into account duration, frequency, intensity, volume, and rest. The TSAC Facilitator may need to adjust the variables, depending on the training and operational status of the tactical athlete.

Duration   Program duration refers to the block of time, typically given in weeks, when the program is implemented. Structuring training around four weeks (plus or minus two weeks) (45) is advised, and the programming should vary in volume and intensity. Once the duration of training has been completed, a short transition period can be spent performing various training methods. See chapter 10 for an in-depth discussion of periodization.

Frequency   The training frequency of an agility development program can range from one to six times per week. The TSAC Facilitator should consider several training variables when developing an agility program and should incorporate training that develops the physical characteristics that will make tactical athletes as effective as they can be (i.e., strength, power, speed, endurance, body composition, coordination) (16). As a matter of practicality, agility training can be implemented two to three days per week and combined with additional fitness methods (11, 16). Because agility is a coordinative ability, shorter training sessions performed more frequently may be better tolerated by people unaccustomed to this style of training. Additionally, shorter, more frequent training bouts may allow the individual to focus on technique while minimizing the effects of fatigue. For instance, performing relatively short practice sessions as part of a dynamic warm-up may be effective for improving movement quality and agility technique.

Intensity   Intensity refers to the quality of movement or "the effort with which a repetition is executed" (20). Using the general adaptation model as a guide, agility development programming should begin with low intensity and high volumes of work. A beginner may not be able to tolerate relatively high volumes of agility training, so progressing slowly is reasonable. An introduc-

tion to fundamental drills and quality of movement is a priority.

Volume   Volume of training is "the amount of work (repetitions × sets) performed in a given training session time period" (20). The volume of agility work is indicative of the program goals and should be incorporated into the overall training stressors and methods.

Rest   Rest is the time between sets and reps (16, 20). For optimal agility training, fatigue should be minimized. This warrants longer rest intervals between sets and repetitions. For example, the recommended work-to-rest ratios for shorter agility drills that stress the phosphagen system are between 1:12 and 1:20, whereas drills that target both the phosphagen and glycolytic pathways may require work-to-rest ratios closer to 1:3 to 1:5 (27), as discussed more thoroughly in chapter 3. How fast the tactical athlete dissipates fatigue accumulated during the training session depends on genetics, training tolerance, experience, and environmental factors, to name a few.

Demands Specific to the Tactical Population

Plyometric, speed, and agility training are well-established methods that have been proven to enhance physical qualities. Tactical athletes need fundamental physical capabilities to support their operational competency. The inclusion and management of these training methods will ensure a tactical athlete has the physical requirements that will better prepare her for the variable, unstable, and demanding situations she must perform in. Additionally, a well-trained tactical athlete should have a higher tolerance for operational demands, a greater capacity to resist injury, and an improved resiliency returning from injury if she is trained optimally and to her potential. The TSAC Facilitator should understand how to manage these training methods in a comprehensive program. The interaction of strength and conditioning methodologies, tactical training, stress, restorative capabilities, age, genetics, nutrition, and how the individual responds to training all play significant roles. It is the responsibility of the TSAC Facilitator to monitor and adjust training variables in organized phases or periods of training to optimize training and target the desired effect.

CONCLUSION

Tactical athletes may be placed in situations requiring an array of physical characteristics, including power, speed, and agility. Training these physical qualities can be daunting initially. The deeper the TSAC Facilitator's understanding of the underlying mechanisms and scientific principles of plyometric, speed, and agility training, the greater the opportunity for success of the tactical athlete and the training program.

Key Terms

acceleration
agility
amortization phase
change-of-direction speed
closed drill
deceleration
discrete task
open drill

plyometrics
power
semi-open drill
serial task
series elastic component
speed
stretch–shortening cycle (SSC)

Study Questions

1. When does the amortization phase occur?
   a. between the end of eccentric muscle action and the start of concentric muscle action
   b. between the start of eccentric muscle action and the start of concentric muscle action
   c. between the end of concentric muscle action and the start of eccentric muscle action
   d. between the start of concentric muscle action and the start of eccentric muscle action

2. Which of the following jumps is a low-intensity plyometric exercise?
   a. broad
   b. lateral
   c. squat
   d. triple

3. Which of the following drills develops total body power and emphasizes triple extension?
   a. depth jump
   b. single-leg bound
   c. overhead forward throw
   d. backward overhead medicine ball toss

4. Before participating in lower body plyometric exercises, what is the recommended percentage of body weight that a tactical athlete should be able to lift when performing five squats in 5 seconds or less?
   a. 50
   b. 60
   c. 65
   d. 70

Chapter 14

Aerobic Endurance Exercise Techniques and Programming

Matthew R. Rhea, PhD, CSCS,*D

Brent A. Alvar, PhD, CSCS,*D, RSCC*D, FNSCA

After completing this chapter, you will be able to

- design a warm-up protocol for an aerobic endurance training session;

- describe proper exercise technique and instructional cueing for machine-based aerobic endurance exercises and aerobic endurance activities; and

- design aerobic endurance training programs based on the training status, goals, and demands of tactical athletes.

Aerobic endurance is an important fitness component that fosters health and performance among tactical athletes. The TSAC Facilitator can provide valuable direction to athletes seeking to reduce their risk of cardiovascular disease and improve their ability to execute tactical tasks without undue fatigue (27). This chapter provides direction for selecting aerobic endurance training modalities and designing safe, effective training plans for tactical athletes.

WARMING UP BEFORE AEROBIC ENDURANCE TRAINING

Physical preparation for aerobic endurance training is similar to preparation for resistance training. All of the body systems respond gradually to applied physical demands. Therefore, preparation for exercise should be a gradual, progressive process. The primary goals of a warm-up are to increase body temperature, enhance pliability of soft tissues, and increase metabolic productivity. A short bout (3-5 minutes) of physical activity such as walking or jogging can help stimulate several of these processes. That activity should be followed by flexibility exercises to improve ROM and tissue pliability.

Many tasks in tactical occupations are dynamic (2, 3, 21, 25, 29, 38, 53, 62), making dynamic flexibility exercises important for both exercise preparation and job performance. The warm-up should prepare the entire body for exertion, but special attention should be paid to the shoulder and hip complexes, hip flexors and hamstrings, Achilles tendon, and low back. Tactical athletes should never skip the warm-up for the sake of time or to rush into the exercise portion of a training session.

Key Point

A proper warm-up, including dynamic flexibility exercises, is an integral part of every exercise session.

EXERCISE TECHNIQUES AND CUEING GUIDELINES

Much like resistance training, the selection and use of equipment will affect progress toward training goals. The TSAC Facilitator must be able to evaluate a tactical athlete and provide direction related to the various parameters of aerobic exercise. The knowledgeable facilitator will be able to help athletes achieve fitness goals by making educated decisions regarding techniques and training strategies.

General Considerations for Aerobic Endurance Training

The greatest benefits of aerobic endurance exercise are achieved through consistent, long-term participation. Therefore, it is important that exercisers follow certain steps to ensure their safety and ability to sustain exercise. Each workout session should be preceded by a warm-up that prepares the muscles, joints, and energy systems for exercise. Wearing proper clothing and footwear is also vital to sustainability. Clothing that restricts motion should be avoided so that the body can function properly; however, excessively loose clothing may get caught in equipment, presenting a danger to the exerciser. Clothing should allow heat dissipation in hot and humid environments and provide ample heat retention when temperatures are cold. Proper footwear should always be worn for walking, running, hiking, and sport-related cardiorespiratory exercise. Shoes should provide the appropriate amount of support to the arches and ankles. As shoes wear, support diminishes and the risk of overuse injuries to the feet increases. Footwear should be replaced as soon as support mechanisms begin to wear out.

Tactical Population–Specific Demands

The metabolic demands of various tactical activities include moderate- to very-high-intensity tasks, such as forcible entry, suspect subduing, fire suppression, quick pursuit, close-quarter combat, and lengthy hikes. These activities can last several hours and involve aggressive bursts of energy followed by a period of rest. Body armor, protective clothing, and tactical gear exacerbate the metabolic demands of these activities by 16% to 63% (45). It is clear that tactical athletes must develop several metabolic components in order to safely and effectively perform their duties. The ability to perform moderate- to high-intensity aerobic tasks for long durations, to perform very-high-intensity activities for shorter durations, and to recover quickly between tasks are all characteristics of highly trained and fit tactical athletes.

A variety of training methods should be used to promote positive adaptations in each of these three metabolic components. Varying the training stresses will help promote a wide range of physiological adaptations that elevate metabolic performance and decrease the relative intensity of the tasks demanded of tactical athletes. For tactical athletes, developing high-level fitness makes their tasks less stressful to perform due to a relative decrease in the overall intensity of effort as a percentage of their maximal capacity. When tactical athletes have a low cardiorespiratory capacity, many of the daily tasks in these occupations will result in maximal or near-maximal effort. Therefore, increasing cardiorespiratory fitness is both a safeguard against cardiovascular injury and a way to improve performance (4, 12, 22).

Exercise prescription should consider the aforementioned factors that contribute to occupational specificity (or the specific adaptation to imposed demands—SAID principle), as well as the fitness level, training necessities, and goals of the individual tactical athlete. The SAID principle asserts that training specificity (e.g., biomechanics, neuromuscular and energy system utilization) should be considered when designing the program. The more closely tactical athletes can mimic the activities of their occupation, the better the transference from the training program (36). The remainder of this chapter discusses how to use these steps in designing cardiorespiratory exercise programs for the tactical athlete.

Designing an aerobic exercise program is a five-step process: exercise mode (step 1), training frequency (step 2), training intensity (step 3), exercise duration (step 4), and exercise progression (step 5) (42). Asking specific questions regarding the population being trained and the goals of the training session allows the TSAC Facilitator to determine the appropriate exercise selection, duration, frequency, intensity, and progression. Following this five-step process ensures that appropriate training exercise prescription can be employed and alterations for fitness and occupational preparedness can be achieved.

STEP 1: EXERCISE MODE

Aerobic exercises consist of repetitive movements that stress the oxygen intake, transport, and utilization processes in the body. Exercise that uses large muscle groups can enhance this stress and improve the value of the training session. Many forms of exercise (modes) meet these metabolic conditions, including both machine-based and field exercise modes. Each mode requires the body to move somewhat differently, presenting a unique stress to the muscular and cardiopulmonary systems. Activities such as running, walking, hiking, cycling, swimming, rowing, and skiing, as well as longer interval sports such as tennis, soccer, and basketball, task the cardiopulmonary system to provide energy in an effective and efficient fashion.

Machine-based training is an excellent option for aerobic training because it gives the TSAC Facilitator greater control of the training environment. Altering training intensity on a treadmill is more precise than attempting to determine changes in speed on the road, and maintaining a consistent intensity is much easier when the exerciser does not have to work around traffic or other exercisers. Monitoring volume is also more accurate with constant feedback from the exercise machine.

Although differences in physiological responses to training exist (34), personal preference should be key when selecting a training method because it may lead to increased adherence (7), and a baseline level of fitness is necessary for health and prevention of premature morbidity and mortality (4). That said, specificity needs to be a consideration in training design or recommendations. Many tasks required of tactical athletes involve ambulation, and therefore a greater amount of running may be useful during training.

In terms of establishing a base level of fitness, if a tactical athlete dislikes running, options such as cycling, swimming, and rowing should be considered to enhance adherence to an aerobic endurance program. Of these choices, cycling involves the least amount of muscle mass but involves lower impact forces compared with running. Swimming and rowing involve low-impact forces yet are challenging to the cardiopulmonary system, making them good choices for aerobic endurance activities. For higher levels of fitness for occupational preparedness, specificity of training is necessary (e.g., running to increase running performance and swimming to increase swimming performance). Varying training modes can reduce overuse injuries that might result from extended use of a single modality such as running (26).

Key Point

Choosing the proper exercise mode may lead to increased adherence, but specificity of training should not be overlooked.

Machine-Based Aerobic Endurance Exercises

Aerobic exercise machines provide a convenient, controllable exercise environment and can be useful for developing aerobic fitness among tactical athletes. Exercise equipment also provides many options for introducing movement variations, which may be helpful in overcoming boredom and avoiding overuse injuries. The TSAC Facilitator should be familiar with each mode of training, including how to adjust the machine and the optimal posture or mechanism for using the apparatus, to assist individuals in reaching their training goals. Also, the SAID principle needs to be considered when choosing the activity mode, as will be shown. The following section provides guidelines for the setup, initiation, and cessation of exercise on treadmills, stair-climbers, elliptical machines, hybrid machines, exercise bikes, and rowing machines (42).

MACHINE-BASED WALKING AND RUNNING

TREADMILL

Setup

- Read all of the instructions listed on the console for operating the treadmill, including how to increase and decrease the speed and incline as well as how to stop and start the treadmill belt.
- Attach the security clip to your clothing in a way that will not interfere with your running (arm swing, body rotation, or leg movement).
- Straddle the belt with one leg on either side, but do not touch the belt.
- Start the treadmill and allow it to reach the predetermined warm-up speed.
- Warm up for 3 to 5 minutes to prepare for the exercise session.

Starting the Exercise

- Hold onto the handles to support your body weight and allow one leg to swing freely.
- Allow the midfoot to make contact with the treadmill (pawing the belt) to get a sense of the speed.
- Once you are comfortable with the speed, begin walking or running on the treadmill.
- Keep your body centered in the middle of the belt and toward the front of the machine.
- Avoid holding the handles or display console while running, because it will alter your running gate (backward lean) and could damage the treadmill.

Ending the Exercise

- Reduce the speed of the treadmill to allow for a 3- to 5-minute cool-down. This will prevent blood pooling and increase circulation once the exercise session ends.

- To stop the exercise, step on the platforms on either side of the belt and press the stop or end exercise button as indicated in the instructions.

Treadmills offer an indoor exercise environment with the ability to control and vary walking and running exercise. In a review of the physiological responses to aerobic exercise on various pieces of exercise equipment, Oliveira and colleagues (34) determined that the highest aerobic demands were measured during exercise on treadmills versus any other machine (cycling and elliptical). This makes the treadmill a desired mode of training when attempting to reach high levels of exertion, burn more calories, or stress the cardiopulmonary system. Variations in speed and incline can change the exercise stimulus, allowing for unique training sessions that stress the peripheral muscular components, the central cardiopulmonary components, or a combination of the two. In general, using a treadmill will decrease the hamstring muscle activation because the treadmill is propelling the leg backward, and it will increase quadriceps activation to eccentrically brake the leg and propel the leg forward concentrically (31). In addition, incline running simulates hilly terrain and increases muscle activation in the lower body (such as in the calves and quadriceps), whereas level-ground running at consistent, moderate speeds challenges the heart and lungs with less muscular fatigue in the lower body. Caution should be taken when starting and stopping the treadmill to avoid falls, and athletes should become accustomed to treadmill running before attempting very high speeds. The tactical athlete must be capable of staying in the center of the belt near the front of the treadmill, and safety clips should always be worn in case of an accident.

STAIR-CLIMBER

Setup

- Read all of the instructions listed on the console for operating the stair-climber, including how to increase and decrease the speed as well as how to stop and start the machine (pedals or belt).
- Grasp the handrails and step onto the machine with both feet.
- Make sure both feet are completely on the pedals and are centered.
- Start the stair-climber and allow it to reach the predetermined warm-up speed.
- Warm up for 3 to 5 minutes to prepare for the exercise session.

Starting the Exercise

- Hold onto the handles and begin stepping.
- Make sure the body is upright and not leaning on the machine or backward. Keep the eyes forward. Take deep steps (4-8 in. [10-20 cm]).
- Make sure steps do not touch the floor (too low) or hit the upper limit of the machine (too high).
- Avoid holding the handrails in a way that supports the body weight. The handrails should be for balance only. In addition, the console should not be held while stepping, because this will cause a backward lean and may damage the machine.

Ending the Exercise

- Reduce the speed of the stair-climber to allow for a 3- to 5-minute cool-down. This will prevent blood pooling and increase circulation once the exercise session ends.
- To stop the exercise, step off the machine and press the stop or end exercise button as indicated in the instructions.

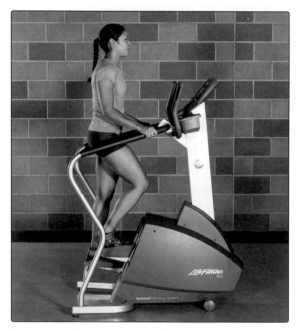

Proper position on a stair-climber.

ELLIPTICAL TRAINER

Setup

- Read all of the instructions listed on the console for operating the elliptical trainer, including how to increase and decrease the speed as well as how to stop and start the elliptical machine (pedals).
- Grasp the handrails and step onto the machine with both feet.
- Make sure both feet are completely on the pedals and are centered, and grasp the two handrails with the body upright and eyes facing forward.
- Make sure the body is upright and shoulders are not rounded.
- The weight of the body should be balanced with all segments of the body directly in line (upper—head, shoulders; lower—hips, knees, and feet).
- The knees should not move past the toes during the movement.
- The feet should remain in contact with the pedals at all times.

Starting the Exercise

- Hold onto the handles and begin pedaling.
- Increase the pedaling rate to get up to the predetermined warm-up speed.
- Warm up for 3 to 5 minutes to prepare for the exercise session.
- Make sure the body is upright and not leaning on the machine or backward. Keep the eyes forward.
- The incline can be increased to more closely simulate running or increase the intensity.
- Using a forward motion will increase the emphasis on the quadriceps, and using a backward motion will focus more on the hamstrings.
- Avoid holding the handrails in a way that supports the body weight. The handrails should be for balance only. In addition, the display console should not be held while pedaling, because this will cause a backward lean and may damage the elliptical machine.

Ending the Exercise

- Reduce the speed of the elliptical to allow for a 3- to 5-minute cool-down. This will prevent blood pooling and increase circulation once the exercise session ends.
- To stop the exercise, slow the pedaling rate until the pedals stop, and step off the machine. Press the stop or end exercise button as indicated in the instructions.

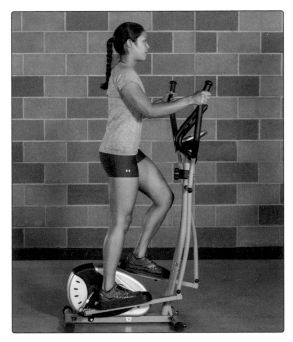

Proper position on an elliptical trainer.

Many varieties of stair-climbers, elliptical machines, and combinations of running and climbing machines (hybrid machines) have been developed, and all present a slightly different movement pattern. Though these machines may reduce the impact forces on the lower body compared with running, the fixed movement path may not be comfortable for some athletes. Because limited individual adjustments can be made on these machines, some exercisers may not feel comfortable using them. Such machines do, however, offer the benefit of working the arms and legs simultaneously, provide an opportunity to reduce impact on the lower body, and provide the ability to add resistance to increase the training intensity or load.

INDOOR CYCLING

EXERCISE BIKE

Setup

- Read all of the instructions listed on the console for operating the bike, including how to increase and decrease the speed as well as how to stop and start the bike.
- Adjust the seat height so that the knee is slightly bent when the pedal is at the bottom of the rotation.
- The foot of the extended knee should be flat against the pedal (parallel to the floor), and the pedal should contact the ball of the foot.
- Adjust the seat so that the knee is over the center of the pedal and the hips do not move during the pedaling stroke.
- Sit upright and tall, keeping a neutral spine with a slight forward lean, and keep the eyes looking forward.
- Adjust the handlebars so that the elbows are bent slightly and the upper arms and torso form an approximate 90° angle.

Starting the Exercise

- Hold onto the handles and begin pedaling to reach the predetermined warm-up speed.
- Make sure the balls of the feet are being used and that they are in contact with the pedals at all time.

- The bullhorn style of handlebars allows for a variety of hand positions:
  - Pronated, with palms facing down, which allows a more upright posture
  - Neutral, with palms facing the grip on the side of the handlebars
  - Racing position, with forearms resting on the handlebars, creating a forward lean
- Warm up for 3 to 5 minutes to prepare for the exercise session.
- Make sure the body is upright and not leaning on the machine or backward. Keep the eyes forward.
- Avoid holding the handles in a way that supports the body weight. The handles should be for balance only. In addition, do not hold the display console, because this will cause a backward lean and may damage the machine.

Ending the Exercise

- Reduce the speed of the bike to allow for a 3- to 5-minute cool-down. This will prevent blood pooling and increase circulation once the exercise session ends.
- Reduce the speed of the pedals until they come to a complete stop, and then dismount the bike (42).

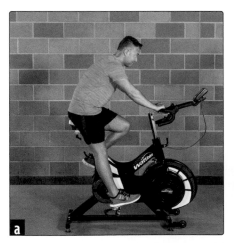 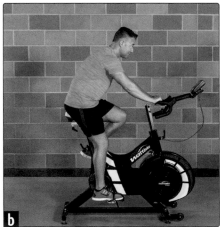 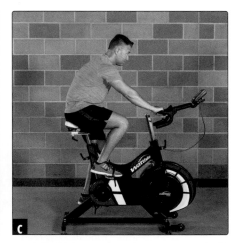

Proper seat height and adjustment: *(a)* leg straight with knee locked and heel on pedal; *(b)* knee slightly bent with ball of foot on pedal; *(c)* with pedal at 12 o'clock, knee is about even with hips and parallel with floor.

INDOOR CYCLING

Similar to other machines, stationary bikes enable indoor exercise year round regardless of climate or location. Machines that allow the addition of resistance during cycling offer the ability to dramatically change the exercise stimulus. However, cycling primarily involves the lower body, which results in less caloric expenditure and lower oxygen demands than running (5, 23, 51). The safety of stationary cycling versus running on a treadmill should be considered, especially among athletes with lower body injuries or balance difficulties.

Seat placement is important in cycling. The seat should be raised to a height that allows for a slight bend in the knee at the point of greatest knee extension. Handlebar and handgrip placement should be in a comfortable position that allows for exercise sessions that last 30 to 60 minutes. If upright bikes cause pain at the seat or handlebars, recumbent bikes may offer a more comfortable exercise position.

Indoor cycling activities generally include periods of higher and lower intensity (sprints and recovery) that mimic many of the HR variations that occur in tactical athletes' occupational activities. The program components of an indoor cycling class can include any style of cardiorespiratory endurance intensity (e.g., long, slow distance; interval; high-intensity interval; and pace/tempo training) and may involve standing and sprinting, simulated hill climbing, and periods of high-intensity riding. Therefore, greater specificity of training is occurring, which makes indoor cycling a good mode of activity.

INDOOR ROWING

ROWING MACHINE

Setup

- Read all of the instructions listed on the console for operating the rowing machine.
- Warm up for 3 to 5 minutes to prepare for the exercise session.

Starting the Exercise

- Starting position:
  - Insert the feet into the straps and tighten them.
  - Keep the back upright and prevent the shoulders and back from rounding.
  - Extend the arms and grasp the handle while flexing the hips and knees so that the shins are approximately vertical.
- Drive—movement phase:
  - Extend the hips and knees while simultaneously pulling the handle to the chest just below the rib cage.
  - Adjust the venting system to increase or decrease the resistance. Opening the vent increases airflow and decreases resistance, whereas closing it decreases airflow and increases resistance.
  - Make sure the body is upright and not leaning forward or backward during the rowing motion. Keep the eyes forward.
- Finish—ending position:
  - The legs should be fully extended (without locking the knees).
  - The torso should have a slight (not exaggerated) backward lean.
  - The handle should be at the rib cage with the elbows flexed.
- Recovery: Move from the finish back to the starting point.

Ending the Exercise

- Reduce the speed of the rowing machine to allow for a 3- to 5-minute cool-down. This will prevent blood pooling and increase circulation once the exercise session ends.
- Reduce the speed until the machine comes to a complete stop, and then dismount the rowing machine.

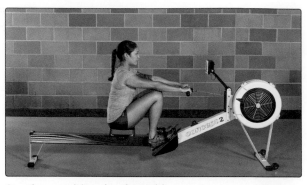

Starting position (and catch)

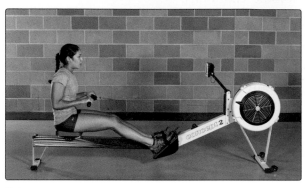

Drive

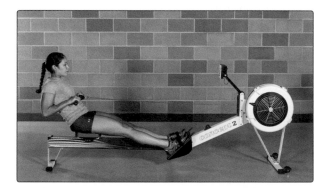

Finish

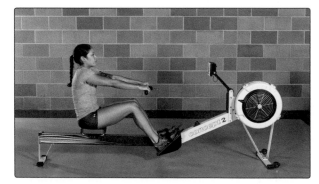

Recovery

INDOOR ROWING

Rowing machines challenge both the upper and lower body musculature, placing higher demands on the cardiopulmonary system compared with exercise that relies solely on either upper or lower body musculature (e.g., arm cranks, exercise bicycles). The rowing motion requires some practice to master, but once an exerciser is comfortable with the cadence, it offers a challenging stress that can stimulate improvements in muscular and cardiopulmonary adaptations. Athletes should avoid leaning too far forward, which places greater repetitive strain on the low back. The trunk should remain fairly stable throughout the entire cadence, with only a slight amount of trunk flexion and extension.

Nonmachine Aerobic Endurance Activities

Aerobic endurance activities such as running, hiking, and cycling are often performed in the outdoor environment (i.e., natural setting, including temperature, weather, and so on). They include many modes of training that can be performed in many locations and environments, often without the need for equipment, which makes training more accessible. The environment can influence training (e.g., weather, traffic), but aerobic exercise in the outdoors may be more enjoyable for some tactical athletes. Although the TSAC Facilitator may have less control over the environment during nonmachine exercise, there are still many ways to assist the tactical athlete in improving fitness.

Running, Walking, and Hiking

Overground ambulation is a natural movement pattern and skill, making this form of exercise fairly easy for most tactical athletes. Generally speaking, walking or running on a treadmill is similar to walking or running overground (46). One main difference is the increased oxygen cost of overground activity. Regardless of the activity mode, overuse injuries are a common problem among runners, especially in tactical populations with a high volume of training (40). Pain in the feet, shins, knees, and hips makes it difficult to perform sufficient walking, running, or hiking to promote the desired improvements in fitness. For tactical athletes who are able to perform this type of exercise without pain, it can be an effective form of aerobic exercise without the need for equipment. In addition, this type of training may be used during occupational training (job training), making it a good choice for carryover (specificity of training).

Proper footwear must be worn during this type of exercise, and caution should be taken when walking or running on uneven surfaces. The type of running shoe that is appropriate for tactical athletes may differ significantly. Research examining injury rates among runners in different types of shoes is inconclusive (33), but if pain arises, a trained professional should conduct an evaluation to determine what footwear is most appropriate.

Swimming

Swimming is a challenging, full-body, low-impact form of exercise. Although it requires a good degree of skill to perform for long periods of time, the stress it places on the cardiopulmonary system is very positive. Improvements in vital capacity (amount of air expelled) and maximal breathing capacity have been shown to be higher in swimmers versus in runners or controls (9). For those who lack the skill to sustain swimming for long periods of time, it may be a good choice for variety from time to time or when performing high-intensity intervals of shorter duration. It has been shown to be a good mode of exercise for improving cardiorespiratory fitness, although to a lesser extent than other forms of cardiorespiratory training (41, 58).

Some concern about shoulder overuse is warranted, especially among athletes who have less-than-optimal shoulder mobility or who are inexperienced (59). As with most exercise modes, overuse injuries are the most prevalent form of injury for swimming, primarily from high-volume training and repetitive strain (specifically in the shoulder) (13). Problems with exercise technique to look for and correct include the following (13):

- The hand crossing the midline when entering the water
- The thumb entering the water first
- The body rolling asymmetrically from side to side
- Breathing only on one side
- The arm crossing the midline during the swim stroke

Cycling

Another low-impact form of aerobic endurance exercise is road cycling. Low-impact forces often enable athletes to exercise for longer periods of time without resulting in overuse injuries to the feet and knees. Safety precautions including wearing a helmet, using reflective devices, and selecting routes with clearly marked bicycle lanes. It may also be difficult for highly trained athletes to sustain the riding speeds necessary to promote continued fitness improvements without introducing higher risks of injury; using alternating periods of high versus low training or intervals may be a better alternative (30).

Although cycling seems to be a simple activity (get on a bike and ride), certain aspects of technique should be addressed, including cadence, foot position, hand position, and bike fit. When getting fitted for a bike, the major concern is trying to get the bony skeleton, rather than soft tissues (i.e., soft perineum, blood vessels, nerves, and other sensitive areas), to support the rider's body weight. This ensures optimal comfort and performance, making the feel of the bike disappear. Following is a brief discussion of bike fitting; however, it is only an introduction. A bike-fitting expert should be consulted to ensure the bike fits properly. The 2013 Medicine of Cycling consensus statement includes recommendations on placement for the pelvis, hands, and feet and how each component of the body should be considered for overall fit and comfort (1).

In terms of the foot and cycling, shoe comfort is a critical starting point. In addition to comfort, shoes should have a small, cycling-specific insole. Cycling shoes can have a modicum of adjustment, and minimizing the accommodations and adjustments is highly recommended. The most common evaluation is making sure that the feet can remain flat during pedal rotations and that there is no pain after a ride. An expert should be consulted for more than minimal adjustments; most clips allow for approximately 6° of movement, which should be more than ample for most riders.

Regarding the pelvis, fit concerns include saddle selection, height, fore–aft position, and tilt. Many types of seats (saddles) can be used in cycling. To optimize comfort and reduce restriction, pressure needs to be primarily in the rear of the seat, resting on the bony pelvis or pubic rami. In terms of saddle tilt and position, a neutral saddle is the most common; however, a slight downward nose can reduce pressure on the front of the seat. Some riders report comfort with a slight upward tilt, which can keep them from sliding off the front of the seat, but this is much less common. The tilt should be only a few degrees if possible. Pain and pressure typically mean there is too much loading on the middle or front of the seat. Seat position can also be adjusted forward and backward. When the seat position is correct, the center point of the knee is directly over the pedal when the leg is at 90° or the 3 o'clock position (see figure 14.1).

Many seat styles are available (including those with holes), but trying the seats to find the most comfortable style is probably the best approach. In addition, the saddle should be in line with the top tube of the bike. In terms of seat height, while sitting on the saddle with the pelvis neutral, the heel of the foot should just touch the pedal when it is at the 6 o'clock position. When the foot is adjusted so that the ball of the foot is on the center of the pedal, there should be a slight bend in the knee (approximately 5°-10°).

Finally, hand position should be considered for comfort and safety. The handlebar position should allow for a light touch or grip while also allowing easy access to the shifters and brakes. In addition, the thumb should always be wrapped around the bars for safety reasons. The handlebars can be adjusted up and down as well as fore and aft. Basic alignment will allow an approximately 15° angle in the elbow and a 90° bend in the shoulder (based on the forward position of the torso). Also, handlebar rotation should allow for a neutral wrist (not flexed or extended) to reduce any impingement. Handlebar height can be adjusted based on comfort, as previously described.

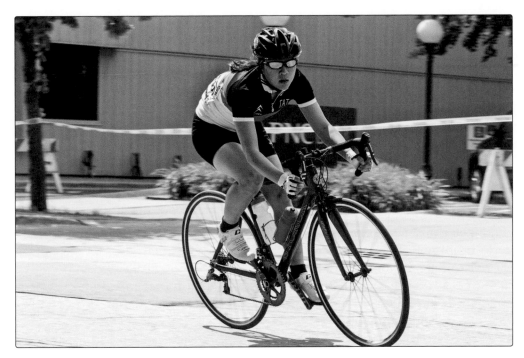

Figure 14.1   Correct bike fit, showing saddle height, fore–aft position, tilt, and handlebar height and rotation, all of which result in appropriate knee, elbow, and wrist positioning.

Many issues arise with an improperly fitting bike, including foot and knee pain, low back pain, shoulder and neck pain, and wrist and hand pain. In addition, suboptimal performance and muscular fatigue can be related to bike fit. It is highly recommended to consult a professional for any pain or discomfort experienced from an improperly fitting bike or equipment.

Pedaling cadence is another important consideration. Pedaling cadence determines power output as well as efficiency. In other words, it determines the speed of the ride as well as how long the rider can continue the ride (maximizing power and minimizing fatigue). Research has shown that a pedaling rate of approximately 80 to 90 revolutions per minute (RPM) seems to optimize power and efficiency (14). At times cadence can reach as high as 120 RPM or higher, but this is quite challenging and typically takes the rider into the LT (lactate threshold). As such, the cycling program can be altered to mimic program variables discussed in the remainder of the chapter.

Aerobic Sporting Activities

Aerobic sporting activities such as soccer, tennis, basketball, and ultimate Frisbee may be more enjoyable than conventional aerobic exercises for some tactical athletes and thus may promote more consistent participation. That being said, the inability to precisely control the workout stress, along with some added risk of musculoskeletal injury, makes this a less-than-optimal exercise mode from a programming perspective. The playing area (field) should be well maintained, and officiating is often needed to ensure safety. Sporting activities are not a replacement for regular cardiorespiratory training unless they can be performed consistently three to five days per week.

STEP 2: TRAINING FREQUENCY

Training frequency refers to the numbers of sessions per day or week for a particular component of fitness, such as aerobic endurance. Interplay of training frequency, duration, and intensity plus the training status of the tactical athlete will determine the efficacy of the programming as well as recovery considerations. The higher the intensity and the longer the duration of the training session, the less frequently the training sessions should occur. In addition, highly trained tactical athletes require less recovery time and therefore may add more training sessions to optimize occupational preparedness. However, lesser trained individuals need additional recovery time to ensure they are prepared for the subsequent workout and to reduce the risk of overtraining and injury. There is an art to the science of this type of exercise prescription that takes time and experience to fully understand, but certain scientific generalizations can be followed to get started. Too much training can lead to injury and illness, but not enough training will fail to optimize the cardiorespiratory training adaptations.

For alterations in cardiorespiratory fitness, it is necessary to train more than two times per week (16, 61). Most guidelines for health advocate three days per week. However, training the same component of fitness more than five times per week can lead to overtraining and injury (22). To maintain the required level of fitness, less frequent training may be required.

STEP 3: TRAINING INTENSITY

For years, MHR (maximal heart rate) has been a key benchmark for identifying appropriate intensity of long, slow distance (LSD) training. A laboratory exercise test would be necessary to determine true MHR, so equations have been developed for predicting it. These include an age-determined equation (MHR = 220 – age) and the more recent and accurate Gellish equation (MHR = 207 – 0.7 [age]) (15). MHR estimation should be used with caution, because the predictions lack reliability (34, 47, 50). An example of how to use MHR to calculate training zones can be found in the box titled "Heart Rate Calculation."

In addition, **heart rate reserve (HRR)**, which is the difference between the maximal and resting HRs, can be used to determine appropriate training zones. Once HRR has been calculated, the Karvonen method using percentages of MRH method can be utilized. As an example of training zones, for LSD training, it has been recommended that training be conducted at approximately 60% to 80% of MHR (12, 43). Lower ranges can be used for those who are less fit (sedentary), whereas higher ranges can be used for people with a higher level of cardiorespiratory fitness. See the box titled "Heart Rate Calculation" for a sample calculation using the Karvonen method.

Another means of estimating training zones is the RPE (rating of perceived exertion) scale (see table 14.1). The RPE has been shown to be an accurate estimate of how hard the exerciser perceives the exertion to be during exercise, even in the tactical environment (6, 19, 54). That stated, there are some concerns about external influences (e.g., age, training status, temperature, pain) limiting accuracy (19, 37). RPE is a scale that uses a number system (from 1-10) to describe how much effort is perceived by the exercises. After familiarization with the scale, exercisers use the numeric rating system to rate how they feel during their exercise session.

Table 14.1 Rating of Perceived Exertion (RPE) Scale

Rating	Description
1	Nothing at all (lying down)
2	Extremely little
3	Very easy
4	Easy (could do this all day)
5	Moderate
6	Somewhat hard (starting to feel it)
7	Hard
8	Very hard (making an effort to keep up)
9	Very, very hard
10	Maximum effort (can't go any further)

Reprinted, by permission, from NSCA, 2012, Aerobic endurance training program design, P. Hagerman. In *NSCA's essentials of personal training*, 2nd ed., edited by J.W. Coburn and M.H. Malek (Champaign, IL: Human Kinetics), 395.

Heart Rate Calculation

Karvonen Method

Formula

- Age-predicted maximum heart rate (APMHR)
- = 220 − age
- Heart rate reserve (HRR)
- = APMHR − resting heart rate (RHR)
- Target heart rate (THR)
- = HRR × exercise intensity + RHR

The calculation should be done twice to determine the target heart rate range (THRR).

Example

A 30-year-old firefighter with an RHR of 60 beats/min is assigned an exercise intensity of 60% to 80% of functional capacity.

- APMHR = 220 − 30 = 190 beats/min
- RHR = 60 beats/min
- HRR = 190 − 60 = 130 beats/min
- Lowest number of the athlete's THRR
- = 130 × 0.60 + 60 = 78 + 60
- = 138 beats/min
- Highest number of the athlete's THRR
- = 130 × 0.80 + 60 = 104 + 60
- = 164 beats/min

For ease of use, divide THR by 6 to get a 10-second pulse interval.

- 138 ÷ 6 = 23
- 164 ÷ 6 = 27

The athlete's THRR is 23 to 27 for a 10-second pulse interval.

Percentage of Maximal Heart Rate Method Using the Gellish Formula

Formula

- Age-predicted maximum heart rate (APMHR)
- = 207 − 0.7 (age)
- Target heart rate (THR)
- = APMHR × exercise intensity

The calculation should be done twice to determine the THRR.

Example

A 30-year-old firefighter with an RHR of 60 beats/min is assigned an exercise intensity of 60% to 80% of functional capacity.

- APMHR = 207 − 0.7 (age)
- = 207 − 0.7(30) = 207 − 21
- = 186 beat/min

(continued)

Heart Rate Calculation (continued)

- Lowest number of the athlete's THRR
- = APMHR × exercise intensity
- = 186 × 0.60
- = 112
- Highest number of the athlete's THRR
- = APMHR × exercise intensity
- = 186 × 0.80
- = 149

For ease of use, divide THR by 6 to get a 10-second pulse interval.

- 112 ÷ 6 = 19
- 149 ÷ 6 = 25

The athlete's THRR is 19 to 25 for a 10-second pulse interval.

Adapted from (42).

Similar to the estimated MHR zone of 60% to 80%, RPE has recommended training zone for altering cardiorespiratory fitness: 6 to 8 on the RPE scale (39).

Another alternative for determining training zones is to simply select a comfortable intensity for LSD. The conversation test is a good way to gauge whether or not intensity is too high. If it is not possible to carry on a conversation with a training partner, the workout intensity is too high for LSD training. The challenge is getting the intensity high enough to be valuable without going too high. It might take some trial and error, but experimenting with various paces can help identify the point at which breathing is not too heavy to carry on a conversation but the training is difficult enough to be classified as exercise.

STEP 4: EXERCISE DURATION

Most recommendations for continuous cardiorespiratory exercise for health-related benefits advocate a minimum of 20 minutes of vigorous aerobic activity per session three days per week or 30 minutes of moderate aerobic activity five days per week (20). These recommendations also advocate for shorter bouts of exercise, such as 10- or 15-minute sessions (20). Exercise duration is often determined by the intensity of the exercise, especially if the intensity is at or above the LT.

Exercise at a lower intensity can be performed for a much longer duration (an hour to several hours) (42).

STEP 5: EXERCISE PROGRESSION

A number of methods have been developed for promoting improvements in cardiorespiratory fitness, including LSD training, pace/tempo training, interval training, and repeated sprints. These methods can be used regardless of the mode of exercise.

Long, Slow Distance Training

Long, slow distance training (LSD) involves higher volume training at a constant pace and can be used to improve general aerobic endurance. Identifying the intensity of LSD is a challenge and will be discussed shortly. The volume of training (e.g., miles or time for a runner, laps for a swimmer) depends on the athlete's current fitness level and training goals. Tactical athletes should start at a volume that is comfortably challenging but not overbearing. Over time, the distance or time can be increased in order to progress. A commonly accepted rule is not more than a 10% increase in overall time or volume (42), but this is not based on research evidence. For instance, in week 1 of a training program, a firefighter completes a 5-mile (8 km) run for an LSD workout. In week 2, that

Table 14.2   Suggested Parameters for Training Methods

Training method	Frequency	Intensity	Duration
LSD	1-2 days/week	Comfortable, sustainable pace, ~70% $\dot{V}O_2max$	30-120 min
Interval training	1-2 days/week	Near-maximal intensity, close to $\dot{V}O_2max$	3-5 min (work:rest ratio of 1:1)
Pace/tempo training	1-2 days/week	At LT, 75%-105% $\dot{V}O_2max$	20-30 min
Repeated sprints	1-2 days/week	Maximal intensity	5-20 sprints
HIIT	1 day/week	Greater than $\dot{V}O_2max$	30-90 s (work: rest ratio of 1:5)
Fartlek	1 day/week	Varies between LSD and pace/tempo training intensities	20-60 min

Adapted from references 10-12, 35, 43, 44, 55, 57, 60.

Table 14.3   Sample LSD Training Program for Tactical Athletes Preparing for an Extended Training Run (6+ mi or 10+ km)

Sunday	Monday	Tuesday	Wednesday	Thursday	Friday	Saturday
15 min LSD	20 min fartlek	Rest	45 min LSD	20 min fartlek	Rest	60 min LSD

Comments:

- Frequency: To help combat overtraining or overuse, the LSD training days are spread out evenly over the week to allow ample recovery.
- Duration: Because the training run could exceed 60 minutes, the duration of the LSD training should approach that time.
- Intensity: To complete the extended LSD sessions, the tactical athlete should run at a lower intensity or training pace.

Adapted from Reuter and Dawes (42).

distance should not be increased more than 0.5 mile (0.8 km), or 10% more than the first week. Injuries often result from rapid increases in total training volume; therefore, a gradual progression should be followed that considers the tactical athlete's current health and fitness and the rate at which the athlete is adapting to the physical stress of conditioning.

Some debate exists regarding how much LSD training should be performed to improve fitness (24). As part of a well-rounded training program involving interval, pace/tempo, or repeated sprints, 30 minutes per training session is a good starting point. As the total length of time increases to 40 to 120 minutes per session, greater benefits will likely result (32). Training volumes of 30- to 60-minutes appear to present the greatest opportunity for adaptation with the lowest risk of injury (12, 44, 55, 57). Table 14.2 suggests training parameters for LSD training, and table 14.3 provides a sample training program using LSD training.

Pace/Tempo Training

Pace/tempo training is similar to LSD in that it is conducted for a set period of time or distance, but it is performed at a much higher intensity (10-12). Exercise pace is based on a certain percentage of a race condition or anaerobic threshold, with workouts designed to improve anaerobic threshold or work rate. This method requires participation in a race or event in order to determine a race pace or the completion of a metabolic test to determine anaerobic threshold. The most feasible method for undertaking this training approach is using a time from a recent event or completing a time trial. Once a race pace has been identified, the same distance can be completed at various percentages of that time (ranging from 75% to 105%). Lower percentages will make the session less intense, and intensities can be altered or progressed over time to add variation in the training stress.

The keys to pace/tempo training are the selected distance or time and the ability to maintain the prescribed pace or intensity. For tactical athletes, this volume should range from 20 to 30 minutes (11). Longer distances and times (i.e., 30 versus 10 minutes) obviously increase the demand of pace/tempo workouts and make the workouts more challenging. Monitoring pace is necessary in order to sustain the appropriate pace throughout the session. Therefore, performing pace/tempo training sessions on a track, in a pool with a clock, or on exercise equipment will make it easier to monitor time, pace, and progress.

As an example, a police officer completes a 10K (6 mi) self-paced race on a treadmill in 48 minutes. Training may then include one pace/tempo workout each week for four straight weeks at 75%, 85%, 95%, and 105%. To calculate the appropriate pace and time for the 75% workout, calculate 25% of the total time (12 minutes) and add that to the pace time. The goal time for the 75% workout then becomes 60:00 minutes. For the 105% workout, subtract 5% from the total time, and the goal time becomes approximately 45:36 minutes. After the four weeks are complete, the officer completes a new pace test in the same manner, and appropriate adjustments for each workout are made based on the new pace time. This might be an appropriate technique for a tactical athlete training for an upcoming fitness test, given the high intensity of many physical assessments, or it might simply be a novel way to increase cardiorespiratory fitness (e.g., LT), provided the tactical athlete has demonstrated sufficient aerobic fitness to use this approach effectively. Table 14.2 suggests training parameters for pace/tempo training, and table 14.4 provides a sample program.

Interval Training

Many tactical tasks involve high-intensity effort followed by active recovery before another effort is required. In these situations, the ability to recover quickly will have significant performance effects. If recovery between work efforts is insufficient, the next effort increases in relative intensity and may present a risk of cardiovascular injury or poor performance. Therefore, the goal is to enhance both work effort and the ability to rapidly recover from the effort. The length of each work segment should range from 5 seconds to 3 minutes based on the tasks required of the tactical athlete (43, 44).

The ability to sustain high-intensity effort for longer periods of time and to recover quickly between bouts of high-intensity work can be developed through **interval training** (10, 12, 35, 44) . Various methods of interval training exist, including high-intensity interval training (HIIT) and fartlek training, which will be discussed later in the chapter. In these methods, the individual performs a high-intensity work segment followed by a period of rest before again performing high-intensity work. This process is repeated for a predetermined number of repetitions to form the workout session. Intervals can be performed in any mode of exercise as long as the work-to-rest ratio can be controlled.

A number of variables can be adjusted to vary interval training from workout to workout and across time. The length of the work segment, the length of the rest period, the intensity of the work segment, and the number of repetitions can all be adjusted to change the interval workout (42). Longer work segments, shorter rest breaks, higher

Table 14.4 Sample Pace/Tempo Training Program for Tactical Athletes for a Timed 3-Mile (5K) Run

Sunday	Monday	Tuesday	Wednesday	Thursday	Friday	Saturday
30 min LSD	15 min pace/tempo run	25 min fartlek run	25 min easy run	15 min pace/tempo run	Rest	45 min LSD run

Comments:

- Frequency: Because pace/tempo runs are stressful, they should be spread out to allow for ample recovery.
- Duration: The pace/tempo runs are shorter than the LSD runs to accommodate the higher intensity.
- Intensity: The pace/tempo runs should be at higher intensity to allow for adaptations and higher respiratory stress to simulate the race pace.

Adapted from Reuter and Dawes (42).

work intensities, and higher numbers of repetitions will each increase the overall workload and stress of the interval training session. Although little research has been conducted to identify the most effective progression in interval training, increases in work segment time, followed by shorter rest periods, and then a gradual increase in the total number of repetitions per workout is a reasonable training progression. Table 14.2 suggests training parameters for interval training, and table 14.5 provides a sample interval training program.

Repeated Sprints

Repeated sprints are designed to stress both high-intensity effort and recovery and are similar to interval training except that for repeated sprints, the intensity during the work segment is always 100%. Because intensity is always maximal, the length of time during the sprint and the amount of recovery are somewhat different than in interval training. To maintain maximal intensity, sprint distance must remain within ranges allowing for maximal effort, generally less than 200 meters (219 yd) or 30 seconds, and recovery periods must be long enough to enable maximal performance on the next repetition (43, 60).

The goal of repeated sprint training is to increase speed and speed endurance in tasks demanding maximal anaerobic effort. This will enable the tactical athlete to perform better on maximal-effort tasks lasting less than 30 seconds, which is a necessary component of job function (21), especially if those tasks must be repeated. Interval training will address the metabolic demands of longer tasks. Repeated sprints should, therefore, be limited to 30 seconds and allow for near-maximal recovery (1-3 minutes rest) (28). Sprints of less than 30 seconds in duration (e.g., 5-30 seconds) followed by moderate rest periods (e.g., 1-3 minutes) are a great way for tactical athletes to build speed endurance and increase cardiorespiratory fitness (17, 56). For longer sprints, lengthier rest periods are needed to allow for near-maximal recovery, whereas sprints of 5 seconds may only require 60 seconds of rest. The athlete's fitness level will dictate how much rest is required. Keep in mind that the goal is not to perform the next sprint in a fatigued state. Interval training will address the need to recover quickly and perform while fatigued. Repeated sprints serve a different purpose—to increase speed and speed endurance in tasks demanding maximal endurance—and the best results occur when fatigue is at a minimum. Table 14.2 suggests training parameters for repeated sprint training.

High-Intensity Interval Training

Similar to repeated sprints, **high-intensity interval training (HIIT)** involves short bursts of high-intensity activity (greater than $90\%\dot{V}O_2max$) with periods of rest between repeated efforts. These sessions can be as short as <30 seconds to as long 4 minutes. HIIT intervals are an ideal way to tax the various energy systems (specifically the anaerobic glycolytic system) and mimic the activities a tactical athlete might encounter in the occupation. Ample recovery between intervals is necessary to ensure adequate recovery. If the rest intervals are too short, the quality of the effort will

Table 14.5 Sample Interval Training Program for Tactical Athletes Preparing for a 3-Mile (5K) Time Trial

Sunday	Monday	Tuesday	Wednesday	Thursday	Friday	Saturday
Rest	5 reps of 0.5 km (.3 mi) intervals at race pace with a 1:1 work:rest ratio	5K (3 mi) easy run	25 min LSD run	HIIT 3 min @ 90% $\dot{V}O_2$max/2 min passive recovery × 3 reps	25 min LSD run	25 min fartlek run on flat course

Comments:

- Frequency: Because interval runs are stressful, they should be spread out to allow for ample recovery.
- Duration: Adjust the duration of the work segments to be between 5 seconds and 3 minutes.
- Intensity: Adjust the intensity level of each work segment to be in proportion to the duration of the work segment.

Adapted from Reuter and Dawes (42).

decrease, and the subsequent risk for injury will increase. Alternatively, if the rest periods are too long, the benefits of ongoing metabolic taxation will likely diminish (42). Table 14.2 suggests training parameters for HIIT, and table 14.6 provides a sample training HIIT program.

Fartlek Training

Fartlek training originates from the Swedish term for "speed play." It is a running style that integrates higher intensity intervals with periods of active extended recovery. For example, while out for an LSD training run at 60% $\dot{V}O_2$max, the runner will sprint the occasional light-pole-to-light-pole distance at 90% $\dot{V}O_2$max and then return to the original training intensity. This can also be accomplished in other modes of exercise, such as swimming or cycling. It is a great way to reduce the monotony of elongated training periods and has the added benefit of increasing $\dot{V}O_2$max, LT, running economy, and fuel utilization (42). Table 14.2 suggests training parameters

for fartlek training, and table 14.7 provides a sample fartlek training program.

Key Point

Fartlek training is a style of interval training that incorporates bouts of higher intensity work (fast running, swimming, or cycling) followed by periods of lower intensity work (slow running, swimming, or cycling). It keeps the training fresh and fun while improving various components of cardiorespiratory as well as performance efficiency.

PROGRAM DESIGN RECOMMENDATIONS

Variation, progression, and periodization of aerobic endurance training are vital to long-term adaptation and fitness (8, 48, 49, 52). Variation of training can be quite simple, involving a rotation of LSD training, intervals, pace/tempo workouts, and repeated sprints. Four metabolic

Table 14.6 Sample HIIT Program for Tactical Athletes Preparing for an Extended Swim (12-Minute Trial)

Sunday	Monday	Tuesday	Wednesday	Thursday	Friday	Saturday
Rest	10 min LSD swim	HIIT 30 s at 95% $\dot{V}O_2$ max 30 s recovery × 8 reps	8 min LSD swim	Rest day (no swim workout)	6 min swim at trail pace	10 min LSD swim

Comments:

- Frequency: Because HIIT swim workouts are stressful, only one is programmed per week.
- Duration: Because swimming can be more intense than cycling or running, work bouts of 30 seconds with 30 seconds of recovery are used.
- Intensity: The swim should be at 95% $\dot{V}O_2$ when completing the work portion of the HIIT session.

Adapted from Reuter and Dawes (42).

Table 14.7 Sample Fartlek Training Program for Tactical Athletes Preparing for a Timed 3-Mile (5K) Test

Sunday	Monday	Tuesday	Wednesday	Thursday	Friday	Saturday
Rest	45 min LSD	30 min fartlek run of hard/easy work on hills and flats	15-min pace/tempo run	30 min LSD run	15 min LSD run	Run test

Comments:

- Frequency: Because fartlek workouts are stressful, only one is programmed per week.
- Duration: The total distance or time of the fartlek training session should equate to the timed-run distance or time.
- Intensity: The run should be close to $\dot{V}O_2$ max when completing the work portion of the fartlek session.

Adapted from Reuter and Dawes (42).

training sessions per week, each using a different method of training, is a great starting point (11). Each week, volume in the four workouts can be increased slightly (<10%) at the same intensity as the prior week. After three to four weeks of this gradual increase in volume, intensity can then be increased at similar rate. Over time, adding workout sessions, increasing the length of each session, and increasing the overall intensity can result in training progression. However, the optimal approach is a periodized training plan that incorporates low-, moderate-, and high-intensity workouts each week with a gradual overall progression in volume and intensity (24). Table 14.8 demonstrates a sample progression and variation of training for tactical athletes.

It is also important to balance high-stress workouts with low-stress sessions (22). As athletes become more highly trained, they are able to safely perform a greater percentage of high-stress workouts. The beginner should perform fewer high-stress workouts; as a general rule, beginners should perform two low-stress workouts for every high-stress session (1:2) with a frequency that considers the individual's fitness, work capacity, and occupational demands (e.g., work schedule). One or two sessions each week should be high-intensity sessions, while the other two to four should be a mixture of low- and moderate-intensity workouts. For highly fit athletes, this ratio can gradually shift to 2:1 in favor of high-intensity training.

Table 14.8 Sample 12-Week Advanced Metabolic Training Regimen

Week	Monday	Tuesday	Wednesday	Thursday	Friday	Saturday	Sunday
1	LSD 30 min	IT 45/90 s repeated 5 times	PT at 75% pace	Rest	Fartlek 20 min	RS 100 m (109 yd) with 2 min rest	Rest
2	HIIT 30/60 s	PT at 95% pace	Rest	LSD 60 min	RS 200 m (219 yd) with 3 min rest	Rest	Rest
3	LSD 45 min	IT 60/60 s repeated 8 times	Rest	PT at 105% pace	LSD 30 min	RS 75 m (82 yd) with 90 s rest	Rest
4	PT at 100% pace	Rest	Fartlek 20 min	Rest	PT at 105% pace	LSD 30 min	Rest
5	RS 50 m (55 yd) with 30 s rest	HIIT 90 s/7.5 min rest repeated 2 times	Rest	LSD 60 min	RS 20 m (22 yd) with 10 s rest	IT 30/30 s repeated 10 times	Rest
6	Fartlek 60 min	PT at 85% pace	Rest	RS 50 m (55 yd) with 30 s rest	LSD 30 min	HIIT 60 s/4 min rest repeated 4 times	Rest
7	Rest	IT 90/90 s repeated 5 times	Rest	LSD 45 min	Rest	PT at 100% pace	Rest
8	Fartlek 30 min	LSD 45 min	Rest	Fartlek 60 min	LSD 60 min	Rest	Rest
9	HIIT 30/120 s repeated 5 times	PT at 105%	RS 30 m (33 yd) with 10 s rest	IT 60/60 s repeated 10 times	PT at 75%	RS 100 m (109 yd) with 30 s rest	Rest
10	LSD 60 min	PT at 95%	Rest	PT at 100%	RS 50 m (55 yd) with 30 s rest	Fartlek 45 min	Rest
11	RS 400 m (437 yd) with 5 min rest	LSD 20 min	HIIT 60 s/4 min repeated 4 times	PT at 95%	Fartlek 60 min	LSD 45 min	Rest
12	IT 20/40 s repeated 20 times	RS 100 m (109 yd) with 30 s rest	LSD 60 min	PT at 105%	Fartlek 45 min	HIIT 60/210 s repeated 4 times	Rest
13	Active rest	Active rest	Active rest	Active rest	Active rest	Active rest	Active rest

F = fartlek training; HIIT = high-intensity interval training; IT = interval training; LSD = long, slow distance training; PT = pace/tempo training; RS = repeated sprints.

Another key component when implementing an optimal metabolic training program for tactical athletes is rest and recovery. As a general rule, for every 12 weeks of training, the athlete should rest from organized training for 1 week. During this week, physical activity is encouraged; however, the athlete should not participate in an organized exercise program and should avoid high-intensity activity. This week is designed to allow the body to fully regenerate following 12 weeks of consistent effort. Over time, this week is important to prevent overtraining and reduce the risk of overuse injuries. Over the course of a 12-week training cycle, an average of two days of rest is recommended for all tactical athletes. Fatigue builds up over time, with overtraining resulting from months of excessive training stress and inadequate rest and recovery, so sufficient recovery must be given.

Training Status and Goals

A common mistake of training programs is to start too quickly, attempting to improve fitness rapidly by performing high-intensity, high-volume training following a lengthy period of inactivity. Tactical athletes who have been inactive should begin slowly and avoid high-intensity exercise until they have progressed through a period of low- and moderate-intensity training. Highly trained athletes who have been consistently training for many years may be prepared for high-volume, high-intensity effort, but they may also be at greater risk for overtraining. Tactical athletes should exercise according to their individual goals. If the goal is to improve overall aerobic endurance, more workouts involving LSD and pace/tempo sessions should be performed. If rapid recovery following high-intensity exertion is the goal, intervals and repeated sprints will have the greatest impact. The TSAC Facilitator should consider both the desired goal and the training status of the athlete and assign the most appropriate mode of exercise—along with the proper progression in training volume and intensity—to ensure safe, effective training.

CONCLUSION

Tactical athletes must prepare for a variety of metabolic demands. Proper exercise volume, intensity, progression, and variation can ensure optimal fitness development while avoiding overtraining. To ensure well-rounded metabolic development, tactical athletes should include LSD, interval, pace/tempo, and repeated sprint training throughout the year.

Key Terms

aerobic endurance
aerobic endurance activities
aerobic exercises
aerobic sporting activities
fartlek training
heart rate reserve (HRR)

high-intensity interval training
interval training
long, slow distance training (LSD)
pace/tempo training
repeated sprints

Study Questions

1. The SAID principle is most closely associated with which aspect of a training program?

   a. specificity

   b. variation

   c. cueing

   d. instruction

2. Which of the following indicates that the seat of an exercise bike is set at the correct height?

   a. The elbows are bent slightly.

   b. The knee is over the center of the pedal.

   c. The upper arms and torso form an approximate 90° angle.

   d. The knee is slightly bent when the pedal is at the bottom.

3. Which of following describes the benefits of a rowing machine?

   a. utilizes upper and lower musculature

   b. maximizes axial loading

   c. allows back to flex and extend through a larger ROM

   d. is simple to master

4. A 35-year-old police officer who has a RHR of 55 beats/min is instructed to perform an exercise session at 70% of his functional capacity. What is the target heart rate range using the Karvonen method?

   a. 130 beats/min

   b. 146 beats/min

   c. 161 beats/min

   d. 170 beats/min

Evidence-Based Approach to Strength and Power Training to Improve Performance in Tactical Populations

Dennis E. Scofield, MEd, CSCS

Sarah E. Sauers, MS, CSCS

Barry A. Spiering, PhD, CSCS

Marilyn A. Sharp, MS

Bradley C. Nindl, PhD

After completing this chapter, you will be able to

- evaluate individual needs for strength and power training to improve tactical performance, and
- provide evidence-based rationale for strength and power training programs to improve tactical performance.

ports such as volleyball, American football, tennis, and soccer require strength and power to execute fundamental movements such as serving, sprinting, jumping, blocking, and interference. Similarly, tactical athletes must possess the strength and power necessary to execute occupational tasks such as negotiating obstacles, evacuating casualties, and breaching entrances, with the additional burden of wearing heavy load-bearing and personal protective equipment. Understandably, muscular strength and power are vital components of tactical physical preparedness that the TSAC Facilitator needs to assess, prescribe, and monitor. This chapter provides an evidence-based approach to muscular strength and power training aimed at improving tactical performance. After completing this chapter, the reader will understand the importance of evaluating job-specific physical requirements, considering individual needs, and integrating strength and power exercises into physical training (PT) for tactical occupations.

OVERVIEW OF OCCUPATIONAL DEMANDS

Strength and power training is necessary for tactical athletes. Tactical occupations commonly encompass tasks that include repetitive lifting, dragging, pushing and pulling, climbing, jumping, and carrying loads, all of which require muscular strength and power (37, 54, 104). The magnitude and frequency of these tasks vary among occupations (20, 38). Therefore, it's important to analyze job tasks (task analysis) and identify job-specific physical demands—especially those that place significant mechanical stress on the musculoskeletal system—to recognize relevant PT outcomes aimed at improving tactical performance (47) and mitigating injuries (45). The nexus of the TSAC Facilitator and the physically prepared tactical athlete is a properly designed PT program incorporating occupationally relevant strength and power exercises.

Before discussing strength and power further, it is important to define the relevant constructs and then explain why these attributes are meaningful for tactical performance. First, **strength** is the ability of the neuromuscular system to produce force. This definition underscores that neural factors (e.g., increased **agonist** activation, improved **motor unit** coordination and synchronization) and muscular factors (e.g., **hypertrophy**) both contribute to improvements in strength following PT (25, 26, 55, 88). Importantly, changes in neural factors explain a disproportionate amount of the initial increase in strength at the onset of PT (25, 26, 55, 64, 88). For this reason, relatively moderate training strategies can initially be prescribed for novices. Most often, strength is operationally defined as **one-repetition maximum (1RM)** performance (i.e., the maximal amount of weight that can be lifted through a full ROM using correct technique for an exercise such as the bench press).

Power equals the product of force and velocity. In more practical terms, power is the ability to rapidly express strength. A vertical jump test illustrates the concept of power: Achieving a high score on a vertical jump test requires one to produce large forces in a relatively short time (~0.3 seconds) (18, 19). Differentially defining *strength* and *power* is critical because they contribute independently and significantly to occupational tasks (35, 48) and because they are different but related physical attributes and thus the optimal strategy for improving each is slightly different. The development of strength and conditioning programs for tactical personnel should include an evaluation of job-specific physical demands that will guide exercise prescription for strength and power (31). Table 15.1 summarizes the parameters of strength and power exercise.

Cross-sectional correlational and longitudinal research studies substantiate the importance of not only aerobic and muscular endurance but also strength and power training to improve tactical performance in both men and women (56, 98). Correlational research indicates that inherent strength and power capabilities of untrained men and women significantly predict **load carriage** performance, or change in the time required to travel 2 miles (3 km) with a loaded rucksack ($r = -0.27 - -0.48$), and **repetitive box lifting (RBL)** performance ($r = 0.47 - 0.77$) (48, 90). As PT progresses, additional improvements in muscular strength and power correlate with improvements in RBL performance ($r = 0.19 - 0.61$) (35, 90). Kraemer et al. (47) performed a six-month study

Table 15.1   Characteristics of Strength and Power Exercise

Characteristic	Strength	Power
Description	Ability of the neuromuscular system to produce force	Ability to rapidly express strength
Frequency	3-5 days per week for each muscle group	1-3 days per week
Volume	3-6 sets per muscle group	80-140 contacts, throws, or catches per session*
Intensity	85%-100% of 1RM (slow tempo)	20%-70% 1RM (fast/ballistic tempo)
Test	One-repetition maximum (1RM)	Vertical jump test

Frequency, volume, and intensity vary depending on the training status of the tactical athlete.

*Foot contacts, upper body catches, and throws (91).

of the effects of four PT programs on military task performance in untrained women. The PT programs were divided into endurance training (ET), calisthenics training (CT), resistance training focusing on total body strength/power (TBP), resistance training focusing on total body strength/hypertrophy (TBH), resistance training focusing on upper body strength/power (UBP), and resistance training focusing on upper body strength/hypertrophy (TBH). Significant improvements ($p < 0.05$) in load carriage (except for the ET group) and RBL were observed for all groups of women pre- to posttraining. However, only the groups that performed resistance training had posttraining values similar to those of untrained men; the ET and CT training groups' posttrain-

ing values were significantly less than those of untrained men (figure 15.1).

Injury mitigation is also an important outcome of a tactical strength and conditioning program, and it can have important implications for physical preparedness. For example, low back pain is common among both the general population and tactical personnel, and it is associated with lower fitness levels (36). A study conducted by Mayer et al. (57) sought to determine whether specific core-strengthening exercises added to firefighters' PT would be beneficial. The researchers found that integrating a 24-week supervised core- and back-strengthening exercise program (twice a week) into the firefighters' (n = 54) PT improved core isometric (12%) and back

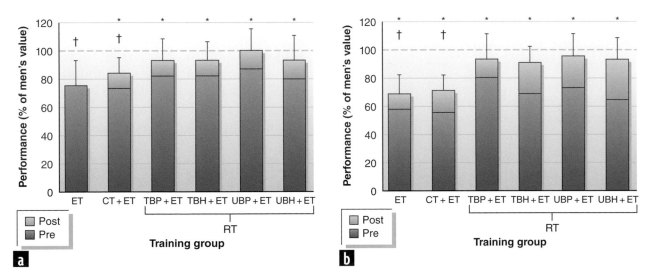

Figure 15.1   Effectiveness of strength and power training for improving military occupational task performance in women. The bars represent women's load carriage *(a)* and RBL *(b)* performance before and after six months of PT. Values are women's performance compared with the performance of untrained men.

Based on Kraemer et al. (47).

muscular endurance (21%) compared with firefighters (*n* = 42) who only performed their usual PT programs (57) (figure 15.2). In summary, research using long-term training interventions confirms the efficacy of integrating strength and power training into PT for both men and women. These improvements are as follows:

- Tactical athletes who perform strength and power training achieve greater improvements in tactical performance than those who do not (90).

- Training interventions that combine strength and power training with aerobic endurance training induce greater improvements in tactical performance than aerobic endurance–only training interventions (47, 50).

- Strength and power exercise during PT allows women to achieve similar standards of tactical performance as untrained men; however, if their training regimen excludes strength and power training, their tactical performance lags behind that of their untrained male counterparts (figure 15.1) (47).

- Integrating a 24-week supervised core- and back-strengthening exercise program (twice a week) into firefighters' (*n* = 54) PT has been shown to improve core isometric (12%) and back muscular endurance (21%) over firefighters (*n* = 42) who only performed standard PT (57) (figure 15.2).

The evidence summarized in table 15.2 clearly supports the inclusion of strength and power training in PT.

Resistance exercise clearly improves strength, power, and tactical performance (33, 35, 47, 50). Augmenting resistance training with **plyometric exercise** (i.e., jump training) can further improve maximal power capabilities (7, 9, 12, 19, 22, 23, 101) (table 15.3). For instance, it has been demonstrated that supplementing resistance training with plyometric exercises induces significant improvements in countermovement jump (CMJ) height, **power output**, and max **rate of force development (RFD)**, all of which influence load carriage performance (19). Supplemental plyometric exercises have also been shown

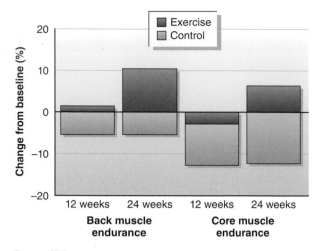

Figure 15.2 Changes in back and core endurance after 24 weeks of supervised worksite exercise among firefighters.

Based on Mayer et al. (57).

to improve muscular endurance and running economy, even in highly trained runners (29, 69, 82, 89, 93, 102). Because plyometric training improves power (7, 19, 22) and running economy (12, 29, 69, 82, 89, 93, 102), performance of tactical activities would also be expected to improve. In 2001, Kraemer et al. (47) demonstrated that six months of **ballistic** plyometric exercises (bounding and jumping) combined with partner-resisted exercises (field exercises) improved squat jump power, bench throw power, squat endurance, 1RM box lifting, and 2-mile (3 km) loaded run time. Conversely, these indices were unchanged in the aerobic training–only group. Supplementary plyometric exercise is thus considered to be a potentially effective method for improving tactical performance.

Key Point

Reviewing the needs analysis will aid in determining the plyometric exercise prescription. As with resistance training, applying the principle of specificity ensures that exercise reflects training status and occupational physical requirements. Supervision to ensure plyometric exercises are executed with the correct technique is highly recommended.

Table 15.2 Peer-Reviewed Publications Comparing Various PT Interventions for Improving Military Occupational Task Performance

Authors	Subjects	Duration	Intervention	Change in 2-mile (3 km) LC time	Change in 5 min RBL performance
Harman et al. (33)	CIV men	8 weeks	CT + ET	−3.5 min[a]	N/A
			RT + ET	−3.8 min[a]	N/A
Hendrickson et al. (35)	CIV women	8 weeks	CON	−2.6 min[a]	+6 boxes[a]
			ET	−4.6 min[a]	+8 boxes[a]
			RT	−4.5 min[a]	+11 boxes[a]
			RT + ET	−4.7 min[a]	+10 boxes[a,b]
Kraemer et al. (47)[e]	CIV women	26 weeks	ET	+0.6 min	+7 boxes
			CT + ET	−2.6 min[a]	+10 boxes[a]
			RT (TBP) + ET	−3.2 min[a,c,d]	+15 boxes[a,c,d]
			RT (TBH) + ET	−2.1 min[a,c]	+15 boxes[a,c,d]
			RT (UBP) + ET	−3.6 min[a,c,d]	+15 boxes[a,c,d]
			RT (UBH) + ET	−3.3 min[a,c,d]	+16 boxes[a,c,d]
Kraemer et al. (50)	AD men	12 weeks	ET	−0.1 min	N/A
			RT (TB)	−1.3 min	N/A
			RT (TB) + ET	−3.6 min[a]	N/A
			RT (UB) + ET	−3.1 min[a]	N/A
Sharp et al. (90)	AD men	12 weeks	CON	N/A	−3 boxes
			RT	N/A	+13 boxes[a,b]

Values represent absolute change in performance from pre- to posttraining.

AD = active duty; CIV = civilian; CON = control group (no intervention); CT = calisthenics training; ET = endurance training; LC = load carriage (change in the time required to travel 2 miles [3 km] with a loaded rucksack); RBL = repetitive box lifting (change in the number of weighted boxes lifted onto a platform in 5 minutes); RT = resistance training; TB = resistance training focusing on the total body; TBH = resistance training focusing on total body strength/hypertrophy; TBP = resistance training focusing on total body strength/power; UB = resistance training focusing on the upper body; UBH = resistance training focusing on upper body strength/hypertrophy; UBP = resistance training focusing on upper body strength/power.

[a]Significant ($p < 0.05$) improvement compared with corresponding pretraining value.

[b]Significantly ($p < 0.05$) greater improvement compared with the CON group.

[c]Significantly ($p < 0.05$) greater improvement compared with the ET group.

[d]Significantly ($p < 0.05$) greater improvement compared with the CT group.

[e]Study used a 10-minute RBL task; results were divided by 2 to estimate 5-minute RBL performance.

Table 15.3 Physical Performance Parameters Improved by Plyometric Training

Performance parameter	References
Maximal power capabilities	7, 9, 12, 19, 22, 23, 101
CMJ height Power output Max RFD	19
Running economy	29, 69, 82, 89, 93, 102
Squat jump power Bench throw power Squat endurance 1RM box lift 2 mi (3 km) loaded run	47

To date, there is sparse research on the most effective prescription of **intensity**, **volume**, and **frequency** of plyometric exercise. Further research validating the effectiveness of this training modality in tactical populations is needed. See chapter 18 in the NSCA's general guidelines for plyometric exercise prescription and associated safety considerations (77).

PT sessions can combine strength and aerobic exercise in a single session; this is known as concurrent exercise training. Although limited research suggests that concurrent training may cause an interference effect (i.e., aerobic exercise following resistance exercise will negate strength improvements) (10), emerging studies suggest that much depends on nutrition (74, 80). Regardless, concurrent training has been shown to elicit greater improvements in load carriage (50) and RBL (35) performance compared with either training mode performed in isolation. However, factors such as the specific tasks, task duration, order of training modes, and length of the intervention will also influence physiological outcomes (40). A benefit of concurrent training is the ability to target multiple fitness components (i.e., strength, power, aerobic and muscular endurance, **mobility**, **speed**) during a single training session while also minimizing the time to complete the session.

Firefighting

Firefighting is a physically demanding occupation that includes a myriad of emergency and rescue tasks (e.g., climbing ladders, lifting and carrying equipment, rescuing casualties, moving over slippery and uneven terrain) (83). The effectiveness of a fire company relies upon the fitness of the firefighters, who must be physically prepared to conduct moderate- to high-intensity tasks (often repetitively) while wearing heat-retaining, heavy turnout gear and carrying heavy equipment (SCBA, charged hose lines) (5). High aerobic and anaerobic work capacities combined with strength and power training in a suitably designed PT program form the foundation of physical preparedness for firefighters (62).

Law Enforcement

Law enforcement personnel are challenged by unpredictable physically demanding events that can escalate to the point where specific physical capabilities are required to effectively react and respond; physical fitness is therefore an important component of job safety and performance (13). As first responders, law enforcement personnel typically are the first to arrive at emergencies. They protect the public and apprehend criminals, all of which can entail unpredictable, life-endangering situations (e.g., domestic incidents, traffic stops, arrests, foot pursuits) (13). These activities can stress physiological capacity and require varying degrees of muscular strength and power (14, 79).

Previous analyses of police tasks observed that the majority of physical activities were critical and often required brief periods of near-maximal effort (13). Anderson et al. (8) reported that police officers in British Columbia were either constantly or frequently performing the following during work shifts: stair-climbing, pulling and pushing, bending and squatting, and lifting and carrying. The officers also performed occasional running, climbing up and down objects, dragging, and leaping and jumping at medium to maximum effort. Additionally, Pryor et al. (79) followed a SWAT team in order to develop an occupational physical task list as part of a physical demands analysis. They found four main physical tasks helped establish physical fitness requirements for SWAT operators:

1. Operations in SWAT gear
2. Operations within the perimeter of approach
3. Tactical entry and maneuvers
4. Man-down drills

Individual physical fitness tests found deficiencies in core body strength, flexibility, aerobic capacity, and muscular power (compared with age- and gender-normative data) among this group of SWAT operators. To remediate these deficiencies, PT prescription included exercises for improving core strength, power, and flexibility plus selective aerobic exercise so that muscular strength could be maintained. These studies provide evidence for the integration of strength and power exercise into law enforcement PT.

Military

The modern battlefield is a hostile, volatile environment that presents many physiological challenges (67). Warfighters must be physically prepared to conduct military tasks and battle drills (e.g., dismounted operations involving carrying heavy loads, negotiating obstacles, reacting to direct or indirect fire, hand-to-hand combat, and so on) in hostile and austere environments (3). Physical preparedness for warfighting tasks thus requires a high level of physical fitness (2). Military tactical performance can be operationally defined in numerous ways. Previous studies have assessed occupational abilities using tests involving load carriage, obstacle courses, repetitive or maximal box lifting, rushes under fire, and simulated casualty recovery (33, 35, 47). The isometric handgrip test is also often used as a simple, expedient surrogate test for upper limb muscular strength (86, 103). A 5 m (5.5 yd) rope climb has also been evaluated as an upper body power assessment for Tunisian commandos (21). For the purposes of this chapter, military tactical performance is operationally defined as load carriage and RBL performance because these are representative occupational tasks common to many of the studies cited herein.

OPTIMIZING OCCUPATIONAL PERFORMANCE

An examination of tactical occupations, specific duty requirements, and diverse individual physical abilities illustrates the uniqueness of tactical performance optimization. It is difficult to address variables such as occupational fitness requirements, job tasks, and individual fitness status using a one-size-fits-all PT program (49). Therefore, specific occupational demands must be analyzed so that the strength and power exercise prescription translates into improved job

performance. The TSAC Facilitator can accomplish this analysis by evaluating the physical demands of the occupation. This assessment, which is part of the needs analysis, generally includes a movement analysis (body movement patterns and muscle involvement), physiological analysis (muscular strength, muscular and aerobic endurance, power, and hypertrophy), and injury analysis (common sites for musculoskeletal injury) (91).

Needs Analysis

A needs analysis is a multistep process that includes an evaluation of the job tasks and physical requirements of the occupation plus the individual's fitness status (91). For example, establishing evidence for occupationally relevant performance goals and outcomes can be done with a task and movement analysis of activities such as load carriage, ladder climbing, forced entry, victim rescue, and reaction to enemy contact. The analysis will also include the frequency and intensity of the actions, environmental conditions, clothing, and equipment load (24). Figure 15.3 provides an example of a movement analysis that uses a box lift. The box lift is performed in two phases. During the first phase (figure 15.3a), the tactical athlete lifts the box from the ground to approximately waist height. The primary movements are **concentric** hip extension, concentric knee extension, and **isometric** handgrip exercise. An appropriate exercise to train phase 1 of the box lift is a deadlift (figure 15.3b), which uses similar movements and muscle actions. During the second phase of the box lift (figure 15.3c), the tactical athlete presses the box onto a platform. The primary movements are concentric shoulder **flexion** and concentric elbow **extension**. An appropriate exercise to train phase 2 of the box lift is an incline chest press (either standing or using an inclined bench) (figure 15.3d). Job-specific physical criterion can be identified once this process is complete. Chapter 8 further discusses testing, and chapter 9 covers the needs analysis in greater detail.

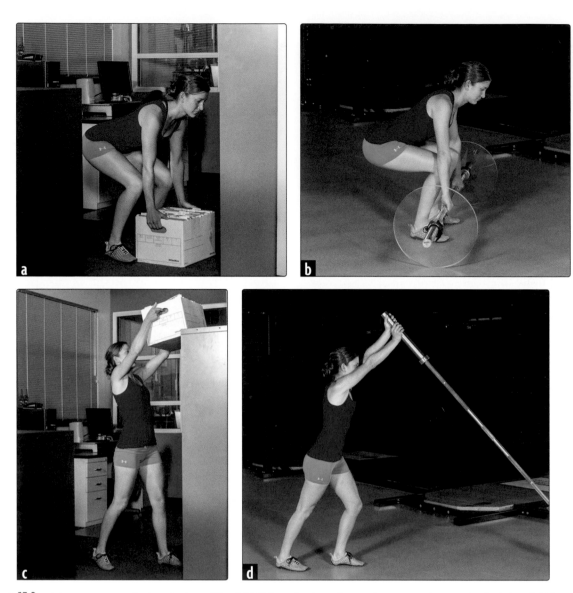

Figure 15.3 Movement analysis of a box lift. *(a)* Lifting the box from the ground to waist height. *(b)* The deadlift trains the muscles used in the first phase of the lift. *(c)* Pressing the box onto a platform. *(d)* The landmine shoulder press trains the muscles used in the second phase of the lift.

Physical Fitness Requirements

Research on task analysis has reported that muscular strength and power are predominant fitness components used during tactical and emergency operations (e.g., evacuating casualties, negotiating obstacles, subduing hostile combatants, forcibly entering buildings) (63, 83, 98). The job-specific physical criteria established by the needs analysis will determine the extent and degree to which attributes of muscular strength and power are required (31, 38). However, strength, power, and **general physical preparedness (GPP)** (i.e., overall fitness) are undoubtedly requisites for all tactical occupations (41, 83, 97). Therefore, fitness testing that assesses overall health status (e.g., body composition, $\dot{V}O_2$max, flexibility) as well as job-specific physical criteria may provide a more accurate interpretation of an individual's job suitability (98).

Fitness Assessment

Please refer to chapter 8, which covers testing and evaluation in greater detail. Selection of occupationally relevant fitness tests should reflect the physical criteria necessary for safe and effective job performance (31). For example, if job requirements include tasks such as advancing a charged hose line or physically subduing and containing combative suspects, then the testing protocol should include task simulations that measure muscular strength and power related to those tasks (15). Job-simulation tasks must

- incorporate the physically demanding critical aspects of the occupational task,
- be individual rather than team tasks, and
- be scored with a continuous grading scale (i.e., not pass–fail) (72).

Examples include timed load carriage tests (35, 43) and RBL tests that consist of repetitively lifting loaded boxes onto a platform within a specified period of time (35).

Relevance and Necessity

Information gleaned from the fitness assessment will indicate the tactical athlete's general physical preparedness and ability to perform job-specific tasks. Appropriately administered JSTs (job-specific tests) provide greater face validity than general fitness tests (used for predictive value) and are likely to be better accepted by the workforce (30). However, general health screening is important for identifying the health status and risk factors of personnel (13, 96).

Gaps Identified From the Assessment

Identifying physical performance deficiencies upon review of the fitness assessment will provide rationale for PT goals and outcomes (31). As a result, individualized PT programs can be designed to improve specific fitness components, such as muscular strength and power, and prepare tactical athletes for successful completion of testing protocols and the physical rigors of the occupation (47, 87).

Training Goals

The goal-setting process provides an opportunity to set physical conditioning benchmarks, as well as identify stressors that can negatively affect recovery and general physical preparedness (16, 28, 92). By nature, tactical occupations present unique challenges (e.g., extended work hours, inadequate nutrition, sleep deprivation) that may require periodic modifications to the PT program in order to mitigate overtraining (49, 92). For these reasons, goals can be a motivational tool for charting progress toward established benchmarks, mitigate injury by establishing predetermined milestones, and encourage adherence to the PT program (81).

PT goals should focus on maximizing physical capacity to safely and effectively execute job-specific physical tasks and maintain health (28, 81). Without goal-oriented direction and supervision, there remains the possibility that PT will diverge from an optimal to a suboptimal training strategy and increase the risk of injury (17, 52, 59, 87). Goal setting for physical performance is especially important for military accession and attendance at advanced training courses, which often have stringent criteria for physical fitness (e.g., SWAT, tactical paramedic) (15, 66). Information regarding physical standards and normative data of both candidates and incumbent personnel can be valuable for determining a relevant exercise prescription (15). By helping to establish occupationally relevant PT goals, the TSAC Facilitator can improve health, mitigate injury, maintain occupational relevancy, and prepare individuals for selection and accession.

APPLYING PRINCIPLES OF STRENGTH AND POWER TRAINING

Resistance exercise improves strength, power, and tactical performance (35, 47, 50, 59, 87, 90). This has been demonstrated in exercise programs utilizing multiset exercise constructs (47, 50, 90, 107). However, the optimal number of sets per exercise for strength and power development is a point of contention among scientists (51, 68). The NSCA guidelines recommend the following multiset principles (table 15.4):

Table 15.4 Volume Assignments Based on Training Goal

Training goal	Goal repetitions	Sets[a]
Strength	≤6	2-6
Power[b]	1-5	3-5
Hypertrophy	6-12	3-6
Muscular endurance	≥12	2-3

[a]These assignments do not include warm-up sets and typically apply to core exercises only (11, 46).

[b]Based on weightlifting-derived movements (clean, snatch, and so on). The load and repetition assignments shown for power in this table are *not consistent* with the %1RM–repetition relationship. In nonexplosive movements, loads equaling about 80% of 1RM apply to the two- to five-repetition range. Refer to the discussion of assigning percentages of 1RM for power training for further explanation.

Adapted, by permission, from NSCA, 2016, Program design for resistance training, J.M. Sheppard and N.T. Triplett. In *Essentials of strength training and conditioning*, 4th ed., edited by G Haff and NT Triplett (Champaign, IL: Human Kinetics), 463.

- 2-6 sets for strength
- 3-5 sets for power
- 3-6 sets for hypertrophy
- 2-3 sets for muscular endurance

Ongoing research is aimed at identifying a dose–response relationship between resistance exercise intensity, volume, and frequency and improvements in tactical performance (15).

Moderate to heavy training loads (i.e., loads that induce momentary muscle failure within 3-12 repetitions) have been shown to improve tactical performance (47, 50, 107). Previously published movement analysis research (47, 50, 60, 90) suggests that a program with multijoint lower body (e.g., deadlift, squat) and upper body (e.g., bench press, pull-up) resistance exercises (performed before single-joint and small muscle group exercises) is ideal for this population. For females, research (47) indicates that upper body–only resistance training induces improvements similar to total body resistance training in RBL performance. This implies that upper body resistance exercises are particularly important for improving tactical performance in women.

The amount of rest between sets can affect acute exercise performance (84, 105) and, ultimately, strength gains following long-term training (76, 85). In general, research indicates that inter-set rest intervals should be between 2 and 5 minutes for strength and power training (76, 85, 91, 106). Ultimately, to determine rest intervals the TSAC Facilitator should consider the load for each set of an exercise rather than applying general guidelines.

Key Point

Prescribing inter-set rest periods will depend on the percentage of 1RM being lifted, size of the muscle group (e.g., leg versus shoulder muscles), number of repetitions, training status of the tactical athlete, and goal of the exercise (i.e., strength, power, hypertrophy, or muscular endurance). For example, 12 repetitions of biceps curls (i.e., 67% of 1RM) may only need a 1-minute inter-set rest period, whereas 4 repetitions of squats (90% of 1RM) may need 4 to 5 minutes of rest (24, 91, 95). In this example, the volume (12 repetitions) of biceps curls is assigned for hypertrophy. Thus, the rest intervals are less than that prescribed for the squat exercise, which is directed at strength development and uses heavier weight and fewer repetitions. Moreover, the squat is a multijoint exercise that uses large muscles and requires longer rest intervals at a given volume in comparison to the single-joint bicep exercise.

For additional information, see previously published studies on resistance exercise intervention and tactical performance (4, 35, 47, 50, 71, 90, 107) and the current NSCA guidelines on resistance exercise training.

Rationale for Program Design

Tactical athletes require job-specific physical abilities for safe and effective occupational performance. The PT program should be designed to improve health and general physical preparedness, reduce the risk of injury, and, most importantly, strengthen the physical capacity to perform occupational duties. These considerations will provide the rationale for program design.

Firefighters

Firefighters operate in conditions that can significantly burden physiological capacity. Being prepared to perform physically demanding tasks (e.g., climbing, crawling, carrying heavy loads) in austere conditions (e.g., extreme heat, wildland firefighting, frigid water extraction) wearing protective firefighting equipment requires a well-designed PT program (59). Numerous firefighting occupational tasks physiologically stress the anaerobic energy system, which reinforces the PT objective to improve anaerobic work capacity (5). As an example, tasks of moderate to high intensity such as hoisting and pulling a hose, raising a ladder, forcibly entering structures, and dragging or carrying victims all require muscular strength and power (5). Interestingly, absolute maximal strength has been positively correlated with upper body muscular endurance, a fitness component required for many firefighting tasks. Naclerio et al. (65) conducted a study using 14 firefighter recruits to investigate the influence of muscular strength and power on muscular endurance. Using the bench press exercise, the recruits performed a progressive strength exercise test followed by a maximum-repetition endurance test. The study found that maximum strength and absolute power were significantly related to upper body muscle endurance. This suggests that improving absolute maximal strength can have a positive impact on muscular endurance. PT programs that integrate strength and power exercise should expect coinciding improvements in muscular endurance.

Firefighters must sustain a high level of general physical preparedness to meet the physical and environmental challenges that they confront. Exercise tests need to be valid representations of the physiological stress incurred during firefighting tasks and must be reliable in their metrics. Rhea et al. (83) studied 20 firefighters to determine the correlation of various exercise tests that measured muscular strength and endurance, anaerobic endurance, and aerobic capacity with firefighting occupational tests (hose pull, stair climb, simulated victim drag, and equipment hoist) (83). Firefighting task performance was highly correlated with muscular strength and endurance and with anaerobic endurance.

Two periodization training models are applied to program design: undulating and traditional. In 2008, a study compared the physical performance outcomes of firefighters who performed nine weeks of either an undulating or a traditional periodized program (75). The standard periodization model consisted of three-week mesocycles, each dedicated to a fitness component (e.g. strength, hypertrophy). The undulating program alternated training variables each session. At the end of the study, both groups responded well to the training programs. However, greater improvements in upper and lower body muscular strength, power, vertical jump, and JSTs occurred in the undulation training group. Undulating load and volume, if appropriately periodized, may have fewer limitations compared with traditional periodization for firefighters with variable work schedules.

Law Enforcement

Law enforcement personnel engage in a broad range of critical activities (e.g., making arrests, pursuing suspects on foot, physically subduing suspects) that necessitate a high level of physical fitness. Law enforcement agencies use physical assessments, usually during recruitment and initial training, to measure physical competencies predictive of job-related task performance. These tests typically consist of running, jumping and climbing over obstacles, pushing and pulling implements, and lifting or dragging a dummy casualty (8). In 2001, Anderson et al. (8) evaluated the occupational requirements of police work in the interest of validating a recruit physical ability test used in British Columbia. The tactics that the majority of officers routinely used during critical incidents involved pushing, pulling, controlling or wrestling and dragging, and lifting below shoulder level. Indubitably, critical incidents that involve the physical control of a target require strength and power. Field tasks are important considerations in program design and need to be included in police physical ability testing (6, 79).

Military

Improvements in coordination mediated by neural factors are responsible for the improvements in muscular strength during the first one to three months of exercise training (25, 26, 55, 64) (figure 15.4). Resistance exercise considerations and recommendations differ for tactical personnel who do or do not have previous experience with resistance exercise (i.e., trained versus untrained tactical athletes) (tables 15.5 and 15.6). Figure 15.4 represents concepts originally established by Sale (88) and shows that the rapid improvement in strength at the onset of training is primarily due to neural factors (e.g., increased agonist activation, improved motor unit coordination and synchronization). Because of this, relatively low-load, low-volume resistance exercise protocols can induce substantial improvements in strength among untrained tactical athletes (1). The relatively modest loads and volume would theoretically reduce the likelihood of injury as well.

To illustrate this, Harman et al. (33) used previously untrained men to compare the effectiveness of a calisthenics training regimen (i.e., the U.S. Army's Physical Readiness Training [PRT] regimen, which the Army implemented in 2010) (44) against a traditional resistance exercise regimen for eight weeks. At the end of the study, both groups had comparable improvements in 1RM strength, vertical jump, and load

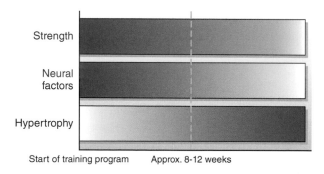

Start of training program   Approx. 8-12 weeks

Figure 15.4 The rapid improvement in strength at the onset of training is primarily due to neural factors. Following two to three months of training, most of the further strength gains are due to muscular factors (i.e., hypertrophy). At this point, heavier loads and greater volumes appear to be required for further performance improvements (47, 88).

carriage performance (33). This supports the use of calisthenics during the initial weeks of a PT program to improve strength, power, and physical performance.

After this initial period, traditional resistance training with heavier loads is needed for further improvements in strength, power, and occupational task performance. This was demonstrated in a study by Kraemer et al. (47) in which female volunteers were randomly assigned to one of six training groups (four resistance exercise groups, one calisthenics-based exercise group, and one aerobic endurance–only exercise group) for six months. At the conclusion, the resistance exercise interventions resulted in greater improvements in strength, load carriage, and RBL than the calisthenics or aerobic endurance groups.

Collectively, these data imply the following (33, 47):

1. Calisthenics improve strength, power, and physical performance during the initial stage of training (i.e., initial two to three months).

2. Long-term (i.e., greater than two or three months) improvements in strength, power, and tactical performance are best achieved using a traditional resistance exercise program.

Key Point

In untrained tactical athletes or people returning from an injury, substantial improvements in physical performance can be achieved through bodyweight resistance and calisthenics during the initial two to three months of training. Progression to machine and free weight resistance and power exercise will be necessary for further improvements.

Program Considerations

PT program design should consider variables such as the size of the training group, ability level, environment and terrain, and equipment (60, 73). Teaching complex strength and power movements is best conducted in small groups for greater supervision. This will improve the ability to analyze, reinforce, and modify lifting technique and ensure a greater level of safety. Space and location (indoor or outdoor) will further dictate the PT format.

Equipment

Access to traditional fitness equipment is often limited or nonexistent, especially when conducting PT with large groups (2). To overcome equipment limitations, task-specific exercises using occupational equipment (e.g., hoses, sandbags, flak vests) can be included. For example, a 12-week functional exercise program performed by firefighters who used available firehouse equipment improved completion rates of a simulated fireground test and anthropometric measures (70). Harman et al. (33) used combat-relevant tests to compare two 8-week exercise training protocols. One group performed total body weight-based workouts, running, interval training, agility training, and progressively loaded 8 km (5 mi) rucksack marches. The other group followed the U.S. Army's standardized PT program (stretching, calisthenics, movement drills, sprint intervals, shuttle running, and distance runs). Both groups significantly improved 3.2 km (2.0 mi) loaded (32 kg [71 lb]) run or walk time, 400 m (437 yd) loaded (18 kg [40 lb]) run time, obstacle course with load (18 kg [40 lb]) time, and casualty (80 kg [176 lb]) rescue time.

Elastic bands have become a popular alternative to free weights and machines for strength training. Several studies have evaluated characteristics such as RFD, peak power, force, and kinematics using elastic bands versus free weights (39, 61, 94) and have reported increased muscle activity, including power, force, and peak velocities,

Table 15.5 Considerations for Training Physically Unconditioned Tactical Athletes

Considerations	Optimum resistance exercise training	
Be aware of susceptibility to injury and delayed-onset muscle soreness.	Choice of exercises	Primarily multijoint
Focus on technique.	Order of exercises	Most important exercises first
Use low to moderate intensity and volume.	Intensity	Load that allows 8-12 repetitions per set with moderate effort
Caution and supervision should be used when participating in commercialized exercise programs and when the number of sets or the duration of rest intervals exceed functional capacity.	Volume	1-3 sets per exercise
	Rest intervals	2 min between sets*
	Frequency	2-3 days per week

*Rest interval reflects hypertrophy volume assignment (8-12 repetitions).

Table 15.6 Considerations for Training Physically Conditioned Tactical Athletes

Considerations	Optimum resistance exercise training	
Gradually increase intensity and volume.	Choice of exercise	Primarily multijoint
Generally, heavier loading can be prescribed.*	Order of exercises	Most important exercises first
Utilize program variation or periodization.	Intensity	Load that allows 3-12 repetitions per set with maximal effort
Reduce training when physical demands are high (e.g., field training, combatives, load carriage).	Volume	2-4 sets per exercise
	Rest intervals	2-5 min between sets
	Frequency	2-3 days per week

*Use the two-for-two method to determine when to increase an exercise load: If the tactical athlete can complete two repetitions over the repetition goal for an exercise for two consecutive workouts, the load can be increased (5%-10%) for the following workout session (11, 91).

particularly during **eccentric** contraction with band use. Elastic bands are light, portable, and easily modifiable for a variety of physical abilities and exercises, making them an effective alternative to free weights.

Safety

Strength and power training is relatively safe to perform (32). However, untrained or deconditioned people, including those returning from an injury, are at increased risk for musculoskeletal injury or reinjury if exercise progression occurs too rapidly (45, 78). Therefore, measures to mitigate musculoskeletal injury should be enacted. This can be accomplished by prescribing two to three months of calisthenics training (e.g., the U.S. Army PRT regimen, described in detail at www.armyprt.com) and introducing relatively light-load, low-volume resistance training before progressing slowly to heavier loads or higher volume.

Tactical occupations include activities (e.g., field training exercises, advanced training schools, extended missions) that can collectively overburden the capacity for recovery and result in an increased risk of overuse injury and burnout (16, 27, 53, 73). Frequently reviewing mission requirements will help attenuate any deleterious outcomes from excessive stress (53). Erring on the side of caution and reducing exercise intensity or frequency during periods of strenuous tactical-related responsibilities may be required (49).

Commercialized training programs have grown in popularity among tactical personnel. These programs are generally characterized by physically and metabolically demanding circuit workouts consisting of resistance, plyometric, and interval running exercise (42). These programs appear to address real-world demands due to their functional design. However, when participating in commercialized training programs, beginners and deconditioned tactical athletes should use caution and follow the guidelines presented herein and summarized in tables 15.4 and 15.5. If highly conditioned individuals choose to participate, they should do so under the guidance of a TSAC Facilitator or certified fitness professional.

Oversight

A certified fitness professional or TSAC Facilitator should ensure safe and appropriate PT that incorporates strength and power training. This includes teaching and evaluating exercise technique, intensity, volume, frequency, and exercise progression (60). Supervised exercise programs have been shown to enhance long-term improvements in strength and power compared with unsupervised programs (58). Goal setting, motivation, and psychological reinforcement are additional benefits to participation in a supervised exercise program. Coutts et al. (17) examined the benefits of supervised resistance training versus unsupervised and observed that after 12 weeks of resistance training, the supervised group had improved strength and power and had completed significantly more training sessions than the unsupervised group. It was suggested that the higher motivation and competitiveness facilitated by the trainer helped to shape the observed improvements.

Supervision also improves accountability. This was demonstrated by improved performance among firefighters voluntarily participating in a 12-week exercise program in either a supervised or control group (70). Prior to the program, the firefighters completed a simulated fireground test, and no differences in completion rate were observed between the two groups (supervised: 82%; control group: 78%). After the 12-week exercise program, the supervised group performed significantly better on the simulated fireground test than the control group (100% vs. 56%). This study and others demonstrate the utility of a supervised PT program for improved fitness and tactical performance.

CONCLUSION

Strength and power training improve tactical performance and may mitigate injuries. The design of the strength and power training program will depend on factors such as fitness status, occupational requirements, equipment, and supervision. Calisthenics-based exercise training (e.g., U.S. Army PRT) or relatively moderate-load resistance exercise training (i.e., loads that allow 8-12 repetitions per set with moderate effort, one to three sets per exercise, and 2 minutes of rest between sets) should be conducted for the first two to three months of training. Progressing to multijoint lower body (e.g., deadlift, squat) and upper body (e.g., bench press, pull-up) resistance exercises is recommended for further gains in muscular strength, power, and endurance (upper body training is especially important for women). This phase of training is prescribed as two to three nonconsecutive days a week using moderate to heavy training loads (i.e., loads that allow 3-12 repetitions per set with maximal effort), two to four sets per exercise, and 2 minutes of rest between sets for optimal improvements in tactical performance.

Key Terms

agonist
ballistic exercise
concentric
eccentric
extension
flexion
frequency
general physical preparedness (GPP)
hypertrophy
intensity
isometric
load carriage

mobility
motor unit
one-repetition maximum (1RM)
plyometric exercise
power
power output
rate of force development (RFD)
repetitive box lifting (RBL)
speed
strength
volume

Study Questions

1. Augmenting resistance training with which of the following types of training will have the greatest positive impact on countermovement jump height?

   a. plyometric

   b. aerobic

   c. flexibility

   d. mobility

2. Concurrent training could be beneficial for tactical athletes for what primary reason?

   a. targets multiple fitness components

   b. maximizes time to complete session

   c. separates resistance and aerobic endurance training

   d. focuses on a specific fitness component

3. A tactical athlete performs 10 repetitions of an exercise for 5 sets. What is the training outcome with this rep and set combination?

   a. strength

   b. power

   c. hypertrophy

   d. muscular endurance

4. What type of periodization program might be the most beneficial for a firefighter with a variable work schedule?

   a. traditional

   b. undulating

   c. triphasic

   d. linear

Chapter 16

Care and Rehabilitation of Injured Tactical Populations

Danny McMillian, PT, DSc, OCS, CSCS, TSAC-F

After completing this chapter, you will be able to

- discuss how the phases of rehabilitation from an injury are related to the tissue healing process;

- describe a typical return-to-function time frame;

- develop a training program for a currently or previously injured tactical athlete through collaborative discussion with other allied health professionals;

- identify common acute and chronic injuries and risk factors for injury in fire and rescue, law enforcement, and military populations;

- recognize the signs and symptoms of overtraining and overtraining-related injury; and

- define the scope of practice of the TSAC Facilitator regarding injury care and rehabilitation.

Timely and effective injury care has long been appreciated in traditional sport, and such care is no less important in tactical populations. In fact, the **sports medicine model** of injury care (athlete-centered care by a multidisciplinary team) (4) has been proposed as a means for improving management of the similar needs of tactical athletes (8, 45). This chapter reviews what is known about traditional injury care and highlights factors that are unique to tactical populations.

COMMON INJURY PREVALENCE AND RISK FACTORS

Injuries and physical impairments are a fact of life for most tactical athletes. The varied and rigorous physical nature of tactical duties, combined with operations that are often conducted in harsh environments, predisposes the tactical athlete to injury risk. Once injured, the tactical athlete is predisposed to subsequent injury unless **rehabilitation** restores full functionality. This chapter focuses on musculoskeletal injuries because they are amenable to the interventions of the tactical strength and conditioning team.

Injuries have been cited as the biggest health problem of the military services (31). In 2006, there were 743,547 injuries among nondeployed military service members in the United States. To provide some context, for every 1,000 service members tracked for one year, 628 sustained a musculoskeletal injury (24). Over 80% of the injuries were considered overuse. The knee and lower leg (22%), lumbar spine (20%), and ankle and foot (13%) were leading body regions. TSAC Facilitators should target the prevention of such injuries, with the expectation that many can be eliminated, as has been observed with strategies including slower progression of running distance, reduced total running volume, running groups based on ability, and greater variety of training exercises (e.g., multiaxial, neuromuscular, proprioceptive, and agility exercises). Those interventions have reduced the incidence of injuries by 52% in men and 46% in women (35).

More detail on discipline-specific injury prevalence and risk is provided in other chapters, but it is notable that firefighters are 3.8 times more likely to suffer a musculoskeletal injury than private-sector workers (62). Just over 50% of fireground injuries are musculoskeletal and include sprains, strains, dislocations, and fractures (50, 67). Although many of these injuries are likely the inevitable consequence of harsh conditions and extreme movement requirements, optimizing the tactical athlete's movement skills and work capacity will reduce the risk.

Lack of general fitness is also a significant component of injury risk. In a study of Minnesota police officers, those with the highest self-reported fitness levels were less likely to experience sprains, back pain, and chronic pain than those who considered themselves less fit. Officers who were the most physically active were about a third as likely to report back pain and less than half as likely to report chronic pain as those who engaged in less activity. Officers with a body mass index (BMI) greater than 35 were three times more likely to report back pain than those whose BMI fell in the normal range, defined as 18 to 25 (46).

Studies of military populations have also shown that lower rates of exercise participation before military service and decreased performance on fitness assessments are predictive of injury (31, 34, 35, 36). Fortunately, strength and conditioning professionals are effective at improving general fitness. Greater utilization of such professionals by the tactical professions should reverse the injury trends noted previously.

Finally, previous injury is consistently cited as a risk factor for future injury (21, 36, 59, 68, 74). Leaders of tactical units should ensure that individuals are screened for injury risk factors that are specific to their duties as well as for any past injuries that might compromise physical performance. Individuals deemed at risk of injury should be evaluated by the appropriate medical or rehabilitation experts.

Key Point

Injuries are common in the tactical population and predispose individuals to subsequent injuries. Members of the tactical sports medicine team must be aware of past injuries and provide comprehensive rehabilitation and performance training to mitigate the risk of future injury.

PHASES OF TISSUE HEALING

Injuries may be classified as traumatic or overuse. Both types have unique tissue characteristics that influence their management.

Traumatic Injuries

The body's initial response to physical injury, or trauma, and the associated tissue damage is to create an **inflammatory response** that limits further tissue damage and sets the stage for healing. Classic signs of inflammation are redness, swelling, pain, heat, and loss of function. The inflammatory response, also known as the acute phase or the inflammatory phase, generally lasts a few days, but signs of inflammation may persist for weeks depending on numerous factors, including the severity and location of the injury, effectiveness of the initial injury management, and individual response. The acute phase of an injury requires a protection phase of rehabilitation (33). Treatment objectives during this phase are to minimize pain and swelling, protect the injured site from further damage, maintain motion as long as it does not interfere with **tissue healing**, and maintain conditioning.

A useful acronym to guide treatment during the inflammatory phase is PRICEM (protection, rest, ice, compression, elevation, motion). This acronym is a variation on the traditional RICE (rest, ice, compression, elevation) method of treatment and indicates the need for protection and motion (as indicated) in addition to the other components of RICE. Although clinicians and researchers acknowledge the scarcity of quality evidence supporting the use of RICE, its use in sports medicine is widespread and generally accepted, with the caveat that clinicians must weigh the risks and benefits for each individual (4, 40, 70).

Recommendations for early motion after injury are increasingly supported by quality evidence (22, 29, 32). Such early motion, appropriately prescribed by medical or rehabilitation specialists, promotes optimal healing while preventing atrophy and loss of tissue extensibility. Leaders of tactical athletes should have systems in place for applying the PRICEM principles immediately after injury. TSAC Facilitators should recognize that protection of the injured tissue and motion of the affected region are potentially conflicting principles; thus the obligation to coordinate care with the medical or rehabilitation staff to best apply PRICEM.

TSAC Facilitators should also be aware of the pervasive use of nonsteroidal anti-inflammatory drugs (NSAIDs) in tactical populations and the need to communicate with the medical providers when such use might be contraindicated. Despite the lack of strong evidence to support their effectiveness, the short-term (<5 days) use of NSAIDs is widely accepted when excessive inflammation causes symptoms after injury (22, 60). However, the use of NSAIDs for chronic conditions and recent injuries without excessive inflammation likely carries more risk than benefit (6, 22). Adverse effects of NSAIDs are usually associated with their prolonged use and most commonly involve the gastrointestinal, cardiovascular, and renal systems (22).

Though short-term, low-dose use of NSAIDs does not appear to delay the healing of soft tissue, their use does inhibit bony healing (9). Their long-term use is associated with harmful effects to cell growth and metabolism (22). For tactical athletes concerned about negative effects of NSAIDs on performance, it is unlikely that the occasional use of NSAIDs will negatively affect muscle growth. However, long-term use might limit muscle growth due to negative effects on satellite cell activity (60).

Toward the end of the inflammatory response, new cells (such as fibroblasts, which ultimately produce collagen) move to the site of soft tissue injury and begin the repair phase. This phase of healing corresponds with the controlled motion phase of rehabilitation and generally lasts two to three weeks (32). As with the inflammatory phase, the length of the repair phase depends on the severity and location of the injury, effectiveness of prior rehabilitation, and individual factors (22, 33). During this phase, the objectives are to gradually restore full motion, begin progressive resistance training, initiate neuromuscular control exercises, and restore conditioning that might have been lost during the protection phase (33).

Although the repair phase of healing normally finishes within a few weeks, injured tissues will continue to remodel for months (63). The quality of the ultimate outcome depends in large part on the quality of training during the remodeling phase. This phase of healing corresponds to the **return-to-function phase** of rehabilitation. The primary objective is to progress all modes of training to a level that is commensurate with the tactical athlete's physical requirements. Appropriate rehabilitation for traumatic injuries based on the stage of healing is summarized in table 16.1.

During all phases of tissue healing, it is important for the TSAC Facilitator to closely collaborate with medical and rehabilitation personnel to ensure that physical training does not compromise recovery. As discussed later in this chapter, it is not within the TSAC Facilitator's scope of practice to evaluate and manage injuries.

Key Point

> Matching the phase of tissue healing to the appropriate phase of rehabilitation is necessary to avoid excessive stress to healing tissue and provide the optimal stimulus for repair.

Overuse Injuries

Overuse injuries occur when the cumulative stress applied to tissues of the body exceeds their ability to adapt to the stress. Common overuse conditions include tendinopathy, stress reaction or fracture, and patellofemoral pain syndrome (8).

Such conditions occur frequently among tactical athletes, especially in the military, where distance running for conditioning is associated with lower extremity overuse (6).

Two primary factors contribute to the excessive tissue stress associated with overuse injuries: **training errors** and **movement impairments** (6). Training errors occur when the volume or intensity of training is excessive for the individual. The most commonly documented training error has been excessive frequency and duration of distance running (69). For example, distance running more than three times a week or for longer than 30 minutes has been associated with an increase in overuse injuries (58). Limiting the frequency and duration of distance running is most likely to benefit novice runners (5).

Movement impairments contribute to overuse injuries when one or more links in the kinetic chain lack the mobility or stability required for a given task. The **kinetic chain** refers to the linked influence on movement performance that one area of the body has on another. For example, lack of mobility in the hips and thoracic spine might require movement of the lumbar spine beyond its safe zone to perform a lift or complete a tactically relevant task. Some trainers have used the terms *victim* and *culprit* to describe kinetic chain relationships associated with injury. In the current example, the lumbar spine is the victim of the

Table 16.1 Phases of Rehabilitation for Traumatic Injuries Based on Stage of Healing

Stage	Rehabilitation objectives and activities
Inflammatory (acute)	Protection phase • Protect the injured site from further damage. • Minimize pain and swelling. • Maintain motion as long as it does not interfere with tissue healing. • Maintain function of uninjured areas. • Maintain general fitness.

Repair (subacute)	Controlled motion phase
	• Apply controlled stress to align the healing tissue.
	  • Begin low-load ROM and stretching, progressing as tolerated.
	  • Begin low-load resistance training in a relatively shortened position; gradually progress loading and lengthening as tolerated.
	• Begin neuromuscular control activities.
	• Maintain general fitness.

Remodeling (chronic)	Return-to-function phase • Achieve an occupationally specific level of strength and endurance. • Ensure neuromuscular control of occupationally specific movements.

Based on Kisner (33).

limited mobility of the hips and thoracic spine (the culprits).

Overuse injuries might affect bones, joints, muscles, tendons, ligaments, and even skin (e.g., blisters) (4). This section focuses on tendon and bone overuse injuries because they are common in tactical populations and their management reflects the general care for overuse conditions.

Tendinopathy is the broad term to describe tendon problems. However, distinction should be made between pathology that is primarily inflammatory (tendinitis) and primarily a matter of degeneration (tendinosis). Tendinitis usually presents with the signs of inflammation; therefore, treatment with PRICEM is indicated. Tendinitis can usually be traced to a recent increase in training volume or intensity.

Tendinosis is a more difficult condition to treat. It occurs when degenerative changes are noted within the tendon, and it is normally associated with more than two months of symptoms. The rehabilitation professional must correct biomechanical and training errors that contributed to the tendinosis. Concurrently, the rehabilitation professional must also prescribe exercises that promote tendon resiliency (57, 64). Successful treatment often takes months to restore full function (63). Unsuccessful treatment leaves the tactical athlete with chronic pain and impaired performance or cessation of the provocative activities.

Bone stress injury (BSI) is the other major category of overuse injury. BSI represents the inability of bone to withstand repetitive mechanical loading, resulting in structural fatigue and localized bone pain and tenderness (73). It occurs when the cumulative effects of weight-bearing activity and physical training exceed the individual's capacity to manage the skeletal stress. BSI is a process that begins with stress reactions, which can progress to stress fractures and ultimately fractures. People with low levels of fitness are particularly vulnerable to BSI when beginning or progressing a fitness program (28, 36).

The primary symptom of BSI is activity-related pain with a gradual onset (28). Early in the process, the pain is often mild and diffuse. Unlike mild tendinopathy, the pain of BSI does not decrease with a warm-up or continuation of the weight-bearing activity (73). If such activity continues after the onset of symptoms, the BSI will progress and symptoms will become more severe and localized (73). Early in the process of BSI, symptoms abate when weight bearing ceases. However, in the later stages, symptoms are often experienced at rest.

Ideally, symptoms and signs of BSI are recognized early and activity is modified to decrease bone stress. If the weight-bearing stress is modified appropriately, individuals should be able to maintain fitness without impeding the healing process (31, 73). To assist tactical athletes toward this objective, TSAC Facilitators must plan an exercise prescription that is carefully coordinated with medical or rehabilitation professionals.

CAUSES, SIGNS, AND SYMPTOMS OF OVERTRAINING SYNDROME

In addition to traumatic and overuse injuries, tactical athletes are predisposed to overtraining syndrome due to the cumulative effects of a demanding work environment and the physical training required to prepare for work-related tasks. Those factors might induce positive or negative adaptations. The following terms and descriptions clarify the range of adaptations with which the TSAC Facilitator must be familiar:

- **Overreaching**, or functional overreaching, occurs when an athlete undertakes excessive training that leads to *short-term* decrements in performance. Recovery from this condition is normally achieved within a few days or weeks of rest. Overreaching is often a planned phase of training that, together with adequate rest, allows for supercompensation, or positive adaptations that elevate the athlete's performance capacity (17).

- **Nonfunctional overreaching (NFOR)** occurs when the intensification of a training stimulus continues without adequate recovery and regeneration. NFOR leads to stagnation and a decrease in performance that continues for several weeks or months.

- **Overtraining syndrome (OTS)** is a prolonged maladaptation of the body and several of its biological, neurochemical, and hormonal regulation mechanisms (17). Diagnosis requires the exclusion of other potential medical pathologies and is often made retrospectively, with full recovery usually requiring months (44).

The physiological markers of overtraining do not always parallel a decrease in performance (65). Such markers include increase in resting HR, decrease in maximal or submaximal exercise capacity, decreases in immunoglobulin A (IgA), changes in the Profile of Mood States (POMS) questionnaire responses, and decreases in the testosterone-to-cortisol ratio. Due to the complexity and diversity of hormonal mechanisms and complications with their analysis, at present no definitive physiological markers are capable of defining OTS (44).

The TSAC Facilitator must be prepared to adjust scheduled training to allow for greater recovery in tactical athletes exhibiting symptoms and signs of overtraining. The primary treatment is rest. Because other pathology might mimic overtraining, early referral for medical evaluation is recommended.

MAINTENANCE OF TRAINING STATUS DURING REHABILITATION AND RECONDITIONING

To meet individual needs in tactical organizations, physical readiness training (PRT) events and the level of participation in those events must be varied. For larger organizations, separating PRT into two categories allows leaders to provide the appropriate level of training for individuals at various levels of physical readiness, including tactical athletes who are recovering from injury.

As the name implies, the purpose of **foundational phase PRT** is to lay the foundation upon which functional (tactical) physical performance is built. People who are new to the organization, have physical or medical restrictions, are returning from physical restrictions, or are chronically unfit should be in this stage. Foundational PRT should not include activities with known injury risk, such as obstacle courses, tactical foot marches, or runs over 30 minutes (6, 31, 34, 35, 36, 56). Additionally, gut-check hybrid workouts that demand high degrees of power and endurance should be reserved for the functional phase.

In addition to improving general fitness, foundational PRT activities are designed to improve movement quality. A study with firefighters comparing a conventional fitness program with a movement-guided fitness program found that while both groups improved fitness, only the movement-guided group improved motor control of occupational tasks (18). These findings highlight the importance of optimizing movement quality along with fitness and the potential impact on the safety and effectiveness of tactical athletes.

Preventing Nonfunctional Overreaching and Overtraining Syndrome

Following are recommendations to prevent NFOR and OTS (3, 30, 44):

- Use an individualized, periodized program, with integration of recovery methods into the program.
- Monitor the tactical athlete with comprehensive testing integrated into the program.
- Look for early warning signs:
  - Unusual fatigue
  - Mood changes
  - Elevated HR and blood pressure
  - Diminished quality of sleep
  - Occurrence of illness or injury
  - Menstrual changes
- Educate the tactical athlete:
  - Best nutritional practices
  - Stress management
  - Best sleep practices
  - Early warning signs of overtraining
- Keep a training log that includes notes on the following:
  - Training volume and intensity
  - Duration of training
  - Weight fluctuation
  - Rating of well-being
  - Rating of sleep quality
  - Comments on training
  - Illness or injury

Trainers working with injured individuals in the foundational phase should be trained by and work closely with rehab professionals. They must be familiar with appropriate modifications to traditional exercises (see the later section Modification of Exercises to Allow Injured Individuals to Continue Training). Organizationally defined performance standards should be met before tactical athletes move from this phase to the functional phase.

Key Point

Restoring optimal movement quality, as well as fitness, is an important objective after injury.

Functional phase PRT gets the unit fully ready for its mission-based physical requirements. To ensure readiness for this phase, TSAC Facilitators should be familiar with the following return-to-sport guidelines that have been effectively used with sport athletes (4):

- Observation of time constraints for soft tissue healing
- Pain-free, full ROM
- No persistent swelling
- Adequate strength and endurance
- Good flexibility
- Good proprioception and balance
- Adequate cardiorespiratory fitness
- Skills regained
- No persistent biomechanical abnormality
- Psychological readiness
- Proper training form

Foundational PRT activities will remain a large part of the functional PRT program. The two groups can train together as long as there is a check in place to prevent people in the foundational phase from exposure to training events that exceed their current capabilities.

Training Objectives for Each Phase of Rehabilitation

After injury, both physical training and tactical performance training must be modified so as not to exceed the individual's decreased physical capacity (see table 16.1). Awareness of the stages of healing, as described previously, allows the TSAC Facilitator to select appropriate physical challenges.

In the initial period after injury, the primary objective is protecting the injured tissue from further damage. Because the injured tissue might not tolerate stress, training activities primarily target adjacent areas with the intent of maintaining their functionality. For example, a tactical athlete with an acute ankle sprain will normally tolerate single-leg activities on the uninjured leg, as well as most trunk and upper extremity exercises. Cardiorespiratory conditioning is maintained with activities that reduce or eliminate stress through the injured ankle (e.g., bicycling, swimming or deep-water running, using an upper body ergometer). Even in the acute phase of healing, some motion and loading at the injured site might be indicated (33). However, during this period of tissue vulnerability, the decision to move or immobilize is made by medical or rehabilitation personnel.

After the inflammatory stage of healing, the injured tissues begin to repair. To optimize function of the repairing tissues, rehabilitation applies controlled motion stresses. The objective is to provide a stimulus that aligns new fibers in a manner that is similar to the tissue in its uninjured state (33). Training activities should be pain free and the motion well controlled, either through passive restraint of unwanted motion or the individual's ability to stabilize moving segments. Though the tactical athlete might report stiffness, it should reduce gradually within the session if the tissue is ready for the load applied (33).

When novel activities or new levels of ongoing activities are initiated, both the TSAC Facilitator and the athlete must monitor the response over the next 48 hours. If pain, swelling, or stiffness increase during this time, the tissue loading was excessive, indicating the need to treat those symptoms and reduce the training load. When progress stops prematurely or a setback occurs, the TSAC Facilitator should coordinate further care with the rehabilitation staff.

Even when the tactical athlete appears to tolerate a progressive training load, rehabilitation staff and the TSAC Facilitator must cautiously progress activities and tissue stress, sticking with a scientifically supported progression rather than relying on the tactical athlete to report problems such as pain (64, 73). In the controlled motion phase of rehabilitation, it is often wise to focus on the quality of movement rather than the volume and intensity of training.

When injured tissues are fully repaired, the next stage involves a long period of remodeling. The objective of rehabilitation becomes a return to full function. Normally during this phase a transition is made from rehabilitation to performance training. Clear communication between the TSAC Facilitator and the rehabilitation staff is essential to ensure that the tactical athlete is ready to begin and progress performance-based training. When planning progression, consider the following factors in light of the tactical athlete's unique performance requirements (it is generally best to progress only one factor at a time):

- **Excursion:** Excursion involves increasing ROM about the joints of the injured body part. Tactical athletes commonly encounter tasks that demand controlled mobility through a large ROM. Increase the excursion of movements in small increments, ensuring proper form and pain-free execution throughout.

- **Speed:** During initial rehabilitation, the speed of movement is often slow in order to ensure adequate neuromuscular control and technique. However, many tactically relevant movements require quick reactions. Such reactions are best trained in a controlled environment with the supervision of a performance specialist. If excursion of a movement has been progressed previously, it is often best to decrease excursion before adding speed. When control of the new rate of movement is demonstrated, then excursion can be added again.

- **Load:** Many tactical athletes encounter significant loads in their duties. As with speed, traditional rehabilitation might not progress loads to an occupationally relevant degree. Therefore, it is incumbent upon the TSAC Facilitator to optimize the training load in consultation with medical and rehabilitation specialists. Because strength deficits and imbalances are commonly cited as factors that predispose a person to injury (37, 51, 73), restoring adequate strength is a major

concern when considering readiness to return to duty.

- **Volume:** For resistance and neuromuscular control training, the volume of training reflects the total number of repetitions for a given period of time. For endurance training, mileage or minutes may be used to measure volume. Increasing the volume of training, along with increasing strength and movement efficiency, will lead to a greater work capacity.

- **Complexity:** Many tactical tasks require a high level of movement skill, meaning that a substantial degree of neuromuscular control is needed to complete the task. The tactical athlete becomes better prepared for such tasks by progressing the complexity of movement during rehabilitation and performance training. Means of increasing movement complexity include decreasing the base of support (e.g., narrowing the stance), moving in multiple planes and on uneven surfaces, and reacting to a changing environment. For example, complexity can be added to a simple agility drill of weaving through cones in the gym by adding tactical equipment, moving outdoors to rougher terrain, placing the cones at asymmetrical intervals, and directing the tactical athlete to react to sight or sound.

Modification of Exercises to Allow Injured Individuals to Continue Training

Although the harmful effects of disuse on muscle size and strength are well documented, recent evidence shows that such effects begin to occur with as little as five days of disuse (71). Clearly, it is in the tactical athlete's interest to continue training to the extent possible after injury. Mobility is also frequently compromised after injury; however, the rehabilitation staff members usually direct restoration of mobility during the postinjury period. Therefore, the focus of this section is on preserving strength and motor control after injury. Though a full discussion of resistance training for the tactical athlete is covered in other chapters, it is instructive to note at this point the distinction between isolated and integrated resistance training.

Following injury, the goal of resistance training is to prepare tactical athletes to manage all of the loads they will encounter during tactical and performance training and their duties. Most often those loads are managed through the coordinated effort of multiple muscle groups working in more than one plane. Thus, **integrated resistance training** must be a prominent part of a tactical athlete's strength preparation.

However, **isolated resistance training** is indicated when a muscle or muscle group lacks the force production capability to perform its natural role in the kinetic chain. For example, when landing on one leg during running, gravity promotes a collapse of the pelvis on the unsupported side. If the hip-stabilizing muscles of the stance side (primarily the gluteus maximus and medius) do not exert adequate force, the stance knee will be at risk for excessive strain (52, 75). For people with this problem, isolated training of the gluteal muscles is likely an important component of their rehabilitation. When adequate force production of the gluteal muscles is established, it is time for more complex, integrated exercises that more closely mimic functional tasks. Isolated resistance training to restore optimal function of links in the kinetic chain spans both rehabilitation and performance. Tactical athletes benefit when personnel in both disciplines (rehabilitation and tactical training) collaborate to consistently define physical training objectives and parameters.

In addition to resistance training to preserve muscle mass and function after injury, the TSAC Facilitator must also promote optimal motor control and efficiency, especially as training activities become more integrated. Efficient movement is a constant give-and-take between mobility and stability, with each segment of the body and its unique movement capabilities influencing all the other segments. When mobility and stability are in balance, and all segments are synchronized, movement is optimal and potentially powerful. When they are not, the result is often injury or suboptimal performance. The discussion that follows will offer suggestions for modifying PRT for the injured tactical athlete. The specific exercises presented are just a few examples of possible interventions. As long as the performance specialist understands tissue stress, the stage of tissue healing, and the tactical athlete's physical demands, many other training interventions may be used.

Region-Specific Exercise Modifications

Exercise modifications for the injured tactical athlete often require accommodations at multiple body regions. However, the following section is provided as a starting point for planning.

Foot and Ankle   Injuries to the foot and ankle often require weight-bearing restrictions. In addition to the numerous options for open kinetic chain training to maintain strength and motion in other regions, there is evidence that closed kinetic chain exercises involving the uninjured lower extremity might improve balance and lower extremity function on the injured side (23). Figure 16.1 shows a simple single-leg rotational exercise, initially standing on the uninjured leg. To increase the motor control challenge, vary the direction, excursion, and speed of the reach. Also include leg reaches and swings, heel raises, and squats. Ensure adequate control of the trunk and the stance leg. Later, when the injured side is cleared for weight bearing, the same exercises are then indicated for both lower extremities. At that time, another strategy to improve balance and lower extremity function is to spend time barefooted. Doing so will likely provide better proprioception for the CNS, possibly leading to better motor control (43).

Injuries to the foot, ankle, and lower leg often compromise ankle dorsiflexion (10). Consequently, the restricted ankle joint limits squatting and many other functional exercises (2, 61). Figure 16.2 shows one strategy to accommodate the lack of ankle dorsiflexion—using a strap so that the tactical athlete can shift the center of gravity posterior relative to the base of support. Notice that the tibias are essentially perpendicular to the ground, reflecting little if any dorsiflexion. Use of the straps should be modulated to appropriately load the injured or restricted ankle. This modification also demands less contribution from muscles crossing the ankle; therefore, people with muscular strains around the ankle are more likely to tolerate squatting when it is assisted. Box squats and front squats also promote posterior displacement of the center of gravity, thus demanding less of the ankle joint.

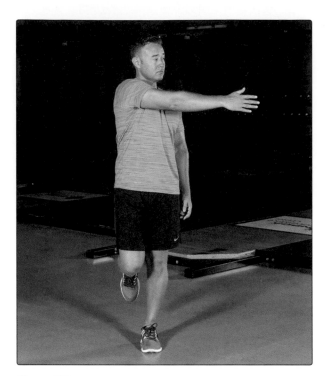

Figure 16.1 Single-leg rotational reach.

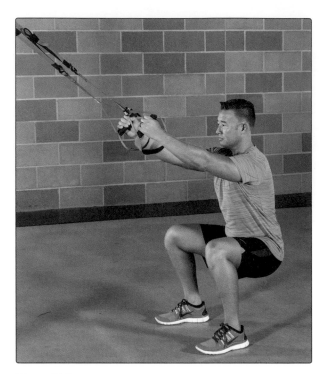

Figure 16.2 Strap-assisted squat.

Knee Injury to the knee has the potential to profoundly affect function, and many strength and conditioning exercises are limited accordingly. Modifications are designed to limit knee forces (usually by restricting flexion in the closed kinetic chain) while maintaining functionality of segments above and below the knee. Figure 16.3 shows a single-leg T-stance that uses assistance from a stick to modulate forces to tolerable levels. This exercise promotes motor control of much of the kinetic chain while keeping knee forces low. Note that the knee is slightly flexed and the trunk is in a neutral alignment. The assisted squat shown in figure 16.2 and similar variations are often well tolerated in the controlled motion phase.

When the tactical athlete is ready to progress, squats and other closed chain activities are introduced, though TSAC Facilitators must consider the mechanical effects (13, 61). If the knee is vulnerable to increasing compressive loads at the patellofemoral or tibiofemoral joint, squat depth and knee flexion must be limited accordingly. Modifying a squat with 130° of knee flexion to 60° reduces tibiofemoral compressive forces by over 30% (47). This reduction in squat depth might best serve people with patellofemoral pain, meniscal injury, or degenerative lesions of the joint.

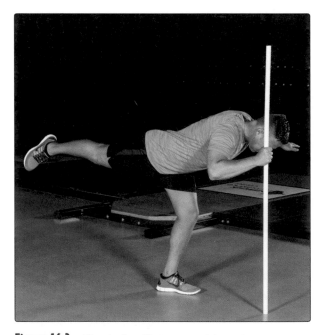

Figure 16.3 Single-leg T-stance with assistance.

Shearing forces at the knee are also a consideration, especially for people with compromised cruciate ligaments. The reduction in squat depth to 50° to 60° knee flexion is also indicated for posterior cruciate ligament (PCL) compromise, with some evidence that the leg press exercise places less strain on the PCL than squatting (12). Although shearing forces to the anterior cruciate ligament (ACL) are highest at 15° to 30° of squatting, the compressive forces of weight bearing and coactivation of the hamstring and quadriceps muscles prevent significant ACL strain (13, 61). However, open kinetic chain exercises for the quadriceps, such as the seated knee extension, create potentially harmful strain to the ACL, especially from 45° to 0°. Therefore, the exercise is generally restricted to 90° to 45°, usually beginning eight weeks after reconstruction (20). The TSAC Facilitator should continue to coordinate care with the appropriate medical and rehabilitation staff when training tactical athletes after surgery.

Knee problems are often related to dynamic malalignment. Most commonly, the knee drifts medially during functional loading activities, such as running or squatting. Figures 16.4 (facilitated box squat) and 16.5 (facilitated split squat) show the use of elastic bands to facilitate activation of the lower extremity muscles (primarily at the hip) that align the knee.

Hip   Injuries to the hip are less common than injuries to the ankle and knee, but they can be just as debilitating (24). Most muscle strains around the hip joint resolve with proper post-injury care and restoration of optimal kinetic chain function through rehabilitation. Such cases seldom require ongoing exercise modification. However, a chronic hip condition that is increasingly recognized in tactical populations is femoroacetabular impingement (7). Symptoms usually present when the hip is flexed greater than 90°, especially if internal rotation is a component motion. Modifying exercise and occupational activities to avoid those positions alleviates symptoms in many people (72). The TSAC Facilitator should modify exercise to limit squat and lunge depth while ensuring lower extremity alignment. Additionally, optimizing the posterior chain and stability of the pelvis and trunk are indicated.

Insufficient hip mobility is a common problem affecting the kinetic chain. Rotating sufficiently at the hips is a key component of many tactical tasks (e.g., getting up and down from the ground, climbing, negotiating obstacles, grappling). When hip motions are limited, the body will try to complete the task by finding motion somewhere

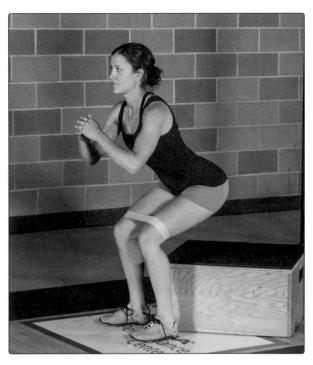

Figure 16.4   Facilitated box squat.

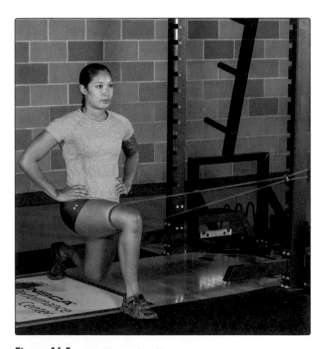

Figure 16.5   Facilitated split squat.

else—usually the low back—creating excessive strain (15). The incorporation of several hip mobility exercises in the daily warm-up routine should help improve hip mobility. High-value hip mobility exercises include dynamic stretches of the hip flexors, tensor fascia latae, and piriformis. If there is pain or a lack of progress, the TSAC

Facilitator should refer the tactical athlete to medical or rehabilitation professionals.

Spine Injuries to the spine, as well as low back pain unrelated to a known injury, are common in the general and tactical population (24). Even with a seemingly complete recovery, recurrence is common (42). Because the spine is involved in nearly all functional movement, it is critical that tactical athletes learn to train and protect it.

Although most tactical athletes are familiar with exercises such as planks and bridges and consider them core exercises, developing neuromuscular control of the trunk and pelvis is not just a matter of performing those exercises. When teaching any lift or movement, TSAC Facilitators should promote awareness of the core's role in force transmission. Tactical athletes should learn to set the trunk in a neutral position (the low back is neither arched excessively nor flattened but somewhere in between) and engage the core (cinching up the trunk and pelvic muscles without losing the neutral position or inhibiting breathing). They should also learn to modulate muscular forces to avoid excessive activation, which can not only limit performance but also create pathological strain to healing tissues (42).

During the early stages of recovery from a spinal injury, substituting single-leg activities might provide an effective stimulus for maintaining lower extremity functionality while keeping spinal loads light. The single-leg T-stance with assistance (figure 16.3) is an example that primarily works the posterior kinetic chain. The wall plank with exercise ball and alternating leg lift (figure 16.6) shows the use of an unstable surface to increase trunk muscle activation, primarily targeting the anterior kinetic chain.

The TSAC Facilitator should be aware that unstable surfaces are a double-edged sword: Although they might meet the intent of increasing muscular activation, such activation might excessively load healing tissues (42). The hanging knee raise shown in figure 16.7 is often well tolerated by people with back conditions, perhaps due to the lack of axial loading of the spine. Note that the neutral position of the spine is maintained.

The wall plank and hanging knee raise (figures 16.6 and 16.7) target stability primarily in the

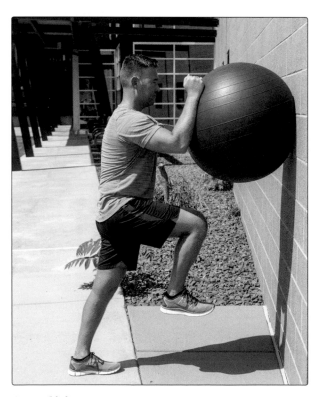

Figure 16.6 Wall plank with exercise ball and alternating leg lift.

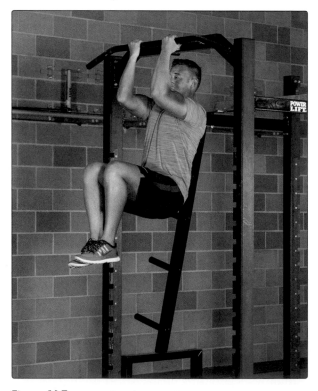

Figure 16.7 Hanging knee raise.

sagittal plane. To target the frontal and transverse plane, consider the exercise shown in figure 16.8, the sidestepping crouch with elastic resistance. With the elastic band held close to the body, the resistance is primarily in the frontal plane. When the elbows are extended, the forces move significantly toward the transverse plane. Ensure alignment of the spine and lower extremity in all three planes.

Triplanar exercises for the trunk are a natural progression once the tactical athlete has demonstrated effective exercise performance and tolerance of uniplanar challenges. Figure 16.9 shows one such exercise, the diagonal plate swing. The trunk remains aligned, with flexion occurring at the hip and the rotational component occurring at the hip, thoracic spine, and shoulder girdle.

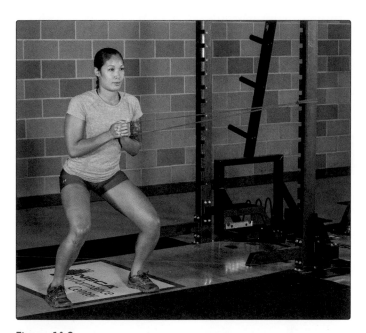

Figure 16.8 Sidestepping crouch with elastic resistance.

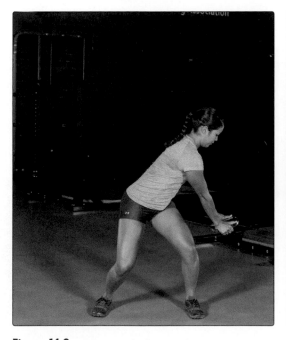
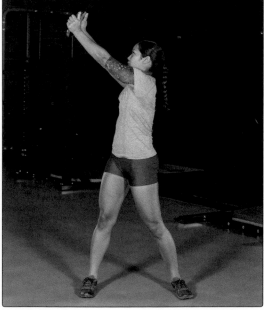

Figure 16.9 Diagonal plate swing.

To ensure that the tactical athlete can not only generate stabilizing force but also modulate muscular activation to promote skillful movement, consider the medicine ball wall throw (figure 16.10). Note the alignment of the trunk and left lower extremity for loading. Muscular activation should be high near this position and then decrease quickly as weight shifts to the right lower extremity during the follow-through. After follow-through, the quick return to the catch position is associated with increasing muscular tension in preparation for the load. The tactical athlete should be encouraged to coordinate this exercise with diaphragmatic inhalation to increase intra-abdominal pressure for the catch and then exhale during the throw and follow-through.

In the return-to-function phase of rehabilitation, traditional lifts such as the squat, deadlift, and clean may be resumed, beginning with relatively light loads and ensuring the natural curve of the low back is not lost during the lift. For deadlifts, use the hexagonal bar to keep the load close to the spine (see figure 16.11), thus reducing stress to that area (66). Do not add an external load to the squat unless form with bodyweight squatting is optimal. The TSAC Facilitator should take a conservative approach to load progression and consider the front squat (see figure 16.12) as the primary technique in the return-to-function phase because it is associated with lower stress to the lumbar spine (19).

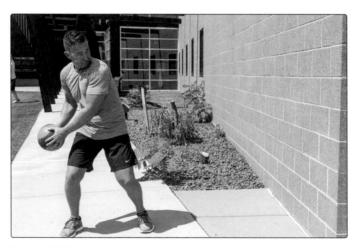

Figure 16.10   Rotational medicine ball wall throw.

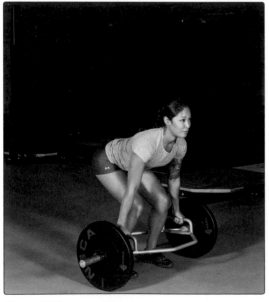 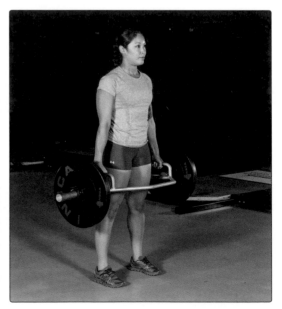

Figure 16.11   Deadlift with hexagonal bar.

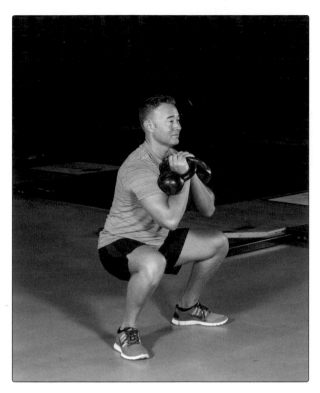

Figure 16.12   Front squat with kettlebells.

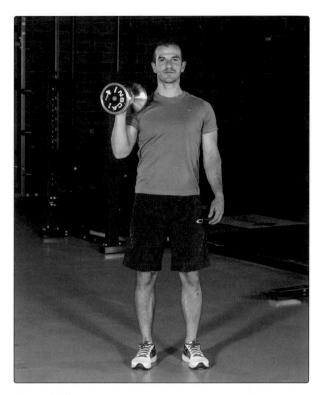

Figure 16.13   Starting position for dumbbell press in the scapular plane.

Shoulder   Efficient use of the shoulder demands mobility and stability of the articulation between the scapula and the thorax. The scapula serves as the base of support for upper extremity movement. If it is not in the right place at the right time, or if it shifts too easily under load, then excessive strain is transmitted to the shoulder joint.

Although optimizing motion and stability of the scapula is a rehabilitation concern, TSAC Facilitators should recognize the role of the scapula and observe for optimal mechanics during all activities. Once scapular mechanics are sufficient, traditional upper body exercises may begin. Frequently, pressing movements must be modified to accommodate shoulder pathology. Dumbbells or kettlebells are usually preferable to the barbell in pressing movements because they allow the movement to occur in the scapular plane rather than the frontal plane. Note the arm and dumbbell angle in figure 16.13.

For people who experience a painful arc of motion during pressing activities (usually 60°-120° and commonly diagnosed as impingement [38]), the push press allows the weight to move through the range with minimal shoulder strain.

Once the weight is overhead and aligned, many tactical athletes with shoulder conditions tolerate a variety of total body exercises such as the single-arm overhead split squat, shown in figure 16.14. For such overhead exercises, the elbow is straight and the head and spine are aligned perpendicular to the ground. The TSAC Facilitator should also monitor overhead exercises for excessive elevation of the scapula. Common cues are "pack the scapula" or "place your shoulder blade in your back pocket." However, those cues should not be used until the arm is fully overhead; otherwise the exerciser might not achieve sufficient upward rotation of the scapula.

Anterior instability is another common shoulder problem for tactical athletes (54). The primary precaution is to avoid horizontal abduction and external rotation (high-five position). The dumbbell floor press (figure 16.15) uses the floor to limit horizontal abduction, although bench-pressing with a barrier on the chest achieves a similar effect. People with anterior shoulder instability should avoid behind-the-neck presses or pulldowns; this is a sound precaution for shoulder protection in general (11, 55).

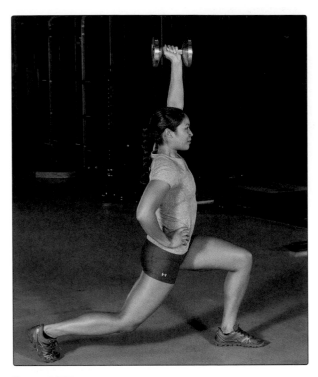

Figure 16.14 Single-arm overhead split squat.

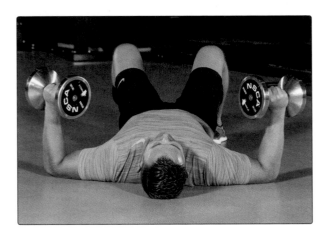

Figure 16.15 Dumbbell floor press.

Posterior instability of the shoulder is less common (54). The primary precaution is to prevent forces that drive the arm posteriorly. Pressing movements require excellent control of the scapula, which should be trained during rehabilitation. Initial pressing activities are modified, using only a wide grip to promote a congruent position of the humerus and scapula.

Using a cable system to train reciprocal push–pull movements can train rotation of the entire kinetic chain (see figure 16.16). Note the weight shift and rotation of the hips, pelvis, midback, and shoulder girdle. Very little motion occurs in the lower back. This exercise is also effective for training neuromuscular control of the shoulders. The TSAC Facilitator should cue the tactical athlete to lead with retraction of the scapula (and follow with the arm) on the pulling side. On the pushing side, care is taken to ensure that the hand does not lag behind the forward rotation of the pelvis, trunk, and shoulder girdle. Note also in figure 16.16 that adjustment of the pulley height and direction of the hand movement should be considered in light of the tactical athlete's unique needs. For example, some individuals will better tolerate a lower finishing position of the pushing arm compared to that shown in figure 16.16.

The following suggestions are offered to tactical athletes looking to manage shoulder problems:

- Carefully consider the volume and intensity of pressing movements. Although the bench press is a staple of resistance training in tactical populations, large compressive and shearing loads are common (14). The TSAC Facilitator and the tactical athlete must perform a risk-to-benefit analysis. It is best to train pressing movements that contribute to function and are modified to accommodate individual restrictions. Always use strict, mechanically correct form, and choose a conservative progression of volume and intensity.

- The clean and jerk, snatch, and overhead squat are commonly performed by tactical athletes, but they come with some risk to the shoulders and spine (14). Master the coordination of those lifts with feedback from an exercise professional and quality reps with a light weight. If the tactical athlete does not demonstrate effective technique using a lightweight stick or bar, loaded overhead movements should not be attempted.

- Kettlebell get-ups may be used in the functional phase to integrate stability of the shoulder, core, and legs. As with any complex movement, approach the learning process with the intent of achieving mastery part by part and in due time, not in minutes. While developing technical mastery of the exercise, keep the load modest and avoid a high level of fatigue (27).

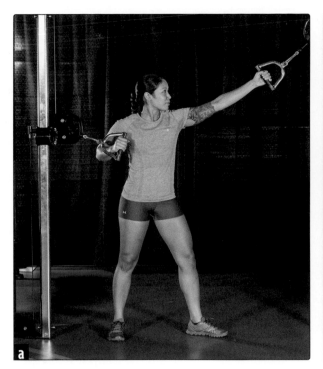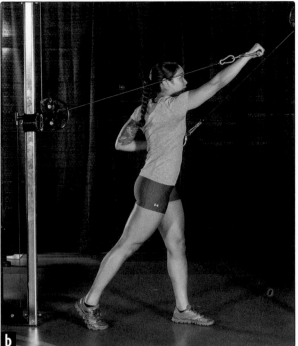

Figure 16.16   Reciprocal push–pull: *(a)* starting position; *(b)* final position.

Key Point

The skillful use of exercise modifications often allows tactical athletes to maintain a considerable degree of fitness and functionality during injury recovery. Collaboration between the TSAC Facilitator and rehabilitation professionals ensures that modifications are appropriate.

Common Options for Aerobic Endurance Training While Injured

Tactical professions vary in their endurance demands. Wildland firefighters and infantry forces must have a high level of both aerobic and anaerobic endurance. Police officers are more likely to need anaerobic endurance. All tactical professionals benefit from being in optimal condition. Following an injury or movement impairment, tactical athletes might be unable to perform their customary fitness activities. Rehabilitation and performance specialists working with injured tactical athletes must not only find alternative ways to maintain fitness while recovering, but they must also guide the progression of conditioning activities once the tactical athletes are cleared for return to their normal duties.

Aquatic Training   Aquatic training is effective for maintaining or improving conditioning while minimizing weight-bearing stress to healing tissues (16). Swimming is of course an option, but so is running at various depths, including deep-water running. For running workouts, the stride rate is reduced by the resistance of the water. So, running in the water might make for a stronger stride, but recovery of speed will likely require speed drills out of the water.

Biking   If sufficient ROM of the hips and knees is available, biking is an option for maintaining aerobic endurance while weight bearing is limited. Unlike swimming, biking allows for a rapid cadence. However, the physiological and biomechanical aspects of biking might limit its transferability to walking and running tasks (58).

Stepper and Elliptical Machines   Because there are numerous models of stair-stepper and elliptical machines, each with different stride characteristics, it is difficult to make summary recommendations for their use. The upright posture associated with these machines likely increases their transferability to walking or running, though to date no research has tested that theory.

Rowing Compared with many other endurance activities, rowing offers more of a stimulus to trunk and upper extremity endurance. Similar to biking, the seated posture of rowing might limit its transferability to walking and running tasks.

Varying Aerobic and Anaerobic Endurance Training It is important for most tactical athletes to train for full-spectrum endurance. A common fault among injured tactical athletes is to perform only steady-pace sessions for their cardiorespiratory training. Neglecting high-intensity workouts during recovery from injury compromises anaerobic fitness and leaves the tactical athlete unprepared for duties that require repeated bursts of high-intensity effort. The simple solution is to vary the duration and intensity of conditioning sessions over the course of five to seven days: an aerobic session at a steady pace and relatively long duration; an anaerobic session of repeated short-duration, high-intensity efforts; and a tempo session of moderate to high intensity at a steady pace (HR is maintained at about 85% of max). Such workouts are commonly used by runners and cyclists (see chapter 14) but can easily be adapted to the injured tactical athlete training in the pool or on the machines discussed previously (see the earlier section Common Options for Aerobic Endurance Training While Injured).

For tactical athletes who must return to running following an injury, a systematic approach to running progression is necessary to allow optimal bone and soft tissue responses to the new stress of running (73). Although numerous such programs exist, the following guidelines and table 16.2 show a phased return to running that is commonly used in the military and is consistent with the principle of progressive tissue stress (73). The intent is to safely progress running to a common military run of 30 minutes. Guidance for the tactical athlete is as follows (73):

- Begin the program only if able to walk 30 minutes without symptoms at a moderately challenging pace.
- Begin each session with a few minutes of walking or other form of dynamic warm-up before beginning the running portion of the workout.
- Perform no more frequently than every other day. Do not run two days in a row. During phases 4, 8, and 12 (noted with an asterisk in the table), rest at least two to three days between running sessions.
- Perform at a sustainable pace on a level surface.
- Stop if experiencing increased pain, swelling, or stiffness. Such symptoms might not arise until the day after running. Do not run again

Table 16.2 Sample Return-to-Run Progression

Level	Run (min)	Walk (min)	Repetitions	Total time (min)
1	1	5	5	30
2	2	4	5	30
3	3	3	5	30
4*	4	2	5	30
5	5	1	5	30
6	10	5	2	30
7	12.5	2.5	2	30
8*	15	15	1	30
9	17.5	12.5	1	30
10	20	10	1	30
11	22.5	7.5	1	30
12*	25	5	1	30
13	27.5	2.5	1	30
14	30	0	1	30

*Schedule two to three days of rest between run days.

until these symptoms are gone, and then resume running at the last phase in which running was pain free. Discuss with medical and rehabilitation professionals when in doubt.

- Try each phase at least twice; progress only if there is no increased pain, swelling, or stiffness. If there are no setbacks, the program will last about four months.

- After phase 14, if greater running distance is desired, progress gradually by no more than 10% per week.

Monitoring Progress of Injured Individuals Through Functional Assessment

Evaluation of the injured tactical athlete is an ongoing process. Every training session and subsequent recovery period provides an opportunity to assess whether the physical stimulus is eliciting the desired response. When rehabilitation progresses to the return-to-function phase, the TSAC Facilitator then selects functional assessments that give insight into the tactical athlete's readiness for unrestricted duties. Although there are many such tests, few have strong evidence to support their use (25, 26).

The single-leg hop for distance shows moderate responsiveness to changes during rehabilitation and thus might be used to gauge progress after lower extremity injuries (26). There is also moderate evidence that the single-leg hop for distance and the hexagon hop give insight into ankle stability; therefore those tests should be considered after ankle injury (25). In the same analysis of the literature on performance tests, only performance on the Star Excursion Balance Test (SEBT) performed in three directions (anterior, posteromedial, and posterolateral) was associated with injury risk (25). The SEBT is a relatively expedient way to evaluate multicomponent function of the lower extremities. Value is likely added when tests such as the SEBT are considered in conjunction with demographics and injury history (39).

Given the lack of valid and responsive functional assessments, the TSAC Facilitator must frequently take a practical approach to assessing function. The varied physical demands of the tactical professions often require the TSAC Facilitator to go on-site to observe occupational tasks and evaluate the tactical athlete's execution and response to the task in light of previous injury pathomechanics (53).

GUIDELINES FOR INJURY CARE AND REHABILITATION

When working with injured tactical athletes, TSAC Facilitators must be keenly aware of the risks associated with physical training in light of the injury. Because injury evaluation and management is outside their scope of practice, TSAC Facilitators must collaborate with rehabilitation professionals in order to best serve injured tactical athletes.

Scope of Practice of the TSAC Facilitator

TSAC Facilitators might work with injured tactical athletes at any point during the recovery process. The design and implementation of strength and conditioning activities for the injured tactical athlete are guided by the phase of healing and readiness for tissue stress, as established by medical and rehabilitation professionals. Rehabilitation objectives and activities are presented in table 16.1.

During the acute and subacute phases, TSAC Facilitators must be keenly aware of the vulnerability of injured tissue to mechanical stress and design activities accordingly. When in doubt, the TSAC Facilitator communicates directly with medical or rehabilitation professionals. The strength and conditioning objectives during these phases are to maintain general fitness and functionality of uninjured areas. When injured tissue is ready for mechanical stress, medical or rehabilitation professionals will prescribe the appropriate application of stress through an exercise prescription. The TSAC Facilitator may supervise the execution of the plan.

During the return-to-function phase, the TSAC Facilitator continues to follow guidance from medical and rehabilitation professionals. Additionally, the TSAC Facilitator must now consider directing activities toward the occupational demands of the tactical athlete.

Scope of Practice of the Physical Therapist and Allied Health Professionals

Although the term *physical therapy* is often used to describe a range of therapeutic measures delivered by a variety of sources, physical therapy is limited to the care and services provided by or under the direction and supervision of a physical therapist. It includes the following (1):

- Examining individuals with impairment, functional limitation, disability, or other health-related conditions in order to determine a diagnosis, prognosis, and intervention
- Alleviating impairment and functional limitation by designing, implementing, and modifying therapeutic interventions
- Preventing injury, impairment, functional limitation, and disability, including promoting and maintaining health, wellness, fitness, and quality of life in all populations
- Engaging in consultation, education, and research

In the United States, 50 states and the District of Columbia (DC) allow physical therapists to evaluate patients without a physician's referral, and 48 states and DC allow physical therapists to evaluate and treat, under certain conditions, patients without a referral from a physician.

Athletic trainers, under the supervision of a physician, also provide injury care and rehabilitation. The National Athletic Trainers' Association (NATA) Board of Certification requires that athletic trainers are educated, trained, and evaluated in five major practice domains (48):

1. Prevention
2. Clinical evaluation and diagnosis
3. Immediate and emergency care
4. Treatment and rehabilitation
5. Organization and professional health and well-being

Interprofessional Collaboration

Many factors will determine whether the tactical athlete recovers fully from injury or experiences a decline in performance and remains at risk for further injury. Managing these factors demands a team approach. Ideally, medical doctors and physician's assistants manage the medical and primary care needs; physical therapists and athletic trainers provide musculoskeletal care and rehabilitation; and strength and conditioning specialists, including TSAC Facilitators, plan and direct progressive physical training programs that are best suited to the unique demands of tactical athletes as they recover from injury and return to full duties.

Unfortunately, tactical athletes may not have direct access to each of these professionals, making it imperative that team members are broadly cross-trained in the other disciplines and aware of the occasional need for referral. For example, physical therapists and athletic trainers must be well versed in the essentials of strength and conditioning, and strength and conditioning specialists must understand injury management and rehabilitation principles and refer to the appropriate professional as needed.

Although the focus of this chapter has been the care of injured tactical athletes, gaining better control of injury and overtraining is widely recognized as an important objective for rehabilitation and performance teams working with tactical populations. To better control injuries, a 2008 U.S. Department of Defense injury prevention work group reviewed the medical literature and presented several recommendations to the military services (69). Two recommendations are particularly pertinent for TSAC Facilitators: Prevent overtraining, and perform multiaxial, neuromuscular, proprioceptive, and agility training. These particular recommendations are directed at the military services; however, their application to other tactical populations is likely valid. Effective implementation of the recommendations will often require the interprofessional collaboration described previously.

CONCLUSION

The greatest risk factor for injury is a previous injury, suggesting that rehabilitation of the initial injury is often inadequate to restore full functionality. Rehabilitation and performance professionals restore full functionality by optimizing motion, force production, neuromuscular control, and muscular and aerobic endurance. Such rehabilitation often takes months to complete; therefore, tactical athletes are best served by a long-term approach that is communicated clearly from the beginning. Throughout the process, the tactical athlete's training background, injury history, and job-related physical requirements must guide the rehabilitation choices. Frequent and effective communication between members of the rehabilitation and performance teams ensures that the tactical athlete hears one message and makes a seamless transition from injury rehabilitation to peak performance.

Key Terms

bone stress injury (BSI)
exercise modifications
foundational phase PRT
functional phase PRT
inflammatory response
injuries
integrated resistance training
isolated resistance training
kinetic chain
movement impairments
nonfunctional overreaching (NFOR)

overreaching
overtraining syndrome (OTS)
overuse
rehabilitation
return-to-function phase
scope of practice
sports medicine model
tendinopathy
tissue healing
training errors

Study Questions

1. What is the biggest health problem in the military services?

   a. PTSD

   b. injuries

   c. diabetes

   d. stroke

2. Which stage of healing for traumatic injury rehabilitation involves low-load ROM and stretching exercises?

   a. inflammatory

   b. repair

   c. remodeling

   d. return-to-function

3. Which of the following is NOT a warning sign of overtraining?

   a. mood changes

   b. elevated heart rate

   c. decreased blood pressure

   d. diminished quality of sleep

4. A firefighter has suffered an ankle injury and is currently undergoing rehabilitation. When the athlete is back to weight-bearing activities, what exercise will promote posterior displacement of the center of gravity and therefore less stress on the ankle joint?

   a. lunge

   b. front squat

   c. heel raise

   d. box jump

Chapter 17

Physiological Issues Related to Fire and Rescue Personnel

Katie Sell, PhD, CSCS,*D, TSAC-F,*D
Mark Abel, PhD, CSCS,*D, TSAC-F,*D
Joseph Domitrovich, PhD

After completing this chapter, you will be able to

- describe the physiological and biomechanical occupational demands, injury risks, environmental exposures, and occupational stressors experienced by fire and rescue personnel;

- discuss the fitness requirements and recommendations for fire and rescue personnel;

- design fitness programs by applying training principles and approaches to improve and maintain fitness in fire and rescue personnel across disciplines, subdivisions, professional statuses (cadets versus incumbents), and fitness levels; and

- analyze case-specific and problem-centered scenarios.

Firefighters perform a multitude of duties in diverse environments. These settings include metropolitan and rural areas as well as military, public, private, and industrial arenas, many of which require specialized training. Fire and rescue personnel may be members of professional, volunteer, contract, seasonal, or combination departments, responsible for "providing rescue, fire suppression, emergency medical services, hazardous materials mitigation, special operations, and other emergency services" (82). The **National Fire Protection Association (NFPA)** estimates that there were approximately 1,140,750 volunteer and professional firefighters in the United States in 2013, with approximately 69% considered volunteer (55). According to the U.S. Bureau of Labor Statistics, the number of paid firefighters is expected to grow by 19% to approximately 367,900 firefighters by 2018 (126). The NFPA uses the following definitions to describe the work of structural and wildland firefighters:

- **Structural firefighting** encompasses "the activities of rescue, fire suppression, and property conservation in buildings or other structures, vehicles, rail cars, marine vessels, aircraft, or like properties" (82) and involves professional and volunteer firefighters.

- **Wildland firefighting** covers "the activities of fire suppression and property conservation in woodlands, forests, grasslands, brush, prairies, and other such vegetation, or any combination of vegetation that is involved in a fire situation but is not within buildings or structures" (79). It uses Type 1 firefighters (e.g., smoke jumpers, hotshots, rappellers) and Type 2 firefighters (e.g., hand crews).

CRITICAL JOB TASKS FOR FIREFIGHTERS

Firefighting is a physically demanding occupation requiring optimal physical fitness. In recognition of the importance of physical fitness and health to fire and rescue personnel, the governing agencies that oversee fire services have released guidelines and recommendations for implementing comprehensive **wellness** programs for professional and volunteer firefighters that emphasize regular exercise and physical conditioning. These include the *Joint Labor Management Wellness-Fitness Initiative* of the **International Association of Fire Fighters (IAFF)** and **International Association of Fire Chiefs (IAFC)** (63), *Fitness and Work Capacity* of the **National Wildfire Coordinating Group (NWCG)** (110), *Health and Wellness Guide for the Volunteer Fire and Emergency Services* of the **U.S. Fire Administration (USFA)** (128), and Heart-Healthy Firefighter Program of the **National Volunteer Fire Council (NVFC)** (www.healthy-firefighter.org). Additional resources are presented throughout this chapter.

Physiological Demands

When designing physical training programs, TSAC Facilitators must consider which energy systems are stressed during structural and wildland firefighting tasks. A comprehensive description of the typical job tasks for structural and wildland firefighters can be found in *NFPA 1582: Standard on Comprehensive Occupational Medical Program for Fire Departments* (81) and the NWCG's *Fitness and Work Capacity* (110). Additional information may be sought for descriptions of job tasks for specialized teams (79, 80, 84).

Both structural and wildland firefighters perform a variety of tasks that stress all three energy systems. Table 17.1 summarizes several structural and wildland firefighter job tasks and the primary energy system that each task utilizes. Research regarding the cardiorespiratory demands of structural firefighting indicates that performing fireground tasks results in oxygen uptake levels that are 63% to 97% of maximum (122, 129, 132) and HR values between 84% and 100% of maximum (26, 122, 132). Not only are these physiological demands present during firefighting tasks, but HR and oxygen uptake may remain elevated for an extended period of time following work (often exceeding 30 minutes) (94), consistent with the established excess postexercise oxygen consumption effect (49). The minimum aerobic capacity for performing structural fireground rescue tasks should be 42 ml·kg^{-1}·min^{-1} or 12 METs (range: 39-45 ml·kg^{-1}·min^{-1}) (15, 51, 82, 91, 122). Peak blood lactate values range from 6 to 13 mmol/L when performing fireground and rescue tasks (51, 129), suggesting a high degree of anaerobic stress.

The energy expenditure that occurs during wildland firefighting tasks varies from approximately 17 ml·kg^{-1}·min^{-1} (or 2.5 kcal/min) for light tasks to >30 ml·kg^{-1}·min^{-1} (or >10 kcal/min) for highly demanding job requirements (e.g., uphill hiking with a pack) (29, 110). Wildland firefighters must often sustain these tasks for prolonged periods of time on consecutive days, depending on the duration of the wildfire assignment, suggesting a need for aerobic fitness and LT levels higher than in the average population (8, 110).

Biomechanical Demands

Common tasks for structural firefighters include carrying equipment (figure 17.1), advancing and operating hose lines (figures 17.2-17.4), climbing stairs with equipment (figure 17.5), setting ladders, victim dragging and searching (figure 17.6), forcibly entering spaces (figure 17.8), and doing other salvage and overhaul tasks (51, 62). Common tasks for wildland firefighters include building fire lines using various hand tools such as a Pulaski tool or dust hook (figure 17.9), packing heavy or light loads, hiking in wildland terrain with load and in adverse conditions, chainsawing (figure 17.11), chopping wood, and performing various emergency responses (e.g., fast escape from fire to safety zone, victim assistance) (29, 110). Several wildland firefighting tasks may be specific to certain crews, such as tree–land rappels performed by smoke jumpers.

A biomechanical analysis of common structural and wildland firefighting tasks is provided in table 17.2. Many of the tasks performed by structural and wildland firefighters are performed in the sagittal plane, use multiple joints, engage major muscle groups of the upper and lower body, use dynamic muscle contractions, and involve some degree of proximal stability. However, many chopping and digging motions also involve rotation and movement in an oblique (or diagonal) plane. These tasks may differ across departments or disciplines within a department depending on primary responsibilities, equipment used, and geographical location (73, 95). Physical fitness characteristics associated with structural and wildland firefighting tasks include upper body strength and endurance, torso strength and endurance, lower body power and endurance, flexibility and mobility, and joint stability (especially ankles, knees, hips, core, and shoulders) throughout the entire body (8, 26, 77, 84, 101, 110, 113).

Occupational Demands

Firefighters wear fire-resistant clothing, often called **personal protective equipment (PPE)**, to help protect the body from the by-products of combustion (embers, sparks, heat, smoke, and gases) and radiant heat exposure (60, 81). This PPE may vary across firefighting disciplines but generally consists of a bunker coat and pants, boots, helmet, face mask, gloves, face and neck

Table 17.1 Physiological Assessment of Structural and Wildland Fireground Tasks Classified by Primary Energy System Used

Energy system	Structural firefighter tasks	Wildland firefighter tasks	Relative intensity	Relative duration
ATP-PCr	• Hose pull • Ladder raise • Hose hoist • Forcible entry • Lifting/lowering objects	• Rescue tasks • Tree felling (ax)	High	Short ATP-PCr: 0-10 s
Glycolytic	• Load carriage • Victim drag	• Packing heavy loads • Using hand tools	Moderate	Moderate Glycolytic: 30-120 s
Oxidative	• Load carriage • Stair climb • Crawl/search • Hose operation • Salvage • Overhaul	• Hiking with light loads • Chainsawing • Shoveling • Stacking wood	Low	Long Oxidative: >120 s

Adapted, by permission, from M.G. Abel, K. Sell, and K. Dennison, 2011, "Design and implementation of fitness programs for firefighters," *Strength and Conditioning Journal* 33(4): 31-42.

Common Tasks for Structural Firefighters

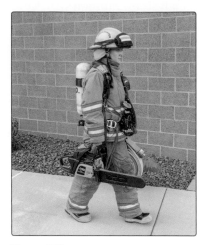

Figure 17.1 Structural firefighter carrying equipment.

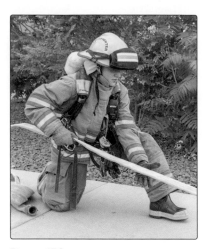

Figure 17.2 Structural firefighter completing a kneeling hose pull.

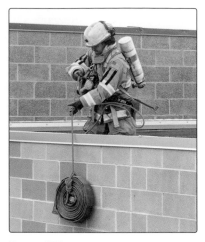

Figure 17.3 Structural firefighter performing a hose hoist.

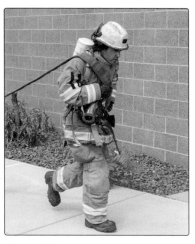

Figure 17.4 Structural firefighter performing an upright hose pull.

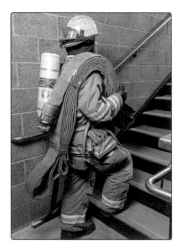

Figure 17.5 Structural firefighter performing a stair climb with a hose bundle.

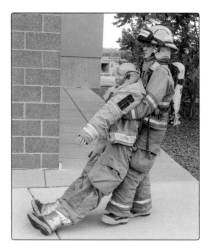

Figure 17.6 Structural firefighter performing a victim drag.

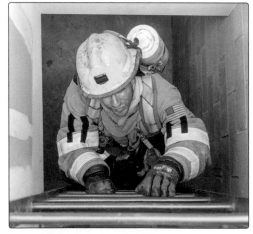

Figure 17.7 Structural firefighter gaining access through a scuttle hatch for roof operations.

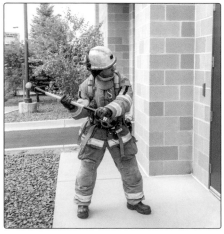

Figure 17.8 Structural firefighter performing a forcible entry using a sledgehammer.

Common Tasks for Wildland Firefighters

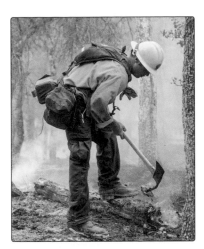

Figure 17.9 Wildland firefighter building a fire line with a Pulaski hand tool.

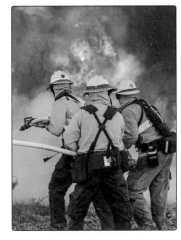

Figure 17.10 Wildland firefighter operating a hose line in arduous conditions.

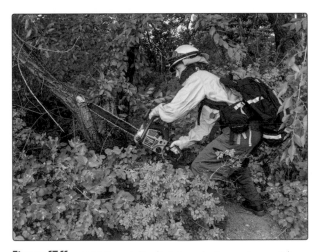

Figure 17.11 Wildland firefighter chainsawing with load.

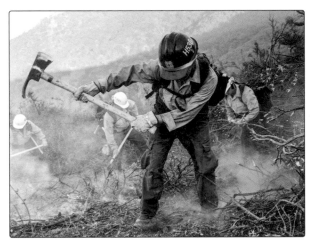

Figure 17.12 Wildland firefighter with pack in personal protective equipment.

shroud, and **self-contained breathing apparatus (SCBA)** (79, 81, 83, 89) (figure 17.1). For structural firefighters, the PPE and SCBA weigh approximately 22 kg (49 lb). SCBA packs with a carbon filter typically weigh 9.5 kg or 21 lb, although this may vary depending on whether a 30-, 45-, or 60-minute cylinder is used; other PPE weigh approximately 11 kg (24 lb) depending on differences in design and material (83). Wildland firefighters must carry their own supplies for the work shift in a gear pack. These packs typically weigh 10 to 22 kg (22-49 lb) with water, safety equipment, and any required special items. Along with their standard pack, wildland firefighters carry chainsaws (11 kg, or 24 lb), extra water

(18 kg, or 40 lb), extra fuel (7-22 kg, or 15-49 lb), and other firing devices (7 kg, or 15 lb). All gear and body weight for a 20-person crew must be below 2,320 kg (5,115 lb), which equates to a maximum of 25 kg (55 lb) of gear per person (89). However, several pieces of equipment that must be lifted or maneuvered can weigh up to 40 to 45 kg (88-99 lb) (e.g., hose packs, water bags) (110). The positioning of PPE may also vary depending on the firefighting discipline.

PPE are designed to protect the wearer from environmental hazards, but there must be a trade-off with internal hazards, primarily heat stress produced by the body. An important consideration that affects the metabolic demands of firefighting

Table 17.2   Biomechanical Analysis of Fireground Tasks and Suggested Exercises to Enhance Task Performance

Task	Muscle and joint action	Plane of motion	Exercise
Stair-climbing with hose pack, hiking with load	• Isometric contractions of rectus abdominis, obliques, and transversus abdominis • Static scapular retraction • Static shoulder abduction and elbow flexion • Unilateral hip, knee, and ankle extension	Sagittal	• Lunge with unilateral kettlebell • Step-up with unilateral kettlebell
Hose hoist	• Isometric contractions of rectus abdominis, obliques, and transversus abdominis • Hip and trunk flexion and extension • Scapular protraction and retraction • Unilateral horizontal shoulder abduction and elbow flexion	• Sagittal • Frontal • Transverse	• Upright unilateral cable or kettlebell row • Good morning • Glute-ham raise
Walking hose pull	• Isometric contractions of rectus abdominis, obliques, and transversus abdominis • Static scapular retraction and elbow flexion • Unilateral hip, knee, and ankle extension	Sagittal	• Sled pull • Split squat • Plank
Kneeling hose pull	• Isometric contractions of rectus abdominis and transversus abdominis • Scapular protraction and retraction • Horizontal shoulder abduction and elbow flexion • Isometric contractions of hip and knee	Transverse	• Kneeling unilateral cable row • Hip hinge • Back extension
Equipment lift and carry	• Isometric contractions of rectus abdominis and transversus abdominis • Static scapular retraction • Unilateral hip, knee, and ankle extension	Sagittal	• Farmer's walk • Deadlift
Ladder raise	• Hip flexion and extension • Static scapular retraction • Shoulder flexion with elbow extension	Sagittal	• Turkish get-up • Lunge with unilateral dumbbell shoulder press
Forcible entry, tree felling, digging fire line	• Dynamic contractions of rectus abdominis, obliques, and transversus abdominis • Static scapular retraction • Hip and shoulder rotation with elbow extension	• Transverse • Sagittal	• Wood chop • Sledgehammer swing on tire
Search	• Isometric contractions of rectus abdominis and transversus abdominis • Contralateral shoulder and hip flexion and extension	• Sagittal • Frontal	Quadruped progression
Victim drag	• Isometric contractions of rectus abdominis, transversus abdominis, and erector spinae • Static scapular retraction, shoulder flexion, and elbow flexion • Unilateral hip, knee, and ankle extension	Sagittal	• Tire drag • Split squat • Reverse lunge with kettlebell
Breach and pull	• Isometric contractions of rectus abdominis, transversus abdominis, and erector spinae • Shoulder flexion and extension • Extension and flexion of ankle, knee, and hip	• Sagittal • Frontal	• Lat pulldown • Dumbbell front raise • Back squat

Adapted, by permission, from M.G. Abel, T.G. Palmer, and N. Trubee, 2015, "Exercise program design for structural firefighters," *Strength and Conditioning Journal* 37(4): 8-18.

tasks is the weight of the PPE and ventilatory limitations presented by the SCBA. For instance, Dregar et al. (32) and Dorman and Havenith (31) demonstrated that oxygen uptake is significantly higher while working at submaximal intensities in PPE with an SCBA versus in exercise clothing. In these studies, aerobic capacity decreased by 17% and 12%, respectively, while working at maximal levels in PPE with an SCBA versus in exercise clothing. Although carrying the external load of PPE and an SCBA increases the metabolic demands of work (42, 115), it appears that the resistance of breathing through the respirator and impairment of thoracic excursions caused by the SCBA harness may also promote decrements in aerobic capacity (32, 34).

In addition, the **load carriage** associated with the PPE (including SCBA for structural firefighters) may affect gait mechanics, balance, mobility, fatigue, movement patterns, and injury risk (58, 92, 117, 118). During a functional balance test (simulating firefighting movements such as crawling and walking on uneven ground) of firefighters with an average of five to six years of experience, wearing PPE decreased balance (especially in the presence of an overhead obstacle), decreased performance time, and increased errors during the test (e.g., contacting a rigid obstacle, placing a hand on the ground to maintain body control) (60). PPE may affect balance by altering center of gravity (dynamic shifts in weight during body movement), imposing an increased and bulky load, and limiting both mobility and peripheral vision (SCBA face mask) (60, 119).

The heavier boots worn by both structural and wildland firefighters may negatively influence gait mechanics by increasing rate of fatigue, restricting foot pronation and normal foot motion, and increasing flexing resistance and gait instability. Research suggests that the altered gait performance may increase risk of movement errors, foot misplacements, slips, trips, and falls and consequently increase risk of injury (92, 103). The magnitude of this impact on gait and metabolic cost is influenced by the type and weight of boot, as well as the weight of the air pack and other PPE (92, 103, 119). For example, research suggests that firefighters wearing heavier boots have an increased metabolic cost (typically 5%-12% greater cost for every 1 kg [2 lb] increase in boot weight) and are more likely to trip over obstacles (24).

Key Point

> Structural and wildland firefighters face different physiological, biomechanical, and occupational demands that may influence physical fitness programming.

ENVIRONMENTAL, OCCUPATIONAL, AND EXPOSURE CONCERNS

Many environmental factors may affect firefighter health and performance, including thermal stress (hot or cold), variable terrain, noise and air pollution, altitude, and of course fire. Given that firefighters respond to emergency situations regardless of the weather, it is important to understand how these factors affect physiological responses, work efficiency (e.g., physical training emphasis), and firefighter safety (e.g., appropriate recovery).

Thermal Stress

Thermal stress is one of the primary environmental factors that structural and wildland firefighters experience on a regular basis. Thermal stress may be created by the increased metabolic demand of contracting muscles during physical work, increased heat storage due to PPE, and ambient heat produced by the fire or weather (116). Not surprisingly, the magnitude of exercise and thermal strain may also vary depending on proximity to the fire line and responsibilities during a fire assignment. Previous research has recommended an exposure time of no more than 25 minutes when suppressing fire in temperatures of 100 °C (212 °F) and thermal radiation limits of 1 kW/m, and further time limitations have been proposed for temperatures above these limits (46). In the western United States, the typical fire season is May to September. The ambient conditions during western wildland fires may include temperatures above 32 °C (90 °F) and can be over 100 °C (212 °F) with relative humidity below 20%.

Cold thermal stress can also present physiological challenges to structural and wildland firefighters. What constitutes extreme cold ambient temperatures will vary across regions and may depend on the acclimatization of the firefighters in a given region. Firefighters are at risk for **hypothermia** (body temperature below 95 °F [35 °C]), frostbite, chilblains, and trench foot when operating in colder ambient temperatures and wet conditions (54). Cold, dry air also increases the risk of dyspnea. Given the risk of exposure to hazardous conditions, firefighters must wear the appropriate PPE during operations, whether in cold or hot ambient conditions. Although PPE is designed to protect the firefighter from heat stress, the clothing may increase the risk of cold stress when wet, especially if the clothing under the turnout gear is drenched with sweat (54). Severe hypothermia can increase fatigue, decrease coordination, and impair judgment (7, 23), which can have fatal consequences for a firefighter.

Physiologically, humans respond to cold exposure with an increase in heat production through a shivering response. Additional physiological responses include vasoconstriction of peripheral blood vessels to redirect blood flow to internal organs (decreasing blood flow to the limbs), as well as increases in oxygen consumption, HR, SV, cardiac output, and blood pressure (23, 134).

Thermal Balance Equation

Heat balance is critical in maintaining physiological function. During work, over 70% of potential muscle energy is given off as a heat by-product (19). This exothermic reaction can produce up to 400 kilocalories of heat per hour during typical firefighting tasks (110). The storage of heat during physical work can be examined by the components in the following thermal balance equation (50):

$$S\ (W \cdot m^{-2}) = M \pm W - E \pm K \pm C \pm R$$

where S = heat storage, M = metabolism, W = mechanical work produced by the body, E = rate of heat loss due to evaporation, K = conduction, C = convection, and R = radiation.

Factors Contributing to Thermal Balance

Metabolism appears to have the greatest effect on increasing body temperature during exercise, whereas evaporation is the primary method for decreasing body temperature (50). When thermal balance is achieved, heat storage is zero. This is an optimal situation because the amount of heat produced is equal to heat lost. Significant correlations have been found between percent body fat, metabolic rate, and HR in firefighters performing physical activity in PPE (8). Increased levels of body fat increase potential heat storage, especially when exposed to hot ambient conditions, because body fat serves as an insulator, impeding heat dissipation (8).

PPE decreases the ability of the body to decrease heat storage (see the box titled "Effects of Multiple Layers . . ."). The addition of clothing PPE can increase heat storage depending on the physical properties of the clothing material and its ability to dissipate heat. As important as PPE is as a barrier between the external environment and the firefighter's body, it creates an internal environment in which sweat pools on the skin and collects on the protective gear, therefore decreasing the body's ability to dissipate heat (23, 25). The partial pressure of water increases when water vapor is not able to dissipate through clothing (45, 90). This increase in partial pressure decreases the ability of sweat to evaporate off the skin and lower skin and body temperature. Skin temperature can act as a regulator of exercise (106), and therefore allowing sweat to evaporate from the skin to maintain a moderate temperature is critical for maintaining performance.

Thermal stress increases the demands placed on the cardiovascular system. Specifically, there is a competing demand for blood flow between the contracting skeletal muscles and through vasodilation of cutaneous blood vessels attempting to dissipate heat (116). Profuse sweating decreases blood plasma volume, which decreases venous return and subsequently SV (116). Likewise, warm thermal stress causes a redistribution of blood flow to cutaneous vascular beds and also reduces SV. Thus, perspiration and redistribution of blood flow—independently or collectively—may decrease SV and consequently increase HR in order to maintain cardiac output (116). Increases in core temperature have been noted during short-term and repeated exposures to fire suppression activities. Romet and Frim (102) evaluated active firefighters for 24 minutes in a burning structure and noted a 1.3 °C (2.3 °F) increase in core temperature as well as HRs above 150 beats/min. Horn et al. (59) demonstrated average core temperature increases of 1.9 °C (3.4 °F) during repeated bouts of firefighting activity over a 3-hour period, even with breaks greater than 30 minutes. Negligible increases in core temperature occur in firefighters working outside the burning structure (102). If the thermal stress remains and physical effort continues, the increases in HR to maintain or increase cardiac output will no longer be sufficient if SV is compromised. Ultimately, these factors increase cardiovascular and thermoregulatory strain, which may increase the risk of **hyperthermia** (body temperature greater than 99.9 °F or 37.7 °C) and heat illness, especially in a hypohydrated state (**hypohydration** occurs when there is insufficient water in the body) (86).

Effects of Multiple Layers of PPE on Physiological Heat Stress

A study completed at the University of Montana Human Performance Lab tested the effects of single versus multiple layers of PPE used in wildfire suppression. The study reported that after 3 hours of exercise in a heat chamber (38 °C [100 °F], 30% relative humidity), there was a significant increase in body temperature between the two types of single layers (SL-I, SL-II) and the double (DL) layers. During the double-layer trial, five out of the nine subjects had to be removed due to core temperature reaching 40 °C (104 °F) (28). Firefighters must take precautions to reduce the impact of heat-related stress during occupational assignments and training, including physical training (30).

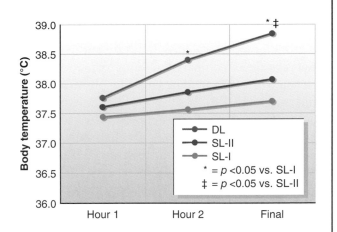

Figure 17.13 Effects of single and multiple layers of PPE over time in a heat chamber.

Tactical Considerations and Countermeasures

In addition to ambient conditions (e.g., windchill, air temperature, humidity), research suggests that several factors increase the risk of both heat and cold stress in firefighters, including improper attire, exhaustion and fatigue, lack of physical conditioning, and predisposing factors such as hypertension, diabetes, and asthma. For example, higher aerobic fitness levels may attenuate the negative effects of hypohydration on cardiovascular responses when exercising (76). Merry et al. (76) demonstrated that aerobically trained subjects experienced significantly less HR drift than untrained subjects during a 40-minute cycling bout at 70% of $\dot{V}O_2$peak. Furthermore, firefighters with higher levels of aerobic fitness may be able to acquire and sustain the benefits of heat **acclimatization** (23). Although different people will adapt at varying rates of acclimatization, research suggests that most will acclimatize after 10 to 14 days of consecutive heat exposure (16). Therefore, it would be beneficial to build in an acclimatization period before the fire season for wildland firefighters or following a period away from firefighting. In addition, given the aforementioned research suggesting that firefighters with higher aerobic capacity may tolerate thermoregulatory strain (heat and cold stress) more readily than firefighters who are less fit, training to improve aerobic fitness is important in helping to maintain thermal balance.

If firefighters have experienced thermal stress, the TSAC Facilitator may need to modify or postpone conditioning practices, because the firefighters' work capacity may be reduced and they may need to be monitored for adverse signs or symptoms. For example, as a result of the physiological response to cold ambient conditions, power output may be reduced, and insulation strategies such as layered clothing may increase energy expenditure. Combined with the increased need for urination during cold conditions, firefighters may be at increased risk of fluid loss and dehydration. Consequently, TSAC Facilitators should be aware of any risk management plans within the department to reduce the incidence of heat or cold stress injury, and they should recognize that overall physical conditioning may need to be reduced until the firefighters have been cleared to return (22, 54).

Altitude

Altitude provides a unique environmental challenge, especially to wildland firefighters. The decreased barometric pressure, particularly the partial pressure of oxygen, reduces the pressure gradient that aids in the binding of oxygen to hemoglobin. This produces a decreased saturation of arterial oxygen levels. As a result, performing tasks at submaximal levels at altitude, especially over 5,000 feet (1,524 m; considered low to moderate altitude), increases ventilation rate and HR while decreasing SV compared with performance at sea level (75, 110). At high levels of physical exertion, maximal HR is reduced (11) due to an increase in parasympathetic activity. After an acclimatization period, red blood cell production increases (polycythemia) to help offset the effects of the reduced barometric pressure (133). Unfortunately, it is not possible to entirely offset the effects of altitude. Therefore, firefighters should acclimate by gradually progressing workloads upon exposure to higher altitudes to avoid decreased performance and risk of altitude-induced illness (110).

Altitude Illness

Acclimatized firefighters working below 5,000 feet (1,524 m) most likely will not experience significant decreases in work capacity. Elevations higher than 5,000 feet (1,524 m), especially for unacclimatized firefighters, may increase the rate of fluid loss and reduce work capacity as previously explained. However, elevations higher than 8,000 feet (2,438 m) may further increase the firefighters' risk of altitude illness (110), especially if they ascend too rapidly (insufficient time to acclimatize) or are inadequately acclimatized prior to ascent. Illnesses associated with high altitude include acute mountain sickness (AMS; fatigue, headache, lack of appetite), pulmonary edema (HAPE; fluid accumulation on the lungs and brain), cerebral edema (HACE), and retinal hemorrhage (HARH; causes irreversible visual defects). AMS symptoms often appear several hours after initial exposure, and rest and gradual acclimatization to reduce the chances of reoccurrence is recommended. HAPE, HACE, and HARH are all life threatening and require immediate descent to a lower altitude, supplemental oxygen, and medical attention (20, 23).

Tactical Considerations and Countermeasures

Reports suggest that there is an increased risk of death or injury during physical training when acclimatization is lacking and instructors or trainers are undertrained (36). Acclimatization should be built into the program. Research suggests that acclimatization should follow a rate of one week of training per every 1,000 feet (305 m) above 5,000 feet (1,524 m) in elevation (110). Firefighters can accomplish this by living at similar altitudes in which they may be operating, sleeping in barometric chambers or tents ("live high, train low" approach), or using resistive breathing devices to assist with training (33). People who have increased fitness tend to acclimatize quicker, have greater tolerance for hot and humid conditions and physical effort, and thus have decreased risk of heat illnesses (30). However, depending on whether the firefighter has been exposed to the working environment (heat, humidity, altitude), acclimatization may or may not have occurred (especially if the employment is seasonal or contractual), which will have implications for the person's work capacity in the field and in the training room and should be accounted for in the program.

Even an acclimatized firefighter who has been operating at elevated altitude may need more rest before engaging in further exertion, such as physical conditioning, due to greater fatigue compared with operating at low altitude. TSAC Facilitators should also be aware that working at higher altitudes may influence dietary needs (e.g., higher carbohydrate intake, increased need for fluids), which may further influence the timing of any planned physical training (111). Therefore, physical conditioning should be encouraged but under the supervision of a TSAC Facilitator, who can help make any necessary modifications to the program (including recommending rest) given the status of the individual firefighter.

Key Point

Acclimatization to the environmental conditions (e.g., altitude, hot ambient conditions) in which firefighters are operating and training may influence work capacity.

Uneven and Slippery Terrain

Wildfires are often located in mountainous regions, where the terrain is unpredictable, may vary across the fire season, and is frequently steep, uneven, and unstable (18, 110). Firefighters responding to structural fires may have to navigate difficult terrain such as narrow passages and uneven surfaces while carrying or operating equipment (67, 81). Regardless of the type of firefighter, navigating unpredictable and slippery terrain may increase the risk of injury. When on fire assignment, wildland firefighters typically sleep on uneven ground in either large fire camps with other resources (e.g., caterer, shower unit) or in small crews with minimal resources (usually what is in their pack or vehicles). Sleeping on this type of terrain may interfere with sleep, which may increase physiological recovery time from the previous day of work (110).

Tactical Considerations and Countermeasures

The high number of injuries related to fire suppression activities (17) supports the concept that exercise movement patterns should mimic occupational tasks and movement patterns (2, 47). The majority of strains and sprains experienced by all firefighters occur in the lower extremity (17, 66), suggesting that a major emphasis should be placed on lower extremity movement mechanics, muscular strength, and stabilization. Table 17.3 provides examples of exercise choices related to job tasks. Exercises that necessitate stabilization prior to movement are fundamental to a fitness program emphasizing movement pattern optimization, ankle stability, balance, and injury risk reduction. Furthermore, these exercises help optimize neuromuscular facilitation, movement efficiency, postural control, and force production through the entire kinetic chain, and they decrease the risk of compensatory movement mechanics, thus decreasing the risk of injury. This may not necessitate an isolated stability or core training program. Although exercise machines are useful for developing confidence and generally place

Table 17.3   Indoor and Outdoor Resistance Training Exercises Arranged by Fireground Task

Task	Indoor	Outdoor
Walking hose pull	• Deadlift • Squat • Lunge • Step-up	Weighted sled pull—forward, backward, lateral
Ladder raise	• Lunge with dumbbell shoulder press • Overhead squat • Turkish get-up	• Ladder raise • Squat with overhead medicine ball throw • Walking dumbbell lunge with dumbbell shoulder press
Equipment carry	• Lunge with dumbbell • Step-up with dumbbell • Dumbbell farmer's walk	Farmer's walk with 5 gal (19 L) buckets of water or sand
Victim drag	• Deadlift • Squat	• Mannequin drag • Tractor-tire drag
Stair climb with hose	• Deadlift • Squat • Lunge with barbell	• Stair-climbing with weighted vest or hose • Tractor-tire flip
Hose hoist	• One- or two-arm dumbbell upright row • Dumbbell bent-over row	Weighted hoist from tower
Search	Crawl with weighted vest	Crawl with weighted vest
Breach and pull	• Cable pulldown with straight bar • Upright dumbbell raise • Lat pulldown • Pull-up	Pull-up
Forcible entry	Cable/resistance band wood chop	Sledgehammer swing on tire
Kneeling hose pull	• One-arm kneeling cable row • One-arm bent-over dumbbell row	Hand-over-hand kneeling weighted hose or sled pull
Hose operation	Large-rope stability exercises	Large-rope stability exercises

Reprinted, by permission, from M.G. Abel, T.G. Palmer, and N. Trubee, 2015, "Exercise program design for structural firefighters," *Strength and Conditioning Journal* 37(4): 8-18.

less stress on the body, free weight and closed chain structural exercises may also bring about increased neuromuscular activation through the kinetic chain (14). In table 17.3, many of the exercises that partially or fully resemble common tasks are closed chain structural exercises requiring some degree of spinal loading and stabilization.

Hazardous Exposures

In addition to fire suppression, firefighters may be called upon to respond to emergency situations involving unknown agents, hazardous or industrial material spills, or conditions with poor air quality, such as vehicle fire suppression (43, 84, 108). Despite wearing an SCBA and PPE, firefighters may still be exposed to "toxic fumes, irritants, particulates, biological (infectious) and nonbiological hazards, and/or heated gases" (81). The NFPA estimated that firefighters experienced approximately 25,700 exposures to hazardous situations in 2010 alone (67). Between 2003 and 2006, smoke inhalation at structural fires accounted for 5% of the minor injuries and 3% of the moderate to severe injuries experienced by firefighters (66). Asphyxiation and smoke inhalation were the cause of eight deaths in wildland firefighters between 1999 and 2008 (37), and they accounted for approximately 9% of the injuries experienced at wildfires between 2003 and 2007 (17).

Smoke

Smoke is a by-product of combustion. During complete combustion, natural wood products break down into carbon dioxide (CO_2) and water. However, complete combustion rarely occurs. The main health hazards in wood smoke are carbon monoxide (CO) and particulate matter (PM) (100). Carbon monoxide competes for the same binding site as oxygen on hemoglobin (resulting in carboxyhemoglobin, or COhB, when bound), therefore decreasing the amount of oxygen available to active tissue (19). The hazard of carboxyhemoglobin levels above 5% is increased cardiac output, causing an unnecessary increase in cardiovascular strain (70). Particulate matter may have cardiovascular and pulmonary health consequences after long periods of exposure (10). The levels of exposure during wildfire suppression are typically below OSHA (Occupational Safety and Health Administration) permissible exposure levels (PELs), but about 5% of the time, levels of these hazards are above PELs. The average carbon monoxide exposure during wildfire suppression is 4 parts per million (ppm) (100). This exposure is well below the level required to elicit any dramatic increases in carboxyhemoglobin. However, a recent study of wildland firefighters in Portugal found exposure to gaseous pollutants and PM to be much higher than the recommended limits (78), suggesting that magnitude of exposure may vary from location to location.

Noise

Depending on location and occupational duties, firefighters may be subject to potentially hazardous noise. For example, civilian or active-duty firefighters working in the U.S. Air Force may be regularly exposed to aircraft noise in addition to engine and siren noise (57). Further research is needed to examine the effect of this exposure on hearing loss and work capacity; current research suggests that siren and equipment noise levels are not higher than acceptable guidelines (6, 125).

Tactical Considerations and Countermeasures

The TSAC Facilitator should be able to recognize signs and symptoms of respiratory issues and understand how to modify or postpone planned exercise sessions until symptoms of exposure to particulate matter, carbon monoxide, and other pollutants are no longer present. Acute signs and symptoms may include reduced exercise capacity, increased shortness of breath, unusual coughing, chest tightness, burning or teary eyes, and difficulty breathing during low-intensity activities. The long-term effects of exposure to these hazards may include problems such as atherosclerosis, inflammation, and oxidative stress (87, 112). Acute and long-term effects of exposure to pollutants may also be exacerbated by exercise or physical endeavors (such as firefighting without SCBA). During increased physical exertion, a firefighter demonstrates increases in ventilation, which may also increase respiratory uptake of toxins (112). As with many aspects of programming for firefighters (and other tactical athletes), building a good rapport, as well as communication and trust, between the firefighters and the TSAC Facilitator may also promote willingness on the part of the firefighters to express when they are feeling diminished respiratory function. Be aware that these issues may need to be reported to department health and safety supervisors (87).

Shift Work and Unpredictability of Job Assignment

Structural firefighters typically work in shifts, usually with one day on duty and one or more consecutive days off duty. The on- and off-duty duration (days and hours) may vary across departments and fire duties, but firefighters typically work extra hours responding to emergencies. Seasonal firefighters, such as in some divisions of the U.S. Forest Service (USFS), may also have schedules that mimic shift work but with minimal days away from firefighting duties and any days not in the field spent on base preparing for the next assignment. A wildland firefighter's typical work shift is 12 to 16 hours but can be more than 24 hours during initial attack operations (when firefighters are first suppressing a fire). During large fires, wildland firefighters typically work 14 days, but they may work up to 21 days before having a rest day. The highest energy expenditures are in the afternoon, when the environmental conditions are most arduous, requiring these firefighters to pace themselves throughout the day (56).

For structural firefighters, the unpredictability and complexity of job assignments also makes it difficult to predict the duration of each shift. An emergency response may take several hours or several days. These factors, coupled with the fact that firefighters respond to an emergency situation regardless of the time of day, may add up to an irregular work schedule, disturbance of appetite and digestive processes, disruption in normal sleep patterns, sleep deprivation, and fatigue (7, 74).

Circadian Disturbances

Over 24 hours, physiological variables such as HR, rectal temperature, and oxygen uptake demonstrate rhythmic fluctuations, known as a **circadian rhythm**, thought to be driven by biolog-

ical clocks (20). Circadian rhythms are thought to affect physical performance, and unexpected disruptions to sleep patterns and increased physiological demands placed on the body during the night as a result of shift work may consequently affect work capacity and recovery (110).

Tactical Considerations and Countermeasures

Various governing organizations and departments recommend that structural firefighters be allowed to exercise while on duty to help maintain fitness (84). However, the exercise mode, intensity, duration, and timing should take into consideration the unpredictability of emergency calls and thus the possible need to recover prior to a fire or rescue response. It has been demonstrated that resistance-trained firefighters' simulated work efficiency decreased by 9.6% 10 minutes after a bout of circuit training (five resistance exercises, 10 repetitions per exercise, two rotations of the circuit) (27). Despite the negative effects of exercise-induced fatigue, resistance-trained firefighters still maintained superior work efficiency postexercise compared with untrained firefighters who were not fatigued (27). Similarly, it has been reported that a heavy resistance training session (four working sets of five resistance training exercises, 5RM loads, 2 minutes of recovery between sets) decreased simulated firefighter work efficiency by 7% 10 minutes postexercise. Work efficiency returned to baseline levels by 24 hours postexercise (4).

In summary, resistance training does have a negative impact on simulated work efficiency immediately after exercise, and those deleterious effects subside between 10 minutes and 24 hours postexercise. Based on these findings, it seems reasonable for firefighters to train during low-volume emergency call times or just before the end of a shift; hydrate before, during, and after training; and consume adequate carbohydrate and protein to enhance recovery. Furthermore, to enhance physical fitness while minimizing the negative effects of exercise-induced fatigue, firefighters should use the progression principle and progress conservatively from lower to higher training intensities and volumes. In addition, although regular physical activity may help improve immune function (131), acute strenuous exercise bouts may depress immune function and require longer recovery time (52).

Given the increased risk of and susceptibility to infections, potential compromise in work efficiency and recovery times, and potentially hazardous work environment, this research suggests that the timing of high-intensity exercise bouts needs to be carefully selected, and exercise prescriptions need to be flexible to accommodate reductions in intensity and other programming variables to complement, not compete with, the recovery process. For example, high-intensity resistance training exercise sessions may be more appropriate for off-duty days. Table 17.4 shows a sample training program for a structural firefighter on a one- to three-day shift schedule that attempts to accommodate the potential residual effects of shift-work fatigue and fluctuations in physical work capacity.

INJURY AND ILLNESS RISKS IN FIREFIGHTERS

The following section summarizes current research on several conditions for which firefighters have shown an increased susceptibility. A comprehensive description of medical conditions

that might interfere with job performance can be found in chapter 9 of NFPA Standard 1582 (81). As with the general population, predisposition or vulnerability to these health issues may be influenced by age, gender, prior health, presence of associated risk factors, smoking, lifestyle behaviors, **obesity**, improper use of PPE (e.g., wearing PPE designed for structural firefighting in response to a wildfire), and physical fitness (8, 12, 110). Fire departments with stricter fitness requirements have a lower incidence of cardiac disease (37, 128).

Given the physical demands of firefighting, illness and injury are highly disruptive to job performance. The economic consequences of injury to firefighters can be numerous and may include medical costs, insurance costs, absenteeism and lost productivity, psychological counseling for emotional distress (for those involved in a traumatic incident), and time spent investigating safety concerns and the mechanism of injury.

Cardiovascular Disease or Cardiac Event

Heart attacks have been the leading cause of death in volunteer and structural firefighters for the past two decades (40, 135). Although the number

Table 17.4 Sample Program for a Structural Firefighter on a 24-Hour Work Shift Followed by 72 Hours Off

	Mon On shift	Tues Off shift	Wed Off shift	Thurs Off shift	Fri On shift	Sat Off shift
Warm-up	Off[a]	5-10 min aerobic exercise; dynamic stretching	5-10 min aerobic exercise; dynamic stretching	5-10 minutes aerobic exercise; dynamic stretching	Off[a]	5-10 min aerobic exercise; dynamic stretching
Session		Submaximal workout Examples: • Tempo run <75% max effort • Cross-training (e.g., basketball)	Moderate- to high-intensity circuit training: • Work:rest ratio = 30:30 s (2-3 rotations) • Bent-over rows • Lunges with medicine ball rotation • Push-up • Kneeling sled pull • Chain drag • Dumbbell shoulder press Alternatives:[b] • High-intensity training with compound lifts • High-intensity interval training	Low-moderate intensity (submaximal) workout		Submaximal workout
Cool-down		• Walk 5 min • Static stretching	• Walk 5 min • Static stretching	• Walk 5 min • Static stretching		• Walk 5 min • Static stretching

[a]May need to modify program if department policy allows for exercise on shift (usually 60-90 minutes per shift depending on length).

[b]If firefighter is not experiencing considerable fatigue and has fulfilled necessary prerequisite competencies for intermediate or advanced resistance training.

of on-duty deaths as a result of sudden cardiac death decreased in 2013 compared with previous years, heart attacks accounted for 42% of on-duty deaths from 2009 to 2013 (41). The prevalence of **cardiovascular disease** and cardiac events is higher in on-duty volunteer firefighters relative to their professional counterparts (41, 128). Between 1998 and 2008, sudden cardiac death (due to overexertion, stress, and related medical issues) accounted for the second highest proportion of deaths in firefighters responding to wildfires (i.e., forest, brush, and grass fires) (37). However, these numbers have decreased since then, with all reported on-duty wildland firefighter fatalities in 2013 being the result of other causes (41).

Between 2001 and 2010, 11.3% of all on-duty firefighter deaths (108 deaths) occurred during training-related activities, of which 30 of the deaths (27%) occurred during physical training. Of the 108 training-related deaths, 30 occurred during physical fitness testing, of which 24 were due to sudden cardiac death and 3 were due to stroke (39). These cases included volunteer and professional structural and wildland firefighters (taking the pack test for wildland firefighting qualification) (36). Not surprisingly, the relative employment ratio is much lower for firefighters who have diagnosed heart disease versus those returning from a shoulder, back, or knee injury (107).

Stress and overexertion are the risk factors most highly correlated with both fatal and nonfatal cardiac events in firefighters across all disciplines (17, 37). As previously indicated, active firefighting places a high degree of physical stress on the body (e.g., lifting heavy equipment or light tools for multiple repetitions; experiencing increases in HR, adrenaline, and body temperature), and it requires optimal functioning under stressful situations that involve strategic or tactical decisions that may affect the safety of others. The nature of shift work means that firefighters may also need to respond to an emergency situation from a dormant state (i.e., responding to a firehouse alarm while sleeping). Furthermore, firefighters are often the first professionals on the scene of an emergency, which makes the stressful physical and emotional response difficult to avoid and over time may lead to an accumulation of physiolog-ical and psychological stress (e.g., posttraumatic stress disorder, or PTSD) if no action is taken to mediate its effect on overall wellness. These risk factors have been supported in the literature that has suggested cardiac events are more likely to occur during engagement in on-duty strenuous activities versus nonemergency situations (120). However, firefighters with preexisting hypertension, cardiovascular disease, left ventricular hypertrophy, obesity, and adverse lifestyle behaviors (e.g., smoking, poor fitness) have a higher risk of cardiac incident than firefighters without these predisposing factors (120, 121, 135).

Overweight and obesity rates in career and volunteer structural firefighters have been documented as high as 50% to 70% and 19% to 43%, respectively (68, 99). High percent body fat, body mass index (BMI), and waist circumference, as well as increasing age, may negatively affect simulated fireground performance (77), risk of injury, and absenteeism (65, 98). Of the firefighters suffering sudden cardiac deaths between 1996 and 2012, 63% were obese (135). The odds of filing workers' compensation claims are nearly three times higher for firefighters with a BMI over 30 kg/m² versus those with a normal BMI (69). Baur et al. (12) found that 68% of a large cohort of 768 overweight and obese male career firefighters underestimated their weight categories, a trend that increased by 24% with each BMI unit. This mismatch between perceived and actual body weight may influence the readiness and perceived need to engage in a regular fitness program.

Key Point

Cardiovascular disease risk reduction is an important goal for many firefighter wellness programs given the prevalence of cardiac events and disease in professional and volunteer firefighters.

Heat-Related Illness

As previously indicated, thermoregulation is one of the biggest issues confronting firefighters across all settings, and it has influenced policy on PPE and rehydration practices. Studies have shown that ambient conditions with an elevated heat index can increase the risk of **heat-related illness** (heat cramps, heat exhaustion, and even heatstroke and rhabdomyolysis) during strenuous occupations. A full description of the signs and symptoms can be found elsewhere (86). It is important to remember that heat-related disorders can occur at any temperature or humidity, especially while wearing PPE (16) (figure 17.14). During 2013, 2,080 reported injuries in firefighters were attributed to thermal stress, with 1,385 occurring during fireground assignments and 400 occurring during training (68). It has also been proposed that other injuries related to overexertion, slips, trips, and falls may have been influenced by thermal stress coupled with wearing PPE during occupational tasks (44). Between 1979 and 2011, the NFPA reported seven deaths from heatstroke in firefighters working on wildland fires (38); however, 255 cases of heat- or dehydration-related illness were reported in wildland firefighters between 2000 and 2011 (86). Furthermore, many cases demonstrating early possible symptoms of heat-related illness (e.g., hyperthermia, headaches, nausea) may

go unreported because firefighters believe such symptoms are part of the job and want to avoid punitive repercussions (86).

Heat-related stress is not just a problem during emergency responses. During 1996 to 2005, 3 deaths during physical training were the result of heatstroke (36), and of the 30 firefighter fatalities during physical fitness training between 2001 and 2010, 3 cases were due to hyperthermia (39). As previously indicated, heat intolerance may also increase cardiovascular strain, placing firefighters at increased risk for cardiac issues (116). Heat tolerance and recovery time are affected by multiple modifiable risk factors, such as prior history, known risk factors, physical fitness, and acclimatization to environmental conditions and PPE (35, 108).

The National Institute for Occupational Safety and Health (NIOSH) considers heat-related illness to be a **sentinel health event** (85), suggesting it is a preventable condition that indicates preventative strategies were inadequate (105). Recovery strate-

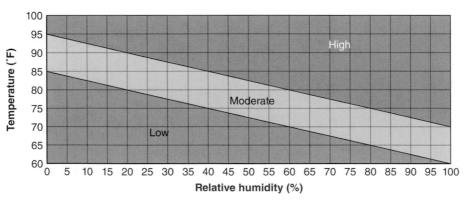

Heat Stress Chart

When heat and hard work combine to drive the body temperature up, the temperature-regulating mechanism begins to fail and the worker faces serious heat stress disorders. This dangerous—often deadly—combination of circumstances can be avoided by monitoring the environment with simple measurements of temperature and humidity. This chart can help alert individuals to dangerous heat stress conditions.

Extreme heat stress conditions. Only heat-acclimated individuals can work safely for extended periods. Take frequent breaks and replace fluids.

Watch for changing conditions. Heat-sensitive and nonacclimated individuals may suffer. Increase rest periods and be sure to replace fluids.

Little danger of heat stress for acclimated individuals. Lack of air movement, high radiant heat, and hard effort can raise danger.

Figure 17.14   Heat stress chart.

Adapted from B.J. Sharkey, 1997, *Fitness and work capacity*, 2nd ed. (Missoula, MT: National Wildland Fire Coordinating Group NFES 1596), 29.

gies such as whole-body precooling and hand and forearm immersion in cold water have been shown to reduce physiological strain in hot ambient conditions with elevated thermal stress (8, 9), but many of these approaches have limited feasibility and take a long time to take effect (130), which limits their application for firefighters looking to sustain work capacity.

Infectious Diseases

Firefighting assignments, especially those related to wildland fires, often necessitate groups of individuals living in close proximity for multiple days. This close proximity coupled with the aforementioned environmental stressors (e.g., dietary changes, physical demands, exposure to toxins) may increase the risk of infection and disease (74, 81). In 2010, the NFPA estimated that volunteer and structural firefighters had approximately 11,200 exposures to infectious diseases (67).

Musculoskeletal Injuries

Injury rates vary depending on departmental responsibilities and the nature of the emergency response (e.g., fire suppression versus medical emergency or nonfire response) (17). However, the NFPA estimates that close to 71,875 firefighter injuries occurred in the line of duty during 2010 (67) and 65,880 in 2013 (68). Often these numbers are based on survey data that may not include injuries reported to certain federal or state agencies (66). This section summarizes many of the injuries that firefighters have shown an increased susceptibility to during the last few years.

The majority of injuries are minor and may require no or minimal recovery time; however, firefighters are also susceptible to debilitating injuries that may require considerable rehabilitation time (if they are not career ending). The leading injuries in all firefighters between 2004 and 2006 are sprains, strains, and muscle pain (128), although the number of injuries has fluctuated over the last 10 years (67). The primary causes of injury on the fireground are overexertion; slips, trips, and falls; and contact with (being struck by) an object (17, 67, 68). However, a significant number of strains and sprains occur when operating, pulling, lifting, or carrying equipment. From 2003 to 2006, 52% of all minor injuries and 51% of all moderate to severe injuries were related to occupational tasks such as handling hose lines or using hand tools (66). The most commonly injured areas between 2003 and 2011 were the leg and foot and the arm and hand, followed by the trunk (including lower back), shoulder, and neck (17, 68). The most common sites for sprains and strains were the lower extremity, followed by the trunk, shoulder, and neck. The most common sites for dislocations or fractures were the arm or hand, leg or foot, and head (66), although these sites may change across firefighting disciplines (17, 18). These findings suggest that injuries are not isolated to one region of the body.

Firefighters had a greater predisposition to strains and sprains (or these conditions were further exacerbated) if they had a prior related condition (127, 128). These preexisting conditions are termed *cumulative trauma disorders* or *ergonomic-related disorders* and may include conditions such as back pain and joint, ligament, or tendon issues such as tendonitis (127). Other contributory factors include fatigue, decreased flexibility or mobility, and biomechanical challenges caused by changes in center of gravity due to PPE and carrying or operating equipment (44, 67, 74). Firefighters may also be susceptible to muscular imbalances, especially those related to strength and mobility (109), possibly as a result of unilateral occupational tasks. During shifts involving many hours of moderate to hard work, or multiple-day assignments involving repetitive fire suppression activities while wearing PPE, firefighters may experience high levels of fatigue. As fatigue increases, attention to detail may decrease, compromising movement patterns and increasing risk of injury from tripping over obstacles or using equipment improperly (74). In addition to fatigue, poor visibility, cold ambient sleeping conditions, and uneven terrain have also affected injury rates during night hours (66).

A recent study found that over a five-year period (2004-2009), approximately one-third of injuries experienced by firefighters and rescue personnel occurred during physical fitness or exercise-related training (96). In this study, many injuries also occurred at the beginning of the work shift, possibly due to the physical training and conditioning that frequently occurred at that time of the day (96).

OPTIMIZING FUNCTIONAL FITNESS

To develop an optimal training program for a structural or wildland firefighter, the TSAC Facilitator must first conduct a needs analysis and determine the physical fitness and health status of the firefighter. Then population-specific training goals that also address individual needs must be established.

Physical Fitness Requirements and Testing

Several assessments of physical job-performance competency are mandatory for firefighters across disciplines, but these are required for candidates only, municipalities that are using it to hire applicants (e.g., CPAT), or prior to seasonal work (e.g., pack test). A full description along with passing criteria for the CPAT and the pack test can be found in the box titled "Physical Fitness Assessments for Firefighters." It is not mandatory to reassess performance on these tests following graduation from the fire academy (for structural firefighters) or during the fire season (for wildland firefighters) unless department policy includes a reassessment protocol. For structural fire departments, the implementation of physical fitness testing, individualized or group training, or physical fitness standards is the prerogative of individual departments. According to the Wellness Fitness Initiative (WFI), a wellness program is meant to "be a positive individualized program that is non-punitive" (63). Although definitive fire-specific recommendations do not exist for all associated physical fitness attributes, it has been reported that the minimum aerobic capacity for performing structural fireground rescue tasks is 38 to 45 ml·kg^{-1}·min^{-1} (51, 91), which is equivalent to 11:40 to 13:30 minutes for 20- to 29-year-old men or women on a 1.5-mile (2.4 km) run (5).

When structural firefighters are performing an aerobic capacity test in exercise clothing, the recommended maximal oxygen consumption may be higher than the minimal recommended level for completion of firefighting tasks. This addition accounts for the attenuation in maximal oxygen uptake due to the PPE and SCBA (32). For wildland firefighters, more specific physical fitness recommendations have been generated for specific divisions of wildland firefighters (110). For example, the third edition of *Fitness and Work Capacity* (110) recommends interagency hotshot crews and rappellers be able to complete the 1.5-mile (2.4 km) run in 10:30 minutes, but smoke jumpers are *required* to complete the same test in 11 minutes. These run times indicate maximal oxygen consumption levels beyond those of the aforementioned wildland firefighter tasks but promote an adequate level of *sustainable fitness*, defined as the workload that can be maintained throughout the day (104, 110). Smoke jumpers are also required to perform seven pull-ups, whereas it is recommended that hotshots and rappellers be able to complete two and four pull-ups, respectively, during a test to fatigue. It is also recommended that all three of the aforementioned crews be able to bench press their body weight and leg press 2.5 times their body weight (110). TSAC Facilitators should be aware of the latest fitness requirements for the firefighting department they are working with (both recommendations or requirements put forth by governing bodies such as the IAFF or NWCG and standards and policies established by individual departments) and keep up to date on the latest publications of testing protocols that accompany these standards.

Resources published by governing organizations will help guide professional practice in working with fire and rescue personnel, and they may enhance collaboration between the TSAC Facilitator and union representatives and fire department administrative personnel. Overall wellness is beneficial for fire and rescue personnel and is well supported by virtually every governing agency in the profession of fire and emergency rescue. The IAFF, IAFC, NVFC, NFPA, and USFS all suggest that a physical fitness program be incorporated in a comprehensive wellness program that includes education on nutritional practices, lifestyle behaviors, psychological well-being, and so on. This may require interaction, teamwork, and collaboration between experts in several disciplines and may include

Physical Fitness Assessments for Firefighters

Candidate Physical Ability Test

The Candidate Physical Ability Test (CPAT) was developed by the IAFC and IAFF in the late 1990s to ensure that candidates meet the minimal requirements for occupational-related physical capability. Tasks in the CPAT include the stair climb, hose drag, equipment carry, ladder raise and extension, forcible entry, search, rescue, and ceiling breach and pull. These tasks are performed in sequence without rest. A pass–fail time has been established at 10 minutes and 20 seconds.

Research on the CPAT indicates that it significantly stresses both aerobic and anaerobic energy systems. On average, oxygen consumption during the CPAT was 36.6 and 38.5 ml·kg^{-1}·min^{-1} for women and men, respectively (132). The high anaerobic demands of the CPAT were evident as participants produced a respiratory exchange ratio (RER = volume of carbon dioxide produced / volume of oxygen consumed) of approximately 1.0 (132). Sheaff and colleagues (113) supported these findings and reported that absolute $\dot{V}O_2$max and anaerobic fatigue were the best predictors of CPAT performance. These findings indicate that people preparing for the CPAT should progressively develop aerobic and anaerobic endurance and muscular strength over a period of weeks to months, depending on initial fitness status.

Pack Test

The pack test was implemented by fire directors of federal agencies to evaluate the muscular strength and aerobic endurance of wildland firefighters in the field. Although the test does not include all job tasks of wildland firefighters (e.g., constructing a fire line with a hand tool, shoveling dirt, throwing dirt, deploying a fire hose, pulling a charged hose, packing a load), it requires that firefighters pack a 45-pound (20 kg) load over a distance of 3 miles (5 km) in 45 minutes or less. It was determined that this single task correlated to the performance of other wildland firefighting tasks, produced a similar rate of energy expenditure compared with overall job tasks (22.5 ml·kg^{-1}·min^{-1}) (111), and predicted a maximal oxygen consumption rate of approximately 45 ml·kg^{-1}·min^{-1} when completed in 45 minutes (123). This value has been used as the fitness standard for wildland firefighters since 1975 (111). A progressive periodized training program focused on aerobic and anaerobic endurance may help prepare for the pack test.

---

working with or serving as a health and fitness coordinator or peer fitness trainer if the department aligns with suggestions in NFPA Standard 1583 and the IAFF-IAFC WFI.

Enhancing Adherence to Fitness-Based Programs

To promote program adherence, a training program must be implemented with population-specific considerations in mind. A comprehensive preparticipation screening should be conducted to identify any potential obstacles to implementation, instances when further evaluation (such as by a physician) may be necessary, and occupational or motivational factors that may influence the frequency and composition of the optimal training program for individual firefighters.

Preparticipation Screening

Preparticipation clearance is imperative in order to address any medical conditions or diseases that may affect the firefighter's ability to safely participate in job-related requirements or a physical training program. Due to the prevalence of cardiovascular disease and stressful job demands, all firefighters should have regular physical checkups (at least annually) with a physician or medical professional, particularly if they have a known disease, prior to starting or significantly changing a physical training program (5, 81). All personnel should also be encouraged to participate in physical fitness testing on a periodic basis to help guide program design, measure progress, and detect changes in health that may affect work capacity. Note that the confidentiality of all medical information must be respected by any medical or training staff, especially given the implications this information may have for meeting job requirements. Each department will need to develop its own preparticipation screening protocols, but examples of preparticipation forms can be found in the guidelines for implementing the IAFF-IAFC WFI (63) and in the *Fitness and Work Capacity* text (110).

Programming Considerations

Fire and rescue personnel may benefit from different approaches to physical training, and therefore the TSAC Facilitator should take a flexible approach to program design to accommodate individual differences and the combination of occupational demands and personal responsibilities that may affect program implementation. Physical fitness programs should be individualized and developed from the results of physical fitness tests and health evaluations. Occupational tasks are multijoint and multiplanar, suggesting the training program should include the entire body and not be isolated to one region.

Motivation

A lack of physical fitness standards may present motivational obstacles to the implementation and continuation of a fitness program within a fire department. Although it is beyond the scope of this chapter to comprehensively explore motivational psychology, note that the operational differences between firefighters may influence the motivation strategies used to promote adoption and maintenance of a fitness program. For example, some settings may have volunteer, career, seasonal, contract, or even active-duty military-commissioned and civilian firefighters working together, all of whom may be motivated to engage in a physical training program for different reasons. Furthermore, departments may often be composed of firefighting crews used to working as a large group (e.g., interagency hotshot crews) or in small groups or partnerships, and consequently they may feel more comfortable training in a group exercise setting or using a teamwork approach to training versus training independently. Furthermore, firefighters may need to address individual barriers (e.g., time constraints,

personal commitments, lack of motivation, inexperience in optimal exercise approaches) as they engage in a functional training program. Although no one motivational approach will work for all firefighters, goal setting (discussed in the next section) based on individual and departmental needs has been recommended as a motivational tool for firefighters.

Training Considerations

Following the preparticipation screening and fitness assessment, long- and short-term training goals need to be established to help drive training program development and implementation. Training goals will influence, for example, which areas of muscular fitness are a priority for a given firefighter and consequently guide the selection of the appropriate load, volume, and exercise selection.

Training Goals

Physical training for firefighters should reflect health and fitness goals specific to individual and occupational needs. The maintenance or improvement of physical fitness in firefighters may be driven by the following objectives:

- Optimize efficiency of occupational tasks and minimize physical strain so that the burden of work does not exceed the physical work capacity of the individual or create undue fatigue that negatively affects subsequent occupational performance.
- Decrease risk of injury.
- Decrease psychological stress and risk of morbidity and mortality.
- Decrease risk of heat-related stress.
- Decrease absenteeism.
- Prepare for occupational physical ability or fitness tests (e.g., CPAT, pack test).
- Increase energy, stamina, and work capacity.
- Decrease risk of chronic diseases.

Program design and goal setting should be guided by a needs analysis that identifies the occupational demands (i.e., metabolic and biomechanical components), personal health-related goals, and common injury and illness risks, as well as any personal, departmental, and environmental considerations that may influence training objectives and compliance (2).

Key Point

Short- and long-term goals may need to be individualized to each firefighter, although several goals (e.g., decrease risk of injury) may apply to everyone. Goal setting helps drive program development, provide motivation, and improve program adherence.

Exercise Selection

The physiological, biomechanical, and occupational needs of firefighters are important to understand when developing programs to improve the physical well-being of firefighters, particularly when selecting exercises that have a high degree of specificity to the job tasks. Table 17.2 suggests exercises with movement patterns similar to actual occupational tasks for structural and wildland firefighters. These exercises are meant to provide a foundation for an appropriate training program; additional exercises should be included to create a comprehensive training program and provide a movement progression dictated by the technical proficiency of each firefighter. Additionally, recent research supports the use of common equipment found in a firehouse versus conventional exercise equipment for resistance-based exercises as part of a supervised training program—for example, using foam buckets as resistance during farmer's walks, placing a bundled hose line on the shoulder while lunging, or wearing an SCBA while performing squats, lunges, step-ups, and so on. (93).

Muscle imbalances and lack of muscular strength or endurance increase the likelihood of injury as a result of compensatory movement patterns that put additional stress on one or more muscle groups (3, 64). This may be related to physical fitness levels, but occupational tasks (such as those in table 17.2) that necessitate unilateral or bilateral rotational movements involving disproportionate force generation or stabilization, heavy loads, or excessive vibration may predispose people to muscle imbalance or immobility. Muscle instability, imbalance, or weakness may also be associated with increased likelihood of acute and chronic muscle-related injury (71). Long work hours coupled with poor flexibility or weakness in the hamstrings and low back may further magnify muscle tightness during the wildfire season (110). Corrective exercises may help correct imbalances and instabilities, and they may even be incorporated in a preparatory (prehabilitation) routine to activate the targeted muscles and patterns of activation during the warm-up. However, to optimize the benefits of training using many of these job-specific movements, any prerequisite competencies must be demonstrated (e.g., ankle, knee, and hip stability), and correct form must be demonstrated to avoid increasing the risk of injury.

Work-to-Rest Cycles

Work-to-rest cycles for resistance training or aerobic and anaerobic conditioning should be influenced by the training goals and targeted metabolic systems. As discussed previously, structural and wildland firefighters frequently engage in tasks that use the phosphagen system (e.g., ladder raise, forcible entry), glycolysis (e.g., load carriage, victim rescue), and oxidative phosphorylation (e.g., hose operation, hiking with load, stair-climbing) (2). Therefore, a training program for firefighters is likely to include programming that targets each of these pathways. As discussed in previous chapters, the training emphasis—along with factors such as the training status of the firefighter—will influence the recommended work-to-rest ratios. For example, an activity that is targeting the anaerobic pathways may be sustained for 15 to 30 seconds or 1 to 3 minutes, for which a work-to-rest ratio between 1:3 and 1:5 is recommended. On the other hand, activities sustained for greater than 3 minutes (with a work-to-rest ratio of 1:1-1:3) will stress the oxidative pathway to a greater extent (53). The TSAC Facilitator needs to carefully plan a firefighter's training program to incorporate approaches that target the necessary training emphases while also minimizing an interference effect that results in training decrements in one area while improving fitness in a second area of metabolic conditioning or fitness (48, 72) (see discussion later in the chapter).

Program Progression

As with any training program, the TSAC Facilitator must ensure that firefighters demonstrate the prerequisite capabilities before adopting or progressing a training program. This may include demonstrating specific lifting competencies (e.g., bench press body weight before engaging in upper body plyometrics) or simply demonstrating good form on an exercise before load is increased (53). As with sport athletes, program progression can be accomplished in many ways, such as adding load, frequency, volume, or intensity; increasing the complexity of an exercise (e.g., adding rotation to an exercise performed previously in the sagittal plane); or decreasing stability during the exercise (e.g., going from a wide-stance squat to a split squat) (2). For firefighters, the rate of progression, as well as the duration and intensity of an exercise or training session, may need to be modified or planned based on the unpredictability of job demands. For example, if structural firefighters are on successive callouts throughout their 24-hour shift, it may not be wise for them to conduct a training session during that shift, given the high levels of fatigue they experience from the job demands. This may require modification of a training program that had scheduled the firefighters to exercise that day. Fire department policy concerning on-duty training may also affect the frequency of training sessions (2), and the training goals for both structural and wildland firefighters will influence the intensity prescribed for aerobic conditioning and resistance training. These factors should also be individualized to meet the health and job-related goals of each firefighter. See chapters 9 and 10 for a full description of how to prescribe duration and intensity to meet training goals.

Periodization

Periodization may work well for fire or rescue personnel who have specific goals in mind or are on a seasonal schedule. (A comprehensive discussion of periodization can be found in chapter 10.) Figures 17.15, 17.16, and 17.17 outline sample traditional and block periodization training plans for a wildland or structural firefighter. Table 17.5 provides a breakdown of possible microcycles

that could be extended from figures 17.15 and 17.16. Although these would need to be adapted for specific firefighters or departments, table 17.6 provides a sample weeklong program for a wildland firefighter (extending from the periodization model in figure 17.16), and table 17.7 provides the same for a structural firefighter candidate; both focus on anaerobic endurance. In table 17.6, the program includes strength training specific to the occupational demands of firefighting. High-volume (high-repetition) training is performed after the aerobic endurance training. High-intensity activities are performed on days that tax the glycolytic systems. In table 17.7, the days that target the development of high-intensity anaerobic endurance (i.e., glycolytic stress) are followed by low-intensity aerobic work that is used as a compensation activity. The goal is to develop the ability to buffer lactic acid production and remove it quickly, inducing a faster recovery rate. In this example, days that follow HIIT are always followed by compensation training days and activity designed to enhance recovery. Strength and power training days would be incorporated toward the end of the preparatory phase.

Aerobic fitness has important implications for health (e.g., risk of illness) (13), job performance (e.g., physical work capacity), and recovery. It also forms a sound foundation from which to further develop other areas of fitness. As observed in the sample training programs in figures 17.15 and 17.16, aerobic endurance is important to establish in the early stages of a training program. In figure 17.15, aerobic endurance is developed in the transition and early preparation phases (one to three months). This can be achieved with uniform and steady-state methods, such as tempo runs at moderate intensities emphasizing sustained effort for a set period of time (e.g., 30, 45, or 60 minutes), or with more challenging approaches such as interval and LT training. Depending on training goals and status, specific endurance training may be necessary. This type of training coincides with the precompetitive and competitive phases in figure 17.15. The appropriate training method depends on the bioenergetic characteristics of the activity and the individual needs of the tactical athlete. For example, wildland firefighters may consider hiking on unstable terrain and gradually

Table 17.5 Sample Traditional Periodization, Undulating Periodization, and Circuit Training Microcycle Models for Firefighters

	Training goal	Frequency (days/week)	Intensity (% 1RM)	Reps	Sets	Rest period (s)	Mode
Traditional (linear) training program							
Microcycle 1	Hypertrophy	2-3	67%-85%	6-12	3-6	30-90	Machine and free weights
Microcycle 2	Strength	2-3	≥85%	≤6	2-6	120-240	Machine and free weights
Microcycle 3	Power/speed	2-3	75%-85%	3-5	3-5	120-300	Free weights and plyometrics
Undulating training program							
Microcycle 1 (workouts 1-4)	Hypertrophy	4 workouts during microcycle	67-75%	10-12	3-6	30-90	Machine and free weights
Microcycle 1 (workouts 5-6)	Strength	2 workouts during microcycle	85%	6	2-6	120-240	Machine and free weights
Microcycle 1 (workouts 7-8)	Power/speed	2 workouts during microcycle	BW (low-moderate intensity)	5	3-5	120-300	Free weights and plyometrics
Circuit training program							
Microcycle 1	Muscular endurance	2-3	65%-67%	12-15	2-3	≤30	Machine and free weights
Microcycle 2	Hypertrophy	2-3	75%-85%	6-10	2-3	20-60	Machine and free weights
Microcycle 3	Strength	2-3	85%	6	2-3	20-60	Machine and free weights

% 1RM = percentage of one-repetition maximum; BW = body weight.

Adapted, by permission, from M.G. Abel, K. Sell, and K. Dennison, 2011, "Design and implementation of fitness programs for firefighters," *Strength and Conditioning Journal* 33(4): 31-42.

Table 17.6 Sample Microcycle (Transmutation Phase) Exercise Program for a Wildland Firefighter With a Focus on Anaerobic Endurance

	Mon	Tues	Wed	Thurs	Fri	Sat	Sun
Training objective	Anaerobic endurance	Anaerobic endurance	Aerobic endurance	Anaerobic endurance	Anaerobic endurance	Aerobic endurance	Rest
	Lower body	Upper body	Maintenance	Lower body	Upper body	Maintenance	
Warm-up	• Run 5 min • Dynamic stretching	• Run 5 min • Dynamic stretching	• Run 5 min • Dynamic stretching	• Run 5 min • Dynamic stretching	• Run 5 min • Dynamic stretching	• Run 5 min • Dynamic stretching	
Session	Circuit • Sled pull • Tire flip • Lunge • Step-up • Hamstring curl • Lateral medicine ball slam	Circuit • Dumbbell chest press • Seated row • Shoulder press (dumbbell) • Wood chop • Rope swing • Back extension	Weighted hike (80% MHR)	Circuit • Sled pull • Tire flip • Lunge • Step-up • Hamstring curl • Lateral medicine ball slam	Circuit • Push-up • Pull-up • Shoulder press (dumbbell) • Turkish get-up • Superman	Weighted hike (80% MHR)	
Cool-down	Walk 5 min	Walk 5 min	Walk 5 min	Walk 5 min	Walk 5 min	Walk 5 min	
Flexibility training	Static stretching	Static stretching	Static stretching	Static stretching	Static stretching	Static stretching	

introducing load such as carrying weight or tools similar to what they do during the fire season.

However, firefighting tasks require contributions from multiple energy systems, both aerobic and anaerobic. Consequently, circuit and interval training that incorporates various tasks of different intensities, as well as distance runs or hikes, may be recommended depending on training goals, fitness status, and fatigue (from callouts or wildfire assignments) (1, 94). For example, when working with a large group of firefighters

simultaneously, a circuit-based training session is a time-efficient approach that provides similar anaerobic stress and comparable (but slightly lower) aerobic stress compared with structural fireground tasks (1).

Injury and Illness Risk Reduction

Given firefighters' increased risk of numerous illnesses, any physical training program should be combined with a comprehensive wellness intervention that incorporates an annual physical

Table 17.7 Sample Microcycle Exercise Program (Realization Phase) for a Structural Firefighter Candidate with a Focus on Anaerobic Endurance

	Mon	Tues	Wed	Thurs	Fri	Sat	Sun
Training objective	Aerobic endurance	Anaerobic endurance	Active recovery	Rest	Anaerobic endurance	Active recovery	Rest
Warm-up	• Run 5 min • Dynamic stretching	• Run 5 min • Dynamic stretching	• Run 5 min • Dynamic stretching		• Run 5 min • Dynamic stretching	• Run 5 min • Dynamic stretching	
Session	Run (80% MHR)	Work:rest 30:30 s (2 rotations) • Upright sled pull • Push-up • Kneeling sled pull • Victim drag • Shoulder press (dumbbell) • Medicine ball rotation	Elliptical (75% MHR)		Work:rest 30:30 s • Tire flip • Medicine ball throw • Bent-over row • Shoulder press (dumbbell) • 3 × 400 m (437 yd) repeats (1:2 work to rest ratio) • Stationary bike 15 min	Elliptical (75% MHR)	
Cool-down	Walk 5 min	Walk 5 min	Walk 5 min		Walk 5 min	Walk 5 min	
Flexibility training	Static stretching	Static stretching	Static stretching		Static stretching	Static stretching	

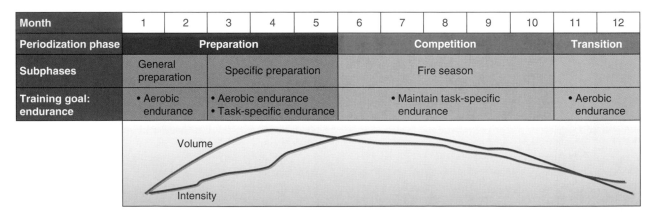

Month	1	2	3	4	5	6	7	8	9	10	11	12
Periodization phase	Preparation					Competition					Transition	
Subphases	General preparation	Specific preparation				Fire season						
Training goal: endurance	• Aerobic endurance	• Aerobic endurance • Task-specific endurance				• Maintain task-specific endurance					• Aerobic endurance	

Figure 17.15 Sample annual traditional periodization model for wildland firefighters.

Provided by Dr. Mark Abel, 2014, *Periodization strategies for firefighters*. Available: http://www.nsca.com/videos/periodization-strategies-for-firefighters.

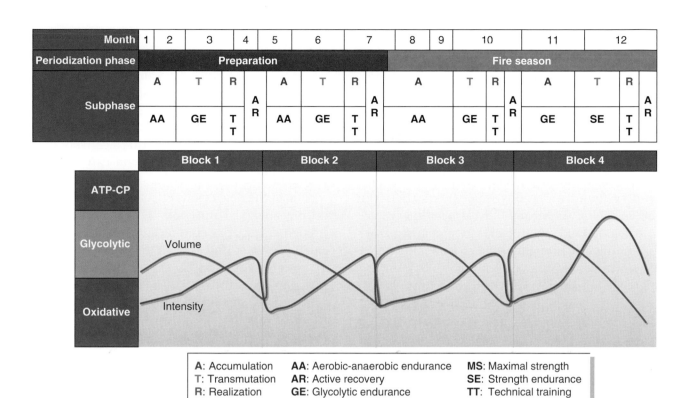

A: Accumulation	AA: Aerobic-anaerobic endurance	MS: Maximal strength
T: Transmutation	AR: Active recovery	SE: Strength endurance
R: Realization	GE: Glycolytic endurance	TT: Technical training

Figure 17.16 Sample annual block periodization model for wildland firefighters.

Provided by Dr. Mark Abel, 2014, *Periodization strategies for firefighters.* Available: http://www.nsca.com/videos/periodization-strategies-for-firefighters.

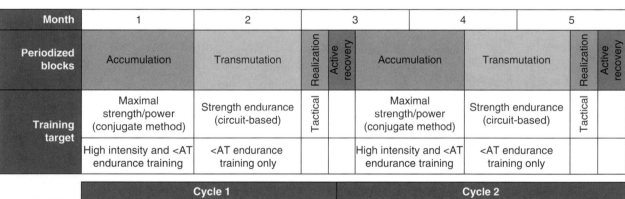

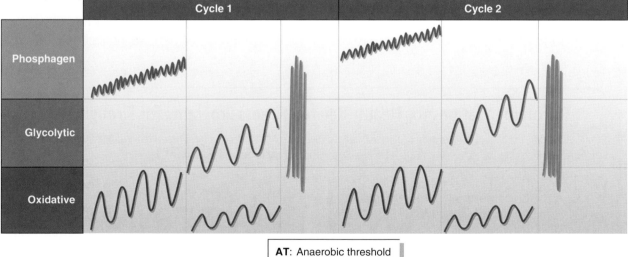

AT: Anaerobic threshold

Figure 17.17 Sample periodization model for structural firefighters (intermediate or advanced lifters).

Reprinted, by permission, from M.G. Abel, T.G. Palmer, and N. Trubee, 2015, "Exercise program design for structural firefighters," *Strength and Conditioning Journal* 37(4): 8-19.

screening to identify health-related concerns and educate the firefighter (and facilitator) about any modifications that should be made to the physical training program (see the box titled "Recommendations for Health-Related Fitness Programs for Firefighters"). Comprehensive guidelines for preprogramming health evaluations and clearance can be found in various NSCA texts (53). The NFPA, NVFC, USFS, and IAFF also outline recommendations and requirements for preparticipation screening and firefighter-related evaluations that cover increased areas of susceptibility during required annual physical exams via various health and safety standards (e.g., NFPA 1582, 1583, and 1051; NWCG's *Fitness and Work Capacity*). In particular, physician clearance is required before returning to duty (including physical training) following an injury or illness that required medical attention or detrimentally affected work capacity (81). These guidelines and requirements recognize the benefits of regular exercise and physical activity for firefighters beyond occupational performance, as well as lifestyle modifications that may improve overall wellness (e.g., smoking cessation, dietary modifications). Physical fitness has numerous implications for managing the physiological and psychological demands of the job.

Recent research suggests that physical well-being is higher in firefighters who have fewer signs or symptoms of depression (21). Mindfulness and resiliency training interventions that apply an integrated approach to physical training and mental toughness may help reduce stress and improve coping in firefighters (114). Physically fit firefighters may have more confidence in their ability to handle stressful situations, decision-making skills, and ability to implement a plan of action (20, 124), especially given the physical nature of firefighting tasks. The TSAC Facilitator should be aware of interventions such as these and the contribution that a collaborative and integrative wellness program can make to firefighter health and fitness.

Due to the deleterious effects of hyperthermia on physiological function, it is important that firefighters practice countermeasures to decrease the risk of heat illnesses on the fireground, after a response call, and during physical training, and stop or modify work (including exercise) if symptoms of heat-related illness persist (110). For example, firefighters may work in pairs and rotate crews to perform fireground tasks to decrease metabolic heat production, an approach that can also be implemented during training. Firefighters should consume fluids with appropriate electrolyte concentrations before, during, and after rehabilitation at the fireground. Reports have shown an increased risk of death or injury during physical training when there was insufficient rest, water was not provided to the exerciser, the trainer failed to recognize the signs and symptoms of injury or illness, or the firefighter was improperly prepared for exercise (e.g., wearing clothing that did not allow sufficient heat dissipation) (36). A TSAC Facilitator should be aware of the hydration status (see chapter 5) and overall preparedness of firefighters before physical training or educate them on the necessary steps prior to training. Wearing proper clothing for training is imperative, as is training in appropriate locations, such as training in an air-conditioned area for rehabilitation. The benefits of acclimatization to

---

Recommendations for Health-Related Fitness Programs for Firefighters

The *NFPA 1583: Standard on Health-Related Fitness Programs for Fire Department Members* (84) suggests that a health-related fitness program should include the following:

1. The assignment of a qualified health and fitness coordinator
2. A periodic fitness assessment for all members
3. An exercise training program that is available for all members
4. Education and counseling regarding health promotion for all members
5. A process for collecting and maintaining health-related fitness program data

thermal stresses and altitude have been discussed earlier in this chapter.

As previously mentioned, TSAC Facilitators should be able to recognize the signs and symptoms of common illnesses and injuries, but they should also be able to identify signs of overtraining syndrome (see chapter 16) and fatigue. Fire and rescue personnel cleared to participate in training may harbor residual effects of various ailments and be susceptible to reinjury, and trainers may subsequently have to work under the direction of a physician or medical health professional. Even though firefighters may be cleared by a physician to rejoin a training program, the facilitator still needs to discuss with them any personal limitations, as well as their specific job requirements, in order to design a safe and functional training regime. Therefore, each program needs to be individualized to meet the firefighter's specific needs. Please refer to chapter 16 for further discussion of this topic.

Regular aerobic exercise may help decrease the risk of cardiovascular disease (e.g., decreases clotting, slows plaque accumulation, strengthens cardiac muscle), improve emotional status, promote a healthy lifestyle, and assist with weight management (5, 128). Higher levels of aerobic fitness have been correlated with a decreased incidence of cardiovascular disease in firefighters, improved lipid profile, and lower blood pressure regardless of BMI levels, but these may improve further with reductions in BMI (13). Research also suggests that firefighters can reduce their risk of injury by up to 14% for every 1 MET (3.5 ml·kg^{-1}·min^{-1}) improvement in aerobic fitness (97).

Additionally, recent research highlights the importance of optimizing aerobic fitness to combat the negative effects of PPE and SCBA on occupational performance (110). The impact of PPE on movement patterns and injury risk is important for the TSAC Facilitator to understand in order to design a conditioning program that helps decrease the elevated risk of injury that comes with wearing PPE. Consequently, facilitators must be aware of changes in PPE use and current guidelines for all firefighters with whom they may be working, especially if firefighters have different responsibilities across changing fire seasons.

PROGRAM DESIGN AND SAMPLE TRAINING APPROACHES

Given the need to individualize training programs, fire and rescue personnel may benefit from a variety of approaches to physical training. The TSAC Facilitator should take a flexible approach to program design to allow for individual differences and the combination of occupational demands and personal responsibilities that may affect program implementation. Physical fitness programs should be developed from the results of physical fitness tests and health evaluations. Occupational tasks are multijoint and multiplanar, suggesting the training program should include the entire body and not be isolated to one region.

Key Program Variables

As suggested earlier in this chapter, many job tasks vary across disciplines. In addition, several other differences may influence the nature of the physical fitness program offered to fire personnel.

Equipment

Fire departments may show considerable disparity in accessibility to fitness training resources, such as equipment and availability of subject experts to help design, implement, and maintain fitness programs. Some departments may have training resources at the fire station, whereas other departments may offer access to a commercial training facility at a reduced cost (especially if the station size does not allow for an on-site training facility). However, some firefighters may not have access to training resources automatically through their fire department affiliation. Firefighters may be able to use equipment found within the fire station (e.g., sandbags, chains, tools) as weights or loads during exercises instead of using commercial exercise equipment (e.g., dumbbells) (84). The advantages and considerations for each approach are summarized in the IAFF-IAFC WFI document (63).

Safety

If training is taking place as part of a department-sanctioned mandatory or optional wellness or fitness program, the department leadership and administration should be consulted to promote communication, collaboration, consistency regarding departmental policies (e.g., time to work out on shift), and resource allotment and to highlight leadership's support. These dynamic variables are important to accommodate in order to design a population-specific, affordable, efficient, safe, and beneficial training program.

Training program supervision or guidance by a trained exercise professional is imperative for optimal prescreening evaluation, safe transition through a training program, and appropriate manipulation of training variables. For example, the program should incorporate education on training practices related to safety (e.g., form) and program benefits.

Oversight

Depending on the department size and setting (e.g., urban or rural, cold or hot climate), as well as the sociological conditions in which the department operates, job responsibilities, biomechanical and metabolic demands, and injury and illness trends may vary considerably. As with many tactical athletes, firefighters may also have multiple demands on their time, which are potentially exacerbated by the recovery time needed following night shifts. Volunteer firefighters (who compose the majority of U.S. fire departments), for example, often have a paid job that occupies a significant amount of their time outside firefighting duties or training.

Numerous fire departments have adopted the 2008 edition of the IAFF-IAFC WFI as the foundation of their wellness and fitness programs, but this is not mandated by either affiliated organization. Although governing agencies (e.g., IAFF, USFS) unequivocally support a wellness program of sorts for all firefighters, the nature of the program is dictated by the administration or departmental leadership and may be influenced by factors such as department size and composition (i.e., seasonal, career, volunteer, or combination) (128). Consequently, fitness program attributes may vary, such as time allowed to work out on shift and amount of financial support for resources (e.g., equipment, education for peer trainers). Fire departments may also have differences concerning personnel responsibilities within

the department, call volume and response roles, leadership and management roles and involvement in training programs, training requirements, union involvement, and interpersonal dynamics between coworkers (88). For example, some departments may have volunteer, career, seasonal, contract, or even active-duty military-commissioned and civilian firefighters working together. Furthermore, departments may often comprise firefighting crews working as a group (e.g., interagency hotshot crews) or as a partnership (e.g., interagency smoke jumpers), which may influence their preferred training environment. These factors will have a significant impact on the feasibility of a training program, access to equipment, motivation, and sustainability.

Program Scenarios

A number of challenges must be considered when designing a training program for structural firefighters. Such challenges include designing a periodized training program that optimizes performance throughout the year (because emergency responses may be unpredictable) yet minimizes risk of overtraining and enhances multiple competing fitness attributes (e.g., aerobic endurance versus muscular strength). Although a traditional periodization scheme may be effective for untrained firefighters or for wildland firefighters who have a defined work season (figure 17.15), it may be less effective for highly trained wildland and structural firefighters or structural firefighters who must respond to unpredictably timed emergencies.

Block periodization is one alternative training strategy that addresses these challenges. Originally designed for Olympic athletes with sporadic competition schedules, it is structured to achieve peak performance multiple times throughout an annual cycle. Block periodization is composed of 5- to 10-week training cycles that allow for frequent evaluation of physiological development. A training cycle is composed of three training blocks, as shown in figure 17.17 (i.e., accumulation, transmutation, realization) (61). Each training block targets a minimal number of fitness attributes to optimize their development. Block periodization is based on sequencing training targets according to their training residuals.

Fitness attributes with longer training residuals are typically stimulated in the accumulation block (e.g., aerobic endurance and muscular strength; 2- to 6-week training phase), fitness attributes with moderate residuals are targeted in the transmutation block (e.g., anaerobic endurance; 2- to 4-week training phase), and fitness attributes with the shortest residuals are targeted in the realization block (e.g., speed and power; 1- to 2-week training phase) (figures 17.16 and 17.17) (61). Therefore, firefighters may optimize development of a fitness attribute during a specified block, but due to the relatively brief block durations, minimal time is spent away from stimulating a given fitness attribute.

In addition, because firefighters must develop most fitness attributes (from aerobic endurance to muscular strength/power) (2), it may be advisable to use complementary training stimuli to improve aerobic endurance and muscular strength throughout the training cycle while minimizing the interference effect. That is, training concurrently for aerobic endurance and muscular strength outcomes has been shown to attenuate strength development (72), and therefore complementary endurance and strength training intensities should be used to minimize this interference effect (48). It appears most efficacious to avoid concurrently training with high aerobic endurance intensities (i.e., >95% of $\dot{V}O_2max$) and moderate resistance training intensities (i.e., 75%-80% of 1RM) (48). Sample resistance training and conditioning microcycles for wildland and structural firefighters that provide suggestions for avoiding the interference effect are illustrated in tables 17.6 and 17.7.

Sample programs to use as templates for developing functional and individualized training programs can be found in the current literature (e.g., 3, 4), NFPA Standard 1583 (84), chapter 8 and appendixes A and C of the NWCG's *Fitness and Work Capacity* (110), and various NSCA texts (8).

CONCLUSION

TSAC Facilitators need to educate themselves thoroughly on the occupational needs of the firefighters for whom they are designing training programs. This increases the likelihood that they will implement exercises and training programs that mimic the movement patterns, train the metabolic needs, and address the areas of injury risk in this population. The TSAC Facilitator also has to consider a multitude of factors in addition to the biomechanical and metabolic needs of occupational tasks. The TSAC Facilitator must become familiar with the firehouse culture and develop effective communication, trust, and collaboration with the firefighters. Program design and implementation must be adaptable to the wide variation in training status throughout a department, the type of training resources that may be available, and the need to prioritize occupational needs and firefighter health over physical training preference. By taking these logistical, sociocultural, and occupational factors into consideration, the TSAC Facilitator will help firefighters manage the occupational demands they face each day and "will protect the most valuable piece of equipment in the Fire Service, the firefighter" (2).

Key Terms

acclimatization
cardiovascular disease
circadian rhythm
heat-related illness
hyperthermia
hypohydration
hypothermia
International Association of Fire Chiefs (IAFC)
International Association of Fire Fighters (IAFF)
load carriage
National Fire Protection Agency (NFPA)

National Volunteer Fire Council (NVFC)
National Wildfire Coordinating Group (NWCG)
obesity
personal protective equipment (PPE)
self-contained breathing apparatus (SCBA)
sentinel health event
structural firefighting
U.S. Fire Administration (USFA)
wellness
wildland firefighting

Study Questions

1. A firefighter must perform activities that use all the energy systems. Which task primarily uses the glycolytic system?
   a. ladder raise
   b. hose hoist
   c. stair climb
   d. victim drag

2. Which of the following exercises is the most beneficial in training a firefighter to raise a ladder?
   a. Turkish get-up
   b. glute-ham raise
   c. farmer's walk
   d. good morning

3. Which of the following increases due to warm thermal stress?
   a. heart rate
   b. stroke volume
   c. blood plasma volume
   d. venous return

4. For structural firefighters who must respond to unpredictably timed emergencies, which periodization program might be the LEAST effective?
   a. nonlinear
   b. sport season
   c. block
   d. traditional

Chapter 18

Physiological Issues Related to Law Enforcement Personnel

Ben Hinton, MSc, CSCS

Sgt. Mick Stierli, BPhysEd, MExSc, CSCS,*D, TSAC-F,*D

Robin Orr, PhD, MPhty, BFET, TSAC-F

After completing this chapter, you will be able to

- describe the physiological and biomechanical occupational demands, injury risks, environmental exposures, and occupational stressors experienced by law enforcement personnel;

- discuss the fitness requirements and recommendations for law enforcement personnel;

- design fitness programs by applying training principles and approaches to improve and maintain fitness in law enforcement personnel across disciplines, subdivisions, professional statuses (cadets versus incumbent), and fitness levels; and

- analyze case-specific and problem-centered scenarios.

The physiological demands of law enforcement have been a polarizing topic for some time. Law enforcement officers are typically sedentary but perform short periods of high-intensity activity, often in life-threatening situations. This chapter addresses physiological issues that TSAC Facilitators should be aware of when working with law enforcement personnel, as well as physical training methods to help mitigate these issues.

CRITICAL JOB TASKS FOR LAW ENFORCEMENT PERSONNEL

The occupational tasks of law enforcement personnel can be unpredictable and highly diverse. These tasks can change daily or even hourly, where, for example, an officer performing desk work may suddenly be called upon to assist with a riot situation or an intoxicated offender in the watchhouse. Given the nature of this work environment, law enforcement personnel face a variety of occupational, physiological, and biomechanical demands.

Occupational Demands

Law enforcement work is complex, and occupational tasks can vary greatly (4, 5, 16, 17, 21, 47, 86, 98). Discrete populations within law enforcement may include police cadets (94), general duty officers (4, 5, 7, 94, 98), traffic officers (47), patrol officers (16, 17, 94), police motorcyclists (47), and specialist units (99). Given this diversity, officers often perform an assortment of occupational tasks. One study investigating the range of tasks officers responded to during their shifts found great variations in the requirements of general duty officers. This study found that the most common occupational tasks completed by 53 police officers were checking bona fides (29%) and responding to domestic disputes (15%); the least common tasks were serving defective-vehicle notices and following up on threatening phone calls (1%) (101). The duration of these tasks also varied greatly, from dealing with theft (mean = 41:28 ± 22:50 min) and persons on premises (mean = 37:13 ± 18:46 min) to responding to domestic disputes (mean = 10:02 ± 02:33 min), driving urgently (mean = 7:45 ± 3:21 minutes), and attending noise complaints (mean = 2:22 ± 2:07 min) (101).

A study investigating officers who spent a long time in their vehicles looked at the tasks performed within the vehicle (68). The study found that, in addition to driving, which made up just over 50% of time in the vehicle, officers also completed paperwork (20% of time) and used a mobile data terminal (approximately 13% of time) (68) while seated in their vehicles.

Within each of these occupational tasks, there is a plethora of physical subtasks. These physical subtasks can range from low-intensity activities such as desk work and general driving to high-intensity activities such as carrying **personal protective equipment** (PPE), running, and jumping (4, 5, 7, 16, 17, 47, 98). Other activities reported by officers include standing, balancing, walking, running, running up stairs, climbing, bending over, squatting, kneeling, lifting, crawling, frisking, dragging, gun loading, wrestling, dodging, and driving urgently (4, 5, 7, 16, 17, 47, 68, 98).

Police officers may typically drive in vehicles and, according to some research, rarely run more than an average of 87 m (95 yd) (range: 5-350 m or 5-383 yd) (5). Anderson et al. (5) acknowledged this; however, the researchers also stated that once the officer gets to the problem, it is necessary to control and remove the problem. Thus, critical incidents observed in the research could last up to 29 minutes. Although the average tasks and requirements of officers are often used as reference, they should be viewed with caution. Consider the example of a police officer who chased an offender a considerable distance on foot across fields and then, when they both became entangled in a fence, fought to retain his weapon as the offender struggled to acquire the firearm (62). Law enforcement officers may be exposed to notable physiological and biomechanical stresses in the range of tasks and the variations in physical subtasks.

Physiological Demands

Considering the diversity of occupational tasks and variations in physical subtasks, it is not surprising that the physiological demands of law enforcement can range from sedentary to highly demanding. Furthermore, the dispersion of less to more demanding physiological tasks may not necessarily be equal. Law enforcement can be a sedentary occupation in general (5, 86). As an example, one study investigating self-reported physical activity during duty hours found that the mean intensity during police shifts equated to the metabolic equivalent (MET) of 1.6, which is essentially equal to sitting (86). This is understandable given the nature of common tasks such as driving a patrol car or doing desk work. However, officers may also have to rapidly respond to situations with dramatically increased physiological demands. Anderson and colleagues (5) suggest that law enforcement work is 80% to 90% sedentary with intermittent points of high-intensity activity. More direct associations between physical requirements and physiological demands can also be seen. When struggling with an uncooperative subject, police officers have been reported to physically push and pull the offender in 93% of incidences, with over 70% of these instances requiring medium to maximal effort (5).

Physiological costs of tasks can be further exacerbated by the external loads law enforcement officers must carry (56). These external loads can range from 7 kg (15 lb) when wearing a general duty belt to around 10 kg (22 lb) or greater when wearing a protective vest (5). This load has been found to decrease officer maneuverability, acceleration, relative strength, and balance while increasing HR, RPE, and oxygen consumption during general and occupational tasks (37).

For specialist police officers, these external loads can be greater. Tactical operations officers, such as **special weapons and tactics (SWAT)** or tactical operations unit (TOU) personnel, may carry loads of around 22 kg (49 lb) consisting of primary and secondary weapons systems, body armor, and communication systems. These loads have been found to decrease mobility (29, 37) and even marksmanship to some degree (26).

Key Point

Heavy loads are an integral part of the police officer's duty belt and PPE. The TSAC Facilitator needs to consider such external loads when conducting a needs analysis.

Occasionally, specialist police officers may be required to perform tasks wearing other forms of PPE, such as **chemical, biological, radiological,** **and nuclear (CBRN) suits**. This form of specialized protective clothing can weigh over 26 kg (57 lb) (19). Not only do these loads impart known physiological loads associated with load carriage, but they also affect thermoregulation (19). When required to perform tasks that included unarmed house entries and crowd control, one study found that not only did HR increase but so did body temperature, and it was body temperature that was a major limiting factor in performance (19). Thermal considerations are discussed later in this chapter.

Although there may be periods of lower intensity or even sedentary work, law enforcement is one of the most stressful and difficult occupations (43). On a daily basis, law enforcement officers experience a broad range of emotionally harrowing events, make decisions under duress, and encounter life-threatening situations, all of which can dramatically alter their physiological state. Examples of situations that may induce a stress-related physiological response include shootings, robberies, and severe motor vehicle accidents (63).

In summary, the evidence suggests that the physiological requirements of law enforcement officers performing daily tasks can range dramatically. Furthermore, these physiological requirements may be influenced by other factors such as stress. Law enforcement officers require the physiological ability to maintain a given task at a low intensity over a period of time and to perform explosively or apply maximal force for short durations.

Biomechanical Demands

One notable concern for the police officer is the need to sustain a posture for a considerable time, most notably sitting in a vehicle. Long periods of sitting and driving in a vehicle are a risk factor for back injuries (13), and the duty belt and protective vest further impede sitting posture (52). The duty belt, for example, has equipment to the rear that may press into the lower back during sitting, causing discomfort and influencing posture (52). Officers may conform to a seated posture that they would not typically select if they were not wearing a duty belt and protective vest (52).

Operating a mobile data terminal within the vehicle (68) further influences movement mechanics. Typically the terminals are to the side of the seat and have little maneuverability (67). Officers have to rotate through their spinal column, already in a compromised position, as well as reach across the body with the arm in order to use the console (67). Although this postural loading may initially be minimal, research suggests that the discomfort felt by officers performing tasks on a terminal while seated increases over time (67).

Key Point

Common activities such as riding in a car can have significant biomechanical implications that the TSAC Facilitator should consider.

Load carriage tasks elicit several biomechanical responses from the body, including changes to the carrier's posture, changes to gait kinematics (e.g., stride length, stride frequency), and changes to ground reaction force (GRF) when walking (8, 56). The most notable changes to posture include increases in forward trunk lean, changes to spine curvature (those who had a small curvature straightened under load, while those with a greater curvature had an increase in curvature), spinal compression, and spinal shearing forces (8, 70, 75). Changes to gait induced by load carriage include changes in the duration of the double-limb support phase, stride length, and stride frequency (55, 59, 84). Finally, GRF has been reported to increase significantly in downward, anteroposterior, and mediolateral directions as the carried load increases (15, 55, 59, 84). These changes to posture, gait, and GRF are influenced by the weight of the load and can increase the potential for injury through increasing spinal and musculoskeletal loads and the total volume of impact forces (15).

Research by Rhea has revealed several biomechanical impacts on task performance when police officers perform specific duties, such as "restraining subjects, close-quarter hand combat, forcible entry, lifting objects and rapidly maneuvering through or around objects" (88). In addition, several observations in this environment are of note. In one observation period, officers were required to perform lifting and dragging movements and physically restrain offenders under the

influence of alcohol and narcotics. These officers were often in poor postural positions enforced by their environment, in this case the size of the watchhouse cells. To maneuver an uncooperative offender through the single-cell doorway, officers were required to twist and reach across their bodies. Likewise, to remove restraints within the cell, officers had to flex forward from the hips with straight legs (the cell walls were directly behind them), flex their spines, and extend their arms to reach the ground while wearing protective vests. Discussions with the officers revealed that going home with an aching lower back and shoulders following a shift in the watchhouse was expected. Other observations have found that officers often have poor posture while carrying protesters who struggle while suspended or develop increasingly kyphotic postures when holding riot shields for a protracted period. With research showing that up to 38% of U.S. police officers have suffered an injury during use-of-force incidents (3), these individual anecdotes provide a personalized insight into the biomechanical stresses placed on police officers completing occupational tasks. These chronic biomechanical stressors could also explain the decrease in trunk mobility found in experienced police officers when compared with younger recruits (81).

Key Point

Law enforcement personnel experience a high level of musculoskeletal injury, and special consideration for injury prevention should focus on use-of-force incidents.

ENVIRONMENTAL, OCCUPATIONAL, AND EXPOSURE CONCERNS

In addition to law enforcement officers' level of physical fitness, environmental, occupational, and exposure concerns can influence the physiological demands on officers. Environmental conditions can affect fluid balance and the ability to maintain thermal homeostasis (core body temperature between 36 °C and 37.5 °C [97 °F and 99.5 °F]). An officer's PPE, such as load-bearing vests or even something as simple as gloves, can inhibit convective cooling during hot days but may be necessary to reduce the risk of death as well as occupational exposures in the line of duty (31). Occupational exposures include, for example, contracting serious illnesses when dealing with infected offenders or persons of interest (61).

Thermal Concerns

Law enforcement officers are, for the most part, sworn to protect life and property, and they can be required to perform their duties in all types of environmental conditions. Depending on their role, officers may wear a range of PPE (e.g., ballistic or stab vests, load-bearing vests, helmets, gloves) as well as their personal weapon systems and appointments, which, as mentioned earlier in this chapter, can weigh 8 to 10 kg (18-22 lb) for general duty officers and up to 22 kg (49 lb) for officers on specialist high-risk duty. The impact of this load carriage has been discussed in physiological and biomechanical contexts, but the thermal impact also warrants consideration given that this load can cover a large percentage of the body.

For example, general duty police officers perform a range of tasks that could increase their susceptibility to thermal-related problems. A common task of these officers in Australia is conducting random breath testing and mobile drug testing on citizens driving motor vehicles. In summer, ambient temperatures can reach in excess of 40 °C (104 °F); more tropical locations may be slightly cooler, around 34 °C (93 °F), but have a humidity level above 80%. Officers are required to stand on the side of the road wearing PPE, weapons, and appointments for extended lengths of time. The radiant heat from the road can be extreme (above 50 °C or 122 °F), especially when the road surface is made of asphalt (bitumen). Rather than wear a duty belt, many police officers opt to wear a load-bearing vest that sits over the torso, holds their equipment, and often also has removable ballistic plates. This vest can increase the likelihood of thermal strain due to the reduced ability to cool the torso, especially when the ballistic plates are in place (69).

Officers in specialist units, such as a SWAT unit, riot unit, or units that require special equipment to perform their roles (e.g., CBRN suits), can be at greater risk of heat-related issues because of the extra equipment they wear (19, 31). SWAT officers may be required to hold a perimeter for extended periods during a siege, and riot squad officers may need to repel a large crowd of civilians to maintain local law and order. Figure 18.1 shows what a SWAT officer usually wears during operational duty. No part of the body is left uncovered in case of, for example, deployment of gas that can affect the skin, eyes, nose, ears, or mouth. Likewise, officers with CBRN duties perform tasks with PPE that limits heat transfer from the body to the environment (19, 31).

The impact of PPE on the heat-induced thermal stress of the wearer is important; research has found that thermal stress can reduce work capability over time. As an example, Snook and Ciriello (92) reported that the ability to conduct work tasks over a continuous period (40 min) was significantly reduced in a hotter environment (27.0 °C [80.6 °F] versus 17.2 °C [63.0 °F]).

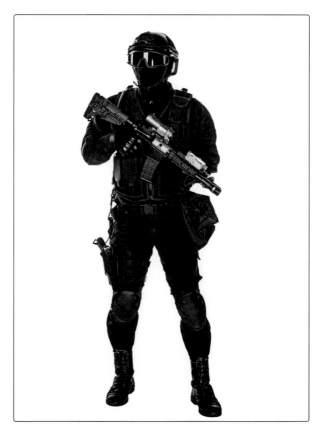

Figure 18.1 Operational uniform and appointments of a high-risk tactical law enforcement officer. Uniform, appointments, and PPE for this type of officer can weigh around 23 kg (51 lb).

Research where officers wore CBRN suits highlights this impact, with officers unable to complete tasks due to heat stress rather than physiological fatigue (19). Furthermore, with evaporation being the primary mechanism of heat loss during physical activity (100) and thus providing the primary physiological defense against overheating (64), the body loses fluid and electrolytes as it attempts to return to a thermoneutral status. An absence of fluid intake, in conjunction with fluid loss through sweating, can increase the potential for dehydration, which in itself has been shown to decrease physical performance (28). Although the focus in this instance is on reduced occupational performance, this prolonged exposure to heat and fluid loss not only reduces work performance but also can lead to heat-related illnesses.

Considerations and Countermeasures

Given law enforcement officers' tasks and their requirement to serve and protect citizens, they often cannot simply stop performing their duties as their heat stress increases, nor can they stop to rehydrate. As an example, an officer involved in holding back a riot cannot simply walk away from the shield wall. Furthermore, prevention is the best method to combat heat-related illness, but it is not always possible for law enforcement personnel. Officers cannot choose the environment, timing, or duration of their tasks. This is not to suggest that heat stress should be accepted, however. Officers and their departments should always take appropriate steps to ensure their own thermal safety whenever possible, such as staying out of direct sun for prolonged periods, sitting in a car with air conditioning when in the field, drinking small amounts of water at regular intervals (400-800 ml [134-27 fl oz]) (1), and consuming a similar volume of sport drink (e.g., Gatorade) interchanged with water when in the sun for over an hour (1).

Heat-related illness or injury in the hotter months can be minimized through heat acclimatization. When acclimatized, an officer's physiological system becomes more efficient at maintaining temperature homeostasis in the environment. Research suggests that heat acclimatization should be conducted over 10 to 14 days (14), although this will vary depending on the degree of climate change and individual factors such as the officer's health and aerobic fitness. Most law enforcement officers will achieve some natural acclimatization through the change of seasons, but acclimatization becomes important for officers who deploy into areas much warmer than their home environment. These officers should try to limit any lengthy exposure to the heat upon arrival and gradually increase time outside over the next 7 days if possible.

For a planned task, such as random breath testing (i.e., DUI checkpoints), countermeasures such as ice vests for the torso or ice scarves for the neck could be used to reduce the likelihood of thermal strain (65). Officers should be educated on hydration, especially in regard to achieving euhydration before these tasks. Weighing oneself at the start and end of a shift measures the amount of fluid lost during the shift or activity. Where possible, work:rest tables for working in hot environments should be available that include planned hydration breaks to allow regular ingestion of water (duties permitting) (74). During longer periods, these water breaks should be interspersed with drinks containing electrolytes in order to prevent hyponatremia (51).

Ensuring staff are appropriately hydrated before their shift begins is a simple way to minimize heat illness. Testing involves each officer producing a small urine sample that can be analyzed using a test strip or refractometer. Officers' **urine-specific gravity (USG)** should be in the range of 0.005 to 0.015. Urine in this USG range is almost clear or a very light yellow. Although urine color can be affected by some medications and foods, the general rule is that the darker urine is, the less hydrated a person is. A person with a USG reading of 0.020 or higher is considered dehydrated.

Hazardous Exposure

No one would deny that a law enforcement officer's job can be hazardous, but few consider the number and nature of hazards in terms of exposure. During an arrest or when responding to a riot, officers can be exposed to a range of bodily fluids, including saliva and blood that may contain infectious diseases (such as hepatitis or HIV). When performing tasks at clandestine drug laboratories, or even at evidence holding areas, officers can be exposed to a wide range of toxic chemicals through either airborne or skin-contact exposure. There is also the chance of exposure to lead when regularly firing or handling ammunition (60), with continued exposure known to cause serious problems such as kidney damage (33). In addition, some locations where an officer is required to conduct tasks repeatedly (e.g., vital asset protection) may contain asbestos, which, if disturbed, can cause mesothelioma (83).

Considerations and Countermeasures

The nature of these hazardous exposures makes them difficult for officers to avoid. Countermeasures typically involve administrative policy (e.g., wearing face shields when attending riots, using protective shields if required to give CPR, wearing a breathing apparatus and gloves when attending suspected drug laboratories, reporting and obtaining blood screening after exposure to bodily fluids such as blood or saliva). However, the unpredictable nature of tasks means that adhering to these policies can be difficult. Likewise, it is often not known whether a building contains asbestos or a suspect is carrying an infectious disease, and this information may only become known months or even years later. Duty of care to take reasonable precautions against the likelihood of exposure is shared by both the law enforcement agency and the individual officers.

Shift Work and Unpredictability of Job Assignment

Law enforcement rosters are usually structured so that officers work a series of shifts (e.g., two 12-hour day shifts followed by two 12-hour night shifts) followed by a block of days off. Night shifts can affect the body's **circadian rhythms** because officers are awake when they would typically be asleep (2). This change in rhythm can lead to a decrease in performance during the night shifts or following day shifts depending on the break between shifts (2, 85). This change in sleep patterns can significantly increase the likelihood of sleep-related accidents during the night shift (45). Anecdotally, people with higher levels of aerobic fitness cope better with the transition from day to night shifts (50); however, shift work has been found to have a negative impact on the desire to conduct physical training (50).

Law enforcement officers generally face a high level of uncertainty upon arriving at a job. A civil conversation between an officer and a civilian can quickly descend into physical violence where nondeadly or deadly force is used. It is critical for law enforcement officers to maintain situational awareness at all times, especially when working as a single unit (e.g., general duty mobile supervisor, highway patrol officer). It is not uncommon for single units to be involved in high-stress, high-risk situations where officer safety is threatened (10). Physiological responses can be heightened to the point where **tunnel vision** and the auditory exclusion effect occur. During high-stress situations, vision can narrow (tunnel vision) so that the person has no peripheral vision. Similarly, auditory exclusion is the temporary loss of the ability to interpret sound. Both effects are caused by overexcitement of the sympathetic nervous system, or the fight-or-flight system.

Considerations and Countermeasures

Shift work and law enforcement go hand in hand. Some work has been done to develop fatigue management policies whereby officers who are at risk of fatigue (e.g., on-call officers who have not had a mandatory period of downtime between shifts, officers with issues outside of work that affect the ability to stay alert on the job) can be assisted or their roles adjusted to mitigate fatigue (e.g., offering alternative duties, giving time to rest on duty, relieving the officer of duty for the shift) (97).

The TSAC Facilitator can also provide educational programming on such topics as sleep and understanding the impact of alterations in shifts. For example, officers can learn about **sleep hygiene**, which is a grouping of behaviors, practices, and conditioning that can be changed to improve sleep. Avoiding napping, limiting alcohol and caffeine, being exposed to natural light, and doing certain relaxation activities right before bed are examples of sleep hygiene (53).

Shift alterations are a common practice in law enforcement (99). One example is the concept of forward versus reverse shift rotations. Rotating forward with the clock versus backward against the clock has a differential effect on circadian rhythms. Specifically, rotating shifts forward (moving from day to evening) is easier than backward (moving from days to midnight) because the body's circadian rhythms are predisposed to such a change. It has been estimated that it takes 4 additional days to adjust to a reverse shift compared with a forward shift (8 versus 12 days) (46, 73).

The TSAC Facilitator needs to encourage officers to treat sleep as a safety and performance issue (97) and find ways to teach officers how to reduce stress, incorporate physical activity, obtain proper nutrition, and avoid excessive caffeine and alcohol. These are all associated with quality sleep (46).

INJURY AND ILLNESS RISKS

Every shift, police officers are exposed to factors that can affect their health and lead to physical injury. It is therefore not surprising that the number and compensation costs of reported injuries for police staff covered by workers' compensation are well above the average of the public sector (96, 98). In addition, over a two-year period, more than 50% of officers who separated from the police force in New South Wales, Australia, separated as medical retirements (96). These separations represent a substantial loss of corporate knowledge and skills in addition to incurring significant financial costs. Such separations also appear to be age related, meaning that older officers tend to have more severe injuries or that the injuries lead to a greater disruption in their ability to work.

In terms of musculoskeletal injuries in police officers, the most common injury sites are the neck, back, ankle, hamstring, knee, and rotator cuff (78, 79, 88). This is not unexpected given the nature of the job tasks. Sitting for long periods in prolonged and altered postures (52), reaching and rotating across the body to operate a mobile data terminal (67), and physically restraining offenders (5) are likely to overstress these body sites. Furthermore, backs, knees, and shoulders are known sites of injuries associated with load carriage (76). An investigation profiling the movement capabilities of new recruits and veteran officers identified a notable decrease in performance scores relating to shoulder mobility, trunk rotational stability, and single-leg movement with age (77). As such, a potential exists to identify structures at risk of injury and implement a risk management strategy to mitigate these concerns. Furthermore, it is possible to retrain injured officers to a movement standard (most notably at the key injury sites) before they return to full-time duties (79). Optimizing the ability of a law enforcement agency to identify an officer's potential for injury and return an injured officer to full duties is vital to capability maintenance.

While musculoskeletal injuries are a regular occurrence in law enforcement, psychological injuries are fast becoming more prevalent and may eventually become the top injury to law enforcement officers. Large numbers of law enforcement officers, especially police officers, are reporting psychological injuries as a consequence of being exposed to regular trauma; extreme situations that officers routinely respond to, such as deceased persons, motor vehicle accidents, and domestic incidents, can result in posttraumatic stress disorder (PTSD) (11). Officers have also developed PTSD as a result of workplace issues such as stress and job dissatisfaction (27). Research has shown that maintaining a suitable level of fitness can build resilience and hopefully reduce the likelihood of suffering from PTSD (38). Similar to musculoskeletal injuries, there is an opportunity to identify officers most at risk of psychological injury in the early stages through basic reporting and programs that use psychologist and exercise interventions to assist officers in their recovery. There are now guidelines on how to best treat and diagnose PTSD in emergency service workers (18); however, guidelines need to be produced to deal specifically with the issues faced by law enforcement personnel.

OPTIMIZING FUNCTIONAL FITNESS

Optimization of functional fitness or occupational preparedness is the primary duty of the TSAC Facilitator. This requires a strong understanding of the physical fitness requirements for the occupation and designing or using tests to measure the fitness level of recruits and officers. The results of these tests can guide exercise prescription and goal setting to optimize adherence to and motivation for the program in order to reduce injury and increase the ability to perform job tasks (both physically and mentally).

Physical Fitness Requirements and Testing

Physical job performance capabilities are a necessity for police officers regardless of job assignment. Unfortunately, many municipalities only test these fitness requirements for entrance into the training academies (e.g., POPAT, FLETC battery of tests) or prior to advancement into a specialized unit such as SWAT. A full description along with sample criteria for the POPAT and FLETC tests can be found in the boxes titled "Peace Officer Physical Aptitude Test (POPAT)" and "Federal Law Enforcement Training Centers (FLETC) Tests." Reassessment of these tests is not typically mandatory after graduation from the training academy unless individual departments have specified policies on testing.

Enhancing Adherence

Enhancing adherence to any program once recruits have graduated from the academy or training center is difficult. The job of a police officer is to be on the street enforcing the law, so allocating time for the officer to undertake physical training on the job can be difficult. The generally sedentary nature of police work does not prepare officers for high levels of activity or even maintain good health.

Education can go a long way toward enhancing adherence to any program. A TSAC Facilitator can be embedded in law enforcement departments or specialist units such as SWAT teams to provide expertise in designing and implementing fitness programs. TSAC Facilitators can provide ongoing education and support to the officers regarding the benefits of a healthy lifestyle for decreasing stress and injuries.

Preparticipation Screening

Before commencing any physical training program, a police officer should be made aware of the risks of the program. Each police department should have an in-depth policy and procedures document that outlines the expectations required of an officer before undertaking a physical fitness program. This preparticipation screening helps identify people with a known disease or signs or symptoms of disease who may be at a higher risk of an adverse event during physical activity (9).

Programming Considerations

Essential physical tasks have been identified in law enforcement (12, 32, 88):

1. Walking
2. Running short and moderate distances in foot pursuit

Peace Officer Physical Aptitude Test (POPAT)

The **Peace Officer Physical Aptitude Test (POPAT)** consists of five tests. These tests are based on a job analysis and are meant to simulate the tasks performed by patrol officers. The tests involve the following:

1. Obstacle course for 99 yards (91 m)—Run a 99-yard (91 m) obstacle course consisting of several sharp turns, a number of curb-height obstacles, and a 34-inch (86 cm) obstacle that must be vaulted.
2. Body drag—Lift and drag a 165-pound (75 kg) lifelike dummy 32 feet (10 m).
3. Chain-link fence—Run 5 yards (5 m) to a 6-foot (2 m) chain-link fence, climb over the fence, and continue running another 25 yards (23 m).
4. Solid-fence climb—Run 5 yards (5 m) to a 6-foot (2 m) solid fence, climb over the fence, and continue running another 25 yards (23 m).
5. 500-yard (457 m) run—Run 500 yards (457 m), equivalent to one lap of a standard running track plus 60 yards (55 m).

Points are allotted based on times for each test. The POPAT is an overall assessment of the candidate's potential as a patrol officer. Each test is weighted based on its importance relative to job occurrence and specificity (6).

3. Climbing stairs and ladders
4. Jumping and dodging obstacles
5. Lifting and carrying objects and people
6. Dragging and pulling objects and people
7. Pushing and pulling heavy objects
8. Bending and reaching
9. Using force of short and moderate duration with subjects
10. Using **restraining devices**
11. Using restraining and control holds
12. Using hands and feet for self-defense or combat
13. Performing **forcible entry**

Considering the variations in task requirements, physiological and biomechanical effects, and risk of injuries discussed earlier, designing strength and conditioning programs for police officers poses unique challenges. Programs should show an understanding of the nature of law enforcement tasks if they are to complement rather than compete with job requirements.

For an officer, having the physical ability to complete critical tasks is paramount to operational success even if such tasks occur infrequently. Most of the time a police officer may not be required to perform a great deal of physical activity (21). However, with the example given previously of an officer running an extended

---

Federal Law Enforcement Training Centers (FLETC) Tests

The FLETC **Physical Efficiency Battery (PEB)** contains five tests to assess candidate fitness: the three-site skinfold test (body composition), Illinois agility run (agility), sit and reach (flexibility), bench press (muscular strength), and 1.5-mile (2.4 km) run (cardiorespiratory fitness). Scores of 75% or higher are necessary in all categories (excluding body composition) to receive a fitness certificate (see the following tables) (30).

PEB Scores (Male)

Age	Flexibility in inches (cm)	% body weight push	1.5 mi (2.4 km) run	Agility run (s)	% body fat
<24	21.70 (55.1 cm)	131.60	10:44	16.19	11.05
25-29	21.23 (53.9 cm)	127.00	11:05	16.40	12.61
30-34	21.00 (53.3 cm)	122.17	11:19	16.70	14.02
35-39	20.70 (52.6 cm)	115.20	11:47	17.0	15.13
40-44	20.00 (50.8 cm)	104.65	12:25	17.5	16.43
45-49	19.50 (49.5 cm)	96.40	13:07	18.10	17.35
50-54	19.20 (48.8 cm)	89.70	13:49	18.60	17.80
55-59	18.25 (46.4 cm)	83.50	14:48	19.25	18.44
60+	17.70 (45.0 cm)	78.68	15:07	20.20	18.6

PEB Scores (Female)

Age	Flexibility in inches (cm)	% body weight push	1.5 mi (2.4 km) run	Agility run (s)	% body fat
< 24	23.30 (59.2 cm)	66.10	13:35	18.31	19.96
25-29	23.00 (58.4 cm)	66.40	13:43	18.59	20.26
30-34	22.25 (56.5 cm)	66.00	14:21	18.90	20.67
35-39	22.00 (55.9 cm)	63.40	14:37	19.38	22.03
40-44	21.75 (55.2 cm)	58.80	15:12	20.00	23.18
45-49	21.25 (54.0 cm)	55.40	16:02	21.09	23.66
50-54	20.75 (52.7 cm)	52.60	17:00	22.19	25.85
55+	20.44 (51.9 cm)	50.00	17:37	22.92	25.05

distance and then fighting to retain his firearm, critical tasks that occur infrequently come with a notable cost of failure.

Conversely, the sedentary nature of the majority of the police officer's duties does little to prepare her for levels of high activity or even maintain physical fitness for the job or general health. The physical activity required while on duty is too infrequent to maintain a high level of fitness; hence, regular participation in a fitness program is essential if officers are to maintain their fitness (91).

Motivation

Long working hours, family commitments, and shift work can have a negative impact on an officer's motivation. This lack of motivation could lead to making poor choices with regard to food and drink while at work or at home. In addition, performing adequate physical activity to maintain health and occupational preparedness can be difficult if activity is not tracked and assessed regularly.

Goal setting and motivation are common issues that are influenced by shift work, and having access to a TSAC Facilitator at the workplace can help overcome these problems. The TSAC Facilitator can assist in developing education packages about creating small, sustainable goals and rewards to increase motivation and adherence. In addition, the TSAC Facilitator can work to establish a wellness program that covers all areas of officer fitness, health, and wellness to ensure an appropriate system of knowledge, support, and accountability is in place to support the officers.

Training Considerations

Most physical fitness programs for police officers are provided at the academy level while the recruit is training to become an officer. These programs are usually based on military-style, one-size-fits-all training approaches (34). The TSAC Facilitator should individualize training programs to take into account age, previous injury history, and the physical qualities required by the officer.

Establishing Training Goals

These training programs typically aim to improve the general physical fitness of the recruit in order to pass fitness tests that are based on measures such as push-ups and sit-ups, and they do not usually take into account the job requirements of a police officer. Once an officer leaves the academy environment, mandatory physical training is generally no longer required, and officers are left to their own devices. Program design thus becomes more difficult for general duty police officers. Unless the department has a mandatory fitness standard, officers have no official reason to conduct any form of physical training, and an officer's drive to maintain or improve her health, well-being, and fitness stems from self-motivation or lifestyle choices.

Because of this, it is important that academy training programs instill proper movement mechanics and fitness components (e.g., strength, muscular endurance, metabolic capacity) that help build the resilience of a police officer for the long term. These programs should provide officers with the knowledge and skills to be able to develop and implement programs for themselves in a way that does not increase the potential for injury. These key factors highlight the need for experienced TSAC Facilitators.

Academy programs are influenced by a variety of factors, from the volume of recruits and their demographics to the number of physical training sessions conducted per week and access to equipment. As such, there is no one-size-fits-all approach for academy programming. Training time at police academies is finite—recruits are required to attend sessions on physical conditioning, defensive tactics, law, and firearms training all within the constraints of an academy schedule. Recruits may have the added incentive to pass a physical fitness standard by the end of the training program.

Exercise Selection

Law enforcement officers need a training program designed for their individual needs and circumstances based on a needs analysis. Proper movement mechanics and a graduated progression in training loads should be enforced to ensure the adaptability and long-term benefits of the training program.

Exercise selection should replicate the movement patterns of critical tasks in law enforcement.

This will enhance the likelihood of exercises in the gym transferring to the operational environment. In general, critical tasks require officers to exert force dynamically while stabilizing themselves. Compound free weight exercises, kettlebells, odd objects, medicine balls, free-moving cable machines, and bands can all be implemented in a training program for law enforcement officers. If TSAC Facilitators do not have access to such equipment, which is not out of the realm of possibility, especially in an academy, they can consider incorporating a movement competency program. As illustrated in the case study, movement competency programs are designed to provide recruits with physical literacy that ensures survival at the academy and promotes physical resilience during active duty (41).

CASE STUDY

Movement Competency Program at New South Wales Police Academy

The following is an example of a movement competency program that was successfully implemented in a large recruit environment. The New South Wales Police Academy produced an average of 250 new police officers every four months between 2012 and 2014. The rationale behind the program was fostering resilience while recruits were training to become police officers. The training aimed to provide a long-term approach to physical development. Because the literature showed that poor movement patterns increase the risk of injuries to personnel (20, 66), movement competencies were developed (see figure 18.2) to ensure that all recruits could meet the standards required to progress in training, thereby ensuring graduating officers were capable of high-quality movement patterns as applied to exercise examples (see figure 18.3).

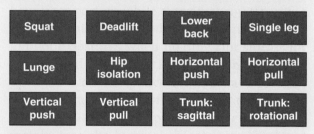

Squat	Deadlift	Lower back	Single leg
Lunge	Hip isolation	Horizontal push	Horizontal pull
Vertical push	Vertical pull	Trunk: sagittal	Trunk: rotational

Figure 18.2 Physical competency streams used by the NSWP Academy.

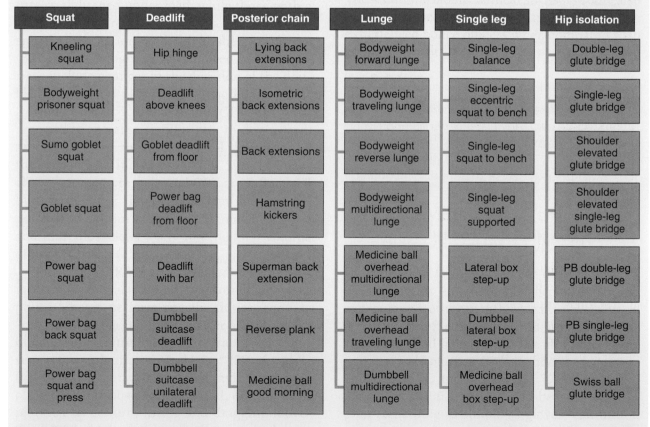

Squat	Deadlift	Posterior chain	Lunge	Single leg	Hip isolation
Kneeling squat	Hip hinge	Lying back extensions	Bodyweight forward lunge	Single-leg balance	Double-leg glute bridge
Bodyweight prisoner squat	Deadlift above knees	Isometric back extensions	Bodyweight traveling lunge	Single-leg eccentric squat to bench	Single-leg glute bridge
Sumo goblet squat	Goblet deadlift from floor	Back extensions	Bodyweight reverse lunge	Single-leg squat to bench	Shoulder elevated glute bridge
Goblet squat	Power bag deadlift from floor	Hamstring kickers	Bodyweight multidirectional lunge	Single-leg squat supported	Shoulder elevated single-leg glute bridge
Power bag squat	Deadlift with bar	Superman back extension	Medicine ball overhead multidirectional lunge	Lateral box step-up	PB double-leg glute bridge
Power bag back squat	Dumbbell suitcase deadlift	Reverse plank	Medicine ball overhead traveling lunge	Dumbbell lateral box step-up	PB single-leg glute bridge
Power bag squat and press	Dumbbell suitcase unilateral deadlift	Medicine ball good morning	Dumbbell multidirectional lunge	Medicine ball overhead box step-up	Swiss ball glute bridge

Figure 18.3 Competency streams with exercise examples.

(continued)

Figure 18.3 *(continued)*

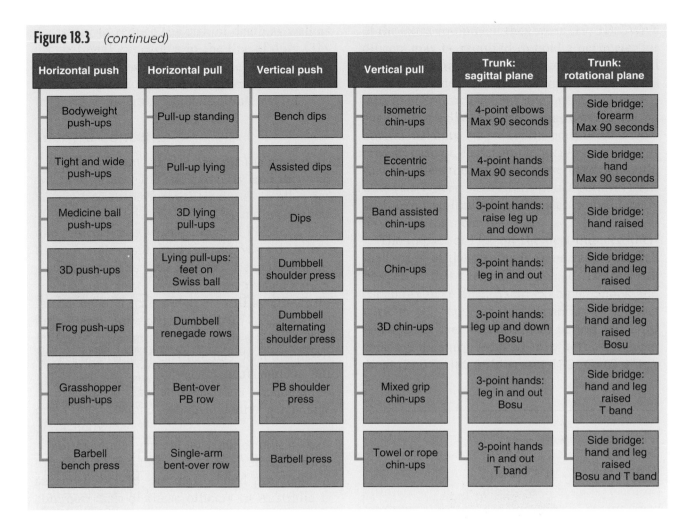

Horizontal push	Horizontal pull	Vertical push	Vertical pull	Trunk: sagittal plane	Trunk: rotational plane
Bodyweight push-ups	Pull-up standing	Bench dips	Isometric chin-ups	4-point elbows Max 90 seconds	Side bridge: forearm Max 90 seconds
Tight and wide push-ups	Pull-up lying	Assisted dips	Eccentric chin-ups	4-point hands Max 90 seconds	Side bridge: hand Max 90 seconds
Medicine ball push-ups	3D lying pull-ups	Dips	Band assisted chin-ups	3-point hands: raise leg up and down	Side bridge: hand raised
3D push-ups	Lying pull-ups: feet on Swiss ball	Dumbbell shoulder press	Chin-ups	3-point hands: leg in and out	Side bridge: hand and leg raised
Frog push-ups	Dumbbell renegade rows	Dumbbell alternating shoulder press	3D chin-ups	3-point hands: leg up and down Bosu	Side bridge: hand and leg raised Bosu
Grasshopper push-ups	Bent-over PB row	PB shoulder press	Mixed grip chin-ups	3-point hands: leg in and out Bosu	Side bridge: hand and leg raised T band
Barbell bench press	Single-arm bent-over row	Barbell press	Towel or rope chin-ups	3-point hands in and out T band	Side bridge: hand and leg raised Bosu and T band

Once the movement competency training program is completed, the recruits are able to move into a strength and power training program. By incorporating strength training into a training program for recruits, police are able to increase their muscle strength and strengthen tendons and ligaments to provide structural integrity to joints. Many of the critical tasks performed by police officers require a certain degree of physical contact or a hands-on approach (e.g., restraining a person, deescalating a situation) using near-maximal strength. This type of physical contact can significantly increase acute injuries if police officers lack strength (22). Though some injuries are unavoidable, others may be preventable or at least reduced in severity with the implementation of a prehabilitation program as part of a strength training program (71). *Prehabilitation* has been defined as a systematic approach to identifying common injuries within law enforcement and designing a series of exercises to minimize their incidence (71).

Strength training has its benefits, but the ultimate goal for law enforcement officers should be converting that strength into power. Strength is the act of overcoming resistance; the greater the resistance overcome, the greater the strength, and as a consequence, the slower the movement (102). Stated another way, strength is the ability to exert force. With no time constraints, it is a matter of how much force can be applied (44). Although strength is an asset, police officers need to be powerful; most of their defensive tactics involve creating distance and space to enable them to employ a tactical option. The short, explosive bursts of activity associated with defense require muscular strength and power (95).

To maximize power training, heavy resistance training needs to be accompanied by explosive exercises (57). By incorporating explosive exercises in their strength training, police officers will be able to produce more force in a shorter time compared with strength training alone. The ability to exert force quickly and combine muscular strength and power has a direct impact on operational success (93).

A resistance training program for officers should develop the strength and power required to successfully complete their critical tasks and reduce the risk of injury while doing so. Every officer should be treated as an individual, and programs with evidence-based recommendations should be developed based on the needs analysis of the officer's occupational role, previous injury history, and training age.

Rest-Work Cycles

The rest provided between sets in a strength training session should be a minimum of 2 minutes. Two to 5 minutes of rest between sets has been shown to allow more repetitions over multiple sets and to produce greater increases in absolute strength. This is due to higher intensities and volume of training as well as higher levels of power in multiple sets with 2 to 5 minutes of rest (42, 48).

A combined strength and power day can be incorporated into a police officer's training program. Where **complex training** or **contrast training** is employed, a heavy resistance load is followed quickly by a biomechanically similar plyometric exercise in an attempt to enhance explosive power (for example, a squat followed by a plyometric box jump). This type of training may be superior to other types of strength and power training, but it may differ from person to person and needs to be individually prescribed (39).

The optimum time period between the heavy loading and subsequent power performance is yet to be determined; however, the suggested rest period between the resistance exercise and the explosive exercise is less than 1 minute (49, 89). This rest period of less than 1 minute was chosen because it most likely replicates the work capacity needed for critical tasks such as crowd control, restraint of violent offenders, or self-defense.

Progression, Duration, and Intensity

Any program for a law enforcement officer should be designed for that individual's needs and cir-

cumstances. Programs should be based on a needs analysis of the occupational role being performed, previous injury history, training age, and evidence-based recommendations. Law enforcement officers with little or no training experience or even an officer who has not exercised for a while might be at a beginning level, where the training program initially consists of one to two sessions a week at a low training stress with exercises that require minimal skill or technique, all while attempting to maximize muscular strength adaptations (48). Such a program could include 6 to 10 resistance training exercises (1 per muscle group) at approximately 60% of 1RM using one set of 8 to 12 repetitions per exercise. This would theoretically optimize the strength outcome while minimizing the duration.

Officers with at least six months of experience might be considered to be at a moderate training level. Their program could consist of two to three sessions per week with a medium training stress and exercises requiring basic skill and technique (48, 82). This might include the aforementioned beginner's training program but with an increased intensity up to 80% of 1RM and increased volume of two to three sets per muscle group (82).

Officers with extensive training experience, generally more than 1 year, would be considered advanced. Their training program might consist of three to four training sessions a week with a high training stress. An officer with an advanced training history is able to complete more difficult exercises that require more skill (48, 82). An appropriate progression from the aforementioned exercise protocol would increase intensity to upward of 80% to 100%, with concurrent increases in volume of three or more sets per muscle group (82).

Proper movement mechanics and a graduated progression in training loads should be enforced to ensure the adaptability and long-term benefits of the training program. Progression should be introduced systematically and gradually once technical requirements of lifts and exercises are met.

Periodization

Periodization involves the manipulation of training variables in a practical, systematic, and sequential manner to stimulate specific physiological adaptations that will improve physical performance (48). See chapter 10 for a more complete discussion of periodization in tactical settings.

In the academy setting, undulating periodization could be used to decrease or increase the physiological demands of the session based on other training being undertaken. For example, if the defensive tactics training has a high physical demand on a particular day, then the physical training session can be manipulated to reduce the total training load for the day. This would be an example of **flexible undulating periodization**.

Flexible undulating periodization can also be used by police officers who have graduated from the academy. Training volumes and intensities can vary depending on whether the training is before or after the shift or on a rest day. On work days, training before a shift might have a power or explosive focus, where quality rather than quantity is the aim and the program is designed to stimulate the nervous system. At the conclusion of a shift, the training session might have a recovery aimed at physical and mental restoration or a postural reset focus. On days off, the officer can focus on hypertrophy and the strength phase of the undulating plan. This ensures that all components of the periodization plan can be completed around the officer's shifts without affecting the ability to perform occupational tasks.

Program Variations

A bodyweight program should be provided if the recruit or police officer is unable to attend or complete a strength training session due to job requirements. This program should be implemented with minimal or no equipment. It should include variations on basic exercises to reduce the number of repetitions performed and increase the intensity of the workout.

A medicine ball program is another alternative to the traditional strength/power training session if, for example, an officer's operational requirements make it impossible to attend and complete a regularly scheduled session. Medicine ball training can also be used as an adjunct to the regular strength and power training session. Medicine ball exercises can be performed with or without releasing the ball (releasing the ball allows for

power movements). Medicine ball throws allow the police officer to release the ball at the end of the ROM, eliminating the need to decelerate the ball in order to remain in control of it. This would be beneficial for police officers, because the ability to exert force earlier and through a greater portion of the movement plays a vital role in almost all critical job tasks. These types of movements are time and force dependent (40).

Prehabilitation and Injury Prevention

The most common nonfatal injuries among police officers are sprains and strains, with the neck, back, ankle, hamstring, knee, and rotator cuff all being predominant sites of injury (87). The training program should account for these types of injuries by focusing on physical resilience and injury prevention.

Another way to ensure injury prevention is to incorporate a movement screen. Movement screening has been shown to have good inter-rater and intra-rater reliability (72, 90). This type of screening could be used to evaluate the effectiveness of training protocols and injury prevention programs. A prehabilitation plan can be provided for officers to follow as they complete their resistance training. For example, the first two days of the program could be split into lower and upper body days where the officers complete upper body strength work and lower body prehabilitation one day and then lower body strength work and upper body prehabilitation the next day.

Typically, if a resistance training session targets the upper body, then lower body and core stabilizer prehabilitation exercises can be performed during rest periods. Conversely, if the resistance training session focuses on the lower body or total body movements (88), then prehabilitation exercises can focus on the upper body (71).

Energy System Training

Although aerobic fitness has a place in the training of police officers, it does not supply the bulk of the immediate energy supply at critical times when officers have to protect themselves or others from injury. Such critical times usually range from 15 to 20 seconds to less than 2 minutes (88).

To increase the specificity of training, methods involving the anaerobic energy system, such as interval training, should be used instead of LSD running. Interval training consists of high-intensity work followed by a low-intensity recovery or rest. This training works both the anaerobic and aerobic energy systems, integrating the energy systems in differing amounts—similar to what may occur in real life—rather than attempting to use each energy system in isolation (35).

Interval training improves the ability of the muscular system to resist fatigue by exposing it repeatedly to bouts of high-intensity exercise (54). Interval training has also been shown to result in greater improvements in running speed than long-distance running alone, especially in sedentary and recreationally active people (58).

Having the ability to resist fatigue during high-intensity activities would assist police officers with many of their critical tasks, such as crowd control, physical restraint, and self-defense. As officers are able to produce the required effort for a longer time, they increase their ability to recover more efficiently after performing the task.

Anaerobic training through high-intensity intervals, strength training, plyometrics, and agility training can elicit specific adaptations in the nervous system. These adaptations lead to greater muscle fiber recruitment, rate of motor unit firing, muscle synchronization, and muscle function, resulting in increased strength and power.

Some of the chronic responses to excessive aerobic endurance training decrease muscle mass, strength, speed, and power, which may increase the number of injuries suffered by police officers. To prevent this from happening, the program should focus on interval running based on the termination velocity of the **30-15 intermittent fitness test (30-15 IFT)** (25). The 30-15 IFT consists of 30-second shuttle runs for 40 m (44 yd) interspersed with 15-second passive recovery periods. The test commences at a velocity of 8 km/h (5 mph) for the first 30-second run and increases by 0.5 km/h (0.3 mi) every 45 seconds thereafter. This continues until the participant can no longer complete the test (24).

Research has shown that recruits who start an academy training program with a lower level of anaerobic and aerobic fitness have a higher chance of sustaining an injury during training (80), as shown in figure 18.4. The recruits who sustained

an injury (group 1) during training ran an average of 10 fewer shuttles on the Multi-Stage Fitness Test (MSFT) than those who did not sustain an injury (group 0). Figure 18.5 shows the dispersion of those recruits who sustained injuries compared with those who were not injured. Whereas 83% of participants who did not perform more than 33 shuttles were injured, only 39% of participants who performed a minimum of 52 shuttles were injured. At the level of 53 shuttles (level 6.1 or 1,040 m [1,137 yd]), the MSFT was able to predict 97.5% of injuries with a false negative rate (i.e., officers who were predicted to suffer an injury but did not) of 2.5%.

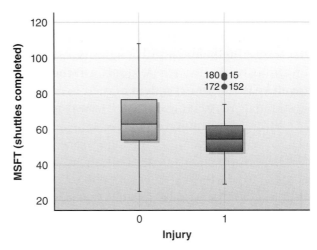

Figure 18.4 Mean ± SD of MSFT results of New South Wales Police Academy recruits who did not sustain an injury (0) against those who did (1).

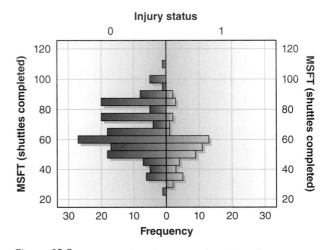

Figure 18.5 MSFT shuttles completed against number of recruits (0 = no injury; 1 = injured).

The problem TSAC Facilitators face is how to improve the energy systems without increasing the risk of injury. Increasing $\dot{V}O_2$ in large tactical groups has previously been achieved using longer distance intervals or continuous running (80). These programs are generally one size fits all, aiming at either the average recruit or the lowest common denominator. This can lead to overtraining or undertraining a large portion of the group, as well as increasing the rate of injuries.

A solution to this problem is to implement individualized running programs or ability-based training (80). As an example, the 30-15 IFT (figure 18.6) is a prescription test that allows individual running programs to be implemented based on termination velocity (23).

At the conclusion of the 30-15 IFT, the recruit's termination velocity is expressed as kilometers per hour. This number is divided by 3.6 to provide a figure that is expressed as meters per second (m/s). This number is then entered into a spreadsheet where running intervals are derived from the following formula (80):

Interval distance = running speed in m/s × % of effort × duration of interval

Ability-based training programs have been shown to reduce the incidence of injury and improve $\dot{V}O_2$ measures when compared to longer intervals and continuous running or control groups (80). When undertaken in the initial phase of training, there was no difference in ability-based training compared to a standardized running program. During this phase, the recruits participated mainly in classroom activities and theory lessons. In phase 2 of training, however, the focus shifted from the classroom to defensive tactics and scenario-based training. In the final physical test, the recruits who completed the ability-based training outperformed the recruits who completed the standardized running programs. This may be due to the added volume and time spent on the standardized program that increased the total training load in comparison to ability-based training (80).

KEY PROGRAM VARIABLES

Key program variables must be considered when implementing a successful and safe program. When designing a program, considerations for equipment, safety, and oversight should be the primary areas of concern. In addition, a thorough needs analysis will help the TSAC Facilitator design and implement a program that has the appropriate level of specificity and individualization necessary to optimize performance and minimize injury risk for the tactical athlete.

Equipment

If a TSAC Facilitator is fortunate enough to be provided with an equipment budget, the purchased equipment should be suited to the requirements of the officers. Low-cost programming can be used to justify additional expenditures. When designing a budget, considerations should include the number of officers who will be using the equipment. In addition, the equipment should cater to a wide range of training experience and necessities. The most important consideration for equipment is safety and oversight required by the style of programming and the complexity of the movement patterns.

Safety

Before using any exercise equipment, all users should be educated on its safe usage. Departments may have certain restrictions around access to exercise equipment or policies that guide use of

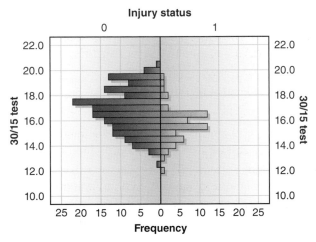

Figure 18.6   Frequency versus 30-15 IFT results of New South Wales Police Academy recruits (0 = no injury; 1 = sustained an injury).

the equipment. If a policy is provided, it must be strictly followed. The TSAC Facilitator should work with the department to craft such policies if they are not in place.

Oversight

If a law enforcement agency has exercise equipment or a gym facility, a specified person such as the TSAC Facilitator should ensure that it is run in a safe and organized manner and that it remains clean and in good working order. If any defects are noted, the equipment should be repaired or replaced.

CONCLUSION

Law enforcement officers are paid to perform critical tasks for the community. If they are unable to complete these tasks, the results could be disastrous for both the officers and the public. Law enforcement officers may perform their duties over careers spanning four decades, and such longevity only increases the importance of proper conditioning.

Although it is accepted that most professions are at risk of some type of injury, organizations that do not respond to these risks and develop a harm minimization policy may find themselves liable for not providing a safe working environment. Almost all activities likely to cause injury have a physical component. Therefore, it is beneficial to help police officers develop the physical capabilities to compete the required tasks. Providing an evidence-based strength and conditioning program for police officers is, in essence, a harm minimization policy. The downstream effect of this approach may even provide protection against indirect causes of injury whereby increased fitness delays fatigue and thus reduces the potential for fatigue-induced injuries (e.g., motor vehicle accidents).

Physical training is a requirement for most law enforcement recruits, yet at the conclusion of the recruit stage, official physical fitness programs and even mandatory requirements typically cease. Furthermore, the typical physical fitness program may not help police officers perform their critical tasks.

To help officers perform their critical tasks, the TSAC Facilitator needs to examine the physiological aspects of the tasks (i.e., needs analysis). By evaluating these tasks, the facilitator can determine which energy pathways and physiological attributes are required for operational success. Then the facilitator can develop a strength and conditioning program to help officers perform these tasks.

By evaluating these critical tasks and then applying current research, the TSAC Facilitator may ensure that police officers have a physical training program that enables them to perform their duties successfully. Such a program will help minimize the officers' risk of injury while enabling them to complete the required tasks that lead to operational success.

Key Terms

chemical, biological, radiological, and nuclear (CBRN) suits
circadian rhythms
complex training or contrast training
flexible undulating periodization
forcible entry
Peace Officer Physical Aptitude Test (POPAT)
personal protective equipment (PPE)

Physical Efficiency Battery (PEB)
restraining devices
sleep hygiene
special weapons and tactics (SWAT)
30-15 intermittent fitness test (IFT)
tunnel vision
urine-specific gravity (USG)

Study Questions

1. The majority of the work performed by law enforcement officers is at what level of intensity?

   a. sedentary

   b. low intensity

   c. moderate intensity

   d. high intensity

2. Which law enforcement unit is expected, at times, to carry an extra 22 kg (49 lb) of equipment?

   a. general duty

   b. motorcycle unit

   c. police academy

   d. SWAT unit

3. When designing a program for law enforcement officers, what is the guideline regarding exercise selection?

   a. replicate the movement patterns of critical tasks

   b. minimize the transfer to the operational environment

   c. limit the use of a movement competency program

   d. focus on the force that is statically used during training

4. Which of the following training modes is the most effective when training an officer to perform periodic anaerobic bouts and resist fatigue?

   a. LSD running

   b. bodyweight movements

   c. interval training

   d. heavy resistance exercise

Chapter 19

Physiological Issues Related to Military Personnel

William Kraemer, PhD, CSCS,*D, FNSCA
LTC David Feltwell, PT, OCS, TSAC-F
Tunde Szivak, PhD, CSCS

After completing this chapter, you will be able to

- describe the physiological and biomechanical occupational demands, injury risks, environmental exposures, and occupational stressors experienced by conventional military and special operations personnel;

- discuss the fitness requirements and recommendations for conventional military and special operations personnel;

- design fitness programs by applying training principles and approaches to improve and maintain fitness in conventional military and special operations personnel across disciplines, subdivisions, professional statuses (cadets versus incumbents), and fitness levels; and

- analyze case-specific and problem-centered scenarios.

The opinions or assertions contained herein are the private views of the authors and are not to be construed as official or reflecting the views of the Army, the Department of Defense, or the U.S. Government.

The diversity of military training and operational situations and their associated physiological demands is daunting. Understanding the physiological issues that are relevant for warfighters can help in the decision-making process when training these tactical athletes. This chapter provides an overview of the many issues related to military operational scenarios, injuries, and physiological demands and the physical training (PT) programs needed to address them.

CRITICAL JOB TASKS FOR CONVENTIONAL MILITARY AND SPECIAL OPERATIONS PERSONNEL

The modern-day military environment is characterized by technological innovation and a broad range of challenges to the warfighter's health. To be effective in combat, military personnel must maintain mission readiness year-round. **Readiness** is defined as "the ability to meet the physical demands of any combat or duty position, accomplish the mission and continue to fight and win" (65). Readiness is the business of the TSAC Facilitator. It is a multifaceted concept that includes physical performance, cardiovascular health, and musculoskeletal health. Optimal PT to prepare warfighters for critical job tasks lies at the core of readiness. It provides the foundation for all other types of training and combat performance. It is a unique concern of military leadership and unites both the performance and injury facets of the TSAC Facilitator's role.

Demands

The demands placed on military personnel are varied and depend on factors such as the physical requirements of the warfighter's **military occupational specialty (MOS)**, the mission of the warfighter's unit, and whether the warfighter is currently deployed. Every service member has a role in the unit's mission and must be ready at all times to fulfill that role during periods of high operational tempo (i.e., frequent deployments) (45, 71). Today's military personnel must have physical fitness capabilities ranging from muscular strength and power to muscular endurance and aerobic capacity. Additionally, military tasks frequently require skill-based capabilities that use flexibility and agility. A thorough understanding of the physiological, biomechanical, and occupational requirements of military personnel will aid the TSAC Facilitator in designing and implementing training programs to enhance warfighter performance.

Physiological Demands

The modern-day operational environment has been characterized as an **anaerobic battlefield** (35, 38). Military personnel often face anaerobic challenges, such as load carriage, sprinting, heavy lifting, repetitive lifting, casualty evacuation, and offensive and defensive maneuvers (16, 24, 38, 39, 66, 68). Many military personnel are required to carry external loads as part of physical fitness training or as part of their MOS. Whereas in earlier conflicts, military personnel often walked long distances carrying much of their equipment, today's wars rarely require long-distance load carriage (i.e., more than 15 miles [24 km]) (16). However, modern-day combat operations continue to require military personnel to carry heavy external loads (38, 49). For most of these anaerobic challenges, strength and power are the limiting factors in how well the warfighter is able to perform the task at hand.

Although the anaerobic challenges faced during combat operations cannot be understated, military personnel also require optimal aerobic conditioning, which enables them to conduct prolonged combat operations at a lower percentage of maximum exercise capacity (lower percentage of $\dot{V}O_2max$) (16). Warfighters frequently face varying mission lengths and operational conditions that necessitate optimal work capacity and the ability to endure protracted missions. This is especially critical when occupational tasks are performed successively, when tasks are performed while carrying external loads, or when tasks are performed while facing other external (operational) stressors (49). Therefore, the modern-day warfighter must not only possess the strength and power capabilities that are required for anaerobic tasks but must also have well-developed aerobic fitness. In short, the warfighter must be a hybrid athlete, possessing a wide range of physiological capabilities related to occupational demands.

Biomechanical Demands

Despite many technological advancements that have improved the ergonomics of load carriage, over the past 150 years there has nonetheless been a sizeable increase in the external loads that military personnel are required to carry (13, 31, 46, 49). For example, during recent conflicts in Afghanistan, U.S. infantry soldiers were routinely required to carry 44 to 46 kg (97-101 lb) (13, 57). Loads may be carried over difficult terrain in unpredictable operational conditions that may require the warfighter to make sudden movements or quickly change direction (38). The addition of a heavy external load adds to the instability of movement and increases injury risk (49, 57, 60). Studies have shown that the majority of injuries among military personnel during deployments are musculoskeletal, with the low back being the most commonly injured body part (57-59).

During deployment, which can last from several months to over a year, military personnel are frequently required to wear PPE such as ballistic vests and helmets, which in total weigh over 14 kg (31 lb) and can be awkward to wear depending on the individual's build (49, 57, 58, 60). Protective equipment is often worn for several hours at a time, in addition to any firearms and external load carried (49, 58). This greatly adds to the total stress placed on the body, increases the effort of locomotion (walking), and increases GRFs exerted on the body during walking or running. Additionally, military personnel must wear protective equipment when riding in military vehicles (i.e., in a seated position or in a cramped environment), which further strains the spine. Not only is protective equipment cumbersome, but wearing it for an extended length of time decreases work capacity. That is, warfighters must exert more effort to perform the same amount of work than they could perform without the addition of protective gear and external loads (49).

Load carriage places a number of biomechanical demands on the warfighter, particularly relating to the spinal architecture and supporting musculature. Load carriage exerts large forces on the lumbar spine as well as the hips, shoulders, and knees (31, 56, 60), and it is one of the largest contributors to musculoskeletal injury, which accounts for 78% of medical discharges from the U.S. military (57, 58). One study found that 80% of injuries in combat arms units were attributable to PT and load carriage (55). Other studies have shown that the majority of injuries during a deployment to Afghanistan could be attributed to dismounted patrols, lifting, body armor wear, and reinjury (58, 59). Additionally, load carriage affects the warfighter's gait and posture (50). When carrying loads, the gait is shortened and the individual compensates for the load by leaning forward (31, 50). This adjustment in posture is related to limb length and upper body strength, and it may be more pronounced in military personnel of smaller stature who have less upper body strength and muscle mass.

In general, larger, more muscular people perform better on load carriage tasks than smaller, less muscular people (31, 50). Load carriage places greater stress on smaller people due to the weight of the external load relative to body mass (16). However, strength training can offset the relative stress of the external load by increasing lean muscle mass, improving upper body strength, and improving the structural foundation (tendons, ligaments, and bones), resulting in improved load carriage (35). Studies have demonstrated that strength training alone can improve performance on military lifting tasks and load carriage, even when load carriage itself is not incorporated into the PT protocol (34). This is an important finding because many units rely on load carriage training as the predominant mode of training for load carriage. Reducing the frequency of load carriage training while incorporating strength- and power-based exercises can mitigate many of the overuse injuries that occur due to excessive running and road marching (27).

Key Point

The warfighter needs to have properly designed resistance training programs that optimize their whole body strength and power capabilities.

Aside from load carriage, military personnel need a variety of skill-based physical fitness capabilities to accomplish occupational tasks (see table 19.1) (45, 65). During military tasks such as offensive and defensive maneuvers, personnel may be required to conduct sudden movements while carrying external loads (38). People who lack agility and flexibility and are unaccustomed to these movements face an increased likelihood of injury. Military personnel may also have to traverse a variety of terrains, such as heavily wooded terrain, swamps, rocky terrain with poor footing, or desert environments with loose, sandy soil. All of these terrain types increase the biomechanical demands of locomotion, which are exacerbated by wearing heavy equipment (49). Military personnel therefore must have good balance, agility, and coordination to be able to withstand these biomechanical challenges (45, 71).

Key Point

A total conditioning program is needed to integrate all the performance capabilities associated with a warfighter's mission demands.

Additionally, many military tasks require jumping and landing, which place further biomechanical demands on the body. Whereas athletes conduct these movements in athletic gear, military personnel perform these activities in boots that are not designed for that purpose. Jumping

and landing are also frequently performed while carrying external loads, which exacerbates the GRF upon impact. Special consideration must be given to circumstances where military personnel face additional physical requirements, such as in airborne units. Jumping and landing from a plane wearing an additional load places a heavy biomechanical demand on the warfighter. Additionally, military personnel assigned to these types of units perform excessive running and road marching, further increasing the likelihood of **overuse injuries** sustained from repeated actions. The prevalence of overuse injuries is high, particularly when combined with high operational tempo and demanding predeployment training cycles (55).

Occupational Demands

Many MOS are found within the branches of military service and have varied physiological demands (3). In general, there are combat and noncombat occupational specialties (3). All military personnel are required to meet minimum fitness standards in order to serve; however, combat occupational specialties are typically more challenging, requiring extensive physical preparation and occupation-specific training.

Table 19.1 Physical Fitness Components and Definitions

Component	Definition
Health-related components of physical fitness	
Muscular strength	The ability of a muscle to exert a maximal force through a given ROM or at a single given point
Muscular endurance	The ability of a muscle to repeatedly exert a submaximal force through a given ROM or at a single point over a given time
Aerobic fitness	The ability of the cardiorespiratory system to continue training (exercising) for extended periods of time (longer than 20 min on average)
Flexibility	The ability of a joint to move through a full ROM
Body composition	The ratio of lean body mass to fat mass or body mass to height
Skill-related components of physical fitness	
Agility	The ability to rapidly and accurately change the direction of the body in space
Balance	The ability to maintain equilibrium while stationary or moving
Coordination	The ability to use one's senses and body parts to perform motor tasks smoothly and accurately
Power	The amount of force a muscle can exert as quickly as possible (force or strength per unit of time)
Reaction time	The ability to respond quickly to stimuli
Speed	The amount of time it takes the body to perform specific tasks (distance per unit of time)

Reprinted, by permission, from M.A. Sharp et al., 2015, "Executive summary from the National Strength and Conditioning Association's second blue ribbon panel on military physical readiness: Military physical performance testing," *Journal of Strength and Conditioning Research* 29(Suppl 11): S216-220.

The demands placed on a soldier in a combat-centric occupation will be much different than those faced by an administrative specialist. For example, an infantryman must be able to perform tasks such as ambushes, offensive and defensive maneuvers, and casualty rescues and must possess the muscular strength and endurance required for extended load carriage (38, 66, 68). On the other end of the spectrum, the military intelligence analyst has few physical demands beyond semi-annual fitness testing and daily unit-level physical fitness training but nonetheless must be prepared for unexpected physical challenges when attached to a combat arms team.

Certain units may have additional physical standards that require a higher level of fitness (e.g., 75th Ranger Regiment, airborne or air assault units). Military personnel assigned to these units are expected to obtain airborne or air assault qualification as part of their training, and they must meet many other physical performance standards. **Special operators**—highly trained personnel who are adaptable, self-reliant, and able to operate in all environments using unconventional combat skills and equipment—face even more demanding requirements. Thus, the occupational specialty, unit of assignment, and mission dictate which physical capabilities are required (35).

Key Point

Careful analysis of military training activities and conditioning programs is needed in order to properly design exercise programs that can prevent overuse injuries or compromise strength and power capabilities of the warfighter. These problems often arise from the excessive use of endurance training.

Some of the occupational tasks that military personnel may perform include lifting and carrying objects, conducting a fireman's carry, and conducting a casualty evacuation (16, 38). Other occupational tasks include performing sprint-type activities (offensive and defensive maneuvers) (38) while carrying an external load, throwing an object (i.e., grenade) a specified distance, jumping and landing safely, maneuvering over terrain and obstacles, low crawling through terrain, quickly changing direction while maintaining balance,

and accurately firing a firearm from various positions or while moving (see table 19.2). Firearm weight, upper body strength and endurance, and prior exercise stress affect the accuracy of shooting and the length of time a person is able to maintain correct firing posture; however, these abilities can be recovered quickly (14).

The addition of a firearm will also affect maneuverability, flexibility, and agility, particularly when carrying external loads (49). Certain occupational specialties expose military personnel to other demands that also have physical implications, such as excessive vibration, jarring, or sitting in cramped environments (e.g., armored military vehicles, watercraft) for extended periods of time.

ENVIRONMENTAL, OCCUPATIONAL, AND EXPOSURE CONCERNS

The warfighter faces short- to long-term exposure to a variety of mission environments. If given enough time, the body can acclimatize to heat and altitude by making adjustments to better tolerate the physiological demands. However, the body does not acclimatize to cold, and protection is necessary in such environments (e.g., shelter, clothing). Understanding environmental challenges can help the TSAC Facilitator prepare military personnel for them; for instance, cardiorespiratory fitness and acclimatization to heat can minimize heat illnesses in training and mission environments (8). Please see the section on acclimatization later in the chapter for additional details.

Thermal Stress

Exposure to heat is a common challenge for warfighters in environments ranging from jungle to desert. Heat exposure can result in different forms of heat illness that reflect the body's inability to adjust to the environment. These illnesses include heat cramps, syncope, heat exhaustion, and heatstroke. They are common not only in mission environments but in training or conditioning scenarios as well (2). Deaths from heat illnesses can be avoided if proper preparation and emergency medical procedures are followed (67). This is especially true for heatstroke, where

Table 19.2 Warrior Tasks and Physical Requirements

Task	Physical requirements
Shoot	
Employ hand grenades.	Run under load, jump, bound, high/low crawl, climb, push, pull, squat, lunge, roll, stop, start, change direction, get up/down, and throw.
Move	
Perform individual movement techniques.	March/run under load, jump, bound, high/low crawl, climb, push, pull, squat, lunge, roll, stop, start, change direction, and get up/down.
Navigate from one point to another.	March/run under load, jump, bound, high/low crawl, climb, push, pull, squat, lunge, roll, stop, start, change direction, and get up/down.
Move under fire.	Run fast under load, jump, bound, crawl, push, pull, squat, roll, stop, start, change direction, and get up/down.
Survive	
Perform combatives.	React to man-to-man contact: push, pull, run, roll, throw, land, manipulate body weight, squat, lunge, rotate, bend, block, strike, kick, stop, start, change direction, and get up/down.
Adapt	
Assess and respond to threats (escalation of force).	React to man-to-man contact: push, pull, run, roll, throw, land, manipulate body weight, squat, lunge, rotate, bend, block, strike, kick, stop, start, change direction, and get up/down. Run under load, jump, bound, high/low crawl, climb, push, pull, squat, lunge, roll, stop, start, change direction, get up/down, and throw.
Battle drills	
React to contact.	Run fast under load, jump, bound, crawl, push, pull, squat, roll, stop, start, change direction, and get up/down.
Evacuate a casualty.	Squat, lunge, flex/extend/rotate trunk, walk/run, lift, and carry.

Adapted from U.S. Department of the Army (65).

immediate whole-body cooling in an ice bath can prevent fatalities (9).

Heat Cramps

Exercise-induced **heat cramps** are muscle spasms that occur when a tactical athlete is exposed to heat during PT or in an operational environment (2, 9, 67). Cramps can be caused by intense exercise (e.g., road march) and can be painful. Muscle cramps can occur even at rest after physical conditioning or a mission. Several factors appear to contribute to heat cramps, including dehydration, electrolyte imbalances, and neuromuscular fatigue. The term *heat cramps* may be a poor description because heat cramps can occur when core temperature is in the normal range. Heat cramps are the most common form of heat illness in the days and weeks of increased training loads, especially in hot environments (4, 67).

Syncope

Heat **syncope** occurs when a person who is in the heat or has just finished an activity feels dizzy or lightheaded or faints (9). It is common in people who have not acclimatized (i.e., natural heat) or acclimated (i.e., artificial heat) to heat exposure (2, 4). Thus, careful exposure to heat in a progressive manner over 7 to 14 days can reduce this common type of heat illness (67). Numerous causes have been identified, including dehydration and issues with blood flow (2).

Heat Exhaustion

Heat exhaustion is difficult to distinguish from heatstroke, which is a medical emergency (9). According to the NATA position stand, heat exhaustion is "the inability to effectively exercise in the heat, secondary to a combination of factors, including cardiovascular insufficiency, hypotension, energy depletion, and central fatigue" (9). Conversely, **heatstroke** is the most severe heat illness. It is characterized by neuropsychiatric impairment elevation in the body's core temperature, usually greater than 40 °C (104 °F) (9, 33). This condition is a product of both metabolic heat production and environmental heat load and occurs when the thermoregulatory system becomes overwhelmed due to excessive heat production (i.e., metabolic heat production from the working muscles) or inhibited heat loss (i.e., decreased sweating response, decreased ability to evaporate sweat) or both (9). When in doubt, best practice is to treat all heat illnesses as heatstroke and implement immediate cooling practices (e.g., ice bath).

Heat exhaustion during exercise can be due to multiple factors, such as heavy sweating, dehydration, sodium loss, and energy depletion (9). It typically occurs in hot and humid environments. Signs and symptoms include pallor, persistent muscular cramps, weakness, fainting, dizziness, headache, hyperventilation, nausea, diarrhea, acute loss of appetite, decreased urine output, and a core temperature that ranges between 36 °C (97 °F) and 40 °C (104 °F) (9).

Exertional Heatstroke

A genuine medical emergency, **exertional heatstroke (EHS)** needs to be addressed immediately. Deaths related to EHS are fully preventable; immediate treatment with whole-body immersion in ice water can eliminate the lethal threat (2, 9). With intense or long-duration exercise, dysregulation of body temperature can occur (i.e., the body is unable to get rid of the heat produced). The heat produced can overwhelm the thermoregulatory system, causing heatstroke. Signs and symptoms of heatstroke include rapid HR (tachycardia), hypotension, sweating (although skin may be dry at the time of collapse), hyperventilation, altered mental state, diarrhea, seizure, and coma (2, 9). Heat-loss mechanisms typically shut down with heatstroke, allowing further elevations in core temperature, and death can occur at core temperatures in excess of 43 °C (109.4 °F) (2, 9). Treatment must focus on rapidly cooling the body—the longer the delay in treatment, the greater the chance of death. Accurate assessment of core temperature is key in timely treatment of EHS. Rectal temperature is the gold standard for assessing core body temperature; other measures have been shown to be inaccurate (17).

Fitness level and age can affect susceptibility to heat illness (2, 9). Sex is not a factor when dealing with heat illness, despite the fact that sweating is triggered at a higher core temperature in women than in men, which results in a delayed sweat response when exercising. Acclimatization and acclimation are vital to mitigating heat stress. Early physiological adaptations take place in 1 to 5 days with improved regulation and control of cardiovascular responses (2, 9, 33). In 5 to 8 days, the body starts to make adaptations that offer partial protection from lethal hyperthermia (i.e., increase in core temperature). By 14 days, most of the adaptations to the heat stress are complete (33):

- Lower core temperature at onset of sweating
- Increased heat loss via radiation and convection (skin blood flow)
- Increased plasma volume
- Decreased HR at a specific exercise intensity
- Decreased core temperature
- Decreased skin temperature
- Decreased oxygen consumption requirement at a given exercise intensity
- Improved exercise economy (the amount of work that can be done per unit of oxygen consumed)

Key Point

Heat illness is completely preventable with proper acclimatization, activity planning (when possible), and hydration protocols. It is also fully treatable if preparations have been made. Thus, symptoms of heat illness should be taken seriously and addressed immediately by cessation of activity, hydration, and whole body cooling—ideally in an ice water bath—if heat exhaustion or heat stroke is suspected.

Cold Exposure

Operational readiness is key to coping with cold exposure. Hypothermia is the major threat to survival in a cold environment. The normal core temperature is about 37 °C (98.6 °F). When the body's temperature drops below 32°C (89.6 °F), physiological systems start to shut down (33).

Environmental temperature can fluctuate widely in the field, going from hot during the day to cold at night. As the external temperature falls, various physiological thermoregulatory mechanisms are engaged to maintain the body's internal temperature. However, although physiological mechanisms can start the adjustment process to help keep the body warm, appropriate clothing or shelter is needed. Additionally, during training and missions, exposure to rain or cold water resulting in wet clothing can speed up heat loss and threaten the ability to maintain thermal balance. Interestingly, because metabolic heat is produced with exercise and protective garments may be very effective (i.e., protective clothing can create a microclimate for the body), it is possible to experience heat illness in the cold (67). Therefore, planning ahead and understanding the training or mission environment are key to adequately preparing the warfighter. Again, one cannot acclimatize to cold environments, so protective garments or shelter must be part of the training or mission planning (33, 67).

Altitude Exposure

Some military missions may involve terrains at altitude. Following are the general classifications of elevations above sea level (44):

- Moderate altitude = 5,000 to 8,000 feet (1,524-2,438 m)

- High altitude = 8,000 to 14,000 feet (2,438-4,267 m)

- Very high altitude = 14,000 to 18,000 feet (4,267-5,486 m)

- Extreme high altitude = 18,000 to 29,028 feet (5,486-8,848 m)

If the altitude is high enough, the ability to perform aerobic activities can be compromised. Again, mission preparation is crucial for such terrains. Most missions do not involve long-term exposure to high altitudes; nevertheless, an understanding of altitude is important for dealing with such environmental demands if they occur.

A common misbelief is that there is less oxygen with altitude. The percentage of oxygen (20.93%), as well as other gases (CO_2 = 0.03%, nitrogen = 79.04%), in the air is the same regardless of the altitude. It is the amount of pressure exerted on each molecule of gas that is different, and this is related to the barometric pressure (mmHg).

As altitude increases, the barometric pressure decreases. Less pressure is involved in gas movement, making it more difficult to extract oxygen from the air in the lungs and transport it to the body's tissues. Oxygen tension, or the partial pressure of oxygen (PO_2), is calculated by multiplying the barometric pressure times the percentage of oxygen in the air. Thus, at sea level (0 feet; standard sea-level barometric pressure = 760 mmHg), there are greater partial pressures in the body helping to move gases from the lungs to the tissues than at an altitude with a barometric pressure of 596 mmHg (2,000 m or 6,562 ft) (33). When less oxygen is delivered to body tissues, a **hypoxic effect** occurs, which is a major challenge of a high-altitude environment.

Key Point

The altitude at which the mission is performed may present challenges to the physiological functions of the warfighter. Prior planning can help prevent potential complications to the health and performance of the warfighter.

As altitude increases, the temperature decreases. Along with lower temperatures, the vapor content of the air is also lower, promoting greater evaporation of sweat from the body, which increases the potential for dehydration, especially with intense physical activity (25, 33). Additionally, greater amounts of solar radiation occur because higher altitudes are a shorter distance from the electromagnetic waves of the sun, which are traveling in a thinning atmosphere. Ultraviolet sunblock is needed to protect exposed skin from the sun's radiation as well. Thus, multiple environmental stressors can occur with increasing altitude, and hydration needs to be monitored. There is no foolproof method for measuring the hydration status of an individual at a single time point. However, USG (urine-specific gravity) or urine color may be used along with observed changes in body mass to get a sense of hydration status (10). Care is needed because one-time measures can produce erroneous results, but catching hypohydration is vital, along with careful adherence to proper water intake (43).

The reduced partial pressure of oxygen in the air at altitude can affect performance in the following ways (33):

- A decrease in the partial pressure of oxygen can reduce the ability of oxygen to reach the body's tissues.

- Exposure to altitude results in several physiological adjustments by the body in an attempt to maintain normal function.

- During exercise at altitude, both ventilatory volume and rate of breathing may increase to help get more oxygen into the lungs.

- At altitude, maximal oxygen consumption, cardiac output, MHR, and SV all decrease, reducing performance capacity.

- Exposure to altitude causes an increase in hemoglobin and hematocrit in the blood, improving the ability to carry oxygen.

- Short performances are not hindered, but bending over at higher altitudes can cause dizziness due to the rapid change in position and hydrostatic pressure.

- Long-duration performances, namely those dependent on aerobic metabolism, are negatively affected by altitude.

A concern at higher altitudes is the development of altitude sickness. The three forms of altitude sickness are mild altitude sickness, **high-altitude cerebral edema (HACE)**, and high-altitude pulmonary edema (HAPE) (19). The symptoms of mild altitude sickness, also called **acute mountain sickness (AMS)**, are highly individual, with some people feeling only minor effects (including headache, nausea, and fatigue), while others are downright sick. Nevertheless, AMS is a warning sign that a person might be risk of more serious conditions. It is caused by a reduction in the partial pressure of oxygen in the air and is a pathological condition that requires medical attention. AMS is of concern because it can lead to HAPE and HACE, which can be life threatening and require immediate medical attention (33). HAPE results in a dramatic, dangerous buildup of fluid in the lungs, which can prevent the lungs from getting air. This deprives the body of oxygen and can be fatal in a matter of hours. Additionally, HACE is a severe form of altitude sickness resulting in increased blood flow to the brain due to low oxygen levels, causing brain damage and death within a few hours.

AMS symptoms include nausea, vomiting, lethargy, dizziness, and poor sleep. HAPE is typically observed after two to three days at altitudes above 2,500 m (8,202 ft). People with this form of altitude sickness are more breathless than those around them, especially on exertion, and exhibit symptoms similar to those of AMS. Additionally, they may experience chronic breathlessness (even at rest), fast HR, blue lips, and elevated body temperature. Symptoms may be confused with a chest infection; coughing may produce white or pink frothy sputum. Symptoms of HACE include severe headache, vomiting, and lethargy that progresses to unsteadiness, confusion, drowsiness, and ultimately coma. People with HACE may have difficulty walking heel to toe in a straight line (this can be used as a test for someone with severe AMS symptoms) and present irrational or bizarre behavior.

Treatment involves removal from altitude, medical care, and rest. Dehydration at altitude can result in a misdiagnosis of altitude sickness, and thus water intake is vital to monitor at altitude and allows for better toleration. Proper hydration guidelines must be followed so as not to drink too much water, which can result hyponatremia, a condition where the concentration of sodium in the blood is abnormally low. This important electrolyte is vital to all cell function and is affected by many factors but can occur with excessively high intakes of water, as has been observed in endurance athletes in training and competition (22).

At what point is altitude an issue? The major effects of altitude are on endurance and appear to emerge at moderate altitudes (around 2,200 m or 7,218 ft) (33). Exposure to altitude requires preparation to minimize these negative effects. Typically, this means the tactical athlete needs to acclimatize to the altitude at which the operational training or mission is to take place. For moderate altitudes, typical strategies involve arriving at the site a week or so before the event or completing the mission at altitude and then leaving right afterward to minimize the exposure to altitude and not allow any negative side effects of altitude to manifest. As noted, care is needed to monitor symptoms during longer missions at higher altitudes because altitude sickness can manifest quickly. At higher altitudes, staging from moderate elevation to allow acclimatization has been used successfully. Short-term acclimatization or acclimation is characterized by altitude exposure of less than one year. Even in shorter periods of three to six weeks, dramatic changes can take place, and warfighters can take advantage of these changes to prepare for combat operations at altitude. (See the U.S. Army Human Performance Resource Center for more information: http://hprc-online.org/environment/altitude.) Long-term acclimatization involves living at altitude for more than three months (33).

Key Point

Altitude exposure can be associated with other environmental hazards and conditions from cold, dehydration, and thermal stressors.

Hazardous Exposure

Hazardous exposure refers to any biological, chemical, mechanical, or physical agent that is reasonably likely to cause harm to humans or the environment with sufficient exposure. While beyond the scope of this chapter, the threat of hazardous exposure during operational missions has been extensively examined, and the reader is referred to Joint Publication 3-11 (26). This document outlines the many challenges of hazardous exposure to the command structure and operational scenarios.

Each wartime mission has involved different hazardous exposures, some known and some unknown at the time (e.g., Agent Orange in the Vietnam War). Hazardous exposures in Operation Enduring Freedom in Afghanistan included the following, according to the U.S. Department of Veterans Affairs (74):

- Dust and particulates, tiny airborne matter that can cause respiratory and other health problems
- Nine infectious diseases associated with Southwest Asia
- Pits left from toxic embedded fragments of roadside bombs
- Shrapnel and other metals that remain in the body after injury

- Radiation exposure from head scans for traumatic brain injury caused by explosions
- Malaria
- Cold injuries from cold, mountainous climate
- Burn pits (waste disposal in open-air pits at military sites)
- Depleted uranium used in military tank armor, jets, and some bullets
- Blast noise from guns, equipment, and machinery
- Rabies (disease transmitted by bite or saliva from an infected warm-blooded animal)
- Heat injuries caused by extremely hot temperatures
- Occupational hazards from working with chemicals, paints, and machinery

Each of these potential exposures can only be mitigated with precautionary steps for prevention, shielding, and treatment. Many of these hazardous insults can affect warfighters throughout their military careers and beyond.

Key Point

A multitude of hazardous exposures accompany various combat and service missions; these need to be carefully assessed and protected against with proper planning, protections, and procedures for avoidance and handling.

Shift Work and Unpredictability of Job Assignment

Shift work varies by military occupation and military service. The goal of most shift work is to optimize performance and reduce chronic fatigue. It is highly related to the MOS skill set, mission requirements, and physical readiness for tasks under varying conditions. As previously noted, the unpredictable nature of mission assignments and demands underscores the importance of physical readiness for warfighters. The TSAC Facilitator must be concerned with MOS-related levels of fitness that can be assessed and quickly attained so that the tactical athlete can successfully perform rapid occupational assignments and task demands. Thus, a flexible program for preparatory activities such as PRT (physical readiness training) must be used where each conditioning session focuses on the warfighter's required physical fitness. Although the TSAC Facilitator is not involved with the development of work schedules for the units, it is helpful to understand certain guidelines that have been set forth (42).

For the tactical athlete, the optimization of each training session is important. Going through the motions in a workout is not acceptable. Determining the warfighter's fatigue level is also important in order to optimize each training session. Optimization has been achieved using a flexible nonlinear training program that allows one to choose the best type of workout or change the workout in midstream if the quality markers of performance are not met (e.g., planned rep number not achieved with prescribed load, running speed not at expected level, height of maximal jump training not even close to 90% of personal best) (37, 40, 41). Thus, monitoring feedback from scales (e.g., session RPE, sleep scales) along with training logs and training partner interactions are vital to optimizing the workouts in a program.

INJURY AND ILLNESS RISKS

Injuries are inherent in the military work environment. It is vital to perform a needs analysis to understand the types of injuries involved and then attempt to mitigate them by improving the fitness and anatomical strength of tissues to withstand forces in the operational environment.

Musculoskeletal Injury Concerns

Military personnel are exposed to wear and tear that can result in injury if the body is not capable of meeting the demands of the job. Injuries can not only affect duty performance and readiness but also have lasting effects on health and increase the expenses of medical care. As mentioned previously, heavy load carriage greatly increases the GRF exerted on the body during locomotion. Due to the biomechanical strain of heavy load carriage and the frequency of military tasks that require repetitive lifting, military personnel typically experience injuries in the lower back and lower extremities (58). Studies have shown that injuries in both deployed and nondeployed military personnel are typically musculoskeletal (58). Exacerbating the problem are PT regimens that focus heavily on aerobic conditioning (16, 48) while neglecting strength and power development, which are necessary for optimal load carriage (35). When the musculature is weak, the spine and connective tissue bear a larger percentage of the external load and are therefore more susceptible to injury.

Key Point

> Musculoskeletal injury is one of the top reasons for loss of duty time and for compromises to mission readiness. Proper prevention with proper design and monitoring of strength and conditioning programs can help to reduce such occurrences.

A heavy emphasis on running frequently results in overuse injuries, particularly among basic trainees, who are not used to high running mileage (16, 48). Injuries typically seen in an athletic population, such as ACL injuries, are also common (64). Many injuries in a military population are preventable with appropriate training and recovery strategies. Stress fractures, for example, are a common overuse injury that can be mitigated through progressive increases in running mileage, adequate rest and recovery, and careful monitoring of the athlete (16, 28, 29). Likewise, studies have shown that the incidence of ACL injuries can be reduced by incorporating training strategies that teach and reinforce proper jumping and landing movements (64). Additionally, once an injury has occurred, strengthening of the surrounding musculature is pivotal in preventing reinjury.

Risk Factors

There are ways to identify and measure risk factors for injury. Research on these factors in both civilian and military populations is extensive and tends to categorize risk factors as either intrinsic or extrinsic, or modifiable or nonmodifiable. Recent comprehensive discussions of risk factors for injury have highlighted the following risk factors (3, 18). The TSAC Facilitator should be adept at identifying and modifying these risk factors when possible.

- Prior level of physical activity
- Injury history
- Smoking or tobacco-use history
- Age and sex
- Command influence and unit culture
- Type of unit and occupational specialty
- Training program frequency and intensity
- Presence and proper use of safety equipment, shoes, and clothing
- Environment, such as weather and surface (ice, snow, rain)
- Athletic skill
- Genetics
- Nutrition
- Menstrual cycle dysfunction
- BMI

Injury Prevention and Treatment

Long-term injury prevention is a top priority for warfighters, health care providers, and U.S. Department of Defense (DoD) policymakers. Preventing injuries from physical activity and occupational task performance is critical in sustaining the health and welfare of the fighting force during an era of high operational tempo and fiscal constraints (20, 48). High injury rates negatively affect combat readiness, and over the long term they can contribute to rising health care costs for service members and veterans. For example, over 45% of Rangers are injured within the first year of training (63), which is similar to injury rates throughout a warfighter's physical career (12, 21). Training and overuse injury rates in other studies of military populations range from 18% to 52% (1, 23).

The team that mitigates the impact of injuries within each unit varies across the services. Over the past few years, the Army's brigade combat teams (BCTs), for example, have included active-duty physical therapists. The intent is for these junior officers to provide both treatment and injury prevention services. However, many units do not have this level of musculoskeletal expertise or any organic physical performance expert. There is currently no MOS for someone who is certified or licensed in the provision of exercise science or with a primary duty of physical readiness and injury control. The TSAC Facilitator may be the only professionally certified physical trainer in the unit and must be able to lead both small and large groups in comprehensive physical fitness training. Involvement of a TSAC Facilitator increases the likelihood that PT will be effective and can have a major impact on injury prevention (7).

In the U.S. Navy, a novel approach to injury mitigation has become part of most Marine installations over the past few years. Sports medicine training rooms in the Sports Medicine and Reconditioning Team (SMART) clinic allow faster access to higher levels of medical expertise for injury treatment, resulting in reduced attrition and reduced referrals to orthopedic surgery (6). The SMART program is not an initiative to prevent injuries; SMART providers engage in treatment once injury has already occurred. Injuries are treated in the sports medicine training room, but they happen on the training field. Placing an expert at the point of injury who can recognize when it is about to happen and who has both the authority and command presence to intervene may be the key to mitigating unintentional injury from PT.

In 2012, the Army relaunched the **Master Fitness Trainer Course (MFTC)** with the intent to place one MFTC-certified active-duty non-commissioned officer (NCO) or officer in every unit from the company (100+ personnel) to the division levels (10,000-20,000 personnel) (69). At its inception, the MFTC provided four weeks of instruction by mobile training teams to several thousand military personnel. More recently, the course has converted to a 40-hour online didactic portion followed by a 93-hour resident, hands-on portion taught over two weeks. Instructors must have TSAC-F certification, and many have a **NSCA-Certified Personal Trainer (NSCA-CPT)** certification or (if they have an undergraduate college degree) **Certified Strength and Conditioning Specialist (CSCS)** certification. The broadest range of certifications is encouraged so that MFTC instructors can teach and speak more authoritatively to a wide range of PT programming.

Master Fitness Trainers (MFTs) can be a vital resource for TSAC Facilitators, providing the military context for planning and implementing PT for the warfighter. MFTs are unit-level experts in the conduct of Army PRT (FM 7-22), and can act as liaisons between the unit and medical personnel to resolve, improve, and optimize physical performance in the unit. They have training in exercise science, anatomy, industrial-scale PT, Army policy and regulations, injury considerations, performance nutrition, recovery, and nonstandardized commercial PT programming. MFTs who are empowered and encouraged by their commands are the closest equivalent in the military services to the TSAC Facilitator.

Key Point

Having professionals with appropriate training and education in a strength and conditioning program can help optimize the physical training of military personnel.

OPTIMIZING FUNCTIONAL FITNESS

As mentioned, optimizing programming for warfighters is vital to achieve the minimal level of physical fitness needed to meet MOS demands. These demands are reflected in both MOS requirements as well as baseline testing, which has recently been a topic of great debate and changes. Thus, the TSAC Facilitator must stay up to date on the testing protocols that are planned for and currently implemented in the various military services.

Physical Fitness Requirements and Testing

Each service requires military personnel to meet physical fitness standards. Resource constraints and DoD policy have resulted in field-expedient physical fitness tests, although the tests do not assess preparedness for a variety of demanding occupational tasks (e.g., lifting and load carriage) (45). Because fitness scores are a part of the warfighter's performance evaluation and can have negative career consequences, fitness tests have traditionally been a key driver of military PT programs (30). Specific testing events vary by service; however, all services test aerobic fitness, muscular strength, and muscular endurance. Each service conducts a sustained run, a sustained upper body

pushing or pulling event, and a sustained trunk flexion event (see table 19.3). Additionally, each service conducts body-fat assessment as part of physical fitness testing. The Marine Corps has an additional testing requirement, the Combat Fitness Test (CFT), which was adopted in 2009. It consists of three anaerobic events that closely replicate combat-specific physical tasks. These CFT tasks replicate movement to contact, movements under fire, and movement away from contact (see table 19.4) (75).

Physical fitness testing is required at least twice per year; however, units may conduct testing at the discretion of the unit commander. Additionally, testing may be a prerequisite for attendance at various military schools. Generally speaking, in a nondeployed setting (when military personnel are at home stations or garrisons), military personnel are expected to meet physical fitness testing standards several times per year, barring special circumstances such as injury or surgery.

Additionally, the U.S. Army developed and validated a test to assess recruits' physical ability to complete basic training for their MOS. Called the Occupational Physical Assessment Test (OPAT), the test consists of criterion standards for the standing long jump, seated medicine ball throw, deadlift, and aerobic interval run. OPAT is scheduled to be fielded as this publication goes to print. In addition, MOS-specific physical fitness tests are currently being examined. Thus, the TSAC Facilitator must keep up with fitness test development for each service and incorporate relevant elements in training programs (e.g., using a deadlift with a trap bar or including standing long jumps in power training).

Currently, no U.S. service has a MOS-specific fitness testing requirement, although the Army, Air Force, and Navy are conducting studies to determine whether Tier 2 occupational fitness tests should be incorporated into the physical fitness assessment for service members (45). Military fitness testing requirements and the physical requirements of the occupational specialty are not one and the same. In fact, the physical fitness tests currently employed by the various services have been found to be ineffective in assessing the fitness components required for many combat tasks (45). The fitness components most needed

Table 19.3 Service-Specific Physical Fitness Test Components

Service	Test sequence		
Air Force (PFA)	1.5 mi (2.4 km) run	Push-ups	Sit-ups
Army (APFT)	Push-ups (2 min)	Sit-ups (2 min)	2 mi (3.2 km) run
Army (ACFT)	3 RM deadlift, standing power throw	Hand release push-up, sprint-drag-carry	Leg tuck or plank, 2 mi (3.2 km) run
Marine Corps (PFT)	Pull-ups (or flexed arm hang option for females); not timed	Crunches (2 min)	3 mi (4.8 km) run
Navy (PRT)	1.5 mi (2.4 km) run	Curl-ups (2 min)	Push-ups (2 min)

Based on Air Force Guidance Memorandum for AFI 36-2905, June 2012; U.S. Department of the Army Field Manual 7-22, October 2012 (APFT), October 2020 (ACFT); Marine Corps Order 6100-13, August 2008; and Navy Physical Readiness Program, OPNAVINSTR 6110.1J, July 2011.

Table 19.4 Marine Corps Combat Fitness Test

Test	Description
Movement to contact	Timed 880 yd (805 m) run in utility uniform and boots
Ammunition lift	2 min lifting 30 lb (14 kg) ammo can over the head, earning 2 points for each number done within the time limit
Maneuver under fire	300 yd (274 m) shuttle run with a variety of combat-related tasks: • 25 yd (23 m) sprint starting from the prone position • 10 yd (9 m) high crawl • 15 yd (14 m) modified high crawl (low then high crawl) • 25 yd (23 m) cone network run • 10 yd (9 m) seated casualty drag • 65 yd (59 m) fireman's carry • 75 yd (69 m) sprint while carrying two 30 lb (14 kg) ammo cans through the same cone network • Grenade throw into a marked circle 22.5 yd (20.5 m) away (add 5 s to total time if missed; deduct 5 s if target is hit) • 3 push-ups • 75 yd (69 m) sprint with ammo cans back to the starting line to finish the event

Adapted from Marine Corps Order 6100.13 W/CH 2, January 2015.

for job performance are muscular strength, muscular endurance, and power (45). Although the physical fitness tests employed by the services are field-expedient, useful assessments of health status, they may not accurately assess the muscular strength and power needed for heavy lifting and load carriage (although these issues are being examined in MOS-specific tests) (45, 61).

It is important for the TSAC Facilitator to be cognizant of the differences in MOS physical requirements and general fitness testing requirements. From extensive discussion with combat veterans, anecdotal evidence suggests that the requirements of the job specialty can far exceed the requirements set forth in baseline physical fitness testing, particularly in the combat arms branches. Such observations have led the military to reexamine fitness testing as it relates to MOS demands. For example, Coast Guard rescue swimmers must pass a variety of swim tests, such as the

500-yard (457 m) crawl swim, 25 m (27 yd) underwater rescue swim, and 200-yard (183 m) buddy tow, as part of regular physical fitness screening (72). Navy SEALs, special warfare combatant-craft crewmen (SWCC), explosive ordnance disposal (EOD) technicians, Navy divers, and aviation rescue swimmers must complete a physical screening test consisting of a 500-yard (457 m) swim, maximum push-ups in 2 minutes, maximum curl-ups in 2 minutes, maximum pull-ups in 2 minutes, and a 1.5-mile (2.4 km) run (events are performed consecutively, with 10 minutes rest between events) (73). The minimum scoring requirements are outlined in table 19.5. However, in most instances, military personnel must exceed the minimum performance standards in order to perform well in these occupations. Additionally, for many combat-centric occupational specialties, the physical requirements are not always outlined in a testable standard.

Table 19.5 Minimum PST Scoring Requirements for Navy SEALs, SWCCs, EOD Technicians, and AIRRs

Event	SEAL	SWCC	EOD	AIRR
Swim (500 yd [457 m]) (min:s)	12:30	13:00	12:30	12:00
Push-ups (maximum reps in 2 min)	50	50	50	42
Curl-ups (maximum reps)	50	50	50	50
Pull-ups (maximum reps)	10	6	6	4
Run (1.5 mi [2.4 km]) (min:s)	10:30	12:00	12:30	12:00

Events are performed consecutively, with 10 minutes rest between each event.

PST = physical screening test; SEAL = SEa, Air, and Land; SWCC = Special Warfare Combatant-Craft Crewmen; EOD = Explosive Ordnance Disposal; AIRR = Aviation Rescue Swimmer.

U.S. Department of the Navy (73).

Key Point

> Fitness testing in the various service branches are part of an ongoing effort to evaluate health status as well as minimum physical fitness needed for military service and occupational skill sets. The testing varies between branches; each TSAC Facilitator should be aware of the testing for the service branch to make sure each warfighter's conditioning program addresses the performance factors tested.

Physical Fitness Training

One of the key issues in military PT is a mismatch between the requirements of the occupational specialty and the manner in which military personnel conduct physical fitness training. Again, military veterans and government researchers in the field have observed that physical fitness training is geared toward preparing military personnel for semiannual physical fitness tests, special military schools with physical prerequisites, and selection and assessment programs for specialty assignments, typically with a heavy emphasis on aerobic exercise. Aerobic conditioning is easy to implement when training large groups, and it builds camaraderie. It can be used to weed out people for assessment and selection courses, and it can be used to toughen military personnel. Moreover, military personnel must have optimal aerobic capacity to be able to sustain physical performance during prolonged mission requirements. A foundation of aerobic conditioning is necessary in developing optimal work capacity in military

personnel and is associated with positive health benefits such as improved cardiovascular health and decreased body fat (16). However, aerobic training often becomes the predominant mode of PT at the expense of strength and power development (30, 48). This leaves military personnel at a sizeable disadvantage when it comes to anaerobic tasks that involve heavy lifting, load carriage, or sprinting.

Many military personnel have inadequate strength and power to meet the demands of their occupational specialty (e.g., repetitive lifting, load carriage). Observation of infantry soldiers in Afghanistan, for example, routinely found that soldiers struggled with heavy external loads, despite having a well-developed foundation of aerobic conditioning prior to deployment (13). The misconception that aerobic endurance is the gold standard of fitness training combined with limited fitness training time propels military personnel to choose exercise that they can complete relatively quickly (e.g., running, HIIT). Though effective, too much volume or frequency might result in overreaching or overtraining syndrome with diminishing fitness returns (52). In addition, an overemphasis on running is detrimental to strength and power development (16). Running and calisthenics fail to stimulate the Type II muscle fibers that must be recruited for strength and power development (35). Even low-load resistance training performed for high repetitions will not result in the strength and hypertrophy adaptations that are necessary for optimal physical performance on anaerobic tasks. Unless strength and power training using appropriate loading schemes are incorporated into the PT plan, military personnel will have underdeveloped strength and power relative to the occupational tasks they are required to perform.

Key Point

> Physical conditioning programs play a vital role in preparing warfighters for the demands of the missions they are involved with. Understanding the relationship of the exercise program to the specific physiological adaptations that result is critical in understanding exercise prescription.

Physical Fitness Requirements During Deployment

Physical fitness standards are quite different during deployment than in a nondeployed setting. Although military personnel are still required to maintain a baseline level of fitness, the unit mission and operational requirements take precedence over PT. PT during deployment is frequently done on an individual basis, depending on operational constraints, availability of facilities, and equipment resources. There are times when the mission demands simply do not allow for optimal PT, which is why it is critical for military personnel to train optimally before the deployment.

When developing a periodized training model for the warfighter, the deployment can be thought of as the in-season period; the idea is to reach peak performance going into the deployment. Ideally, military personnel will maintain their fitness during deployment, but this will be affected by mission constraints, operational tempo, and available resources. Physical fitness testing rarely occurs during deployments; however, once the unit returns home, testing again becomes a priority, with military personnel typically required to pass a test shortly after returning home. This highlights an opportunity for the TSAC Facilitator to implement strength and conditioning strategies to prepare military personnel for testing requirements while minimizing injury risk after several months or more of inconsistent PT schedules during deployment.

Enhancing Adherence

Enhancing adherence to fitness programming requires careful attention to the needs of the warfighter (injury status, movement deficiencies, training goals) and the training cycle of the unit of assignment. The TSAC Facilitator must design flexible training programs that can be implemented around mission training requirements and that factor in the inevitable scheduling constraints. Command support for PT programs is critical for furthering the TSAC Facilitator's efforts in planning and executing purposeful training; it can make the difference in securing resources and time for physical fitness training.

Preparticipation Screening

Screening considerations for the military tactical athlete are much the same as for any athlete: a full medical history, including prior injuries, must be taken into account, and the individual's goals and motivations must be considered. The medical officer should be consulted regarding any contraindications for conditioning activity; as with any athlete, the military warfighter needs to be cleared for conditioning activities and training. For example, a service member may be training for a specific event such as a marathon, an assessment and selection course (e.g., Special Forces Assessment and Selection [SFAS]), or a military school (e.g., Airborne, Air Assault, Sapper School). The requirements of the occupational specialty must be considered—what tasks must the warfighter perform as part of the job? Consideration must also be given to the unit mission—what tasks must the unit perform at home and, more importantly, during deployment? These tasks dictate the physical expectations of military personnel and how the training program should be designed. Identifying any physical deficiencies related to the individual's goals and occupational tasks will assist the TSAC Facilitator in designing a training strategy.

As part of screening, special attention must be paid to the tactical athlete's resistance training history and participation in sport prior to military service. Within the military, there is typically a wide range of athletic ability and history of sport participation. Some military personnel have little to no experience in the weight room, while others come from a background of athletics. Additionally, any movement deficiencies or musculoskeletal imbalances should be identified. Tools such as movement screens can aid the TSAC Facilitator in determining the athlete's functional limitations (47).

The TSAC Facilitator must also consider the warfighter's off-duty activities. Some military personnel participate in sports or athletic pursuits outside of work, which may increase injury risk and will certainly influence the efficacy of the strength and conditioning program prescribed by the TSAC Facilitator. One of the greatest implications of off-duty sport participation is its effect on recovery. Without careful planning and progression, off-duty sport activities can hinder strength and power development, which is crucial to the performance of several military tasks. The accumulation of physical stressors from participating in exercise training programs and intense recreational activities (e.g., off-duty fitness club training, hiking, trail bike riding) in addition to unit activities can lead to overtraining.

These activities are not bad per se; however, the TSAC Facilitator might carefully monitor workouts and use tests for power to ensure there is no interference with planned training goals for physical readiness. This type of overtraining is termed *acute overreaching*. In this acute overreaching, a training variable is emphasized (e.g., more reps, heavier loading, higher frequency of training) and has an acute negative effect on performance. Acute overreaching is of known origin in a training program and used for only a short period of time (e.g., 1-4 weeks). It is used to stimulate supercompensation or a rebound in performance after one removes it and returns to regular training.

When elements are added that are not accounted for (e.g., extra training at a fitness club) or mistakes are made in the program design over a longer time, nonfunctional overreaching can result. The performance decreases can last for weeks or months, and if not corrected or understood, nonfunctional overreaching can lead to overtraining syndrome, which may suppress performance recovery for months. Nonfunctional overreaching and overtraining syndrome may have a negative

impact on job performance both before and during deployment. Not only can off-duty activities limit performance gains, but they also may have negative effects on health. For example, excessive alcohol consumption, smoking, poor diet, and lack of sleep can all increase the likelihood of injury and affect performance and progress in the weight room. Where feasible, a better understanding of the warfighter's lifestyle will help the TSAC Facilitator implement training that is best suited to the individual's needs, correct conditioning program errors, and recommend other lifestyle services available to the warfighter.

Key Point

In today's military, understanding the importance of rest and recovery and preventing overtraining are vital for recovery from missions and long-term health.

Programming Considerations

Programming considerations for the tactical athlete should begin with a needs analysis of the unit mission and the physical demands of the occupational specialty (35). First and foremost, the TSAC Facilitator must have a thorough understanding of the challenges and demands of the tactical athlete's occupational specialty. The requirements of the job, the unit mission, and the individual's training goals and areas of weakness, such as prior injury or musculoskeletal imbalances, provide the basis upon which a strength and conditioning plan can be developed. Physical fitness requirements for military personnel exist along a continuum ranging from strength and power to aerobic endurance performance. All military athletes must develop each component of fitness; however, the extent to which the components are required depends on the occupational specialty and unit mission.

Other programming considerations include the unit's training and deployment cycle. Military personnel face a number of challenges, the biggest of which is being mission ready year-round, ready for deployment at any time. This is especially true for personnel who may deploy frequently throughout the year. Whereas athletes typically have an in-season and off-season, this is not the case with tactical athletes. A deployment can be viewed as the in-season, but military training requirements while at home also require optimal physical fitness. For some military personnel (e.g., operators, combat arms), the demands and stresses of predeployment training (i.e., off-season) can be as demanding as the deployment itself. When possible, as the deployment nears, PT should increasingly mirror the demands during the deployment. For example, occupational tasks that are conducted in tactical gear (e.g., PPE) and with external loads should be progressively included in the PT plan. During the off-season, emphasis can be placed on strength and hypertrophy to build the foundation for more skill-specific work as the deployment nears.

Typically, military units have a predetermined training cycle based on deployment schedules that dictates training requirements that must be completed during the cycle, which will affect the tactical athlete's availability and readiness to train. Most military training priorities will take precedence over physical fitness training, particularly during the months leading up to a deployment. During this time, unit-level PT will be minimal, and time allocated for unit physical fitness training will be sacrificed for other training priorities. In these instances, whether military personnel adhere to a PT program of any kind depends to a large extent on the individual's personal motivation. The TSAC Facilitator can advocate for physical fitness training outside of the normal times allocated for unit-level fitness training (typically 6:00-8:00 a.m.). With command support, it is possible to shift training times to later in the day or to split training times to allow smaller groups access to limited strength and conditioning facilities.

As noted earlier, given the unpredictable nature of military service, programming must be flexible and adaptable to the tactical athlete's schedule. Sometimes military personnel will be unable to adhere to a training plan due to mission constraints. It is not uncommon for last-minute military training requirements to disrupt the warfighter's PT plan. As an example, infantry units are regularly required to perform long-distance loaded rucksack marches that compromise readiness for lower body strength training. In light of these challenges and the need to be ready

for missions year-round, the flexible nonlinear approach is generally better for the tactical athlete compared with traditional linear plans (35). With this approach, as long as the training goals for a given mesocycle are met, adjustments can be made to the training schedule as needed (35, 37). This allows the athlete to maximize training when the military schedule allows. It also facilitates recovery strategies during periods of increased operational tempo or intense predeployment training so as not to push the athlete into an overtrained state, which could contribute to injury risk and have a negative impact on readiness.

Motivation

The availability of strength and conditioning resources varies depending on branch of service and unit of assignment, and military personnel may not be required to seek out strength and conditioning resources that are available on military bases. From our observations over the years, most military personnel are not mandated to train with the strength and conditioning professional, but the resources are usually available to those who seek them out. For the TSAC Facilitator assigned at the unit level, it is important to establish credibility with military personnel assigned to the command—this is the most effective way to motivate military personnel to train. At times, the TSAC Facilitator may be invited to take part in unit PT events or workouts. Military personnel follow the principle of leading by example. Thus, showing warfighters that the TSAC Facilitator is able to perform the same physical tasks that they do, and that the TSAC Facilitator is taking the opportunity to gain an understanding of the military personnel's training environment, aids in establishing the TSAC Facilitator's credibility as a PT expert.

Within a group of military tactical athletes, a variety of factors will influence motivation to train. At one end of the spectrum, military personnel may be minimally motivated to perform only that exercise which is mandatory, as in physical fitness training prescribed at the unit level and semiannual fitness testing requirements. On the other end of the spectrum, military personnel may be highly motivated to conduct physical fitness training on their own, beyond what is required for daily physical fitness training. Some warfighters have specific training goals, such as participating in off-duty physical fitness activities, running a marathon, or participating in another sporting event. Military personnel may also be motivated to attend assessment and selection courses for specialty assignments (e.g., Navy SEAL, Army Special Forces, Air Force Pararescue). Working with many of the elite military units and on various DoD panels, we have observed that military personnel who are in or seeking assignment to specialized units tend to be more invested in maintaining and improving their fitness when compared with military personnel assigned to conventional units. This is due to highly demanding occupational requirements of specialized units.

Key Point

> A deeper understanding of the reasons physical training is important and what is happening to the body with such programs can be vital for increasing a warfighter's internal motivation for improvement.

Training Considerations

At the start of any training program, a facilitator has to develop an overall plan and approach to the program. This process includes individualizing training goals and developing group training programs. This also involves starting with a yearly calendar to fill in known schedules: possible deployments, holidays, fitness testing, and vacations. Plans for environmental acclimatization that might be needed over the year as well as injury rehabilitation protocols can also be assessed.

Establishing Training Goals

When working with military personnel, the TSAC Facilitator will be constrained by missions and deployment timelines. It is rarely feasible to incorporate a perfectly planned program given the typical military schedule. At times, military personnel may only have a month or two to work with the TSAC Facilitator before a deployment or other training event. Many military personnel are hesitant to seek assistance from the TSAC Facilitator due to time constraints or due to familiarity with or preference for other training methods. The TSAC Facilitator must be flexible in working with whatever time frame the individual has available, even if it is less than optimal. This reinforces the idea that training goals should be achievable even when working in small windows of time, and it increases the likelihood that the warfighter will seek out coaching assistance in the future. Perhaps most importantly, within small military teams, buy-in mostly occurs at the grassroots level. Therefore, if the TSAC Facilitator is successful in helping one or two people, it can motivate other team members to seek out coaching assistance.

As with any PT program, the TSAC Facilitator should perform a needs analysis of the warfighter's MOS and the physical fitness tests used by the military service. Each MOS may have different job tasks in the operational environment, but all will be tested with the specific service's own physical fitness test. The program goals need to reflect the needs for each fitness component (e.g., aerobic conditioning, strength, power, flexibility) and movement capability required for the MOS. Then an individual analysis needs to be done to allow the TSAC Facilitator to focus on specific elements that need immediate attention due to the short time frame many warfighters have available. Thus, priority training along with individualized training programs for short-term, intermediate-term, and long-term attainment need to be addressed, keeping in mind that the warfighter's fitness testing must not be compromised by a lack of attention to testing specifics (e.g., need for power if a standing long jump is used for fitness assessment).

Training goals might be organized based on the typical periodization time frame of a microcycle (2-4 weeks), mesocycle (8-12 weeks), and macrocycle (one year). This allows the TSAC Facilitator to understand what can be accomplished and whether a longer time line of contact with the warfighter is possible so that training goals can be modified over each cycle, building a macrocycle plan. Additionally, when soldiers process to a new duty station, it is important to supply a report of what they have done and the plan they've been using so they can continue training at the next duty station.

Here are some points to consider when developing training goals for warfighters and their unit. Ultimately, conditioning goals are individual processes, with formal military fitness testing being the group activity. Realistic goals must be set for conditioning programs; individual genetic potential will influence every parameter measured. Although units can have goals for the whole team, everyone should be able to contribute to unit goal setting. When setting goals, keep the following factors in mind:

- The MOS specifies the required tasks beyond general fitness levels assessed in military testing programs.
- Military unit demands and operational missions may vary.
- The more fit a soldier is, the less improvement can be gained. One might then work on a maintenance program for some variables.
- Various training times are needed to reach a given physical fitness or body development goal. Some goals, such as loss of body fat, also involve other interventions, such as diet behaviors.
- Use training logs and internal testing to determine if the program is working. If not, design changes are needed.
- The availability of equipment or program elements is an important consideration.
- Set goals that are attainable based on the individual and then monitor them. What you measure, you have to manage!

Exercise Selection

Exercise selection is related to the movements and body functions that are targeted for improvement with training. In the weight room, select whole-body exercises that represent the functional ability of the body to produce force and power from the standing position or the closed kinetic chain. With adequate technique training and monitoring, whole-body exercises such as squats, power cleans, and deadlifts, along with bench presses and seated rows, can be at the core of the weight training program. Next, choose exercises for the upper and lower body with attention to exercising the front and back of a joint (e.g., front and back of

arm, or biceps and triceps). Whole-body exercises also include running, swimming (service dependent), cycling, jumping, sprinting, agility training with breaks in the straightforward movement, backward running, and balance training. Flexibility training and movements from functional movement screens can also be used to improve movement capabilities. Care must be taken when using novel exercises such as tire flips and other strongman lifts to make sure technique is clearly understood and monitored.

Exercise-to-Rest Cycles

The amount of rest needed to optimize workout performance can be examined from both within and between workouts. Shorter rest periods within a workout place greater demands on anaerobic metabolism and can affect the pH and acid-buffering mechanisms. Workouts with shorter rests are used to enhance buffering capacities and improve anaerobic tolerance, but they only need to be performed twice a week. Too many of these workouts, including HIIT workouts, can lead to overreaching or overtraining. For resistance training, allow 48 hours between workouts, but 24 hours can be used if the exercise angles are changed in the workout. Although endurance training can be done each day, it is necessary to periodize the intensity and volume of exercise. Again, exercisers need to be carefully monitored for recovery and overtraining. From anecdotal observations, many high-performance warfighters are overtrained but get used to the feeling of being tired, creating a new normal. With more advanced blood marker testing (e.g., cortisol and creatine kinase levels), this can be addressed. Session RPEs and other scale monitoring for fatigue and sleep can help with program adjustments and counsel (11).

Progression, Duration, and Intensity

In resistance training, the progression of intensity is based on the loading range in a program. The goal is to improve maximal strength and power and the resistance or intensity over a training cycle that can be used for a given range of repetitions. With percentages of 1RM, the training weight increases as strength increases. Thus, the resistance or intensity used for a 3RM to 5RM training zone should be heavier in week 12 than it was in week 1, and the resistance used for 12RM to 15RM is also higher in week 12 than in week 1. Progress within the training zone or as the 1RM gets higher. If the 1RM goes up, then, for example, the 80% load will also go up. If the exerciser can do 7 reps in a set that was targeted for a 3RM to 5RM zone, increase the weight to allow only that number of repetitions for the load. Using RM zones often requires trial and error on each set for an exercise. For percentages, many use the Epley formula:

$$1RM = (0.033 \times \text{reps} \times \text{weight lifted}) + \text{weight lifted}$$

Each muscle group and exercise will have a ceiling for absolute gains based on the person's genetics (e.g., number of muscle fibers, muscle fiber types, limb lengths, tendon lengths). The slowing down of gains in a workout log or strength test often reflects such limits if training program design is appropriate and the person works hard (15).

Progression in endurance training can follow a periodized format that varies the integration of tempo training and volume of distance run (54). Progression involves careful modulation of the volume of running, pace of runs, and distance covered based on the individual's toleration of the training. Understanding what distances are needed to complement aerobic function in order to support load carriage and military testing protocols is vital to setting optimal training goals (36).

Nonlinear Periodization

The objective of **periodization** is to optimize adaptations while allowing rest and recovery from the exercise stressors. It allows for manipulations to enhance both acute and chronic exercise training adaptations. In short, periodization is a process of varying workout stressors and allowing recovery to take place. As mentioned in chapter 10, the origins of periodization are related to the work of Canadian endocrinologist Hans Selye, who created the concept of **general adaptation syndrome (GAS)**. In GAS, if the stressor is not removed after a given period of time, the organism dies or, in the case of exercise training, experiences decreased performance. From this concept and after many years of modeling successful athletes, the periodized training program was developed in the Soviet Union and Eastern Bloc countries. The concept has exploded over the past 50 years, and a host of periodization models have been developed based on both theory and science (5, 37, 51).

This chapter will introduce a differential model of periodization termed **nonlinear periodization** and more specifically **flexible nonlinear periodization**. Each of the styles or approaches to periodization has its own distinct advantages, but for military interfaces, flexible nonlinear periodization offers the greatest *flexibility* in optimizing each workout in the short-term training frames typical of military schooling and duty cycles (8-12 weeks) (37). In this model, a nonlinear plan is developed for a mesocycle, and then the ability to do a planned workout is determined at the time of the workout (daily microcycles). If the workout cannot be performed at the level of quality prescribed, the exerciser defaults to another workout or a rest day.

Nonlinear Periodized Model   More recently, nonlinear periodized training programs have been developed to maintain variation in the training stimulus (66). Nonlinear periodized training is a way to easily implement the program around schedule or competitive demands (37). The nonlinear program allows for variation in the intensity and volume within each week of the training program (e.g., 16 weeks). The change in the intensity and volume of training varies within the week. Following is an example of a nonlinear periodized training program over a 16-week mesocycle:

Microcycle 1: 5 sets at 60% of 1RM

Microcycle 2: 5 sets at 75% of 1RM

Microcycle 3: 4 sets at 85% of 1RM

Microcycle 4: 5 sets at 90% of 1RM

Microcycle 5: 4 sets at 65% of 1RM

Microcycle 6: 5 sets at 80% of 1RM

Microcycle 7: 4 sets at 85% of 1RM

Microcycle 8: 4 sets at 95% of 1RM

Microcycle 9: 4 sets at 70% of 1RM

Microcycle 10: 5 sets at 80% of 1RM

Microcycle 11: 3 sets at 60% of 1RM

Microcycle 12: 4 sets at 95% of 1RM

Microcycle 13: 3 sets at 75% of 1RM

Microcycle 14: 4 sets at 85% of 1RM

Microcycle 15: 4 sets at 60% of 1RM

Microcycle 16: 3 sets at 100% of 1RM

The nonlinear program can also be organized where a different style of workout is scheduled for each day and the exerciser progresses though them. An alternative is to use the flexible approach mentioned earlier. It is derived from the planned format, but the workout sequence is not set unless the individual is capable of doing the assigned workout. Under extenuating circumstances such as sickness, lack of sleep, or demanding job tasks, the exerciser defaults to a rest day or a workout that can be completed in more optimal manner. Thus, the TSAC Facilitator can better manage the quality of the training. The flexible approach requires attention to workout logs, interactions with exercisers on the training day, and pretests such as a vertical jump test. For example, before a power day, if warfighters cannot achieve at least 90% of their personal best on a vertical jump test, a less intense workout is performed (37). The workouts done successfully are noted as to how well the individual was able to meet the exercise training demands so that the target goals of a mesocycle are met. In other words, the TSAC Facilitator assesses whether the workouts in the plan can realistically meet the training goals (e.g., whether there are enough heavy workouts to optimize strength).

The following protocol uses a four-day rotation with one day of rest between workouts. A rotational sequence for two days or three days per week could also be used.

The flexibility comes in when, for example, the warfighter cannot perform in the 4RM to 6RM training zone with the same intensity as the prior workout with this RM zone. Then the workout is changed to a lighter one or a rest day. Optimal performance of a set is the key factor in a program; going through the motions is not acceptable for optimal training and improvement.

The variation in training is much greater within the week. In the sample protocol listed previously, intensity ranges from 1RM sets to 15RM sets in the week cycle. This span in training variation appears to be as effective as linear programs. Typically, power training workouts are done with Olympic-style lifts with submaximal loading to promote total body power.

Unlike in traditional periodized programs, the components of muscle size and strength are both trained within the same week. Additionally, nonlinear programs attempt to train different resistance loads within the same week. Thus, the exerciser is working on two neural activation patterns within the same 7- to 10-day period of the 16-week mesocycle.

In this program, the nonlinear planned model rotates through very heavy, heavy, moderate, and light training sessions. If exercisers miss the Monday workout, they can repeat it and then continue on. Thus, you may have a group doing all types of loading programs on a given day. A mesocycle is complete when a certain number of workouts are completed (e.g., 48) rather than using training weeks to set the program length.

Again, the primary exercises are typically periodized, but a two-cycle program can also be used to vary the small muscle group exercises. For example, with the triceps pushdown, the exerciser could rotate between the moderate (8RM-10RM training zone) and the heavy (4RM-6RM training zone) cycle intensities. This would provide the hypertrophy needed for such isolated muscles of a joint while also providing the strength needed to support heavier workouts of the large muscle groups.

In summary, different approaches can be used to periodize a training program. Linear and nonlinear programs appear to accomplish the same effect and are superior to constant training programs. Flexible nonlinear periodization appears to be an ideal style of programming for various military populations. However, the key to any workout programs success is variation, and different approaches can be used over the year to meet this training need.

Key Point

Flexible nonlinear periodization uses daily assessments to determine the appropriateness of the assigned workout. If the assigned workout cannot be done optimally, the training defaults to a workout that can be done optimally. For example, a power workout has been planned for the noon workout, but a 10-mile run was done in the morning; with the residual fatigue that would accompany such a run, a power workout is not possible during the workout time.

Acclimatization

It is possible to improve performance in both heat and altitude from gradual exposure to the environmental stress over time. However, little if any cold acclimatization occurs, and proper clothing and shelter are required. **Acclimatization** refers to exposure to the natural environment. This is in contrast to acclimation, which is exposure to an artificial environment such as a heat or altitude chamber (33).

Heat acclimatization guidelines have been extensively developed by the U.S. Army (67). According to Fleck and Kraemer (15), the earliest adaptations to heat occur in 1 to 5 days with improved regulation and control of the cardiovascular system. This means there is an expanded plasma volume, reduced HR at a specific exercise intensity, and improvement in the autonomic nervous system to assist in the redistribution of blood flow in the capillary beds in the active musculature. In 5 to 8 days, the crucial regulation of body temperature improves, which is vital for protection against lethal hyperthermia. The acclimatization response depends on the environment; for example, does the acclimatization take place in a hot, humid environment or a hot, dry environment? Adaptations include an increased sweat rate, the onset of sweating at lower elevations in body temperature, and sweat gland adaptations (more dilute sweat), depending on the type of environment. Three to nine days is when conservation of sodium chloride (NaCl) takes place during heat acclimatization. NaCl losses in the sweat and urine will decrease, which results in better maintenance of extracellular fluid volume. By 14 days, most of the changes are complete, including the following (15):

- Lower core temperature at the onset of sweating
- Increased heat loss via radiation and convection (skin blood flow)
- Increased plasma volume
- Decreased HR at a specific workload
- Decreased core temperature
- Decreased skin temperature
- Decreased oxygen consumption at a given workload
- Improved exercise economy (amount of exercise performed per unit of oxygen consumed)

Altitude acclimatization is also possible (70). Short-term acclimatization to altitude occurs from altitude exposure of less than one year. Even with three to six weeks of exposure to altitude, dramatic acclimatization can occur. This appears to help oxygen utilization (e.g., increased hematocrit) and performance for endurance activities. Long-term acclimatization refers to people who were born or have lived at altitude for longer than a year. Most warfighters must gain short-term acclimatization in order to perform optimally at higher altitudes.

Injury Rehabilitation

In some units, the TSAC Facilitator is located with physical therapists, athletic trainers, or MFTs. TSAC Facilitators must stay in their lane, so to speak; they are not medical professionals, and diagnosing or treating injuries or diseases is outside their scope of practice. However, they are key players in the medical team of experts and contribute in many ways to injury prevention and rehabilitation programs. Establishing good working partnerships with the medical team can be a sizeable advantage in providing the best care possible and motivating military personnel to train. This is especially important when working with people recovering from injury. Military personnel who have sustained an injury are motivated to return to full duty in most cases, but they may also be skeptical about their progress and the ability of the physical therapist or strength and conditioning professional to help them achieve their goals. The stronger the treatment team, and the earlier a working relationship is established with the warfighter (both before and after injury), the greater the warfighter's motivation to train and work with the rehabilitation or strength and conditioning team when injured. Military personnel of higher fitness levels may be more motivated to train once standard rehabilitation exercises are no longer challenging. Here, the TSAC Facilitator is in a unique position to provide well-designed programming that challenges the individual while taking the injuries into consideration (53). Working with the medical personnel, physical therapist, or athletic trainer can assist the TSAC Facilitator in designing a program that further aids the individual's recovery without exacerbating existing injuries.

Adherence

Some military personnel will not adhere to the training protocols designed by the TSAC Facilitator due to their preference for their own training methods or the misconception that more is better. The best approach is to be patient and educate the person over time as to why recovery and progression, including rest days, are necessary for performance gains. This will not happen overnight. Once the tactical athletes begin to see positive effects, they are more likely to adhere to the training program. At other times, adherence issues are related to competing military training requirements. In this situation, the TSAC Facilitator must be flexible in shifting or redesigning workouts based on the tactical athlete's availability and readiness to train. Although this is not an ideal situation, adjusting training to accommodate the needs of military personnel will greatly influence their motivation to train.

PROGRAM DESIGN AND SAMPLE TRAINING APPROACHES

The principle of specificity requires training to mirror the demands of the occupational specialty. To best prepare for the physiological demands of load carriage, military personnel should train using complex, multijoint movements, with an emphasis on upper body and lower body strength and power development, in addition to posterior chain development. Given the heavy emphasis on load carriage and the high incidence of associated lower back injuries, developing a strong core and posterior chain is pivotal to improving performance of military tasks and preventing injury. Additionally, upper body strength and muscle mass are contributing factors in load carriage performance (16). Studies have shown that strength training can greatly improve performance on military physical tasks (34), and specifically load carriage, even when load carriage is not incorporated in the training plan.

Although military tactical athletes have good overall fitness levels compared with the general population, they may be lacking an adequate strength and power foundation, and they may have limited experience training compound, multijoint movements (e.g., squat, bench press, deadlift) and power exercises (e.g., power clean). For this reason, the TSAC Facilitator will likely have to allocate time for teaching and reinforcing correct technique when implementing resistance training programs. If military personnel are conducting off-duty PT on their own or are involved with commercial programs, the TSAC Facilitator may have to reteach movement patterns or incorporate exercises to correct movement deficiencies. Based on anecdotal experiences, it is thought by military and research professionals that weak gluteal and hamstring muscles are common in military athletes due to the heavy emphasis on running combined with tightness in the hip flexors and quadriceps dominance. These issues must be addressed because strong gluteal musculature and hip extension capability (power) are critical to strength and power development. Furthermore, well-balanced musculature around all sides of a joint not only improves athletic performance but also has been observed to reduce injury risk, particularly overuse injury or injury related to load carriage.

Military physical readiness doctrine outlines the principles of "train to standard" and "train to fight" (65). Mastery of various physical tasks enables a warfighter and thus the unit to perform the mission effectively. Accordingly, training should be tough, realistic, physically challenging, and safe. The PT program should focus on the tasks associated with combat—lifting and loading weapons, reacting to and evading contact, evacuating casualties, moving under fire, navigating across uneven terrain from one point to another, performing individual and team movements, and performing combatives (see table 19.6). The TSAC Facilitator can refer to these physical tasks to gain a general understanding of common warfighter tasks and the physical capabilities needed to perform them. This will be helpful in developing training programs to meet the warfighter's needs.

Table 19.6 PRT Component Matrix, Including Warrior Tasks and Battle Drills

	Warrior tasks						Battle drills	
PRT components	Use hand grenades	Perform individual movement techniques	Navigate from one point to another	Move under fire	Perform combatives	Assess and respond to threats (escalation of force)	React to contact	Evacuate a casualty
Strength								
Muscular strength	X	X	X	X	X	X	X	X
Muscular endurance	X	X	X	X	X	X		X
Endurance								
Anaerobic endurance	X	X	X	X	X	X	X	X
Aerobic endurance		X	X			X		X
Mobility								
Agility	X	X	X	X	X	X	X	X
Balance	X	X	X	X	X	X	X	X
Coordination	X	X	X	X	X	X	X	X
Flexibility	X	X	X	X	X	X	X	X
Posture	X	X	X	X	X	X	X	X
Stability	X	X	X	X	X	X	X	X
Speed	X	X	X	X	X	X	X	X
Power	X	X	X	X	X	X	X	X

Muscle strength and power are necessary fitness components for the performance of all warrior tasks and battle drills, highlighting the importance of anaerobic PT for basic infantry tasks.

Reprinted from Mala et al. (39).

Key Program Variables

Previous literature has described the acute program variables that can be manipulated in a strength and conditioning program to attain various athletic goals (62). In short, exercise choice, exercise order, amount of load, type of load (e.g., accommodating resistance, regular weight), intensity (e.g., sets and reps, volume), and rest periods all influence the adaptations to resistance training (35, 62). These variables can be manipulated to result in the desired outcomes. For example, optimal strength development requires heavy loading in the 1RM to 3RM range, and within a given strength-based workout, one must use longer rest periods of 2 minutes or more to maximize force production. Some experts even advocate 3 minutes or more (15). A hypertrophy-based protocol allows for loading in the 6RM to 12RM range combined with moderate rest periods of 30 to 90 seconds. On the opposite end of the spectrum, when conducting metabolic training, shorter rest periods are appropriate. However, loading must be adjusted because the force needed to lift heavy loads cannot be maintained with short rests.

Care must be taken with metabolically demanding workouts because of their taxing nature and the catabolic hormonal environment that results (35). Cumulative exposure to catabolic hormones can create a hormonal environment that is counterproductive to optimal strength and power development. Two to three metabolic workouts per week are generally enough to maintain metabolic adaptions to exercise (35). Incorporating more than that can yield counterproductive results, particularly when combined with frequent endurance exercise and other demanding military training.

Manipulation of acute program variables (e.g., exercise choice, loads, rest periods) ensures that military personnel develop the necessary strength and power foundation while allowing for optimal recovery. With military athletes in particular, the demands of the profession and the need to be mission ready year-round necessitate optimal recovery from exercise stress. Varying exercises and loading over the course of the training program ensures optimal development and maximizes recovery, thereby reducing the risk of nonfunctional overreaching, a common occurrence with intense training. Another factor that influences the choice and order of exercise is an assessment of the athlete's strengths and weaknesses. Weak body parts can be trained early in the workout to emphasize weak or lagging muscle groups, and manipulation of the acute program variables can ensure that appropriate emphasis is placed on lagging areas.

Equipment

Equipment resources and facilities vary from location to location. This depends to a large extent on which branch of service TSAC Facilitators are supporting and whether they are working with a conventional or nonconventional unit. Typically, conventional units are larger, with fewer resources available relative to the number of military personnel. Nonconventional military personnel, assigned to smaller units, typically have more adequate resources, both in terms of military personnel relative to the amount of equipment and funding available for purchasing equipment. In the best-case scenario, the TSAC Facilitator will have access to a full weight room, conditioning equipment, indoor turf, and indoor and outdoor space similar to what would be available at a collegiate strength and conditioning facility. In situations where the TSAC Facilitator is working with a team of tactical athletes, this is typically the case. However, the TSAC Facilitator may initially have limited equipment and space or may need to train a number of military personnel at once that exceeds the space and equipment available. Again, the TSAC Facilitator must be flexible in working with the resources available and take advantage of opportunities to advocate for and influence future equipment purchasing decisions, which are typically made at the command level.

Effective strength and endurance training is not cheap. However, units that have effective training understand that across the career of a service member, the dollar per warfighter-year cost of the equipment is low. This means, for example, that if a warfighter uses a $10 kettlebell for 10 years, the cost of that kettlebell is $1 per warfighter-year. If 10 service members use it throughout those 10 years, the cost is $0.10 per warfighter-year. If 100 service members use it, the cost is $0.01. Whether purchasing simple kettlebells or high-end antigravity treadmills, the cost of equipment and facilities pales in comparison to the health care costs associated with improper PT. In spite of this, equipment purchases most likely will be driven by initial cost.

Safety

The TSAC Facilitator must take certain factors into account to ensure the safety of the military personnel. First and foremost, fitness level and injury status will influence how warfighters should train, including the intensity with which they can safely exercise, modifications that must be made depending on injury status or existing movement deficiencies, and the degree of supervision and coaching that is required for safe progression. Additionally, the TSAC Facilitator must be aware of outside factors that can influence safety in the weight room, such as military training events, particularly in hot, humid weather; nutrition and hydration status; and auxiliary factors such as quality of sleep and recovery status. All of these factors will influence the ability to train safely. Thus, careful attention to these factors and knowledge of the warfighter's lifestyle (i.e., how well the TSAC Facilitator knows the athlete) will ensure safe progression of exercise and avoidance of injury.

Additionally, as with all athletes, exercises that are more technically complex should be performed with light weight until proper technique is learned, and progression of loading should be incremental, depending on the skill and strength level of the athlete. When the warfighter is fatigued from military training or other operational factors, care should be taken in implementing technically complex movements that are centrally fatiguing. At a minimum, coaches should be certified in first aid, CPR, and AED use, an AED should be on site, and all coaching staff should be trained in the emergency procedures of the strength and conditioning facility.

Coaching Resources

There are no full-time coaches to develop and lead physical fitness programs for military teams. Although military personnel are considered tactical athletes, they are not required to train under the guidance of a coaching staff, unlike professional or collegiate sport athletes. Currently, the delivery of training is the business of the NCO, who receives guidance, resourcing, and intent from the commander. To varying degrees, the services train their NCO leaders in the execution of PT through professional military education and additional skill courses, such as the MFTC. There are no requirements for nationally recognized PT certifications. Only a few installations support commercial certifications.

At the time of this writing, the TSAC Facilitator has no formal doctrinal or regulatory support within the U.S. military system. Those few TSAC Facilitators who are employed by the military are civilian contractors or government employees. The TSAC Facilitator certification is much more likely to be an adjunctive certification earned by a health care professional, strength and conditioning coach, MFT, or service-specific equivalent. Therefore, for the time being, the responsibility for PT and injury control lies with the command, and associated duties are delegated to medical personnel. These medical personnel are sometimes organic to the unit (part of the unit's personnel structure), but more typically they work in medical treatment and gyms on the installation and serve a much broader population than a single tactical unit.

Program Scenarios

No one-size-fits-all strength and conditioning program exists that will be appropriate for all service members. As mentioned, optimal programming must address the physical requirements of the military personnel's occupational specialty and the unit's mission, and it must factor in constraints such as competing military training requirements that must be prioritized in a given training cycle; military personnel's availability, readiness, and motivation to train; and special considerations for the individual's goals, strengths, and weaknesses. Personal factors, such as home life or disrupted sleep schedules, will also affect training outcomes. To implement a program that is not only effective but is one that military personnel can adhere to, the TSAC Facilitator should maintain flexibility in the program design, such as using the flexible nonlinear approach or short training blocks of three to four weeks with adequate recovery and deloading periods. Chapter 10 provides more information on periodization and sample programs that can be used as a starting point for developing a training program for a military population, and other publications also provide examples (35, 37, 38).

A sample training program for a Ranger unit is provided in table 19.7. This program incorporates a resistance training schedule using a flexible nonlinear program. The TSAC Facilitator can then change the programs related to circuit training, strength, power, endurance, or combat-related training. The key is to make the program work with the operational demands and time constraints of the MOS and the unit in order to train the elements needed for combat readiness, including anaerobic endurance, cardiorespiratory function, and strength and power for demanding tasks, as discussed in detail elsewhere (23, 30). The program shows what might be done on base and then during predeployment, deployment, and postdeployment. Using knowledge of program design from this book and others will allow the TSAC Facilitator to develop programs in response to individual and unit demands during these three periods of military service.

Recommended Readings

Due to the vast amount of information available, it is not possible to provide extensive details on all topics covered in this chapter. Table 19.8 lists recommended references for the TSAC Facilitator working with the military.

Table 19.7 Sample Training Program for a Ranger Unit

	Sunday	Monday	Tuesday	Wednesday	Thursday	Friday	Saturday
				Sample Program			
On base							
Resistance training	Rest	Acid–base workout* 3-4 sets at 8RM-10RM Circuit workout 8-10 muscle group exercises 1-2 min rest between sets	Strength workout 85%-90% of 1RM or 4RM-6RM zone 5 major muscle groups 3-4 min rest between sets	Rest	Repeat Monday workout circuit	Repeat Tuesday workout	Rest
Endurance training	Rest	Rest	Interval training	Rest	30-40 min continuous run at 80%-85% MHR	Rest	Rest
Combat-related training	Rest	Rest	Rest	Offensive/defensive maneuvers in uniform and boots	Rest	Rest	Rest
Predeployment							
Resistance training	Rest	Power workout Olympic lifts 50%-70% 1RM (4-6 sets of 2-3 reps) Plyometrics 2-3 min rest between sets	Rest	Strength workout 3RM-5RM zone or 85%-95% of 1RM (3-4 sets) Major muscle groups 3-4 min rest between sets		Repeat Monday workout	
Endurance training	Rest	Rest	Interval training	Rest	30-40 min continuous run at 80%-85% MHR	Rest	Rest
Combat-related training	Rest	Offensive/defensive maneuvers, full uniform body armor, helmet, boots, and rifle	Rest	Offensive/defensive maneuvers, full uniform body armor, helmet, boots, assault pack, and rifle	Rest	Offensive/defensive maneuvers, full uniform body armor, helmet, boots, assault pack, LBV (load-bearing vest), and rifle	Rest
Deployment							
Resistance training	Rest	Power exercises	Rest	Strength workout	Rest	Circuit workout	Rest
Endurance training	Rest	Rest	30 min continuous run at 80% MHR	Rest	30 min continuous run at 75% MHR	Rest	Rest
Combat-related training	Rest	Rest	Rest	Offensive/defensive maneuvers, intermediate load uniform, boots, assault pack, body armor, LBV, helmet, and rifle	Rest	Rest	Rest
Postdeployment							
Resistance training		Active rest				Active rest	
Endurance training			20 min low-intensity run at 50%-60% MHR		20 min low-intensity run at 50% The impact of work-matched interval training on MHR		
Combat-related training		Retrain individual and squad movements				Retrain individual and squad movements	

*An acid–base workout increases buffering capacity when an intense workout lowers the pH.

Table 19.8 DoD and Service-Specific Regulatory Guidance for PT Programs

Service/organization	Publication date	Publication
DoD	November 2, 2002	Department of Defense Instruction 1308.3
Air Force	June 2012	Guidance Memorandum for AFI 36-2905, Fitness Program
Army	September 19, 2014	Army Regulation 350-1, Army Training and Leader Development, RAR
	October 26, 2012	Field Manual 7-22, Army Physical Readiness Training
Marine Corps	August 1, 2008	Marine Corps Order 6100-13
Navy	July 1, 2011	OPNAVINSTR 6110.1J, Navy Physical Readiness Program

Based on Department of Defense Instruction 1308.3, November 2002; Air Force Guidance Memorandum for AFI 36-2905, Fitness Program, June 2012; U.S. Department of the Army Field Manual 7-22, October 2012; Marine Corps Order 6100-13, August 2008; and Navy Physical Readiness Program, OPNAVINSTR 6110.1J, July 2011.

CONCLUSION

The military provides an environment of extraordinary opportunity and challenge for the TSAC Facilitator. The defense of a nation in a resource-constrained era gives the skilled facilitator the chance to offer massive value. The TSAC Facilitator is the unit's fitness expert. In this role, the TSAC Facilitator can drive physical readiness through fitness enhancement and injury mitigation. With command support, radical improvements in warfighter physical readiness become possible. Though the training environment of a Navy SEAL may be very different than that of an infantry soldier, one constant is the need for flexibility in designing real-world programs under constraints ranging from the individual's readiness to train to the unit's deployment schedule. A thorough understanding of the warfighter's training needs and goals, occupational requirements, and lifestyle will ensure that the TSAC Facilitator can provide optimal training support to the tactical athlete or unit, thereby maximizing physical performance across a range of tasks and enhancing readiness for mission demands.

Key Terms

acclimatization
acute mountain sickness (AMS)
anaerobic battlefield
block periodization
Certified Strength and Conditioning
    Specialist (CSCS)
flexible nonlinear periodization
general adaptation syndrome (GAS)
hazardous exposure
heat cramps
heat exhaustion
heatstroke

high-altitude cerebral edema (HACE)
hypoxic effect
Master Fitness Trainer Course (MFTC)
Military Occupational Specialty (MOS)
nonlinear periodization
NSCA-Certified Personal Trainer (NSCA-CPT)
overuse injuries
periodization
readiness
special operators
syncope

Study Questions

1. When designing a program for military personnel, the TSAC Facilitator must consider which of the following first?
   a. injury history
   b. unit mission
   c. training goals
   d. aerobic fitness

2. Which of the following environmental conditions does the body NOT acclimatize to?
   a. hot
   b. cold
   c. humid
   d. dry

3. Which of following is the best procedure to implement immediately if someone is showing signs of heatstroke?
   a. ice bath
   b. extra electrolyte intake
   c. gradual cool-down session
   d. decreased sun exposure

4. As the body adapts to exercising in the heat, which of the following changes occurs approximately nine days into training?
   a. expanded plasma volume
   b. conservation of sodium chloride
   c. improvement in the autonomic nervous system
   d. reduced heart rate at a specific exercise intensity

5. If a warfighter's 5RM for the back squat is 250 pounds (114 kg), what is the estimated 1RM (rounded down to the nearest pound)?
   a. 258 lb (117 kg)
   b. 287 lb (130 kg)
   c. 291 lb (132 kg)
   d. 412 lb (187 kg)

Chapter 20

Physical Training to Optimize Load Carriage

Paul C. Henning, PhD, CSCS
Barry A. Spiering, PhD, CSCS
Dennis E. Scofield, MEd, CSCS
Bradley C. Nindl, PhD

After completing this chapter, you will be able to

- describe the history of and current trends in load carriage for fire and rescue, law enforcement, and military populations;
- discuss the physiological and biomechanical demands imposed by load carriage; and
- design training programs to optimize load carriage.

The opinions or assertions contained herein are the private views of the authors and are not to be construed as official or as reflecting the views of the U.S. Army or the Department of Defense.

Tactical athletes are often required to perform a myriad of physical tasks (e.g., negotiating obstacles, crawling, climbing, marksmanship) while carrying loads (**load carriage**) that weigh 80% or more of their body weight (16, 45). In comparison to unloaded work, significantly greater demands will be imposed while performing physical activities such as patrolling or repetitive material handling with donned tactical equipment that may include firefighting turnout gear, SCBA, and ballistic vests (18, 74, 83). Work demands can be further exacerbated by austere environmental conditions. Strength, power, and agility are important considerations of **mobility** (the ability to move one's body in a straight line, in multiple directions, or while negotiating obstacles), **reaction time** (the interval of time between a stimulus and response), and maneuverability—whether on the battlefield, in a foot pursuit, or at a fire. Injury mitigation is another important aspect of the PT program: Lost duty days due to injury will negatively affect a unit's mission readiness.

IMPACT OF EQUIPMENT LOAD ON BIOMECHANICAL DEMANDS

Operating under conditions of load carriage can compromise safety and increase the risk of musculoskeletal injury during times of fatigue or inadequate physical conditioning (36, 59, 62, 79). Circumventing adverse outcomes requires knowing the physiological and biomechanical responses to load carriage and incorporating appropriate PT program design and evaluation aimed at the specific requirements of the tactical athlete. This chapter provides the TSAC Facilitator with precepts for PT program design aimed at load carriage optimization.

History of Load Carriage

Modern warfare often requires service members to carry a considerable amount of equipment and supplies during dismounted movement. As figure 20.1 shows, the external loads carried by soldiers of various militaries throughout history have not

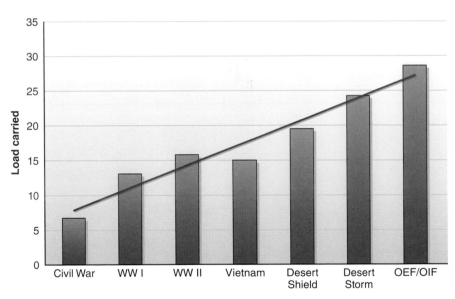

Figure 20.1 External loads (kg) carried by U.S. soldiers throughout major conflicts.

OEF/OIF = Operation Enduring Freedom and Operation Iraqi Freedom.

Reprinted, by permission, from B.C. Nindl et al., 2013, "Physiological Employment Standards III: Physiological challenges and consequences encountered during international military deployments," *European Journal of Applied Physiology* 113(11): 2658.

always been as heavy as the loads carried by modern soldiers. Although soldiers have become stronger and larger than their earlier counterparts (22), their loads have also progressively increased since the time of the British Crimean War at the start of the

Industrial Revolution (45). Advances in technology have driven the need for soldiers to carry weapons and equipment for the purposes of firepower, protection, and communication, resulting in a linear increase in load carriage weight over time.

Table 20.1 Loads Carried by Duty Position in a Light Infantry Unit in Afghanistan

Duty position	Fighting load (kg)	Approach march load (kg)	Emergency approach march load (kg)
Rifleman	29	43	58
M203 grenadier	32	48	62
Automatic rifleman	36	50	64
Antitank specialist	31	45	59
Rifle team leader	29	43	59
Rifle squad leader	28	43	58
Forward observer	26	41	58
Forward observer radio/telephone operator	27	39	54
Weapons squad leader	28	45	60
M240 machine gunner	37	51	60
M240B assistant gunner	32	55	67
M240B ammunition bearer	31	53	65
Rifle platoon sergeant	28	41	54
Rifle platoon leader	28	42	53
Platoon medic	25	42	54
Radio/telephone operator	29	45	No data
Mortar section leader	26	50	68
Mortar squad leader	28	58	65
60 mm mortar gunner	29	49	61
60 mm mortar assistant gunner	25	55	No data
60 mm mortar ammunition bearer	24	46	No data
Rifle company communication chief	31	50	No data
Fire support officer	25	42	No data
Fire support noncommissioned officer	24	41	65
Sapper engineer	27	43	60
Company executive officer	27	42	No data
Company first sergeant	29	41	57
Company radio/telephone operator	29	44	59
Rifle company commander	30	44	50
Average	29 (63.9 lb)	46 (101.4 lb)	60 (132.3 lb)
Current U.S. Army doctrine recommendation	22 (48.5 lb)	33 (72.8 lb)	—

Based on Dean (16).

Key Point

Advances in technology have increased the loads that tactical operators must bear.

Numerous research efforts throughout history have embarked on developing strategies to improve soldier mobility. The aim of this work focused on determining acceptable soldier loads based on physical capability and operational necessity (3, 5, 14). Previous research also examined the applicability of specialized load carriage systems (e.g., front-end carriage system compared with back and shoulder systems) (5, 70, 76).

In 1987, the U.S. Army Development and Employment Agency (ADEA) proposed five ideas to reduce load weight and improve soldier mobility (3). One of these recommendations was the development of PT programs to enhance soldiers' physical capability for load carriage. Since this recommendation, several scientific efforts have investigated the effects of PT on load carriage.

Recent evidence demonstrates that soldiers are currently carrying the heaviest loads in history (45). In a landmark study by Dean (16), the researchers deployed into theater (Afghanistan) with a light infantry brigade (Task Force Devil, 82nd Airborne Division) and recorded the loads carried in combat. This research provided invaluable data on actual loads carried by various duty positions within the infantry. The total loads carried by soldiers in duty positions of a light infantry unit are displayed in table 20.1. For example, the average fighting load, approach march load, and emergency approach march load for a rifle squad leader were 62.4 lb (28.3 kg), 95.0 lb (43.1 kg), and 128.4 lb (58.2 kg), respectively (16).

Task Analysis for Various Tactical Populations

An accurate representation of load carriage stress can only be determined by evaluating occupational physical requirements and tasks through a **needs analysis**—a multistep process of evaluating job tasks and physical requirements plus the individual's fitness status (described comprehensively in previous chapters) (57). A movement task analysis is also included in this process (56). For example, establishing evidence for occupationally

relevant performance goals and outcomes can be done with a task and movement analysis of load carriage and other physically demanding activities (e.g., victim rescue, ladder climbing, reacting to enemy contact). The analysis will note the frequency, intensity, environmental conditions, clothing, and equipment load common to various tactical athletes (21). The information gathered from the task analyses provides a framework for the PT program.

Key Point

A needs analysis is highly recommended to understand the specific requirements of the tactical operator, thereby allowing appropriate exercise programming.

Critical Job Tasks Requiring Load

As reported by previous research (67, 80), load carriage requirements vary among occupations and specific job requirements. Military tactical performance has previously been assessed using tests involving load carriage, obstacle courses, repetitive and maximal box lifting, rushes under fire, and simulated casualty recovery (30, 31, 46). These warfighting tasks require the ability to move effectively while wearing load-bearing equipment. However, job requirements dictate the frequency and weight of equipment load worn by warfighters. Combat arms personnel can expect to wear load-bearing equipment more frequently than those serving in combat support (32, 71). In general, all service members must be physically prepared to conduct common warfighter tasks wearing assigned equipment (1, 34).

Firefighting often requires the wear of PPE while performing physical tasks. Physical conditioning should be driven to optimize performance of firefighting tasks in donned field gear. Firefighting will likely involve moderate- to high-intensity tasks (e.g., handling charged fire hoses), be repetitive, and last for extended durations while wearing turnout gear and SCBA equipment (2). Therefore, a basic knowledge of load carriage (and its implications on occupational task performance) is needed. Park et al. (63) conducted a study using 24 male firefighters to examine the effect of SCBA size and weight on gait performance. Equipped with one of four SCBA configurations, the firefighters completed three conditions (no obstacle, 10 m [11 yd] stationary obstacle, or 30 m [33 yd] stationary obstacle) while walking at either normal or fast speeds. The study found that SCBA bottle weight (mass), obstacle height, and walking speed, but not bottle size, significantly affected gait. In fact, wearing heavier bottles resulted in 42% of the firefighters contacting the taller obstacle, thus increasing the risk of tripping. The heavier bottles also resulted in greater forces in the anterior–posterior and vertical directions of the trailing leg, indicating a higher likelihood of slipping. An assessment of PPE weight, such as SCBA bottles, should be conducted as part of the risk assessment to mitigate injury.

Police respond to an extensive array of critical incidents (e.g., traffic stops, arrests, domestic disputes) that may require the application of physical force and great physical effort. PT for law enforcement must aim to improve overall fitness and optimize the ability to execute physically demanding occupational tasks identified by the task analysis. In 2001, Anderson et al. (4) evaluated the occupational requirements of police in British Columbia and found that the majority of officers routinely used tactics during critical incidents that involved pushing, pulling, controlling or wrestling and dragging, and lifting below shoulder level. Approximately half of the police officers rated these activities as difficult or requiring maximum effort. As these tasks are performed, special consideration should be given to body armor and ballistic vests, which can weigh on average 10 kg (22 lb).

Load Carriage and Movement Patterns

The success of firefighting, police, and military operations greatly depends on the mobility of personnel (61). Not only do units need to deploy quickly, personnel need to overcome challenges presented by the burdensome loads worn, which can potentially increase fatigue, reduce mobility, and hinder effectiveness. As an example, the body armor worn by tactical athletes can negatively affect body mechanics. Sell et al. (79) examined differences in postural stability during single-leg jump landings among 36 subjects, with and without body armor. They observed that wearing body armor reduced postural stability, potentially

increasing the risk for lower extremity injury. Based on these findings, the researchers recommend integrating body armor exercises into the training program in order to improve dynamic postural stability and injury mitigation.

The risk assessment should identify hazards such as slipping, tripping, and falling. The hazards of wearing PPE are further compounded when operating in environments with limited visibility, where reliance on proprioception is all that much more important. A literature review of the impact of load carriage on mobility was published in 2014 (13). The authors defined *mobility* as "the physical movement of a person in a straight line, multidirectional, or negotiating obstacles over distance." All of the studies included in this review found that as load increased, mobility decreased. As load increased, decreases in speed were apparent from increases in time to complete obstacle courses and road marches, even to the extent that some subjects were unsuccessful in their attempts to negotiate obstacles. Dempsey et al. (17) also reported decreased mobility among men wearing stab-resistant body armor (SRBA) in a series of mobility tasks. Strategies to optimize occupational task performance while carrying external loads are PT objectives the TSAC Facilitator will manage and monitor when working with tactical athletes.

Key Point

The TSAC Facilitator is responsible for prescribing an appropriately designed and progressive PT program incorporating load carriage and mobility exercises that reflect job-specific tasks.

Responses of Bone, Muscle, and Connective Tissue to Job Tasks Under Load

Many of the most detailed literature reviews and epidemiological studies fail to include load carriage variables as risk factors for injuries (13). It is paramount for medical units to understand the typical discomforts and injuries associated with job tasks under load so they can be prepared to recognize, treat, and even prevent such problems (41).

Previous research demonstrates that the upper limb is susceptible to short-term injuries, including soft tissue damage and trapped nerves or blood supplies while conducting load carriage activities (11). During an acute road march (one hour) while carrying 24 kg (53 lb), the hip region was rated significantly more comfortable than any other region, and the foot was rated significantly less comfortable than any other region (10). This suggests the foot is an area of concern. This is in agreement with research on a 100-mile (161 km) road march over five consecutive days carrying 47 kg (104 lb) (73). Foot pain was the second most frequent injury and also the largest single reason for limited duty days in this population.

In addition, shoulder pain has also been associated with load carriage (11). Shoulder discomfort may begin at the onset of the load carriage activity, with a gradual increase in pain rating over the duration of the load carriage activity (11). Based on subjective perception of discomfort or pain, along with skin pressure studies, the tolerance of mechanical loads by the shoulder tissues seems to be a major limiting factor of load carriage (11). When assessed with other load-bearing sites, the shoulders were found to be more vulnerable to skin and subcutaneous soft tissue damage when subjected to sustained loading (11). In addition, it is suspected that trapped nerves in the shoulder or reduced blood supply to the arms and hands may cause sensory loss in the hands and failure to fully abduct the arms (11). Using open MRI, Hadid and colleagues (27) were the first to quantify internal soft tissue deformations in the shoulder during load carriage. Applying their model reveals that a load of 25 kg (55 lb) under static conditions may result in compression and tensile strains that are potentially injurious to the brachial plexus (causing functional decrements in the arms and hands).

PHYSIOLOGICAL AND BIOMECHANICAL DEMANDS OF LOAD CARRIAGE

Regardless of tactical occupation, executing the mission will likely require some level of physical exertion while wearing load-bearing equipment. Austere and dangerous environments will further compound the difficulty of task performance. A substantial amount of energy is required to overcome the additional weight of load-bearing equipment compared to performing the same tasks in an unloaded condition. Three energy pathways within the body (phosphagen, glycolytic, and oxidative pathways) contribute to a tactical athlete's physical performance. Both work intensity and duration factor into the primary energy system contributing to a given occupational task.

Association Between Aerobic Power and Load Carried

Previous research has demonstrated that load carriage has a significant impact on physiological, metabolic, and performance variables. Quesada et al. (68) demonstrated that HR and oxygen consumption ($\dot{V}O_2$) increased linearly with an increase in loads of 0%, 30%, and 50% of body mass during simulated road marches, indicating greater physiological stress as loads get progressively heavier. Beekley et al. (7) showed similar trends in HR, $\dot{V}O_2$, RER, RPE, and ventilation (VE). Therefore, they investigated the metabolic responses to heavier loads of 30%, 50%, and 70% of LBM in a fit population during simulated road marching (30 minutes of road marching at 6 km/h [4 mph]) and demonstrated systematic increases in $\dot{V}O_2$, HR, and VE with increased loads at the same velocity of road marching. Figure 20.2 shows the linear increase in the metabolic response of $\dot{V}O_2$ to increasing loads. These results coupled with previous data suggest that HR and relative energy cost are fairly linear for 0% graded marching at 6 km/h (4 mph) (7).

Collectively, these studies demonstrate that performing physical tasks with load carriage increases metabolic and physiological stress concomitant with decreased performance.

Increases in Energy Expenditure as a Function of Load Carried

As demonstrated so far in this chapter, humans expend considerably more effort to walk when carrying a load. There is a progressive increase in metabolic energy expenditure concomitant with increases in load weight, body mass, locomotion

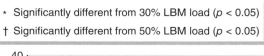

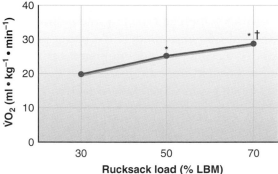

Figure 20.2 Relative oxygen cost to increasing loads on flat terrain at constant speed.

Adapted, by permission, from M.D. Beekley et al., 2007, "Effects of heavy load carriage during constant-speed, simulated, road marching," *Military Medicine* 172(6): 593.

speed, percent grade, and terrain (40). Gait kinematics do not change nearly as much as energy expenditure, which suggests the energetic cost appears to be less due to an altered gait pattern than to the effort of transporting the load itself. As load increases, there is a pronounced rise in joint moments and forces as well as **electromyography (EMG)** activity of muscle in the lower limbs and trunk (40). EMG is a technique in electrodiagnostic medicine for evaluating and recording the electrical activity produced by skeletal muscles.

Energy expenditure increases in a systematic manner with increases in body mass, load mass, velocity, and grade during acute bouts of treadmill exercise (9). One study examined the energy cost (kcal) of treadmill walking during loaded (1 kg [3 lb]) and unloaded conditions (74). Energy expenditure during the loaded condition was significantly greater than in the unloaded condition, and moderate pace walking resulted in an increase in energy expenditure approximately three times (126 kcal/h versus 42 kcal/h) that of slow walking during the loaded condition. The authors of this study concluded that wearing body armor increases the potential for physical exhaustion and impairs the performance of physical tasks during sustained operations (74).

The effects of military load carriage on energetics have been studied for almost a century (45).

The majority of previous studies have concluded that absolute energy expenditure increases linearly as a function of the military load carried (68, 74) up to 70% of soldiers' LBM (7). It has also been shown that this linear relationship of load and energy expenditure exists at the most common military walking speeds (60). Data presented by Grenier et al. (26) on walking energetics are consistent with those reported in the nonmilitary literature (6). The energy expenditure per kilogram of load carried is equal to the energy expenditure per kilogram of body weight up to approximately 30 kg (66 lb). When carrying heavier loads, humans become much less efficient; therefore, the energy expenditure per kilogram of load increases abruptly (52).

Common Injuries Associated With Load Carriage

A study conducted by Mullins et al. (55) used 11 untrained males to determine if prolonged load carriage is associated with lower limb injury, particularly in new recruits. The men walked on a motorized treadmill for 120 minutes at 5.5 km/h (3.4 mph), 0% grade, carrying 22 kg (49 lb) distributed on the body by a weight vest, combat webbing, and replica firearm. The study found that although there were increases in physiological demands, there were no functionally relevant changes in biomechanics (minor increase in step length). A study by Huang and Kuo (33) examined body center of mass and joint work in 8 adults walking at 1.25 m/s (1.37 yd/s) with varying backpack loads of up to 40% of body weight and demonstrated that the increase in metabolic cost was predominantly due to the work about the knee and ankle. However, this finding may depend on the position and manner in which the load is carried, as well as individual variances in load accommodation strategies (35) that affect ground reaction forces.

Excessive military loads have altered battle tactics and led to soldier deaths in previous conflicts (53). For example, during World War II, soldiers drowned due to excessive loads while conducting the assault on Omaha Beach (53). During the 1983 U.S. invasion of Grenada (Operation Urgent Fury), loads of up to 120 lb (54 kg) caused such extreme fatigue in soldiers that 10-yard (9 m) rushes were followed by 10- to 15-minute recovery periods prior to conducting each additional 10-yard rush (20). Evidence suggests that soldiers are currently carrying more weight than ever before (45); thus, the likelihood for injuries and casualties caused by load carriage may seriously affect mission readiness (58).

Foot blisters are the most common load carriage injuries, caused by friction between the sock and skin from boot pressure on the foot (11). Foot blisters can be a limiting factor if not treated appropriately and can progress to more serious problems, such as cellulitis or sepsis. Regular PT with loads causes skin adaptations that reduce the probability of blisters (44).

Stress fracture, another common injury, occurs from repetitive overloading of bone tissue. Stress fractures are common in military recruits (25) and have also been reported in trained soldiers (37). In fact, 60 stress fracture cases were reported in one infantry unit during a 483 km (300 mi) road march (19). The lower extremities (i.e., tibia, tarsals, metatarsals) are the most common areas affected (12). Again, stress fractures are more likely to occur with repetitive overloading of the bones where the bone remodeling balance is upset, causing bone remodeling to be outpaced by bone stress and fatigue (45).

Knee pain is another common abnormality associated with fatigue during prolonged marching distances (41). Dalen, Nilsson, and Thorstensson (15) reported a 15% incidence of knee pain during their load carriage study. Various disorders are associated with knee pain, making it difficult to diagnose. Disorders such as patellofemoral pain syndrome, patellar tendonitis, bursitis, and ligamentous strain can arise from an abrupt increase in load carriage intensity or duration (45).

Lower back injuries can present a significant problem during load carriage and are associated with longer distances (41). Similar to the knee, lower back injuries are difficult to define because the pain might result from trauma to an assortment of structures, including the spinal discs, ligaments connecting the vertebral bodies, nerve roots, and auxiliary musculature (45). Heavy loads are a risk factor for back injuries due to changes in trunk angle, which can stress back muscles (72).

A disabling injury associated with load carriage is rucksack palsy (8). It is postulated that rucksack palsy occurs from the shoulder straps of a backpack or the top portion of individual body armor, which can cause a traction injury of the C5 and C6 nerve roots of the upper brachial plexus. Symptoms include numbness, paralysis, cramping, and minor pain in the shoulder girdle, elbow flexors, and wrist extensors (45).

The monetary cost of injuries that result from excessive load carriage is only a portion of the total costs incurred by an organization. Duty days lost due to injury reduce a unit's mission readiness and, in some cases, preventable injuries can deplete medical resources that are limited in certain theaters (77).

PRACTICAL CONSIDERATIONS FOR TRAINING PROGRAMS TO OPTIMIZE LOAD CARRIAGE

The following section reviews the current literature on strength and conditioning for load carriage and provides recommendations for enhancing the tactical athlete's ability to maneuver successfully under loaded conditions. Over the last 20 to 25 years, there has been a push to develop optimal PT strategies aimed at conditioning soldiers to endure load carriage tasks. Research outcomes have broadened the knowledge base for imposed physiological demands during load-bearing work. Two decades of research suggests that a combination of resistance training, aerobic, and specific load carriage exercise are most effective for improving load carriage performance (24, 29, 38, 46, 49, 85, 86).

Current Fitness Level

The operational success of a tactical unit depends on the physical readiness of tactical athletes within that unit. Within short notice, tactical athletes may be required to march with supplies and equipment, often over rugged terrain, underscoring the need to be physically adapted to the demands of load carriage tasks. To select the people best suited for missions with heavy load carriage, it is essential to predict prolonged load carriage capability using substitute tests. Many organizations use aerobic fitness tests to predict occupational fitness, but such tests are not sensitive enough to predict prolonged load carriage capability (52). **Occupational fitness** is the fitness level required for a certain occupation (e.g., swat, fire and rescue, military).

Past research has clearly shown that non–load-carrying aerobic fitness tests impose a bias against heavier personnel (81). Therefore, body mass, body composition, or both may be important criteria when looking to improve the sensitivity of a fitness test for load carriage. A high LBM strongly correlates with absolute maximal oxygen uptake ($\dot{V}O_2$max) and predicts load carriage performance. In addition, body fat has been shown to impair load carriage (28). As load increases and athletes become less efficient, a high absolute $\dot{V}O_2$ (ml·min^{-1}) reserve is essential for heavy load carriage tasks (52). Lyons, Allsopp, and Bilzon (52) demonstrated that expressing body composition as a ratio of LBM to **dead mass** (i.e., fat mass + external load) resulted in strong correlations with the metabolic demands (%$\dot{V}O_2$max) of a 40 kg (88 lb) load carriage task. Physiologically, the more LBM a person has that can carry the dead mass, the lower the relative demands of the task will be.

Key Point

I RM is crucial for predicting successful load carriage performance.

Although conducting loaded marches that simulate the operational tempo are ideal for testing load carriage ability (84), loaded marches may not always be feasible; thus, alternative testing methods must be used. Several studies have examined indices of fitness measures, such as **anthropometry** (i.e., study of the measurements and proportions of the human body), muscle strength, muscle endurance, and aerobic power, to best predict load carriage performance (23, 39, 47, 84, 87). Williams and Rayson (84) conducted a study using 148 British Army recruits to determine if simple anthropometric tests together with strength and endurance field tests could be used to predict both load carriage performance at a single point and training-induced changes in load carriage performance using loads of 15 kg (33 lb) and 25 kg (55 lb). This research derived

a regression model to predict pretraining load carriage performance with only a 15 kg (33 lb) load, but it was unable to predict changes in load carriage performance for either weight. The predictor variables used in the final regression model for the 15 kg (33 lb) load were shuttle run time, which was most often used, followed by fat-free mass (FFM) and percent body fat. For the pretraining 15 kg (33 lb) load, the proportion of variance for the prediction model was 81%, and the change in load carriage performance model was 55% for men and 80% for women. The prediction models for the 25 kg (55 lb) load had a proportion of variance of 40% and less than 7% for pretraining and change in performance, respectively. Based on this research, it may be possible to predict pretraining load carriage ability with a 15 kg (33 lb) load using simple anthropometric and physical performance tests, but is not likely possible with heavier loads such as 25 kg (55 lb).

Kraemer et al. (47) conducted a study using multiple regression analysis to determine which independent measures were most predictive for a **load-bearing task** (i.e., 2 mi [3 km], 34 kg [75 lb] military rucksack carry) in 123 civilian women. Six variables were included in this study:

1. Thigh muscle cross-sectional area
2. 1RM squat, high pull, bench press, and box lift
3. Maximum push-ups
4. Two-mile run
5. Squat endurance test
6. Explosive squat jump lift

The final regression equation for the load-bearing task included the squat endurance test (SE), 2-mile run (TMR), and body mass (BM) [1831 – 4.28 (SE) + 0.95 (TMR) – 13.4 (BM)] and explained 53% of the variance ($R^2 = 0.53$). This demonstrates that both aerobic capacity and local muscular endurance are vital for load-bearing tasks (47).

Training Programs to Meet Occupational Demands

Numerous studies have examined the influence of types of exercise training programs on load carriage (31, 46, 48, 78, 87). One of the most important concepts for improving load carriage performance is the principle of specificity. **Specificity** is training that is relevant and appropriate to the sport or event for which the individual desires a training effect. Therefore, load carriage tasks should be included in a conditioning program designed to improve load carriage ability (45, 87).

Appropriate application of specificity to load carriage PT was revealed in a study by Patterson et al. (64), who investigated the effects of a 12-week conditioning program (which included circuit and resistance training, running, and load carriage marches) on performance outcomes in soldiers. Although soldiers increased strength and aerobic capacity during the study, load carriage performance did not change significantly. This may be due to two reasons: To minimize any observable effects of training, load carriage was limited to only two sessions throughout the study (weeks 3 and 5), and the longest load carriage march in the study was 30 minutes, which is much shorter than the 15 km (9 mi or 165 minutes) event normally used to assess performance in the U.S. Army. A meta-analysis conducted by Knapik et al. (42) found that the largest overall improvements in load carriage performance occurred when once-weekly progressive load carriage was included in the training regimen (30, 87). This specific training likely involves the skills, energy systems, and muscle groups required for performing this task. It is evident that prescribing progressive load carriage exercise in a strength and conditioning program will develop the skills to enhance performance of this task and condition the muscle groups and energy systems required (69).

Developing strength and conditioning programs to improve firefighter performance is challenging because firefighters routinely perform tasks requiring optimal levels of power, strength, muscular endurance, anaerobic endurance, and aerobic endurance. Limited data are available to provide insight on the most appropriate training programs, but there are a few key findings.

A study conducted by Peterson et al. (65) compared undulated training to traditional periodization for firefighter trainees. The traditional model systematically increased intensity over nine weeks; the program initially focused on improving muscle endurance and hypertrophy, then basic and functional strength, and finally RFD and peak power output. In contrast, the undulated program included daily fluctuations in intensity, volume, and exercise selection to elicit concurrent improvements in muscle endurance, hypertrophy, strength, power, and speed. Both groups improved their 1RM bench press and squat, power output, and vertical jump. Interestingly, the undulated group showed greater improvements in the 1RM bench press and squat, peak power output at 30% 1RM squat, average peak power output at 60% 1RM for squat, vertical jump height, and performance on a firefighter-specific job-task test (65). These findings suggest that over a nine-week training period, undulated training may be a more effective strategy to enhance firefighter task-specific performance compared with linear periodized training.

It is important to use specificity when designing programs for firefighters. TSAC Facilitators should select multijoint resistance and cardiorespiratory exercises that mimic the tasks performed on the fireground. It's also crucial to use the actual equipment (i.e., hoses and ladders) used on the fireground.

Key Point

To get better at load carriage, tactical athletes must train under loaded conditions specific to their respective occupational tasks.

Approaches to Improving Short-Duration, High-Intensity Load Bearing

The tactical athlete requires a certain degree of strength and power for short-duration missions that require high-intensity (heavy) loads. Strength and power training is best facilitated by intensity (load), followed by training frequency (sessions per week) and then by volume (distance). Visser et al. (82) compared a high-intensity (load), low-volume (distance) training program with one of a lower intensity (load) and higher volume (distance) where speed was kept constant. Both training combinations were reviewed against the effects of training frequency (number of sessions per week). Results demonstrated an 18% increase in a load march test in the high-intensity, low-volume group.

Loads were 35% to 55% of body weight for females and 45% to 67.5% of body weight for males, and distances were between 4.0 km (2.5 mi) and 5.5 km (3.4 mi) per session. In addition, the higher frequency condition (once per week) resulted in enhanced performance on the load march test compared with the lower frequency (once every two weeks).

Aerobic Training to Improve Long-Duration, Low-Intensity Load Bearing

Aerobic training alone has been shown to have smaller and more variable effects on improving load carriage. For example, Kraemer et al. (46, 48) examined the influence of periodized resistance training programs on strength, power, endurance, and military occupational performance. The study had six groups of participants: total strength/power resistance (TP), total strength/hypertrophy resistance (TH), upper strength/power resistance (UP), upper strength/hypertrophy resistance (UH), field exercises with minimal equipment (FLD), and aerobic training (AER). Results demonstrated that all groups except the AER group improved their performance on the load carriage task. Additional research (75) supports this finding by showing that aerobic-only training enhances aerobic capacity. Only the load-marching group improved their performance of military tasks. A systematic review of the effects of PT on load carriage performance showed that aerobic training alone had smaller and more variable effects on performance (42).

Strength Training to Improve Mobility During Load Carriage

The fact that load carriage performance has been enhanced with **concurrent training** suggests that combining strength and cardiorespiratory endurance is optimal for load carriage improvement (42). As mentioned, Kraemer et al. (46) examined the influence of periodized resistance training programs on strength, power, aerobic endurance, and military occupational performance. The study selected 93 untrained women who were divided into six groups (TP, TH, UP, UH, FLD, and AER). The TP, TH, UP, and UH groups emphasized both resistance training and 25 to 35

minutes of running, cycling, or stair-climbing for three days a week. The FLD group emphasized calisthenics, dumbbell- and partner-resisted exercises, and ballistic plyometrics. The AER group conducted 25 to 30 minutes of running, with cycling and stair-climbing providing variation for three days a week, and low-volume resistance band exercises (<5 kg [<11 lb]). The load carriage task for all groups was a 2-mile (3 km) time-to-completion event while wearing a 75 lb (34 kg) load. Results revealed that all groups improved their performance on the load carriage task except the AER group. The addition of strength training improved load carriage performance in this study, underscoring the importance of strength conditioning for physically demanding tactical occupations. Interestingly, both studies conducted by Kraemer et al. (46, 48) demonstrated that programs employing either resistance training or aerobic training in isolation failed to make significant improvements in load carriage performance. Therefore, a strength and conditioning program should include exercise specific to all three energy systems.

The TSAC Facilitator should consider two factors when examining studies that suggest load carriage performance can be improved with a concurrent training program that excludes a specific load carriage component. First, subjects with lower initial fitness levels tend to make greater initial gains regardless of training mode, after which specific training is needed to make improvements (87). Second, training for specificity can improve physical performance measures other than those being measured (58). Rudzki (75) published findings in support of this concept by demonstrating that both a run group and load-marching group improved similarly in measures of aerobic fitness, but only the load-marching group improved their performance of military tasks. Table 20.2 provides a comprehensive review of published findings on load carriage performance.

A meta-analysis proposed that periodized resistance training programs may offer greater improvements in load carriage performance than linear resistance training programs (42). The periodized training programs manipulated sets, repetitions, and exercises either in blocks (mesocycles and microcycles) lasting several weeks (30, 46)

Table 20.2 Review of Published Findings on Load Carriage Performance

Authors	Training group and training mode	Training (duration and frequency)	Load carriage task (distance, load)	Mean change in performance time (min) over study
Schiotz et al. (78)	Periodized ($n = 11$)	10 weeks (4 days/week RT; 4 days/week AT)	10 km (6 mi) run with 15 kg (33 lb) load	−7.5
	Constant intensity ($n = 11$) using free weights and machines with equal volume between groups Aerobic training consisting of aerobic intervals, LSD (with and without added weight), and anaerobic intervals			−3.7
Kraemer et al. (46)	UB and LB strength/power RT with AT ($n = 17$)	24 weeks (3 days/week RT; 3 days/week AT)	3.2 km (2 mi) with 34 kg (75 lb) load	−3.4
	UB and LB strength/hypertrophy RT with AT ($n = 18$)			−4.0
	UB strength/power RT with AT ($n = 18$)			−3.8
	UB strength/hypertrophy RT with AT ($n= 15$)			−3.4
	Field training ($n = 14$)			−2.7
	AT only ($n = 11$)			0.4
Williams et al. (86)	Modified basic training ($n = 52$) consisted of strength training, endurance training, agility, material handling, sports, circuit training, and swimming	10 weeks (40 min sessions, 7 days/week)	2 mi (3 km) with 15 kg (33 lb) and 25 kg (55 lb) load	−1.9 −4.1
Kraemer et al. (48)	$N = 35$	12 weeks (4 days/week RT; 4 days/week ET)	2 mi (3 km) with 44.7 kg (98.5 lb) load	
	RT + ET			−3.5
	UB +ET			−3.1
	RT only			−1.25
	ET only			−.016
	Resistance training consisted of free weight hypertrophy/strength training Endurance training consisted of long-distance runs and sprint intervals			
Harman et al. (30)	WBT ($n = 17$) Resistance training, running, backpack hiking, intervals, agility drills	8 weeks (5 sessions/week)	2 mi (3 km) with 32 kg (71 lb) load	−3.8
	SPT ($n = 15$) Military movement drills, stretching drills, intervals, ability group runs, shuttle runs			−3.5
Hendrickson et al. (31)	UB and LB RT only ($n = 12$) Periodized resistance training with weights	12 weeks (3 days/week)	2 mi (3 km) with 33 kg (73 lb) load	−4.5
	AT only ($n =12$) Running 20-30 min mixed interval training			−4.6
	UB and LB with AT ($n = 11$) same as described in first two groups RT followed by AT			−4.7
	No training ($n = 8$); maintained normal recreational training			−2.6

UB = upper body, LB = lower body; RT = resistance training; AT = aerobic training; ET = endurance training; LSD = long, slow distance training; WBT = weight-based training; SPT = standardized physical training.

or in an undulating manner with weekly or even daily alterations in intensity and volume (31). On some days, higher weight and fewer repetitions were prescribed to emphasize strength, and on other days, lower weight and more repetitions were prescribed to emphasize muscular endurance. In addition, different exercises for different muscle groups were prescribed on different days. It is likely that the emphasis on different components of fitness (strength and muscular endurance) combined with the greater variety of trained muscle groups may have provided an advantage in improving load carriage performance (42). Linear resistance training programs that added resistance (i.e., weight) throughout but didn't change the number of sets and repetitions and exercised the same muscle groups throughout the program were more restrictive. Although still effective for recreationally active men, these programs appeared to result in somewhat lower performance gains (42).

Frequency of Weight Carried

Visser et al. (82) examined the impact of various training doses on load carriage capacity, which were analyzed against the effects of training frequency (number of sessions per week). The higher frequency (once per week) training groups made significantly greater improvements in the physical performance outcome measures than the lower frequency (twice per month) groups. These findings suggest that improvement in load carriage performance occurs from at least one session per week of specific load carriage tasks.

Another study (76) examined two 11-week conditioning programs for recruits: One group (run) performed endurance running, load carriage, and other conditioning activities, while the other group (load marching) replaced all running sessions with load marching. Both groups made similar gains in aerobic fitness, but only the load marching group demonstrated improvements in aerobic fitness together with an increase in walking speed and loads carried. These results suggest that the load carriage regimen needs to be at an intensity (load and speed) that is sufficient to stimulate adaptations necessary for significant improvements in aerobic fitness and load carriage.

It is evident that when designing strength and conditioning programs to enhance load carriage performance, the training intensity (load and speed) of load carriage is a key factor. Therefore, the TSAC Facilitator should use loads that the tactical athlete will carry in real-world situations.

Recommendations for Program Design

When designing strength and conditioning programs to improve load carriage, loaded marching should be conducted at least two times a month (43, 45), with enhanced improvements demonstrated when frequency increases to once a week (42). However, this frequency may vary depending on training intensity (load, speed) and training volume (time or distance). To stimulate aerobic adaptations, the intensity (e.g., load, speed) of the training must be sufficient enough to elicit a training response. When prescribing high-intensity load carriage training, the potential for injury with long-term, high-intensity load carriage training should not be overlooked (45).

The TSAC Facilitator is responsible for designing strength and conditioning programs with the specific requirements that mirror the tactical athlete's tasks regarding the distance (or time) of prescribed load carriage tasks against both intensity and outcome requirements. For example, tactical athletes may require short-duration, high-intensity sessions to develop explosive, anaerobic ability (e.g., as needed under direct fire or climbing a flight of stairs to put out a fire) in addition to PT sessions that are longer in duration to optimize the physical and mental endurance needed for dismounted patrols or fighting long-duration forest fires (58). The tactical athlete will benefit from strength and conditioning programs that incorporate upper body strength training and aerobic exercise along with load carriage training.

TSAC Facilitators are charged with designing effective, evidence-based strength and conditioning programs that facilitate all aspects of physical adaptation, including progressive overload, injury **prehabilitation** (strength training to prevent injuries) and mitigation, and recovery. The following practical guidelines are an evidence-based summary of research that demonstrates improvements in load carriage and are to be used when designing and prescribing strength and conditioning programs to improve load carriage performance.

- Once-weekly progressive load carriage (42)
- Progressive increase in the intensity of loads to meet tactical requirements (58)
- Progressive increase in load carriage volume (duration or distance) to meet tactical requirements (58)
- Resistance training performed with free weights and machines at least three days per week, moving from high repetitions (12+ reps) with less weight (muscular endurance) to lower repetitions (3-6 reps) with heavier weight (strength) and working up to three sets per exercise (46, 48)
- Aerobic training with progressive increases in distance (running 20-30 min based on HR two times per week) and interval training with progressive decreases in rest (about once per week) (82)

Table 20.3 provides a sample monthly training template that TSAC Facilitators can use as a guide when designing strength and conditioning programs to enhance load carriage performance by tactical athletes.

The mission success of a unit is based entirely on the performance of the tactical athletes, who often have to react and maneuver in austere environments while under loaded conditions. Firefighters often endure prolonged operations under stressful environmental conditions and under load, while law enforcement members must also maneuver and react quickly under loaded conditions (e.g., SWAT). TSAC Facilitators have the important task of ensuring that the strength and conditioning programs they prescribe are based on sound research and are appropriate for the tactical athletes they are coaching.

CONCLUSION

This chapter has provided a historical perspective of load carriage and an explanation of the types of loads that tactical personnel may carry. Furthermore, the physiological demands of load carriage have been discussed to provide a sense of the metabolic costs and decrements in physical performance that accompany load carriage tasks. Finally, a review of the literature examining the most effective methodologies in strength and conditioning prescription for the purpose of enhancing load carriage performance will provide the TSAC Facilitator with a foundation on which to design appropriate, evidence-based training programs. By applying the principles and guidelines set forth in this chapter, the TSAC Facilitator will be able to offer tactical athletes sound guidance in the development of strength and conditioning programs.

Table 20.3 Sample Monthly Training Program to Enhance Load Carriage Performance

	Monday	Tuesday	Wednesday	Thursday	Friday	Saturday	Sunday
Week 1	Strength: upper body (push)	Rest	Strength: upper body (pull)	Aerobic	Strength: lower body	Rest	Aerobic
Week 2	Loaded march	Rest	Strength: combined upper body	Aerobic	Strength: lower body	Rest	Aerobic
Week 3	Strength: upper body (push)	Rest	Strength: upper body (pull)	Aerobic	Strength: lower body	Rest	Aerobic
Week 4	Loaded march	Rest	Strength: combined upper body	Aerobic	Strength: lower body	Rest	Aerobic

Key Terms

anthropometry
concurrent training
dead mass
electromyography (EMG)
load-bearing task
load carriage
mobility

needs analysis
occupational fitness
prehabilitation
reaction time
specificity
squat endurance test

Study Questions

1. As the weight of an externally carried load increases, which of the following changes the least?

   a. gait kinematics

   b. total energy expenditure

   c. metabolic cost of walking

   d. EMG activity of the leg muscles

2. Which of the following is the most common load carriage injury?

   a. knee pain

   b. foot blisters

   c. rucksack palsy

   d. stress fractures

3. Which of the following types of tests is not sensitive enough to predict prolonged load carriage capability?

   a. power

   b. strength

   c. aerobic fitness

   d. body composition

4. Which of the following is the most important principle in creating the desired training effect for job relevancy?

   a. specificity

   b. measurability

   c. attainability

   d. variability

5. What is the minimum number of load carriage training sessions that must be included in a tactical athlete's program to see improvements in load carriage performance?

   a. one time per week

   b. one time every two weeks

   c. one time every three weeks

   d. one time per month

Obesity

According to the World Health Organization (WHO) (116), a BMI of ≥30 is considered obese. Based on this measure, the prevalence of **obesity** in the general population is increasing worldwide (5). With tactical personnel drawn from the general population, it is not unexpected that obesity levels are having a negative impact on enlistment eligibility. For the U.S. military, the percentage of ineligible recruits due to excessive BMI has more than doubled from 2.8% in 1993 to 6.8% in 2006 (103), with recruits who failed their physicals increasing by 70% between 1998 and 2008 (20, 105). Similar trends were found in emergency responder candidates, with a third being obese on application from June 2004 to June 2007 (110).

Not only does obesity reduce the ability of tactical occupations to generate future personnel, but it is also negatively associated with workplace **absenteeism** following injury (87) and hence productivity. In addition, recent research has shown that 42% of police officers are obese and at risk for cardiovascular disease (15). Another study found 41% of a police officer sample to be hypertensive, 75% to have increased cholesterol levels, and 65% to be clinically obese, all risk factors for cardiovascular disease (108). In a longitudinal study of U.S. firefighters over several years, obesity levels increased from 34.9% in 1996 and 1997 to 39.7% in 2001 (105). These figures are slightly lower in military populations. A study in 2005 of more than 16,000 U.S. military personnel suggested that, although 60.5% were either overweight or obese, only 12.9% were obese; however, this figure had increased by 4.2% since 2002 (103). Obesity is a known risk factor for cardiovascular disease (83), which is a disease of particular concern to tactical athletes (22, 110) due to the strenuous nature of certain tasks and occupational risks (e.g., threat of violence) and their associated impacts on health (22, 82).

Cardiovascular Disease

Cardiovascular disease is a leading cause of mortality in the U.S. population and worldwide (99). Considering law enforcement officers must go from sedentary activity to sudden high-intensity

responses (see chapter 18), it is not surprising that they are twice as likely to suffer from cardiovascular disease as the general population (94). Nor is it surprising that cardiovascular disease is the leading cause of mortality among firefighters while on duty, accounting for nearly half of all mortalities (106). It accounts for only 3% to 6% of all U.S. Department of Defense mortalities, with hostile actions or motor vehicles (both over 20%) the leading causes of mortality in this population (97); however, it is still one of the top five contributors to military deaths (97).

Personal choices regarding **diet**, exercise, and well-being are educable by employers but not controllable. Poor choices in sleep, stress management, meal routine, and circadian cycle disturbances, for example, can contribute to severe cardiovascular incidents and death (17, 113). Further risks come from **metabolic syndromes** or **syndrome X** (a grouping of factors that increase a person's chance of developing cardiovascular disease). Thus, the possibility of mortality from cardiovascular risks significantly increases in tactical personnel exhibiting these habits (6, 113).

Although stress and shift work may contribute to poor cardiovascular health and other conditions, the risk of severe disability or death in firefighting has been attributed to the increased cardiovascular demand of fire suppression and alarm response (52). In the general population, deaths from coronary heart disease are more likely to occur in the morning (46, 97). In firefighters, however, most cardiovascular events are thought to occur within 24 hours of physical exertion at work (52), with research suggesting that 75% of deaths occurred traveling to or from an incident, at the incident itself, or during training (46). With the need for tactical personnel to perform sudden and demanding physical activities, these findings are not surprising. Note that cardiovascular concerns may not necessarily present in a short time period. For example, law enforcement retirees were found to exhibit a greater prevalence of cardiovascular disease compared with their peers in the general population (93). These findings demonstrate a carryover effect of these cardiovascular concerns beyond service time.

Cancer

Cancer (see table 21.1 for examples) is a concern for many occupations; however, the degree of risk may vary among tactical populations. Cancer may be as much as two times more prevalent in the fire service when compared with the general population (24, 89); however, a study of U.S. military personnel found mixed results, with military personnel at greater risk for some types of cancer (e.g., breast, prostate) but lower risk for others (e.g., colorectal) (117). Furthermore, specific tasks may increase the risk of cancer, such as Air Force aircraft desealing and resealing (21). Working in older buildings with structural insulation containing asbestos (an acknowledged cause of cancer) may also increase the risk of cancer (81), particularly if the building is damaged by combat or structural fires (24).

With improvements in technology, protection, and practices, some incidences of cancer, especially respiratory-related ones, have decreased dramatically in the last 30 years, particularly when compared to other occupations at high risk of exposure (11, 18, 24, 89). Some evidence suggests that inadequate PPE, inadequately cleaned fire gear such as hoods, diesel exhaust on turnout pants sitting in the bay, and peripheral smoke during overhaul practices where breathing apparatuses are not worn are the greatest contributors to these conditions (11, 18, 21).

RISK FACTORS REQUIRING WELLNESS INTERVENTIONS

Apart from physical conditioning, there is a need for tactical occupations to incorporate wellness programs (75, 79). Wellness programs are known to decrease fiscal costs for organizations (14), and their importance to tactical athletes extends to postcareer longevity and health for veterans. In fact, veterans are known to be at greater risk of illness and disease (both physical and psychological) (42, 93).

Ameliorating risk factors for chronic illnesses and diseases in tactical populations should be a key focus of wellness programs. These risk factors include **physical inactivity**, stress, tobacco usage, excessive alcohol consumption, **sleep disruption**, and poor **nutritional habits**, as will be discussed in this section.

Physical Inactivity

Because fitness is related to morbidity (49), most health authorities recommend performing three or more weekly exercise sessions (i.e., sessions that are designed to achieve a desired outcome and include dedicated training to increase metabolic demands) (33, 49). Although the need for physical exercise is well acknowledged within both the general and tactical populations, tactical athletes face several barriers to participation. Earlier chap-

Table 21.1 Cancers Common to Tactical Populations

System	Cancer type or targeted tissue
Gastrointestinal and genitourinary	Kidney Bladder Prostate Testicular Colon Esophageal
Female reproductive	Cervical
Endocrinal	Thyroid
Nervous	Brain
Respiratory	Lung Mesothelioma (from asbestos)
Systemic	Multiple myeloma Non-Hodgkin's lymphoma Hodgkin's disease

Based on references 24, 63, 89, 117.

ters have noted that some tactical occupations are quite sedentary. For example, law enforcement officers and firefighters spend a large amount of time sitting doing desk work, driving, or waiting for emergency calls, with only limited (although demanding) tasks requiring physical activity (3, 67). A further complication is found with older officers as they increase in rank and take on more strategic positions that require even less physical activity (104). This decrease in physical activity associated with occupational role is not restricted to rank and age, however. For example, Australian Army personnel working as staff in a training institution reported that their fitness tended to decrease when they served in training environments as opposed to in their operational units due to the logistical and administrative requirements at the training institution (75).

Other work contexts that affect physical inactivity include shift work and unexpected daily tasks. Shift work can decrease sleep quality and in turn increase fatigue (discussed later in this chapter). In addition, research suggests that shift work has a negative impact on the desire to exercise (47). Likewise, tactical personnel may be less inclined to perform physical exercise at the commencement of a shift if they may be required to perform optimally at any time within the shift. For example, a training session that induces leg fatigue could negatively affect the explosive speed of a tactical officer seeking cover or a firefighter moving rapidly up a staircase in a burning structure. At the end of a shift, fatigue, lethargy, and the allocation of time to other priorities (e.g., family, social obligations) can reduce the desire to perform physical exercise. For example, in a study on interventions to reduce cardiovascular risk in law enforcement officers (94), comments collected as part of a focus group included a police officer stating that, given the high daily workload, "All of a sudden, you are done with your shift and it's like you don't want to do much; you just want to crash."

Stress

It is not surprising that work stress is notable in tactical occupations. Firefighters are exposed to the dangers of fighting unpredictable fires. Soldiers may face an enemy who operates outside any laws of armed conflict. Law enforcement officers could be exposed to shootings, robberies, severe motor vehicle accidents, and, similar to firefighters and military personnel, deceased bodies. In addition, tactical athletes may be required to spend extended periods of time away from their families and personal support systems, which increases occupational stress (13). One study suggested that nearly a quarter of military personnel considered time away from family as causing "a lot" of stress (13). And in a population of firefighters, decreased numbers of personnel in a crew or a given shift increased occupational stress (62).

These occupational stresses have far-reaching consequences for tactical personnel. For example, increased occupational stress in tactical populations has been associated with an increased risk of injury (7) and an increased risk of diseases associated with stress (112). Additionally, maladaptive coping strategies may include other health detractors, such as smoking cigarettes and drinking excessive alcohol (40).

Tobacco Use

Smoking cigarettes and chewing tobacco have long been part of some tactical occupations, notably military and law enforcement, for a variety of cultural reasons. Rates of cigarette smoking have been found to increase in these tactical occupations (92, 101), leading to rates that are higher than in the general population (37). Rates can also differ among tactical populations. For example, the smoking rate is higher in Marines than U.S. Air Force personnel (13). Reasons for this higher rate may include both maladaptive coping behaviors to stress (40) and shift work, which is a known risk factor for smoking in a variety of occupations (53). Even within a given tactical population, rates of tobacco use may vary, with research suggesting that lower ranks are more prone to smoking compared with higher ranks (102).

Because of the widely known health risks of cigarette smoking and community education about them, this trend in tactical populations may be changing. For example, in firefighters, smoking tobacco may now be less common than in the general population (45). The main reasons firefighters give for stopping tobacco use are knowing the end result, improving fitness, and becoming more educated on the risks (85). In addition, the decrease in smoking rates may be due to policy at both the state and local levels, such as the restriction of cigarette smoking as a condition of employment and related presumption laws (85). However, smokeless tobacco still has a higher rate in the U.S. firefighter and military populations than in the civilian population (13, 45). These results may be restricted to U.S. populations because smokeless tobacco is less prevalent in other places, such as Australia, where it is banned (4).

Excessive Alcohol Consumption

Alcohol consumption by tactical athletes can vary from the national average to well above (13, 16, 92). Furthermore, two studies noted that although officers may not drink more frequently than civilians, they tend to consume more drinks in a single session (92). As with cigarette smoking, serving in a tactical occupation may increase alcohol consumption (73), particularly as a coping behavior for stress (40). Also akin to cigarette smoking, rates of excessive alcohol consumption are higher in some tactical occupations (e.g., U.S. Marine Corps and Army personnel) compared with others (e.g., U.S. Navy and Air Force) (13). For example, the trends in binge drinking in the U.S. Department of Defense ranged from 39% in Air Force personnel up to 58% in Marines, while professional firefighter rates were similarly high at 56% (16).

Sleep Disruption

Although individual needs vary, the majority of adults require seven to eight hours of sleep per night (96). Insufficient sleep and an accumulation of sleep loss (or sleep debt) have been associated with reduced quality of life, impaired cognitive function (e.g., reduced reaction times, decreased alertness, impaired concentration), and altered mood states (e.g., decreased emotional control, increased anxiety, increased tension) (43, 96). Furthermore, sleep deprivation can cause people to perceptually disengage from their environment and cease to integrate outside information, have diminished situational awareness, and have impaired judgment (96). Sustained wakefulness

for 17 or more hours has been found to decrease cognitive performance to a state equivalent to a blood alcohol content of 0.05% (27). This is concerning given that tactical personnel may be in high-risk situations following periods of limited sleep and thus may be performing with impaired cognitive function. Additionally, research suggests that sleep loss has a cumulative effect. An in-depth study by van Dongen et al. (111) showed that less than eight hours of time in bed led to a progressive increase in sleep debt to the extent where, after 14 days, the subjects performed cognitive tasks at a level similar to people who had not slept for 24 to 48 hours.

Sleep disruption does not just refer to getting three hours of sleep in a night and waking up exhausted. The type of rest must also be considered, especially if the rest occurs while on duty; eight hours of sleep under these circumstances are not the same as eight hours at home. Apart from dozing in a semialtered state and the impact of communal sleep areas and incidental noise, waking once per night on a consistent basis is enough to disrupt the body's natural cycles (34). Chronic exposure to these detractors of restful sleep over the course of a career, especially inconsistent sleep patterns with extra shifts and changes in call load, assignment, and alarm type, can desensitize tactical personnel so that they accept chronic fatigue and its effects as normal (28).

Key Point

Although often overlooked, special attention should be given to sleep patterns in tactical populations.

When subjects in the study by van Dongen et al. (111) were asked every two hours how they were feeling, after two days most stated that they had adapted and were not feeling any additional fatigue even when the cumulative impact of sleep loss increased dramatically (as measured by the Stanford Sleepiness Scale). It appears that people may not be able to accurately rate their level of fatigue, nor may they consider the risks associated with fatigue to be important in light of competing priorities. This lack of insight may contribute to attitudes toward sleep loss where lack of sleep is not seen as a risk and rest is not prioritized over competing activities (36). The consequences of this occupational attitude are highlighted throughout history. For example, soldiers manning forward positions have been known to combat their desire to sleep by pulling pins from grenades and holding down the levers (71). More recently, a police officer suffered a serious road accident after driving to court following nearly 35 hours of work (60). As a final consideration, lack of sleep can affect motivation (41), which feeds into a negative cycle compounding the lack of physical activity.

Nutritional Habits

A multitude of factors affect a tactical athlete's nutritional intake, including shift work, nutrition availability on operations, and so on. Although tactical nutrition is discussed in greater detail in chapters 5 and 6, certain factors related to health and well-being are worth considering here, particularly communal eating and skipping meals. Communal eating increases the transfer of pathogens and subsequent illness. Dirty cookware and cutlery in communal kitchens or sheds in a field are prime examples. In training institutions, food exposure to the elements for extended amounts of time (e.g., over a meal period) and cross-contamination (e.g., sharing a tub of yogurt or carton of milk) can increase the potential for illness (77).

When it comes to good nutritional habits, the tendency to skip breakfast is of notable concern. Breakfast is considered a marker of an appropriate dietary pattern (98) and health quality (8, 69, 100). Missing breakfast may lead to increased obesity (63), increased BMI (19), loss of nutrients that is not regained during the day (69), and reduced mental health (100). An investigation of an officer training unit found that staff members were more likely to miss breakfast than the general population (75). This report also found that, during lunch, many of the staff ate at their desks. Eating lunch at the workplace desk has also been associated with negative health outcomes. For example, sitting at a desk for long periods of time may reduce the amount of daily physical activity. Indirectly, sitting at the desk eating lunch could lead to additional time at the computer, which can increase the risk of repetitive strain injuries (RSIs) (32) and computer vision syndrome (10) and decrease quality of life (50). Interestingly, this culture of eating at the desk may not be related to a lack of facilities. The author noted that one police station had a new kitchen with full cooking facilities and even an enclosed garden that stood empty at lunchtime, with staff eating takeout at their desks and completing reports (75).

Ultimately, poor nutritional habits are prevalent in tactical populations (31, 44, 90). Furthermore, simply making sure healthier food options are available will not lead to optimal nutritional fitness unless personnel make healthy food choices (68). A final consideration lies in the traditional focus in military nutrition on undernutrition. Historically, investigations into soldier nutrition in the military have mainly been concerned with the adverse effects of undernutrition (65); however, an emerging threat to soldier nutrition is overnutrition or overconsumption, resulting in the increased weight concerns (e.g., overweight, obesity) discussed earlier in this chapter (20).

Compounding Effects

Key risk factors associated with chronic illness and disease common in tactical populations have been presented in isolation; however, health and well-being result from a combination of factors. A classic study by Belloc and Breslow (8) identified seven lifestyle habits as the foundation of good health:

1. Moderate exercise two to three times per week (significantly less than today's recommendation of five days per week at a moderate intensity or three days per week at a vigorous intensity [49])

2. Three meals a day at regular times with no snacking

3. Breakfast every day

4. Seven to eight hours sleep

5. No smoking

6. No alcohol

7. Moderate weight

Furthermore, Belloc and Breslow (8) considered these lifestyle habits to be cumulative, meaning that they are related to one another and compounding in nature. These results are not surprising, given evidence suggesting that missing meals is associated with poor sleep quality (1) or that drinking alcohol and smoking cigarettes are associated with stress (92). Although the works of Belloc and Breslow (8) have been criticized for failing to include stress as a measure of health (114), a paper by Morimoto (70) that includes stress measures (subjective stress and work for ≤9 hours per day) likewise lists moderate exercise two or more times per week, seven to eight hours of sleep per night, and daily breakfast as indicators of health.

Because these risk factors may be compounding, risk reduction strategies have the potential to affect multiple risk factors simultaneously. Thus, the impact of wellness programs can be far reaching in both the general population (104) and in tactical populations (82). The SHIELD (Safety and Health Improvement: Enhancing Law Enforcement Departments) program for police officers (57) serves as an example. Rather than targeting a single behavior, the SHIELD curriculum sessions, conducted for 30 minutes once a week for 12 weeks, focused on daily exercise and nutrition, sleep, stress, heavy alcohol consumption, and tobacco usage (57). Improvement in all of these measures was noted and generally maintained for 24 months, with the multipronged approach considered instrumental in the longevity of positive outcomes (57).

OPERATING WELLNESS PROGRAMS FOR TACTICAL POPULATIONS

The aforementioned conditions (i.e. obesity, physical inactivity, smoking) have all been found to affect the health and wellness of tactical athletes as well as the tactical organization itself (66). Apart from the impact on mission readiness and workforce maintenance (66), a substantive cost is involved (23). As an example, tobacco use, obesity, and alcohol misuse cost the U.S. Department of Defense around $3 billion in 2006 (23). In terms of force capability, poor health can lead to increased absenteeism (59, 107). For the tactical organization, not only does absenteeism (67) have a substantive financial cost (e.g., overtime costs of replacement staff [38]), but it can also have an impact on mission readiness (66). For example, in 1997 it was estimated that due to the excess body weight of U.S. Air Force personnel, the organization lost more than 28,000 working days (66). More recently, in 2005 the U.S. Department of Defense blamed moderate to heavy smoking for the loss of 386,000 absentee working days (23, 67).

It is thus not surprising that absenteeism is a leading reason behind the implementation of health and wellness programs (80). In the general population, organizational health and wellness programs have been found to have a positive impact on absenteeism and even workplace satisfaction (80). Positive outcomes of health and wellness interventions have been found in tactical populations as well (91). Examples of successful fitness, health, and well-being programs in tactical occupations range from a health and wellness program in a police force improving fitness and decreasing obesity (48) to a program in a firefighter population improving diet and dietary behavior and decreasing weight gain (35). In a military population, a health and wellness program improved weight loss, eating attitudes, well-being, and overall quality of life (12). Health and wellness programs can provide both short-term and long-term positive effects, such as decreased incidences associated with excessive alcohol consumption and decreased rates of cardiovascular disease (23). These successes are encouraging; however, there are potential limitations to implementing wellness programs and enhancing their long-term success that need to be considered.

Limitations and Considerations for Enhancing Long-Term Success

Numerous limitations can occur across occupations that will affect the long-term success of fitness, health, and well-being programs. Key constraints that are often cited are **fiscal constraints** (54), **cultural challenges** (66, 102) and **leadership investment** (54, 102).

Fiscal Constraints

One notable barrier to tactical organizations is funding (38). Not only may budget affect organizational willingness to participate in a health and wellness program (54), but even free programs may come with indirect costs, such as the cost of paying for personnel to attend sessions and train while on duty (54). However, investing in on-duty exercise programs, facilities, and equipment may actually be cost effective in comparison to the costs associated with absenteeism and medical expenses. In U.S. police officers, an in-service heart attack, a leading cause of mortality in this population (94), may cost anywhere from $400,000 to $750,000 (58).

Cultural Challenges

Even though the need to adopt a cultural change to improve health and well-being may be clear (66), cultural change itself may be difficult. For example, the majority of military establishments may have gymnasiums, but a **culture** of regular physical activity is needed if optimal outcomes are to be achieved (66). Another example, discussed earlier in this chapter, is the new kitchen with an indoor garden at a police station left empty while police officers eat fast food lunches at their desks in order to work. Personnel need to see a tangible benefit (more than just improved cholesterol) if they are to be engaged in cultural change (9).

Another potential cultural challenge is fear of change. For example, less fit personnel may not see the benefits of an exercise program if they have served for many years without it (54). Resistance to change may have little to no impact on the effectiveness of a wellness program (54), and further research in this area is needed. However, although culture may be a challenge, it can also help empower a health and wellness program if the culture is already a healthy one (102). For example, the implementation of a tobacco control program in the U.S. military was found to have indirect support from the culture at a base in Guam. The majority of personnel did not smoke, so the peer pressure of the nonsmoking culture aided the tobacco control intervention (102).

Leadership Investment

Multiple health and wellness programs for tactical populations emphasize that senior leadership investment is vital to the program (54, 74, 102, 115). In fact, strong leadership is often considered a leading factor in the success (74, 115) or failure

(54) of health and wellness programs as well as a contributor to sustaining these initiatives (74, 102). In addition, a health and wellness program may demonstrate to personnel that their employer values them (80), and it is not unreasonable to think that the reverse also applies. Furthermore, poor leadership and leadership change (constant movement of leadership to other positions) could result in low dissemination of well-being programs and thus affect the success of the programs (54).

Role of Governing Bodies and the TSAC Facilitator

Some tactical organizations, like the military, may have formal health promotion doctrines (30), but others may not. Although other successful programs cite the need for organizations to implement these programs (91), governing bodies, particularly for tactical occupations, typically require organizations to implement health and well-being programs (72, 92). For example, following a cardiovascular incident in a firefighter, a NIOSH report recommended that fire departments phase in mandatory wellness and fitness programs to reduce risk factors for cardiovascular disease (72).

It is within the organization's best interest to implement and sustain a health and well-being program, given the ability of such programs to help sustain a workforce (102), decrease costs associated with poor health (e.g., treatments, overtime) (38, 102), reduce absenteeism (80), and increase workplace satisfaction (80). One potential means of circumventing cost concerns while advocating for a health and wellness program could be providing examples of cost-saving benefits from other programs—for instance, the firefighter PHLAME wellness program showed a return on investment as high as 4.6 to 1 (55)—and projecting the potential cost-saving benefits of the program for the organization. Given the aforementioned importance of leadership in program success, TSAC Facilitators need to actively engage and garner support from leadership in order to optimize the dissemination, engagement, and longevity of any proposed programs (55, 59, 79).

Where possible, a health and well-being program should target multiple risk factors because, as discussed earlier, targeting multiple behaviors can have the greatest and longest-lasting impact (57). Multiple approaches could be taken, such as the following examples from previous tactical fitness, health, and well-being programs:

- **Awareness programs:** Use health surveillance systems to motivate personnel to make health behavior changes by showing them progressive changes to their health, allowing for earlier intervention (88).

- **Educational sessions:** Educational sessions can range from tobacco cessation and alcohol moderation programs to stress management and improved sleep programs, either as single entities or, preferably, in an integrated fashion (12, 35, 56, 58, 102). These sessions can take place using currently available websites and helplines (102) or on-site (57, 102), with the on-site option assisting in personnel tracking (102). Educational sessions can be provided not only to operational units and qualified personnel but also to new personnel or even during basic training, where new members can learn about maintaining health and wellness in their new occupation (66).

- **Support services:** External experts can aid in the provision of both education and services. Dietitians (12), physical therapists (12, 78), sport trainers (58), and strength and conditioning coaches (78) all can contribute to health and well-being services. Other professional services that may be of value include those provided by counselors (35, 39), psychologists, and social workers (39). In addition, a team-based, small-unit approach can foster support and accountability within groups (56) where personnel can motivate and check on each other when working toward goals (56).

- **Investing in physical activity:** Where possible, there should be a dedicated investment in increasing physical activity. For tactical athletes, time (58) and motivation (94) are critical barriers to participation in physical activity. An on-duty exercise program not only offers a solution (58) but was recommended by the leadership of one police department as the one program that they unanimously thought should be nationally replicated (58). In addition to formal activities, incidental activity (activity associated with activities of daily living) can

be fostered, perhaps even by setting weekly or ongoing goals, such as walking 10 flights of stairs (12) or 10,000 steps per day (57).

Key Point

To increase efficacy as well as cost effectiveness, wellness programs should be multifaceted as well as focus on multiple risk factors. Programs should include education sessions, support services, and investment in physical activity.

A final consideration is the power of success. Word of mouth in particular is a powerful tool, with the success of some individuals having a leading impact (54, 78). Not only is having members become champions of the cause a leading factor in a program's success (54), but implementation in small teams (e.g., a squad) can encourage involvement and motivation by generating subtle peer pressure and friendly competition, which in turn can guide cultural change (58). In addition, small-unit implementation can make tracking and accountability more effective (58) and act as a pilot program that can lead to a larger program (78) once its effectiveness has been proven. One example of a success story is the Physical Conditioning Optimization Review carried out at an Australian military training institution (76), which is summarized in the case study.

CASE STUDY

Optimizing Fitness, Health, and Wellness Through a Dedicated Optimization Program

In 2007, an Australian military training institution implemented a review to improve the physical conditioning of officer cadets. This review was based on the success of a smaller review at another training institution. Its aim was to investigate lines of inquiry that could influence the physical conditioning of new trainees (76). Some of these lines of investigation included the current physical training and sport programs, management of injured trainees, injury surveillance methods, nutritional and dietary habits, and staff health (76). Following the review, 81 recommendations were made, of which 66 were endorsed and scheduled for implementation (76). Recommendations included increasing physical training sessions provided per week to meet national guidelines, improving nutritional timing and intake, creating a coaching development program, and improving rehabilitation processes.

A noted benefit of the program was continual support from commanding staff, which led to the program being extended for four years (2007-2010). During this time, the project expanded to include a dedicated focus on the health and well-being of staff and reserve populations and addressed issues such as maintaining health and fitness during leave and improving screening and assessment processes. By following through with the program, a number of key benefits were identified, including the ability to evaluate the impact of recommendations, adapt findings as required, and explore emerging topics and trends (76).

The measureable outcomes of this project included a noticeable increase in trainee fitness, which ranged from 5% in general trainees to 158% in candidates preparing to commence training (74). In addition, there was a reduction in lost fitness over the four-week Christmas break by up to 102% (meaning some trainee classes gained rather than lost fitness). Injury rates during the most intensive field phase were reduced by 55%, with the number of trainees failing to complete the training reduced by 50%. Rates of return-to-training following injury rates increased by approximately 43%, and medical discharge rates decreased by approximately 86% ($n = 17$). This achievement was recognized with two safety awards and two safety commendations over the project period (76). In addition, this program has been presented internationally and benchmarked in national strategic documents.

CONCLUSION

Tactical athletes can suffer a variety of common illnesses or diseases. Obesity, cardiovascular disease, and cancer are particularly prevalent in this population. Given the working environment of tactical occupations, risk factors associated with these illnesses and diseases can be more prevalent. Risk factors such as physical inactivity, stress, tobacco usage, excessive alcohol consumption, sleep disruptions, and poor nutritional habits can individually have a negative effect on the health and well-being of tactical personnel. Of greater concern, these risk factors are often found in combination or can be attributed to one another, such as cigarette smoking and excessive alcohol consumption due to workplace stress.

Wellness programs can successfully target these risk factors with an evidence-based approach. With an appreciation of the tactical working environment and its structural, managerial, and cultural factors, TSAC Facilitators can develop, implement, and sustain wellness programs that may have greater repercussions than increasing fitness alone.

Key Terms

absenteeism
body mass index (BMI)
cancer
cardiovascular disease
coping behaviors
cultural challenges
culture
diet
diseases
exercise
fatigue
fiscal constraints
fitness
health

illnesses
leadership
lifestyle
metabolic syndromes
nutritional habits
obesity
physical inactivity
sedentary
sleep disruption
stress
syndrome X
well-being
wellness program

Study Questions

1. At times, law enforcement officers must quickly transition from a sedentary, resting condition to a high-intensity activity. This type of activity change increases the risk for diseases of which type?
   a. CNS
   b. thyroid
   c. cardiovascular
   d. pulmonary

2. Which of the following causes the most significant decrease in cognitive function among tactical populations?
   a. sleep disruption
   b. acute stress
   c. tobacco use
   d. nutritional habits

3. Which of the following are the key constraints often cited for limiting long-term success of fitness, health, and well-being programs in tactical athletes?
   a. fiscal constraints, cultural challenges, leadership investment
   b. fiscal constraints, cultural challenges, commitment issues
   c. leadership investment, availability, injuries
   d. injuries, cultural challenges, political issues

4. Which of the following should be included in a wellness program to improve its cost effectiveness?
   a. education sessions
   b. opt-outs for physical activity
   c. injury rehabilitation resources
   d. single-focus behavioral change classes

Chapter 22

Organization and Administration Considerations

John Hofman, Jr., MS, CSCS
Frank A. Palkoska, MS, CSCS

After completing this chapter, you will be able to

- identify the components of designing and organizing a training facility,
- describe the policies and procedures of managing a training facility, and
- describe strategies to create a safe training environment and reduce litigation.

The opinions or assertions contained herein are the private views of the authors and are not to be construed as official or reflecting the views of the Army, Navy, Marine Corps, Air Force, Department of Defense, or the U.S. Government.

The TSAC Facilitator has many roles and responsibilities. One of the most important roles is the design, equipping, management, and maintenance of the training facility. Design includes new construction, renovation, or the repurposing of an existing building or facility. Equipping the training facility requires analysis of the tasks performed by the tactical athlete, effective utilization of new or existing space, number of tactical athletes to be trained, funding availability, and equipment life cycle and replacement. Facility management is critical in training the tactical athlete. Staff duties, staff supervision, facility usage guidelines, risk management, liability, emergency operating procedures, and program data management are essential tasks of a properly managed training facility, as are facility and equipment maintenance. Regular preventive maintenance of the facility and equipment promotes training optimization, mitigates risk, and ensures a safe training environment for all tactical athletes.

DESIGN

Building a new training facility or renovating or repurposing an existing facility is often a multi-year process from concept to program execution. It is estimated that 800 to 1,000 fitness facilities open each year in the United States (20). This multiyear process is divided into four phases: predesign, design, construction, and preoperation. Timelines are established based on the complexity of each phase. For example, location of the training facility in relation to other training facilities, environmental considerations, ease of access from main thoroughfares, traffic patterns and road closures on military installations, and issues related to utilities such as gas, electricity, water, and waste disposal may all influence the training programs that can be developed and implemented.

Predesign Phase

In this phase, the design committee focuses on four critical tasks. These tasks are derived from an understanding of mission- and job-related tasks performed by the tactical population, such as SWAT, Special Operations Forces (SOF),

conventional military, law enforcement, and fire and rescue units.

Key Point

Adding a TSAC Facilitator to the design committee for a training facility for tactical athletes is recommended due to the facilitator's expertise in the subject.

The four critical tasks in the **predesign phase** are the needs analysis, feasibility study, training facility master plan, and selection of an architectural firm (7). The **needs analysis** identifies essential information related to current and future programs used to train tactical athletes. The needs analysis should answer the following questions:

- What is the mission of the training facility (e.g., tactical athlete training, multiuse shared facility)?
- What category of tactical athlete will use the training facility (e.g., SWAT, special operations, conventional military, law enforcement, fire and rescue personnel)?
- What is the number of tactical athletes that the facility can accommodate per training session, per day, and per week (e.g., SWAT team, fire company, infantry platoon)?
- What is the proximity of the training facility to the user (e.g., fire academy, police station, fighter wing, assault amphibian battalion)?
- What programs beyond strength and conditioning will be conducted within the training facility (e.g., physical therapy, rapid reconditioning, performance nutrition, weight management, resiliency, mental skills training)?
- Who is responsible for operational control, life-cycle replacement, and maintenance of the training facility?
- What are the training facility operating hours (operating hours dictate facility supervision and staffing requirements)?
- What is the training facility operating budget (e.g., facility cost per square foot, manpower costs, utility costs, equipment and life-cycle replacement costs)?
- What is the training facility construction timeline?

- When will the training facility be operational?
- What is the projected life span of the training facility?

The second critical task is the **feasibility study**. Once the needs analysis is complete, the design committee conducts a feasibility study that focuses on the facility requirements. It includes such considerations as cost, location, usage, operating hours, and programs offered. A subcomponent of a feasibility study is a **strengths, weaknesses, opportunities, and threats (SWOT) analysis**. The purpose of a SWOT analysis is to identify strengths and weaknesses internal to the organization as well as opportunities and threats that are external to the organization (15).

The third critical task is development of the **master plan** based on the needs analysis, feasibility study, and SWOT analysis. The purpose of the master plan is to capture the project goals and identify the processes that will be used to meet the project goals. The master plan details the mission of the training facility, strength and conditioning equipment, assessment equipment, physical therapy and rehabilitation equipment, office furniture, information technology equipment, classrooms and classroom equipment, facility care and maintenance plan, and equipment life-cycle replacement plan. The master plan may also include details on alternative uses and expansion of the facility. For example, classrooms could be used to support community programs when not in use. Facility expansion is not a requirement within the master plan but should at least be considered. Consideration should not be limited to simply making the training facility larger; the design committee should also think about adjacent outdoor training areas. Examples include running tracks, rope climbs, obstacle courses, tactical training lockers, small arms ranges, and multiuse fields. The TSAC Facilitator must be cognizant of emerging training techniques and equipment within the strength and conditioning profession. These changes over time may affect the current design of the training facility, and failure to plan may lead to failure in execution.

The fourth critical task is selection of an architectural firm and architect. The design committee selects the architectural firm and architect through evaluative and bid processes. The evaluative process should include a review of credentials, referrals, completed work on similar facilities, experience, and projected cost. The bid process is formal and includes all aspects of the evaluation process. Note that although cost may seem like one of the most prominent factors, it is only one of several that should be considered when the design committee is evaluating bids. Other factors to consider include are the number of years the architectural firm has been in business, experience of the architects, ratings from the Better Business Bureau, and findings from interviews with previous clients and site visits to facilities constructed by the firm.

Design Phase

Depending on the complexity of the training facility, the **design phase** could range from 6 to 12 months. The outcome of the design phase is a detailed architectural blueprint, whether digital or hard copy. Blueprints often include the following (7):

- Site map
- General information
- Existing site conditions
- Site demolition plan
- Site grading and erosion plan
- Life safety plan
- Architectural details
- Plumbing
- Fire suppression
- Mechanical (HVAC, ducting, and control schematics)
- Electrical (power, lighting plan, and information technology plan)

Input from each member of the design committee is critical to the success of the design phase. Complex issues that arise during the design phase that cannot be resolved by the committee may require assistance from outside consultants or experts. One method to ensure that the design process adheres to the established timeline is to conduct periodic reviews with the architectural firm and architect. For example, the architectural firm and design committee may agree on design reviews upon 50% completion, 75% completion, and 100% completion. This method allows both the architect and design committee to address issues that arise during the design phase and allows changes to be made to the blueprints. Examples include compliance with the **Americans with Disabilities Act (ADA)** (1); dedicated, standalone electrical circuits to power specialized training equipment; classroom Wi-Fi; air conditioning; large-door access to move equipment in and out of the facility; break rooms; and expansion of equipment storage areas. The design phase should also address specific training areas along with equipment placement and spacing. Federal, state, and municipal health, safety, fire, and building codes must also be addressed. Nothing is more frustrating to the architect and design committee than unintentional oversights related to these codes. Such oversights often lead to blueprint revisions and may delay the start of the construction phase as well as add financial costs.

Construction Phase

The **construction phase** is the longest phase, typically lasting 12 or more months. The exact length depends on the complexity of the building site and facility being constructed (7). The construction phase typically includes the following:

- Continual review of the master plan to ensure all objectives and requirements established in the predesign phase are met

- Monitoring of project deadlines to ensure the project is not delayed or to support project default penalties against the architectural firm or construction contractor

- Periodic planning committee meetings, including key members of the training facility staff, with the architectural firm and construction contractor to ensure proper execution of the design

Preoperation Phase

The **preoperation phase** focuses on staff recruitment, staff training, and facility operations (7). During this phase, **standard operating proce-**dures (SOPs) are reviewed and revised. Staff-related items that should be included in the SOP are staffing requirements, hiring policies, staff onboarding, procedures for staff development and in-service training, continuing education, certification, and staff conduct policies. Items in the SOP related to training facility operations include prescreening procedures, risk management, emergency procedures, security plan, evacuation plan (fire, inclement weather, mass casualty, and active shooter), equipment maintenance plan, equipment inspection schedules, and cleaning and maintenance plan.

The preoperation phase may also include selecting and ordering office furniture and fixtures (desks, chairs, bookcases, conference tables, classroom tables, and chairs), locker room equipment delivery and setup (lockers, benches, and storage cabinets), and training facility equipment delivery and setup (cardio machines, free weights, dumbbells, kettlebells, selectorized resistance machines, racks and platforms, sleds, and ropes). Some manufacturers may offer staff training during equipment delivery. This training often includes equipment operation, preventative maintenance, and cleaning. In some cases, manufacturers use independent shipping companies to transport equipment. The TSAC Facilitator needs to understand who is responsible for delivery, off-loading, movement into the training facility, and setup. If the shipping company is only responsible for delivery, facility staff will have to plan for equipment and personnel to move the equipment into the facility. If the manufacturer does not provide an equipment assembly team, the TSAC Facilitator may be assigned the duty of equipment placement and assembly. This is also an appropriate time to verify new equipment serial numbers and validate warranty information in the SOP. For a new training facility, the TSAC Facilitator should be included in working the training facility punch list. The punch list summarizes facility shortfalls and repairs that the contractor or builder has to complete before the client accepts the new facility. The punch list may include items such as repairing loose flooring and marred walls, painting touch-ups, and keying doors.

Facility Requirements for Military Training Centers

The U.S. DoD establishes mandatory core standards for military physical fitness centers through DoD Directives (DoDD) and DoD Instructions (DoDI). The DoD Physical Fitness Center Program is the combination of Morale, Welfare, and Recreation (MWR) facilities, fitness staff members, and programs on military installations that contribute to cardiorespiratory, muscular strength, muscular endurance, and flexibility conditioning (24).

The DoD core standards for facilities, programs, equipment, and staffing are specified by military installation and facility. Installation physical fitness centers are expected to meet the following standards (24):

- Installation fitness programs will include fitness assessments, group exercise sessions, equipment orientations, and intermural sport activities.

- Installation fitness centers that meet DoD guidelines will operate a minimum of 90 hours per week.

- Installation fitness programs will include incentive, award, and feedback programs.

- Installation fitness facilities will include a minimum of one basketball court for quarter court play, a swimming pool, a running or jogging trail, and courts and fields on the military installation or within a 15-minute commute.

- Separate group exercise space will be established in accordance with American College of Sports Medicine (ACSM) guidelines and standards for facility design.

- Installation fitness facilities will include a full line of fitness equipment that supports cardiorespiratory, muscular strength, muscular endurance, and flexibility training as determined by military service and industry standards.

- Installation fitness programs will include a preventative maintenance and repair service for all fitness equipment.

- Each installation-level military fitness program will have a professionally certified fitness director with a minimum of an undergraduate degree in a health- or fitness-related field or equivalent professional experience.

The core standards for each fitness facility located on a military installation are as follows (24):

- Military fitness facilities will have designated male and female user locker rooms, restrooms, and showers.

- SOPs for military fitness facilities will include an emergency procedure plan and facility staff training.

- Military fitness facility heating, ventilation, and air conditioning (HVAC) systems should be in accordance with ACSM guidelines and standards for facility design.

- Military fitness facility signage should identify risks associated with facility use.

- Each military service specifies a required user-to-staff ratio to ensure safety and provide users with instruction and supervision.

- Each military facility will have a minimum staff of two personnel during operating hours to ensure coverage for emergency response.

- All military facility staff will be certified in first aid, CPR, and AED.

- Each military facility will have a minimum of one staff member in the training area who is professionally certified; who is familiar with facility operation, safety, equipment maintenance, and repair; and whose duty is to coach, mentor, and supervise.

- Each military training facility will have a designated first aid location.

- Each military training facility will have water fountains or dispensers near exercise areas.

As mentioned, DoDD and DoDI establish fitness facility core standards by installation and facility. The DoD uses the **Unified Facilities Criteria (UFC)** to provide a single service design criteria for fitness centers. The UFC system is prescribed by military standard (MIL-STD) 3007 and provides planning, design, construction, sustainment, restoration, and modernization criteria applicable to military departments, defense agencies, and DoD field activities (26). The UFC acknowledges the program differences in the fitness programs and testing requirements of the various military services. Each service then further specifies criteria to meet its needs.

Key Point

In the United States, the DoD establishes core standards for fitness centers and allows each service to add standards to meets its needs.

Army Physical Fitness Facilities

The Army standard and Army standard design criteria are mandatory for military construction. The standards are based on ACSM guidelines, UFC (UFC 4-740-06, TI 800-01, appendix H), and the technical criteria for U.S. Army Physical Fitness Facilities (PFFs) (5).

The Army operates PFFs worldwide. The Army standard for PFFs was revised to reflect changes in Army PRT (physical readiness training), physical fitness, and recreation. The objective is to gain efficiencies through the use of the existing facilities in order to standardize opportunities across the Army. The Army uses the installation population percentages (military, family member, and civilian workforce) to determine the facility size and total gross square footage. The Army classifies its PFFs as extra small, small, medium, and large (5). The Army standard includes square footage allocations for the following modules: fitness, gym, exercise, structured activities, lockers, showers, latrines, and support.

Air Force Fitness Centers

The Air Force Services Facilities Design Guide (AFSFDG) for fitness centers (21) provides planning, design, construction, sustainment, restoration, and modernization criteria for U.S. Air Force fitness centers. The Air Force fitness facility should facilitate the readiness, fitness, and morale of Air Force members by providing effective, efficient, and pleasant spaces for individual and group exercise, unit physical training (PT), team and individual sports, testing, training and education, and necessary support (22).

Air Force fitness facilities provide dedicated areas to meet requirements specified in the design guide, including areas for the following:

- Fitness equipment
- Unit PT and group exercise
- Fitness testing
- Fitness training
- Intramural, extramural, and varsity team and individual sports
- Administration
- Support
- Health and wellness

The Air Force uses base population percentages (military, family member, and civilian workforce) to determine physical fitness and health and wellness center space allowances and total gross square footage. The Air Force space categories for physical fitness and health and wellness centers are small, medium, large, and mega. Air Force Manual 32-1084 provides tables specifying space allowances for these categories (4).

Navy and Marine Corps Fitness Centers

The Navy and Marine Corps fitness centers facilities criteria (FC) acknowledge differences between Navy and Marine Corps fitness and testing programs. For example, the Marine Corps facilities include space for health promotion and high-intensity tactical training (HITT) programs. The criteria (FC 4-740-02N) provide the minimum requirements for evaluating, planning, programming, and designing Navy and Marine Corps fitness centers (25).

Both the Navy (FC 4-740-02N) and Marine Corps use six classifications to determine fitness center size: extra small, small, medium, large, extra large, and jumbo (25). The Marine Corps adjusts the size of its facility space by using installation population figures and a sizing formula for populations above 3,000 service members. This sizing formula adjusts only the free weight, selectorized resistance equipment, and cardiorespiratory exercise areas. Multipurpose activity fields (running tracks, ball fields, multiuse fields, basketball and tennis courts) may be included as part of the fitness center. FC 4-740-02N (25) offers guidance on the use of an interactive planning spreadsheet for both Navy and Marine Corps fitness centers. The interactive planning worksheet provides space determinations (square footage allocations) for the following fitness spaces: lobby and reception, gymnasium, unit PT and group exercise, fitness spaces, structured activities, locker rooms, support areas, health promotion, and HITT.

Special Operations Human Performance Training Centers

U.S. Special Operations Command (SOCOM) establishes training facility guidelines for its Human Performance Program (HPP), and TSAC Facilitators should make sure they are following the most recent guidelines. Within SOCOM, each component is responsible for managing its own mission-specific program. The component mission-specific programs are as follows:

- U.S. Army Special Operations Command (USASOC)—Tactical Human Optimization, Rapid Rehabilitation, and Reconditioning Program (THOR3)
- Air Force Special Operations Command (AFSOC)—AFSOC HPP
- U.S. Naval Special Warfare Command (NAVSPECWARCOM)—Tactical Athlete Program (TAP)
- Marine Corps Forces Special Operations Command (MARSOC)—Performance and Resiliency (PERRES) program

Facility square footage is based on the number of service members assigned to a supported unit (9). Examples of facility sizes are specified here:

- Small—15,000 square feet (1,394 m²) for units with fewer than 1,000 service members
- Medium—30,000 square feet (2,787 m²) for units with 1,000 to 3,000 service members
- Large—40,000 square feet (3,716 m²) for units with more than 3,000 service members

The differences between conventional military training facilities and special operations training facilities are significant. The purpose of special operations training facilities is to support the HPP to increase physical and cognitive performance, promote rapid recovery from injuries sustained in training or combat, and lengthen the life cycle of service members within special operations (9). These training facilities support the following:

- Physical performance development through training areas for strength, endurance, energy systems, mobility, speed, agility, power, balance, and stability
- Cognitive enhancement through enhanced observation, mental toughness, intellectual ability, creativity, and cultural adaptability training
- Rapid recovery and reconditioning through dedicated health care providers, strength and conditioning specialists, and mental skills specialists
- Lengthening the service member's life cycle through occupational health and safety programs focused on surveillance, advanced training, and protective equipment

A special operations training facility with a small footprint provides the following dedicated areas:

- Office space
- Classroom
- Locker room
- Sports medicine
- Combatives
- Performance
- Hydrotherapy, rehabilitation, and recovery
- Cardio and energy system development
- Speed and agility turf

A special operations training facility with a large footprint provides the following dedicated areas:

- Office space
- Classroom
- Locker room
- Sports medicine
- Combatives
- Research laboratory
- Hydrotherapy, rehabilitation, and recovery
- Performance laboratory
- Cardio and energy system development
- Speed/agility turf

Equipment Requirements

A key responsibility of a TSAC Facilitator is to evaluate and provide recommendations for selecting equipment for the training facility. The evaluation and selection process begins with a thorough review of the needs analysis. There are three phases when selecting exercise equipment: equipment functional criteria development, equipment specifications and effectiveness, and manufacturer business practices evaluation (16).

The TSAC Facilitator should also look at other key planning factors that may assist in the decision-making process (10). Examples include a scaled floor plan, outdoor scaled plan (if equipment is placed outdoors), equipment priority list, current and future budget, and expansion plan. Blueprints are also helpful and provide room dimensions, hallway and corridor locations (traffic flow), electrical outlets, water fountains, and emergency exits.

A scaled floor plan specifies the square footage available by room or area. This is vital when selecting equipment for cardiorespiratory, free weight, Olympic lift, selectorized resistance machine, circuit, bodyweight exercise, stretching, rehabilitation, climbing wall, and assessment areas. A scaled floor plan will also assist with equipment placement, ensure proper traffic flow, and provide safe access between equipment. The same emphasis must be placed on outdoor equipment requirements. Examples of outdoor equipment include training lockers; rope climbs; pegboards; pull-up, dip, and climbing bars; rock-climbing walls; sleds; and obstacles.

The **equipment priority list** is a key planning factor. The needs analysis, budget, and expansion plan for the training facility will affect what is included in the equipment priority list. The equipment priority list specifies equipment type, quantity, manufacturer, warranty, estimated life cycle, and cost. The equipment priority list can be used in the decision-making process when TSAC Facilitator encounters space, budget, or expansion constraints or when additional funding is available.

Conventional Military Training Facilities

The U.S. DoD Physical Fitness Center Program, DoDI, and UFC for fitness centers establish mandatory standards for equipping military physical fitness centers (26). The Air Force, Army, Navy, and Marine Corps establish minimum equipment requirements based on training facility size. Equipment is categorized by the component of fitness trained and includes cardiorespiratory equipment, selectorized resistance training equipment, free weight equipment, fitness assessment equipment (service dependent), functional training equipment, and structured activity equipment.

- The standard line of cardiorespiratory training equipment consists of treadmills, rowers, elliptical machines, cycle ergometers (recumbent, upright, and arm), stair-climbers, Tread-Climbers, and climbing and ladder machines.

- The standard line of selectorized resistance equipment includes leg press; leg curl; leg extension; standing and seated leg abduction; standing and seated leg adduction; standing and seated calf raise; bench press; overhead press; cable lat pulldown; compound row; pec deck or chest fly; arm curl; triceps press; abdominal crunch; back extension; weight-assisted dip; cable crossover; weight-assisted pull-up, chin-up, and dip; and high and low pull machines.

- The standard line of free weight equipment includes a power rack; a Smith machine; a pull-up and dip combination; Olympic, Olympic incline, and Olympic decline benches; an adjustable incline; an incline leg press; a preacher curl bench; a calf raise machine; one set of rubber- or vinyl-coated dumbbells from 5 to 100 pounds (2-45 kg); one set of rubber- or vinyl-coated dumbbells from 5 to 50 pounds (2-23 kg); twin-tier dumbbell racks; an E-Z curl bar; 5-foot (152 cm) and 7-foot (213 cm) Olympic bars; Olympic weight plates up to 45 pounds (20 kg); and one weight tree per two benches.

- Fitness assessment equipment does not have a standard line. Each service uses different assessments. Fitness assessment equipment may include physician scales with height measurement capability, circumference tape measures, sit-and-reach boxes, and functional movement screen kits.

- Functional training equipment is also not defined by a standard line. Each service determines its own equipment list.

See tables 22.1 through 22.5 near the end of the chapter for examples of equipment lists, and see figures 22.1 and 22.2 for examples of Marine Corps and U.S. Army Physical Fitness School (USAPFS) floor plans.

Structured activity equipment is also not defined by a standard line. Each service determines its equipment list. Structured activity equipment includes the following:

- Cycle ergometers (spinning classes)
- Combatives training equipment
- Stretching equipment and mats (yoga)
- Climbing equipment (climbing walls)
- Rackets, balls, and eye protection (racquetball and squash)

Special Operations Training Facilities

SOCOM has established guidelines (baselines) for training facility equipment to support its HPP.

Each service is allowed to tailor its equipment to its mission and program needs. Tables 22.6 through 22.11, found near the end of the chapter, provide examples of equipment for small training facilities (9).

Law Enforcement and Conventional Fire and Rescue Training Facilities

The International Association of Chiefs of Police (IACP) Police Facility Planning Guidelines provide a reference for law enforcement executives, administrators, and consultants in constructing a new facility, renovating an existing facility, or adapting another type of facility to police purposes (8). Municipalities must be in compliance with the National Incident Management System (NIMS) standards for coordinated communication and response in order to receive federal funding.

Because of modern-day issues that require mutual aid—such as active shootings, terrorism,

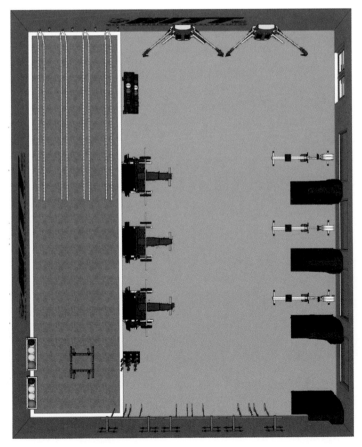

Figure 22.1 Sample layout for a 2,000-square-foot (186 m²) HITT center. This type of facility is required only by the Marine Corps.

Reprinted from Navy and Marine Corps Fitness Centers Facilities Criteria (FC), FC 4-740-02N, Appendix C, page 119.

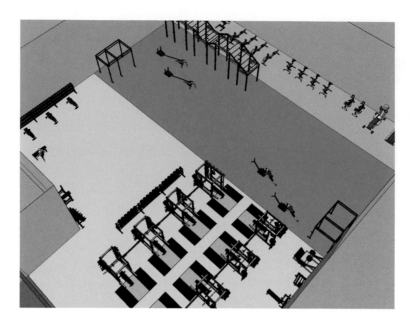

Figure 22.2   USAPFS facility rendering.

Reprinted from Sorinex USAPFS Equipment Rendering ICW US Army Sorinex Equipment Quote No. 4985, Customer No. C01047, November 21, 2014, pages 1-4.

and natural disasters—police, fire and rescue, and other first responders must train together to respond to various situations. Facility design focus is on building multiuse facilities to accommodate joint training of police and fire agencies. Public safety training centers provide integrated training centers for law enforcement, fire and rescue, and emergency personnel. Both police and fire academies may operate out of this training center, and therefore it requires more space and equipment. Following are examples of training facility sizes:

- Large—15,000 square feet (1,394 m²) for academies with more than 60 members
- Medium—10,000 square feet (929 m²) for academies with 35 to 60 members
- Small—5,000 square feet (465 m²) for academies with 20 to 34 members
- Smallest—2,750 square feet (255 m²) for academies with 19 or fewer members

The size of fitness centers within fire and rescue is determined by how many people will be occupying the fire station. The classifications are 1 engine (2-5 people); 1 engine and 1 medic (4-8 people); and 1 engine, 1 apparatus, and 1 medic (6-15 people).

The population of public safety training centers is based on enrollment in the local community college and the hiring needs of the departments. Public safety training centers may provide dedicated areas to meet specific requirements, including the following:

- Administrative offices
- Fitness equipment
- Medical assessment
- Fitness assessment
- Fitness training
- Candidate evaluation
- Offices for medical personnel (physician, registered dietitian)
- Offices for fitness staff, including the TSAC Facilitator
- Community outreach programs such as Police Athletic League (PAL)

The NFPA's 1500 series of standards provides recommendations on health and safety issues when designing a fire station (11). All fire stations in the United States must adhere to the following:

- All police and fire department facilities are considered public buildings and must comply with the ADA (1).

- All fire department facilities must comply with all legally applicable health, safety, building, and fire code requirements (11).

- Fire departments must provide facilities with disinfecting, cleaning, and storage in accordance with *NFPA 1581: Standard on Fire Department Infection Control Program* (12).

- The fire department must prevent exposure of firefighters to and contamination of living and sleeping areas with exhaust emissions (11).

Key Point

All tactical athlete training centers (i.e., conventional military, special operations, police, firefighter, emergency services) must comply with the American with Disabilities Act (ADA).

The following design components should be considered when developing a strength and conditioning facility for a fire or police station (11):

- Location: ground floor

- Ceiling height: 12 to 14 feet (4-5 m) of clearance from low-hanging items, especially within a self-contained power area.

- Flooring: low-pile carpet or rubberized flooring

- Environmental factors: lighting, temperature, air circulation (12-15 exchanges per hour), appropriate sounds levels to hear emergency tones and verbal communication (not to exceed 90 dB).

- Mirrors: should be at least 20 inches (51 cm) off the floor

- Pathway: 36-inch-wide (91 cm) unobstructed pathway that bisects the facility is required by federal law (1)

- Electrical: grounded 110 V or 220 V

- Policies and procedures: guidelines should be effectively and clearly communicated with all members

It is important to examine the types and volume of space rather than just raw square footage when evaluating the needs or considering the adaptive reuse of an existing facility. See tables 22.12 and 22.13 near the end of the chapter for more details.

LAYOUT AND ORGANIZATION

Equipment placement and spacing in a new or recently renovated training facility can be a daunting task. Users of the training facility rarely think about how strength and conditioning equipment is placed or spaced. Equipment placement and spacing is as much a science as it is an art. The science involves not only an understanding of how the equipment is used to optimize human performance but also mathematical calculations for fitting large equipment into defined spaces. This all must be accomplished while adhering to nationally recognized safety standards. The art involves meeting all needs defined in the needs analysis and correctly placing and spacing equipment to ensure efficient and safe training of all tactical athletes.

Nearly all conventional military fitness facilities and large metropolitan law enforcement, fire and rescue, and emergency service departments place strength and conditioning equipment in defined activity areas. **Defined activity areas** are designed around the component of fitness to be trained (e.g., muscular strength, muscular endurance, aerobic capacity, anaerobic power, agility, speed, flexibility, body composition). Defined activity areas include dedicated space for the following:

- Aerobic training machines

- Resistance training machines (circuit training)

- Free weights

- Powerlifting

- Olympic lifting

- Stretching and flexibility improvement

- Warm-ups and cool-downs

- Bodyweight exercise

- Speed and agility

- Structured activities (spinning, yoga, rock climbing)

Guidelines for Placing Equipment

Science, technology, and innovation drive the development of strength and conditioning equipment. Equipment dimensions, shape, power requirements, and relationship to other pieces of equipment; recommended safety areas around the equipment; and traffic flow must all be considered when placing equipment in the facility. Efficiency in training and safety of the tactical athlete and strength and conditioning staff are key aspects of equipment placement and spacing. Following are guidelines for placing and spacing equipment (7):

- Power exercises that require the use of a rack or spotter should not be placed near high-traffic areas (e.g., entrances and exits, water fountains, hallways), windows, and mirrors in order to prevent damage to the facility and to avoid contact with other tactical athletes or strength and conditioning staff.

- Tall strength training machines and equipment (e.g., rack, Smith machine, cable crossover, stand-alone lat pulldown, horizontal ladder or monkey bars) should be placed along walls in accordance with safety and standoff guidelines. When applicable, this equipment should be secured to the floor or wall according to manufacturer guidelines. Tall aerobic training machines (e.g., treadmills, arm ergometers, steppers, ladders, climbers, elliptical trainers) should be placed along walls in accordance with safety and standoff guidelines. Refer to manufacturer installation and safety recommendations when placing and spacing equipment.

- Dumbbells and kettlebells should be placed in single- or double-tier racks designed for this purpose. Dumbbell and kettlebell racks are normally placed along walls in defined areas or may be used to divide activity areas in large rooms.

- Weight trees can be placed along walls or adjacent to plate-loaded machines or equipment. If placed near plate-loaded machines or equipment, a minimum distance of 3 feet (91 cm) should be maintained.

- In free weight areas, a distance of 3 feet (91 cm) should be maintained between bar ends or dumbbells. The intent is to avoid interference between lifters and spotters.

- The bench press, incline bench press, or seated military press requires an area of 90 to 110 square feet (8-10 m²). The squat requires an area of 110 to 130 square feet (10-12 m²). The deadlift is normally performed on a platform. Size of the training area often dictates the platform size; 8 feet (244 cm) by 12 feet (366 cm) is optimal and accommodates the rack. A 4-foot (122 cm) perimeter is recommended on all sides. The total area equates to 144 square feet (13 m²).

- A 4-foot (122 cm) perimeter should be maintained around Olympic platforms.

- The minimum distance between equipment and mirrors is 6 inches (15 cm). Mirrors should be placed a minimum of 20 inches (51 cm) above the floor to alleviate contact with weight plates. If possible, increase this distance to improve ease of supervision, maintenance, and cleaning.

- Selectorized resistance (circuit) training machines are generally placed in order from large muscle group to small muscle group. Another accepted method is to place machines alternating muscle groups (e.g., chest and back, shoulders and lats).

- Multistation machines are often combined with single-station machines. The minimum distance between machines is 3 feet (91 cm). If room permits, increase the distance between machines.

- **Self-contained power areas (SCPAs)** are becoming popular. They conserve floor space, allow multiple users, improve supervision, and permit several exercises to be conducted per rack (10). Typically, each rack is placed on a thick rubber area that is 8 by 14 feet (244 by 427 cm). Distance between racks should be 3 to 4 feet (91-122 cm) or more if space allows. This allows plate removal and storage on or off the rack or adjacent weight trees without interfering with lifters in the adjacent rack. If multiple racks are used, create a center pathway with racks on each side to promote safety and improve supervision.

- Reconditioning equipment such as antigravity treadmills should be on a dedicated electrical circuit in an area that allows for close supervision. A minimum perimeter of 3 feet (91 cm) should be maintained.

- A minimum perimeter of 3 feet (91 cm) should be maintained around aerobic training equipment. This allows for maintenance, supervision, cleaning, and general safety.

- Cycle ergometers and steppers require an area that is 4 feet by 6 feet (122 by 183 cm), or 24 square feet (2.2 m²). Rowers require 4 feet by 10 feet (122 by 305 cm), or 40 square feet (3.7 m²). Treadmills require an area 5.5 feet by 8 feet (168 by 244 cm), or 45 square feet (4.2 m²).

- An area of 7 feet by 7 feet (213 by 213 cm), or 49 square feet (4.6 m²), is recommended for an individual warm-up and cool-down or stretching area. If forward, backward, or lateral movement is used, additional area is required. Many training facilities use turf for speed, agility, and power training. Turf is an excellent multipurpose surface and can also be used for warm-up, cool-down, and stretching activities.

- Traffic flow within the training facility is key to training efficiency, supervision, and safety.

The minimum width of walkways around the perimeter or through the training facility is 3 feet (91 cm). Pathways (traffic flow) need to be in accordance with local, state, and federal code. Strength and conditioning equipment should not be placed in walkways. Entrance, exit, lavatory, and locker room doors should not open into walkways or equipment areas. If possible, a walkway should bisect defined training areas in order to provide unobstructed movement between defined training areas. See table 22.14 near the end of the chapter to assist in determining equipment space requirements, and see figures 22.3 and 22.4 for examples of equipment placement.

POLICIES AND PROCEDURES

Optimizing the performance of tactical athletes requires the right facility, the right equipment, and the right strength and conditioning staff. Exercise science provides the foundation, technology provides the innovation, and training provides the mechanism for success. The TSAC Facilitator must stay in tune with changes in the strength and conditioning field and understand the importance of maintaining relevancy and certification within the profession when addressing

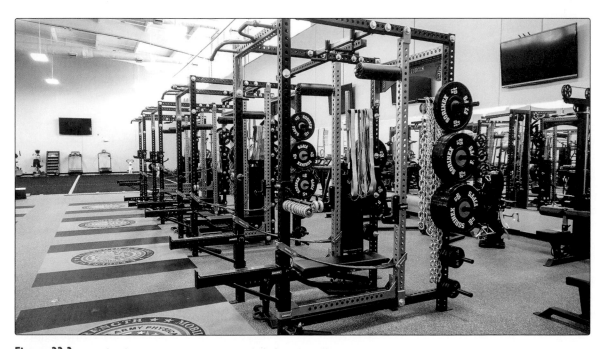

Figure 22.3 Rack placement, spacing, and defined walkways.

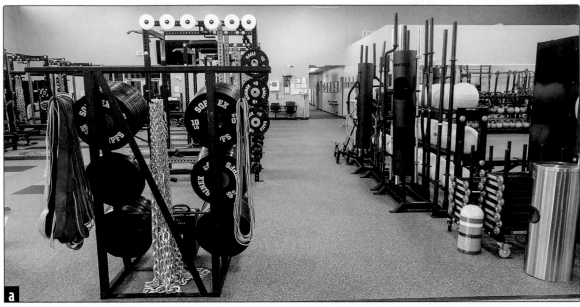

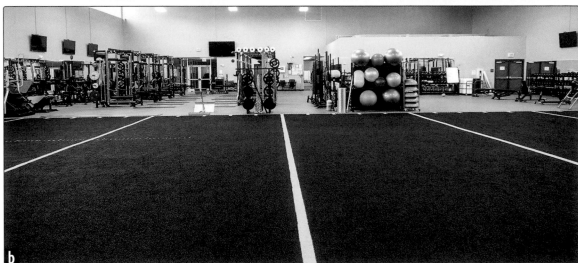

Figure 22.4 *(a)* A walkway should bisect defined training areas; *(b)* turf provides an excellent warm-up and cool-down area.

training center policies and procedures. Defining and clearly communicating the duties and responsibilities of the strength and conditioning staff is key to the efficient operation, maintenance, and effectiveness of the training programs executed in the facility. Policy and procedures should be developed in coordination with labor union and senior administration that reflect a proactive program to sustain longevity. The following resources are available to the TSAC Facilitator to help establish these policies:

- *NFPA 1582: Standard on Comprehensive Occupational Medical Program for Fire Departments*

provides guidelines for medical testing and screening, which simplifies the development of this component. All fitness screenings and medical assessments should be nonpunitive yet mandatory. The purpose of these assessments is to perform health screening, not primary care (13).

- *NFPA 1583: Standard on Health-Related Fitness Programs for Fire Department Members* provides the minimum requirements for the development, implementation, and management of a health-related fitness program (HRFP) (14). It is not intended to establish physical performance criteria, and it is non-punitive.

- Peace Officer Standards and Training (POST) establishes the educational minimum requirements for law enforcement in certain regions across the country. For example, California POST Guidelines for Student Safety in Certified Courses outline the basic guidelines for physical fitness within law enforcement (18).

Staffing Duties and Responsibilities at a Conventional Military Training Facility

The DoD establishes policy, assigns responsibilities, and prescribes procedures for the staffing of conventional military (Air Force, Army, Navy, Marine Corps) physical fitness training centers (23). DoD policy directs that each service establish MWR programs. MWR categorizes physical fitness as one of several programs used to support the accomplishment of the military mission. DoD policy specifies that the service's military physical fitness training centers will be staffed primarily by MWR civilian employees. At times, military personnel serve as staff at military physical fitness training centers in accordance with DoD and service policy. The number of strength and conditioning personnel per physical fitness training center is derived from the mission and size of the facility. Following are examples of positions and job descriptions commonly found at physical fitness training centers on military installations:

- **Fitness director:** This position has oversight of the physical fitness, sport, and aquatic programs. The fitness director works for the MWR director, deputy MWR director, or recreation director. The position requires a degree in fitness or health or equivalent experience. The fitness director should be trained and have working experience in fitness, sport management, and aquatics. Depending on the military service, this position may also be referred to as the *athletic director*.

- **Fitness coordinator:** This position is directly responsible for the physical fitness program on the installation. The fitness coordinator works for the fitness director. The position requires a degree in fitness or health or equivalent experience. The fitness coordinator generally works out of the physical fitness training center and is responsible for the oversight and execution of training programs, equipment, and staff within the facility. Depending on the military service, this position may also be referred to as the *fitness center manager* or *fitness director*.

- **Sports coordinator:** This position is responsible for adult team and individual sports on the installation. The sports coordinator works for the fitness director and must have a degree in sport management or equivalent relevant experience. The sports coordinator plans and programs team and individual sporting events and sport clinics; schedules sport officials; and, when directed, provides assistance to youth sport programs.

- **Aquatics coordinator:** This position is responsible for aquatic programs and pool complexes at the installation. The aquatics coordinator works for the fitness director and must have a degree or related experience in aquatic management. The aquatics coordinator supervises pool operations, aquatic programming, and staff training.

- **Fitness facility coordinator:** This position is responsible for fitness, sport, and aquatic facility operations. The fitness facility coordinator works for the fitness director. This position supervises service staff and is responsible for facility operations. Responsibilities include equipment procurement, equipment accountability, supply purchases, facility maintenance work orders, staff time cards, facility usage counts, and other administrative requirements specified by the fitness director. The facility coordinator allows other facility staff (fitness coordinator, sports coordinator, aquatics coordinator, and fitness specialist) to direct their efforts toward training and programming.

- **Fitness specialist:** This position is responsible for physical fitness training and education on the installation. The fitness specialist works in the fitness facility under the fitness director or fitness coordinator. The position requires a personal trainer certification or degree in fitness or health. The fitness specialist provides customer-focused training recommendations and programming and corrects unsafe training practices.

- **Fitness specialist or group exercise instructor:** This position is responsible for teaching a variety of group exercise classes (e.g., yoga, step, spinning). The fitness specialist works for the fitness director or fitness coordinator. The position requires a personal trainer certification or certification for specialized instruction. This position is often contracted at the installation.

- **Fitness assistant:** This position assists the fitness specialist and group exercise instructor with fitness orientations and corrects unsafe training practices on the facility floor. This position also assists with intramural sport programs and assists with facility maintenance. The position requires on-the-job training in fitness principles and management. The fitness assistant works for the fitness coordinator or sports coordinator.

- **Custodial and outdoor maintenance staff:** These positions maintain and clean indoor and outdoor fitness facilities and complexes. Each installation handles these services in accordance with installation guidelines and operating procedures. Staff requirements may be handled in-house, by contract, or a combination of both. The number of facilities (gyms, pools, sport complexes) and size of installation dictate staffing requirements.

In addition to education and professional certification requirements, fitness training center staffs have additional training and certification requirements specified by each service. Examples include first aid, CPR, basic life support (BLS), AED, handling of potentially hazardous materials (bodily fluids, bloodborne pathogens), Water Safety Instructor (WSI), advanced life saving (ALS), and Certified Pool/Spa Operator (CPO). Within law enforcement and fire and rescue, additional educational and professional training certifications include swift water rescue, hazmat, rescue operations, urban search and rescue (USAR), SWAT, Special Operations Response Team (SORT), mounted units, and K9.

Staffing Duties and Responsibilities at a Special Operations Training Facility

Unlike the conventional military fitness programs and facilities, special operations training programs and facilities initially leveraged an athletic and sports medicine framework with customizations for Special Operations Forces (SOF) and mission-specific requirements. Staffing focuses on three functional areas of expertise: optimizing human performance, rehabilitation, and reconditioning (9). In order to meet program objectives, SOCOM has determined a requirement for expertise in the following areas: strength and conditioning, physical therapy, athletic training, performance nutrition, mental skills enhancement, and resiliency. The SOCOM HPP determines staffing requirements with input from the units. Specific staffing duties and responsibilities are based on the needs of the HPP and the units' mission-specific requirements. The HPP includes the following staff positions:

- **Human performance program coordinator or manager:** This position plans, designs, and implements the strength and conditioning and related programs. The focus is on improving the functional capacity, mitigating the injury risk, and extending the operational life cycle of SOF.

- **Rehabilitation coordinator or manager:** This position manages a full spectrum of screening, diagnostic, and sports medicine services. Along with strength and conditioning professionals, physical therapists, and athletic trainers, the position focuses on rapid rehabilitation and reconditioning of SOF.

- **Physical therapist:** This position applies a full spectrum of screening, diagnostic, and professional physical therapy services. Along with strength and conditioning professionals and athletic trainers, physical therapists focus on rapid rehabilitation and reconditioning of SOF.

- **Strength and conditioning specialist:** This position plans, designs, and implements strength and conditioning programs for SOF. The strength and conditioning specialist also assists the sports medicine staff with the assessment, rehabilitation, and reconditioning of injured SOF.

- **Performance dietitian:** This position is responsible for delivering a comprehensive performance nutrition program designed to support SOF. The focus is on improving nutrition and body composition for optimal performance, rehabilitation, and reconditioning.

- **Athletic trainer:** This position collaborates closely with all HPP staff members. The athletic trainer focuses on treatment of acute and chronic medical conditions involving injuries, functional limitations, and disabilities. Athletic trainers provide an elite level of care, education, and training to SOF who require rehabilitation, reconditioning, or performance improvement.

- **Mental skills specialist:** This position is responsible for conducting SOF-specific mental skills training, which includes key mental components such as focus and concentration, emotional regulation, imagery, pattern recognition and spatial reasoning, situation awareness, and high-speed decision making in an effort to help SOF improve their performance in a wide range of combat skills.

Common Rules for Using the Facility

Training facility guidelines and policies are established to provide tactical athletes and facility staff with SOPs and standards of conduct when using the training facility. Conventional military and special operations facility guidelines and policies are governed by DoDD and DoDI and are typically service specific. Law enforcement, fire and rescue, and emergency services facility guidelines and policies are based on state or municipal statutes and operating procedures. SOPs typically specify operating procedures in order to maintain appropriate order, discipline, and conduct. Facility SOPs encompass topics such as the following:

- Facility hours of operation
- Facility scheduling (mass training or instruction)
- Facility staff (organizational chart)
- Facility floor plan

- Facility orientation
- Facility usage age requirements (military facilities)
- Sign-in or log-in procedures
- Prescreening and clearance procedures
- Personal conduct (etiquette, language, respect, cell phone and personal device usage)
- Training attire (appropriate nonsuggestive clothing, closed-toe footwear)
- New equipment training
- Locker room procedures (storage of personal belongings)
- Equipment safety (spotters, collars, racks, bumper plates, platforms)
- Equipment storage and cleaning
- Outdoor equipment usage
- Food, drink, and supplementation in the facility
- Reporting unsafe acts
- Revocation of facility privileges
- Accident, injury, and incident reporting procedures
- Facility evacuation plan (fire, inclement weather, active shooter, designated accountability rally point)
- AED and first aid kit locations
- Hazardous waste procedures, disposal of blood-soaked towels or clothing, and cleanup of bloodborne pathogens
- Emergency phone numbers
- Visitor procedures

Recommended Insurance Coverage

Conventional military and SOF training facility staff, unlike civilian personal trainers or strength and conditioning specialists, fall under federal guidelines related to liability and indemnification. Law enforcement, fire and rescue, and emergency service personnel often work for municipalities or states that self-insure and provide liability coverage to their employees. However, it is always prudent for facility staff members to confirm that they are covered for **liability** and **indemnification**.

This is especially important for contract employees. If TSAC Facilitators or facility staff members are not covered by their employer, they must purchase personal liability and indemnification insurance to protect against injury and wrongful death lawsuits. Some certifying organizations such as the NSCA provide personal liability and indemnification insurance coverage.

It is important to research the types of coverage. Policies that provide legal defense and payment for any judgment or settlement that may arise from legal action within the limits of the policy are preferred. It is critical to understand the dollar amount paid per incident along with the aggregate limit within a designated policy. The aggregate limit is the maximum dollar amount the insurer will pay to settle a claim within a given period of time, typically one year. An example is $1,000,000 per incident and $3,000,000 aggregate limit. TSAC Facilitators should contact multiple companies for coverage estimates based on where in the country they are employed. Coverage costs vary by state and region.

Procedures for Responding to Emergencies

Conventional military and SOF training facilities have service-specific policies and procedures for responding to emergencies. Law enforcement, fire and rescue, and emergency services have emergency response protocols (policies and procedures) based on municipal, state, and federal laws. The training facility SOP provides guidance, direction, and requirements associated with the execution of facility emergency procedures. Not all emergency situations can be prevented, but that does not mean a plan of action should not be in place for when they do occur. The types of emergencies to plan for are accident and injury, medical emergency, fire, mass casualty, inclement weather, and active shooter. All facility staff members and TSAC Facilitators must be familiar with emergency policies and procedures, understand their responsibilities and duties, and receive emergency response training on a quarterly basis. Two resources to use when developing emergency procedures are the NSCA Strength and Conditioning Professional Standards and Guidelines

(19) and *ACSM's Health/Fitness Facility Standards and Guidelines* (17).

Fitness facilities should have written emergency policies and procedures that are reviewed and practiced on a regular basis (2). Facility emergency response policies and procedures should include the following:

- Preparation for any major emergency situation that may occur. Among these situations are medical emergencies that are reasonably foreseeable with participation in moderate or intense exercise. These include emergencies related to pulmonary disease, such as asthma; metabolic syndrome with conditions that include high blood pressure, high blood sugar, or excessive body fat around the waist; myocardial infarction; sudden cardiac arrest; stroke; exertional heat illness; and orthopedic injuries.

- Rehearsals to deal with emergencies that involve fire, mass casualties, inclement weather, and active shooters, which are less predictable than medical emergencies. Municipalities and military installations typically conduct exercises to rehearse for such emergencies and train military personnel, family members, DoD civilian employees, law enforcement officers, fire and rescue personnel, and emergency response personnel.

- SOPs that provide detailed instructions on how each emergency situation will be handled and the roles that should be played by first, second, and third responders to an emergency.

- Emergency equipment identification through signage and a schematic identifying locations in the facility.

- Contact information for law enforcement, fire and rescue, and EMS. This information must be easily accessible during emergency situations. During an emergency situation, dispatchers will ask for specific information. The TSAC Facilitator should be prepared to provide nature of the emergency, facility address, building and room numbers, and most favorable way for EMS to access the facility.

- Full documentation of the policies and procedures that address staff training and emergency instruction. Policies and procedures should be reviewed on a regular basis. This documentation should include a list of staff professional and BLS certifications and training.

- Emergency and fire evacuation plans. These plans should be posted at multiple locations in the facility. Evacuation plans must include clearly identified staff and tactical athlete assembly and accountability points.
- Emergency drills, including medical, fire, mass casualty, inclement weather, and active shooter drills. These should be scheduled according to military installation, municipal, state, or federal requirements and policies.
- Clearly marked locations of first aid kits and AEDs.
- A directory that identifies the location of key facility personnel, including facility director or manager, strength and conditioning specialist, fitness coordinator, physical therapist, and athletic trainer.

Facilities should have a safety audit that routinely inspects all areas of the facility to reduce or eliminate hazards that may cause injury. The safety audit should also address results of fire, medical emergency, inclement weather, mass casualty, and active shooter drills.

Key Point

Rehearsals that simulate specific emergency situations provide realistic training for both staff and facility users.

Procedures for Recording Injuries in the Facility

Conventional military and SOF training facilities have service-specific regulations or instructions that specify policies and procedures for accident, injury, and incident reporting. Law enforcement, fire and rescue, and emergency services have protocols (policies and procedures) based on municipal, state, and federal laws that specify how accidents, injuries, and incidents should be reported. The facility SOP should clearly identify who is responsible for creating the report; who is

responsible for capturing all information related to the accident, injury, or incident; and what offices and agencies the report is to be filed with. Before a reporting format is adopted, the facility director or manager should obtain a legal review to ensure the report does not violate military regulations or instructions or municipal, state, or federal laws. As part of the risk management process, the facility director or manager, specified facility staff, and TSAC Facilitator should conduct a thorough review of the accident, injury, or incident report. This process is useful and can identify lessons learned that may assist in modifying or revising facility policies and procedures. The TSAC Facilitator and facility staff must be aware that such reports contain **personally identifiable information (PII)**. PII must be protected from unauthorized access or use at all times. Reports should contain the following information (17):

- Type of report (accident, injury, incident)
- Location (name of facility and room or area where the event occurred)
- Date and time
- Name of the individual
- Address of the individual
- Home or cell phone number
- Unit or place of employment
- Work phone number
- Supervisor's name and phone number
- Facility staff present when the event occurred
- Tactical athletes or others who witnessed the event
- Summary of the event, including the type, severity, and mechanism of the accident, injury, or incident
- Whether facility staff provided first aid (specify actions taken)
- 911 activation and whether law enforcement, fire and rescue, or emergency services responded
- Whether the individual was transported to a medical treatment facility (MTF) or hospital; if so, record the name, address, and phone number of the MTF or hospital

- Whether the event meets the criteria for a serious incident report; if so, follow reporting procedures specified in the facility SOP
- Report routing

Key Point

To assist in preventing identity theft, ensure that personally identifiable information (PII) is protected against unauthorized access.

Policies for Handling Evaluative and Performance Data Generated From Programs

Conventional military training facilities have DoD and service-specific policies and procedures for handling PII. Likewise, many states and municipalities also have policies for handling the collection, storage, and reporting criteria of evaluative and performance data. SOF HPPs follow SOCOM-established policies and procedures for the collection and storage of evaluative and performance data. Law enforcement, fire and rescue, and emergency services have protocols based on municipal, state, and federal laws that specify how performance and evaluative data will be collected, stored, and reported. Evaluative and performance data are considered sensitive information because they often include PII. As with all PII, this information must be protected from unauthorized access at all times. Specific policies and procedures should identify who is authorized to collect, handle, store, and report evaluative and performance data. If this information is stored on computers, servers, or external drives, it should be encrypted. If it is stored as a hard copy, it should be kept in a locked container according to agency security policies. Access to this information should be granted only to those individuals who are authorized.

SAFE TRAINING ENVIRONMENT

A high-quality facility always provides a safe environment for its users. It is the responsibility of the TSAC Facilitator and facility staff to create this safe training environment by applying foresight, risk assessment, and preparation. The TSAC Facilita-

tor should be able to respond to any reasonable emergency situation. Managing risk includes identifying dangers and implementing effective policies, procedures, and precautions before the start of a strength and conditioning program. Information that could lead to a potential risk should be disclosed before the start of any strength and conditioning program. Facilities must develop processes to identify and address these factors.

Preparticipation Screening Requirements

A physical examination is important for all members prior to participating in strength and conditioning programs. The TSAC Facilitator should offer a general **preactivity screening** (e.g., Par-Q) or specific preactivity screening tool (e.g., health risk appraisal, health history questionnaire) to all new and current members. This should include a comprehensive health and immunization history. These documents can be found in the NSCA's *Essentials of Strength Training and Conditioning, Fourth Edition.*

All preactivity screening procedures should be quick, simple, and easy to perform; the process should encourage acceptance of the opportunity to participate in the screening. General preactivity screening tools (e.g., Par-Q) help new members determine their level of risk (e.g., low, moderate, high). Members who have been identified (either by preactivity screening or self-disclosure) as having cardiovascular, metabolic, or pulmonary disease or symptoms or any other potentially serious medical concern (e.g., orthopedic problems) and who subsequently fail to consult with a qualified health care professional should be permitted to sign a waiver or release that clearly states they assume the risk and release of liability if they participate in a facility's offerings. If such members refuse to sign a waiver or release, they should be excluded from participation to the extent permitted by law. The TSAC Facilitator should maintain all documents within a locked area in the facility, such as a secure filing cabinet, for at least one year. If the TSAC Facilitator becomes aware that a member has a known cardiovascular, metabolic, or pulmonary disease, two or more major risk factors for cardiovascular disease, or any other self-disclosed medical concern, that member should be advised to consult with a qualified health care provider before beginning a physical activity program.

Checklists and Schedules for Facility and Equipment Maintenance and Cleaning

The TSAC Facilitator is responsible for maximizing the safety, effectiveness, and efficiency of each training facility or station. The facility should adopt a written occupational safety and health policy that identifies specific goals and objectives for the prevention and elimination of accidents and occupational injuries, exposures to communicable disease and illness, and fatalities.

Written policies and procedures should be developed for equipment selection, purchase, installation, setup, maintenance, and repair. Safety audits and inspections of equipment, maintenance, repair, and status reports should be included. Records should include manufacturer-provided manuals, warranties, and operating guidelines, as well as other relevant information (e.g., request for proposals, purchasing, inspections, serial numbers). Establish a daily, weekly, monthly, and annual checklist, such as the following:

- **Daily:** Inspect and maintain all equipment. Place everything in the appropriate setting. Clean floors and mats regularly with industrial-strength products that eliminate methicillin-resistant *Staphylococcus aureus* (MRSA), influenza, H1N1, fungus, and other germs.
- **Weekly:** Clean and disinfect benches with material-safe disinfectant. Clean walls, mirrors, window exits, storage areas, and shelves.
- **Monthly:** Lubricate bars, tighten bolts on machines, and inspect all cardiorespiratory equipment.
- **Annually:** Replace worn upholstery and equipment that is not used.

See figure 22.5 for an example of a safety checklist for exercise facility and equipment maintenance.

Key Point

Regular building and equipment maintenance and cleaning are important aspects of risk management.

Common Litigation Issues and Scenarios in the Facility

TSAC Facilitators have a duty to provide an appropriate level of supervision and instruction to meet a reasonable standard of care and to provide and maintain a safe environment for people under their supervision. These duties also involve informing members of risks related to their activities and preventing unreasonable risk or harm from negligent instruction or supervision. The NSCA provides the following guidelines and recommendations to minimize risk when designing and operating a facility (19).

Assumption of Risk

Assumption of risk is described as voluntary participation in activity with knowledge of the inherent risks. Physical activities, including strength and conditioning, involve certain risks. Members must be informed of these risks, and it is recommended to have members sign a statement to that fact.

Standard of Care

Standard of care is described as what a prudent and reasonable person would do under similar circumstances. TSAC Facilitators are expected to act according to their education, training, and certification status. TSAC Facilitators have a certain degree of care and skill, and they should follow practices that are customary in the strength and conditioning industry. For example, providing a health history questionnaire is a common practice to help identify health risks. If someone is injured and was not provided these documents, the TSAC Facilitator could be found negligent.

Negligence

Negligence is the failure to act as a reasonable and prudent person would under similar circumstances. TSAC Facilitators are considered negligent if they are proven to have a duty to act and to have failed to provide the appropriate standard of care, resulting in injury or damages to another person. An example of negligence would be having a person perform an unfamiliar exercise, such as a back squat, without proper spotting, resulting in an injury.

NSCA's Safety Checklist for Exercise Facility and Equipment Maintenance

Exercise Facility

Floor

- ❏ Inspected and cleaned daily
- ❏ Wooden flooring free of splinters, holes, protruding nails, and loose screws
- ❏ Tile flooring resistant to slipping; no moisture or chalk accumulation
- ❏ Rubber flooring free of cuts, slits, and large gaps between pieces
- ❏ Interlocking mats secure and arranged with no protruding tabs
- ❏ Nonabsorbent carpet free of tears; wear areas protected by throw mats
- ❏ Area swept and vacuumed or mopped on a regular basis
- ❏ Flooring glued or fastened down properly

Walls

- ❏ Wall surfaces cleaned two or three times a week (or more often if needed)
- ❏ Walls in high-activity areas free of protruding appliances, equipment, or wall hangings
- ❏ Mirrors and shelves securely fixed to walls
- ❏ Mirrors and windows cleaned regularly (especially in high-activity areas, such as around drinking fountains and in doorways)
- ❏ Mirrors placed a minimum of 20 inches (51 cm) off the floor in all areas
- ❏ Mirrors not cracked or distorted (replace immediately if damaged)

Ceiling

- ❏ All ceiling fixtures and attachments dusted regularly
- ❏ Ceiling tile kept clean
- ❏ Damaged or missing ceiling tile replaced as needed
- ❏ Open ceilings with exposed pipes and ducts cleaned as needed

Exercise Equipment

Stretching and Bodyweight Exercise Area

- ❏ Mat area free of weight benches and equipment
- ❏ Mats and bench upholstery free of cracks and tears
- ❏ No large gaps between stretching mats
- ❏ Area swept and disinfected daily
- ❏ Equipment properly stored after use
- ❏ Elastic cords secured to base with safety knot and checked for wear
- ❏ Surfaces that contact skin treated with antifungal and antibacterial agents daily
- ❏ Nonslip material on the top surface and bottom or base of plyometric boxes
- ❏ Ceiling height sufficient for overhead exercises (12 feet [3.7 m] minimum) and free of low-hanging apparatus (beams, pipes, lighting, signs, and so on)

Resistance Training Machine Area

- ❏ Easy access to each station (a minimum of 2 feet [61 cm] between machines; 3 feet [91 cm] is optimal)
- ❏ Area free of loose bolts, screws, cables, and chains
- ❏ Proper selectorized pins used
- ❏ Securing straps are functional

(continued)

Figure 22.5 NSCA's checklist for exercise facility and equipment maintenance.

(continued)

❏ Parts and surfaces properly lubricated and cleaned

❏ Protective padding free of cracks and tears

❏ Surfaces that contact skin treated with antifungal and antibacterial agents daily

❏ No protruding screws or parts that need tightening or removal

❏ Belts, chains, and cables aligned with machine parts

❏ No worn parts (frayed cable, loose chains, worn bolts, cracked joints, and so on)

Resistance Training Free Weight Area

❏ Easy access to each bench or area (a minimum of 2 feet [61 cm] between machines; 3 feet [91 cm] is optimal)

❏ Olympic bars properly spaced (3 feet [91 cm]) between ends

❏ All equipment returned after use to avoid obstruction of pathway

❏ Safety equipment (belts, collars, safety bars) used and returned

❏ Protective padding free of cracks and tears

❏ Surfaces that contact skin treated with antifungal and antibacterial agents daily

❏ Securing bolts and apparatus parts (collars, curl bars) tightly fastened

❏ Nonslip mats on squat rack floor area

❏ Olympic bars turn properly and are properly lubricated and tightened

❏ Benches, weight racks, standards, and the like secured to the floor or wall

❏ Nonfunctional or broken equipment removed from area or locked out of service

❏ Ceiling height sufficient for overhead exercises (12 feet [3.7 m] minimum) and free of low-hanging apparatus (beams, pipes, lighting, signs, and so on)

Weightlifting Area

❏ Olympic bars properly spaced (3 feet [91 cm]) between ends

❏ All equipment returned after use to avoid obstruction of lifting area

❏ Olympic bars rotate properly and are properly lubricated and tightened

❏ Bent Olympic bars replaced; knurling clear of debris

❏ Collars functioning

❏ Sufficient chalk available

❏ Wrist straps, belts, and knee wraps available, functioning, and stored properly

❏ Benches, chairs, and boxes kept at a distance from lifting area

❏ No gaps, cuts, slits, or splinters in mats

❏ Area properly swept and mopped to remove splinters and chalk

❏ Ceiling height sufficient for overhead exercises (12 feet [3.7 m] minimum) and free of low-hanging apparatus (beams, pipes, lighting, signs, and so on)

Aerobic Exercise Area

❏ Easy access to each station (minimum of 2 feet [61 cm] between machines; 3 feet [91 cm] is optimal)

❏ Bolts and screws tight

❏ Functioning parts easily adjustable

❏ Parts and surfaces properly lubricated and cleaned

❏ Foot and body straps secure and not ripped

❏ Measurement devices for tension, time, and revolutions per minute properly functioning

❏ Surfaces that contact skin treated with antifungal and antibacterial agents daily

(continued)

(continued)

Frequency of Maintenance and Cleaning Tasks

Daily

❏ Inspect all flooring for damage or wear.

❏ Clean (sweep, vacuum, or mop and disinfect) all flooring.

❏ Clean and disinfect upholstery.

❏ Clean and disinfect drinking fountains.

❏ Inspect fixed equipment's connection with floor.

❏ Clean and disinfect equipment surfaces that contact skin.

❏ Clean mirrors.

❏ Clean windows.

❏ Inspect mirrors for damage.

❏ Inspect all equipment for damage; wear; loose or protruding belts, screws, cables, or chains; insecure or nonfunctioning foot and body straps; improper functioning or improper use of attachments, pins, or other devices.

❏ Clean and lubricate moving parts of equipment.

❏ Inspect all protective padding for cracks and tears.

❏ Inspect nonslip material and mats for proper placement, damage, and wear.

❏ Remove trash and garbage.

❏ Clean light covers, fans, air vents, clocks, and speakers.

❏ Ensure that equipment is returned and stored properly after use.

Two or Three Times per Week

❏ Clean and lubricate aerobic machines and the guide rods on selectorized resistance training machines.

Once per Week

❏ Clean (dust) ceiling fixtures and attachments.

❏ Clean ceiling tile.

As Needed

❏ Replace light bulbs.

❏ Clean walls.

❏ Replace damaged or missing ceiling tiles.

❏ Clean open ceilings with exposed pipes or ducts.

❏ Remove (or place sign on) broken equipment.

❏ Fill chalk boxes.

❏ Clean bar knurling.

❏ Clean rust from floor, plates, bars, and equipment with a rust-removing solution.

Reprinted, by permission, from NSCA, 2016, Facility design, layout, and organization. In *Essentials of strength training and conditioning*, 4th ed., edited by G. Haff and T. Triplett (Champaign, IL: Human Kinetics), 637. Adapted, by permission, from NSCA, 2004, *NSCA's essentials of personal training*, edited by R.W. Earle and T.R. Baechle (Champaign, IL: Human Kinetics), 604-606.

Required Versus Recommended Procedures and Guidelines

It is important to distinguish between *required* and *recommended* because each term has different legal implications (3, 13). A **required procedure** reflects a duty or obligation to meet a standard of care. The requirements set forth in this part may ultimately be recognized as a legal standard of care to be implemented in the daily operation of tactical programs and facilities. A **recommended operating procedure** is developed to further enhance the quality of services provided. Recommendations are not intended to be standards of practice or to give rise to legally defined duties of care, but in certain circumstances they assist in evaluating and improving services rendered.

Standards of Practice

Published **standards of practice** help determine whether a person is negligent in carrying out duties that are recognized as widely accepted practices. Some courts examining these issues in negligence cases have ruled that violations of such professional standards constitute a breach of duty. Published standards of practice can minimize liability exposures associated with negligence and thereby serve as a shield for those who comply with them. They can also be used against those who do not comply with them, potentially increasing liability risks associated with negligence (6).

Methods to Reduce the Risk of Liability and Enhance Safety

Strength and conditioning programs present some level of risk; however, the TSAC Facilitator must proactively identify and mitigate danger. All staff members must be committed to safety within the training environment by requiring appropriate clearance to engage in training, providing adequate instruction, and communicating effectively through words and actions. To reduce the risk of liability and enhance safety within the facility, the TSAC Facilitator should always be aware of the training conditions. It is imperative to develop a safety audit and conduct it on a routine basis. This inspection process will reduce or eliminate hazards that may cause injury. In all cases,

records of each inspection or audit should be kept on file for at least three years. Furthermore, the TSAC Facilitator should encourage staff, tactical athletes, and members to proactively identify perceived hazards.

Risk Management

Risk management refers to the practices, procedures, and systems by which the facility reduces the risk that employees or users will experience an event that could result in harm. Procedures and systems should be in place to reduce or limit exposure to potential liabilities and financial loss. For example, the U.S. Army manages risk through a process known as composite risk management. This process involves five steps:

1. **Identify hazards:** Consider current and future events, environments, and past situations that posed a threat.

2. **Assess the hazards in order to determine risk:** Determine the effect of each hazard based on loss and cost as associated with probability and severity.

3. **Establish controls and make risk decisions:** Establish control measures that alleviate the hazard or reduce the risk. As control measures are established, risk is reevaluated until the risk level is at a point where benefits outweigh costs. The decision rests with the assigned decision-making authority.

4. **Implement controls that reduce or eliminate risk:** Controls must be communicated to all involved.

5. **Supervise and evaluate:** Measure the effectiveness of the controls and adjust or revise as required. Use lessons learned as feedback for future planning.

Risk management levels were developed to assist in the decision-making process. The three levels of risk management are time critical, deliberate, and strategic. The time critical level is used when there is limited time, minimal complexity, or low risk. The deliberate level is used in many workplace environments where group experience produces the best outcomes. The strategic level is used in high-priority situations where additional hazard and assessment tools are required. It is often used for complex, high-risk applications and is time intensive.

The composite risk management process is governed by four principles that are applied before, during, and after the five-step process:

1. Accept no unnecessary risk.
2. Make decisions at the appropriate management level.
3. Accept risk when benefits outweigh costs.
4. Integrate risk management into planning and training at all levels.

Figure 22.6 is a deliberate risk assessment worksheet. The TSAC Facilitator can refer to this form when developing risk management procedures. Instructions for completing the worksheet are located on the third page of the document.

Orientation, Education, and Supervision

All new and current members should be provided with a general orientation to the facility, including the following:

- Basic instruction on the use of the exercise equipment available
- Introduction to a general physical activity regimen that is offered within the facility
- Explanation of the rules and regulations of the facility
- Explanation of the potential risks and hazards for injury
- Explanation of emergency procedures and the evacuation plan
- Introduction to other resources that will help with developing a physical activity program

All participants in a strength and conditioning program must be properly supervised and instructed at all times to ensure maximum safety. Due to the high level of skill associated with tactical occupations, many of the activities implemented in a strength and conditioning program should be coached and supervised. The following supervision principles are recommended:

- Be present at all times.
- Be active and hands on.
- Be prudent, careful, and prepared.
- Be qualified (e.g., accredited degree, TSAC-F credential, CPR, first aid certification).

- Be vigilant.
- Inform all members of safety and emergency procedures.
- Know members' health status.
- Monitor and enforce rules and regulations.
- Monitor and scrutinize the environment.

In addition to the physical presence of the TSAC Facilitator, effective instruction and supervision involve a range of practical considerations:

- A clear view of all areas of the facility and the members in it
- The TSAC Facilitator's proximity to the groups under supervision
- The number and grouping of members (to make optimal use of available equipment, space, and time)
- Age and experience level
- Type of program being conducted

All activities should be planned to meet the recommended guidelines for minimum average floor space allowance per participant (100 ft^2 [9 m^2]), facilitator-to-athlete ratio (1:20), and number of participants per barbell or training station (up to 3) (14).

Emergency Response Policy

Facilities should have written emergency response policies and procedures that are reviewed regularly and rehearsed quarterly. These policies enable the TSAC Facilitator and facility staff to respond to first aid situations and emergency events.

Considerations and Strategies for Training Large Groups

The tactical strength and conditioning program should allow for the optimal number of qualified staff as well as use of available equipment, time, and space. Large training groups are common in tactical populations, and circuit training is often used. It is recommended that facilities do not exceed a 1:50 facilitator-to-athlete ratio; however, this may not be feasible and will be based on the TSAC Facilitator's experience and resources. Novice or special populations engaged in strength and conditioning programs require greater

DELIBERATE RISK ASSESSMENT WORKSHEET

1. MISSION/TASK DESCRIPTION	2. DATE (DD/MM/YYYY)

3. PREPARED BY

a. Name (Last, First Middle Initial)	b. Rank/Grade	c. Duty Title/Position

d. Unit	e. Work Email	f. Telephone (DSN/Commercial (Include Area Code))

g. UIC/CIN (as required)	h. Training Support/Lesson Plan or OPORD (as required)	i. Signature of Preparer

Five steps of Risk Management: (1) Identify the hazards (2) Assess the hazards (3) Develop controls & make decisions
(4) Implement controls (5) Supervise and evaluate *(Step numbers not equal to numbered items on form)*

4. SUBTASK/SUBSTEP OF MISSION/TASK	5. HAZARD	6. INITIAL RISK LEVEL	7. CONTROL	8. HOW TO IMPLEMENT/ WHO WILL IMPLEMENT	9. RESIDUAL RISK LEVEL
[+] [-]				How:	

10. OVERALL RESIDUAL RISK LEVEL *(All controls implemented)*:

☐ EXTREMELY HIGH ☐ HIGH ☐ MEDIUM ☐ LOW

11. OVERALL SUPERVISION PLAN AND RECOMMENDED COURSE OF ACTION

12. APPROVAL OR DISAPPROVAL OF MISSION OR TASK ☐ Approve ☐ Disapprove

a. Name (Last, First, Middle Initial)	b. Rank/Grade	c. Duty Title/Position	d. Signature of Approval Authority

e. Additional Guidance:

DD FORM 2977, SEP 2014

Page 1 of 3

Figure 22.6 Deliberate risk assessment worksheet.

(continued)

Risk Assessment Matrix		Probability (expected frequency)				
		Frequent: Continuous, regular, or inevitable occurrences	**Likely:** Several or numerous occurrences	**Occasional:** Sporadic or intermittent occurrences	**Seldom:** Infrequent occurrences	**Unlikely:** Possible occurrences but improbable
Severity (expected consequence)		A	B	C	D	E
Catastrophic: Mission failure, unit readiness eliminated; death, unacceptable loss or damage	I	EH	EH	H	H	M
Critical: Significantly degraded unit readiness or mission capability; severe injury, illness, loss or damage	II	EH	H	H	M	L
Moderate: Somewhat degraded unit readiness or mission capability; minor injury, illness, loss, or damage	III	H	M	M	L	L
Negligible: Little or no impact to unit readiness or mission capability; minimal injury, loss, or damage	IV	M	L	L	L	L

Legend: **EH** - Extremely High Risk   **H** - High Risk   **M** - Medium Risk   **L** - Low Risk

13. RISK ASSESSMENT REVIEW (Required when assessment applies to ongoing operations or activities)

a. Date	b. Last Name	c. Rank/Grade	d. Duty Title/Position	e. Signature of Reviewer

14. FEEDBACK AND LESSONS LEARNED

15. ADDITIONAL COMMENTS OR REMARKS

DD FORM 2977, SEP 2014

Figure 22.6   (continued)

Instructions for Completing DD Form 2977, "Deliberate Risk Assessment Worksheet"

1. Mission/Task Description: Briefly describe the overall Mission or Task for which the deliberate risk assessment is being conducted.

2. Date *(DD/MM/YYY)*: Self Explanatory.

3. Prepared By: Information provided by the individual conducting the deliberate risk assessment for the operation or training.
Legend: UIC = Unit Identification Code; **CIN** = Course ID Number; **OPORD** = operation order; **DSN** = defense switched network; **COMM** = commercial

4. Sub-task/Sub-Step of Mission/Task: Briefly describe all subtasks or substeps that warrant risk management.

5. Hazard: Specify hazards related to the subtask in block 4.

6. Initial Risk Level: Determine probability and severity. Using the risk assessment matrix (page 3), determine level of risk for each hazard specified. probability, severity and associated Risk Level; enter level into column.

7. Control: Enter risk mitigation resources/controls identified to abate or reduce risk relevant to the hazard identified in block 5.

8. How to Implement / Who Will Implement: Briefly describe the means of employment for each control (i.e., OPORD, briefing, rehearsal) and the name of the individual unit or office that has primary responsibility for control implementation.

9. Residual Risk Level: After controls are implemented, determine resulting probability, severity, and residual risk level.

10. Overall Risk After Controls are Implemented: Assign an overall residual risk level. This is equal to or greater than the highest residual risk level (from block 9).

11. Supervision Plan and Recommended Course of Action: Completed by preparer. Identify specific tasks and levels of responsibility for supervisory personnel and provide the decision authority with a recommend course of action for approval or disapproval based upon the overall risk assessment.

12. Approval/Disapproval of Mission/Task: Risk approval authority approves or disapproves the mission or task based on the overall risk assessment, including controls, residual risk level, and supervision plan.

13. Risk Assessment Review: Should be conducted on a regular basis. Reviewers should have sufficient oversight of the mission or activity and controls to provide valid input on changes or adjustments needed. If the residual risk rises above the level already approved, operations should cease until the appropriate approval authority is contacted and approves continued operations.

14. Feedback and Lessons Learned: Provide specific input on the effectiveness of risk controls and their contribution to mission success or failure. Include recommendations for new or revised controls, practicable solutions, or alternate actions. Submit and brief valid lessons learned as necessary to persons affected.

15. Additional Comments or Remarks: Preparer or approval authority provides any additional comments, remarks, or information to support the integration of risk management.

Additional Guidance: Blocks 4-9 may be reproduced as necessary for processing of all subtasks/ substeps of the mission/task. The addition and subtraction buttons are designed to enable users to accomplish this task.

DD FORM 2977, SEP 2014

Figure 22.6 *(continued)*

Reprinted from Department of Defense, DD FORM 2977, September 2014. http://www.dtic.mil/whs/directives/forms/eforms/dd2977.pdf.

supervision. The following variables should be manipulated by the TSAC Facilitator when developing a strength and conditioning program in a large group setting:

- Exercise or work interval (the duration or distance or number of repetitions executed)
- Exercise order (the sequence in which a set or repetition is executed)
- Exercise work-to-rest ratio (the relief intervals in a set)
- Frequency (the number of training sessions performed in a given time period)
- Intensity (the effort with which a repetition is executed)
- Recovery interval (the time period between repetitions, sets, and exercises)
- Repetition (the execution of a specific workload assignment or movement technique)
- Series (a group of sets and recovery intervals)
- Volume (the amount of work, or repetitions, performed in a given training session or time period)

CONCLUSION

The organizational and administrative considerations associated with a tactical strength and conditioning program are often viewed as less important than program design and the actual training of the tactical athlete. However, facility design; equipment selection, placement, and maintenance; and facility management provide the foundation for the safe and efficient execution of any strength and conditioning program. The four distinct phases of facility design—predesign, design, construction, and preoperation—provide a standardized process whether designing a new facility, renovating a current facility, or repurposing an existing building.

In most cases, the TSAC Facilitator will provide recommendations on equipment selection, placement, and spacing. Resources to assist in this process are available from the federal government, DoD, NFPA, IACP, NSCA, and ACSM. Efficiency in training and safety of the tactical athlete and facility staff are key factors in equipment selection, layout, and organization of the facility.

Training facility guidelines and policies provide SOPs and standards of conduct when using the facility. The facility SOP at a minimum should include a facility mission statement or statements that identify the purpose and guiding principles that govern day-to-day operations of the facility, staff duty descriptions, staff certification requirements, operating rules, risk management procedures, emergency procedures, injury reporting procedures, data-handling procedures, and standards of care.

An important responsibility of the TSAC Facilitator is to ensure the training facility provides an efficient and safe training environment. One method to ensure a safe training environment is to include additional operating procedures in the SOP, such as preparticipation screening requirements; equipment and facility maintenance schedules; an equipment life-cycle replacement plan; daily, weekly, and monthly facility cleaning schedules; a facility safety plan; and a facility usage plan for small, medium, and large groups. Facility organization and administration are essential to properly managing training facilities and enhancing the tactical athlete's training experience.

Key Terms

Americans with Disabilities Act (ADA)
assumption of risk
construction phase
defined activity areas
design phase
equipment priority list
feasibility study
indemnification
liability
master plan
needs analysis
negligence
personally identifiable information (PII)

preactivity screening
predesign phase
preoperation phase
recommended operating procedure
required procedure
risk management
self-contained power area (SCPA)
standard of care
standard operating procedure (SOP)
standards of practice
strengths, weaknesses, opportunities, and
    threats (SWOT) analysis
Unified Facilities Criteria (UFC)

Study Questions

1. Which of the following is the correct order of the phases involved in building, renovating, or repurposing a training facility?

   a. preoperation, predesign, construction, design

   b. predesign, design, construction, preoperation

   c. construction, preoperation, predesign, design

   d. design, construction, preoperation, predesign

2. During which of the following steps in the predesign phase is a SWOT analysis performed?

   a. perform a needs analysis

   b. complete a feasibility study

   c. select an architectural plan

   d. create the training facility master plan

3. Standards for military physical fitness centers are established by which of the following?

   a. U.S. Department of Defense

   b. U.S. Air Force Special Operations Command

   c. ACSM standards for facility design

   d. U.S. Air Force services facilities design guide

4. Which of following is the minimum recommended space to be maintained around self-contained power areas?

   a. 3 feet (91 cm)

   b. 4 feet (122 cm)

   c. 6 feet (183 cm)

   d. 8 feet (244 cm)

5. When cleaning and maintaining a fitness facility, which of the following tasks should be performed monthly?

   a. clean floors

   b. lubricate bars

   c. disinfect benches

   d. replace worn upholstery

Table 22.1 U.S. Army Functional Equipment List

1	Bench, utility	26	Kettlebells—18 kg (40 lb)	51	Plyo boxes—36 in. (91 cm) (steel)
2	Rack system	27	Kettlebells—20 kg (44 lb)	52	Plyo box set—12-36 in. (30-91 cm) (wood)
3	Climbing rope	28	Kettlebells—24 kg (53 lb)	53	Gym timer (wall mount)
4	Knee raise/dip combo station	29	Kettlebells—28 kg (62 lb)	54	Resistance bands—0.5 in. (1 cm) wide
5	Barbell collar set	30	Kettlebells—32 kg (71 lb)	55	Resistance bands—1 in. (3 cm) wide
6	Barbell storage rack	31	Kettlebells—36 kg (79 lb)	56	Resistance bands—1.75 in. (4 cm) wide
7	Barbell straight bar set	32	Kettlebell storage rack	57	Resistance bands—2.5 in. (6 cm) wide
8	Battling ropes	33	Medicine ball—10 lb (5 kg) (hard rubber)	58	Speed/agility ladder
9	Suspension trainer	34	Medicine ball—15 lb (7 kg) (hard rubber)	59	Spring collars
10	Bumper plate sets	35	Medicine ball—20 lb (9 kg) (hard rubber)	60	BOSU balls
11	Bumper plate tree	36	Medicine ball—8 lb (4 kg) (soft)	61	Olympic plate (urethane) pairs—45, 35, 25, 10, 5 lb (20, 16, 11, 5, 2 kg)
12	Chalk bowl	37	Medicine ball—10 lb (5 kg) (soft)	62	Plate tree
13	Cones	38	Medicine ball—12 lb (26 kg) (soft)	63	Step hurdles—6 in. (15 cm) high and 12 in. (30 cm) wide
14	Exercise mats	39	Medicine ball—14 lb (31 kg) (soft)		
15	Dumbbell set	40	Medicine ball—16 lb (35 kg) (soft)	64	Stability balls—18 in. (46 cm)
16	Dumbbell storage rack	41	Medicine ball—18 lb (40 kg) (soft)	65	Stability balls—22 in. (56 cm)
17	Flat bench	42	Medicine ball—20 lb (44 kg) (soft)	66	Stability balls—26 in. (66 cm)
18	Lifting chains	43	Medicine ball storage rack	67	Stability balls—30 in. (76 cm)
19	Glute/ham bench	44	Medicine ball—15 lb (7 kg) (rubber slam)	68	Weight vest—25 lb (11 kg)
20	Ring set	45	Medicine ball—20 lb (44 kg) (rubber slam)	69	Abdominal (core training) mat
21	Jump ropes	46	Half rack (self-standing with pull-up bar)	70	Climbers
22	Kettlebells—10 kg (22 lb)	47	Pull-up and chin-up bars	71	Treadmills
23	Kettlebells—12 kg (26 lb)	48	Olympic bar	72	Rowers
24	Kettlebells—14 kg (31 lb)	49	Plyo boxes—24 in. (61 cm) (wood)	73	Ladders
25	Kettlebells—16 kg (35 lb)	50	Plyo boxes—30 in. (76 cm) (steel)		

Adapted from Department of the Army 10th Mountain Division and Fort Drum combat readiness training facilities and company readiness training areas, Fort Drum, New York, February 6, 2013, pages 16-29.

Table 22.2 U.S. Marine Corps HITT Center Equipment List

Equipment	Item number	Vendor	Number needed
Exercise band—small (32 in. [813 mm])	6428SP	Perform Better	8
Exercise band—medium (38 in. [965 mm])	6428MP	Perform Better	8
Exercise band—large (43 in. [1,092 mm])	6428LP	Perform Better	8
Stretch Out Strap	9251P	Perform Better	15
First Place Competitor hurdle	6921P	Perform Better	6
Dynamax Accelerator II	5043P	Perform Better	4
Dynamax Stout I	5044P	Perform Better	4
Dynamax Stout II	5045P	Perform Better	4
Dynamax Hefty I	5046P	Perform Better	4
Dynamax Hefty II	5047P	Perform Better	4
Dynamax Burly	5048P	Perform Better	4
Dynamax Rack	5059P	Perform Better	3
Sled Dawg Elite	2068P	Perform Better	8
Agility ladder	3561P	Perform Better	8
Saucer cones—set of 12	6526P	Perform Better	6
Saucer cone carrier	6528P	Perform Better	3
Bullet Belt deluxe pack	7649P	Perform Better	12
Plyo-Safe G2 set (black)	5622P	Perform Better	1
Vertimax	2823P	Perform Better	2
Training rope anchor	3018P	Perform Better	2
Training rope holder	3019P	Perform Better	4
30 ft (9 m) training rope (1.5 in. [38 mm])	3226BP	Perform Better	2
30 ft (9 m) training rope (2.0 in. [51 mm])	3229P	Perform Better	2
First Place Medbell (kettlebell)—10 lb (4.5 kg)	2442	Perform Better	4
First Place Medbell (kettlebell)—12 lb (5.4 kg)	2443	Perform Better	4
First Place Medbell (kettlebell)—15 lb (6.8 kg)	2444	Perform Better	4
First Place Medbell (kettlebell)—18 lb (8.2 kg)	2445	Perform Better	4
First Place Medbell (kettlebell)—20 lb (9.1 kg)	2446	Perform Better	4
First Place Medbell (kettlebell)—25 lb (11.3 kg)	2447	Perform Better	4
First Place Medbell (kettlebell)—30 lb (13.6 kg)	2448	Perform Better	4
First Place Medbell (kettlebell)—35 lb (15.9 kg)	449	Perform Better	4
First Place kettlebell rack	P-2693	Perform Better	2
Lifting chain—30 lb (13.6 kg)	1825P	Perform Better	2
Lifting chain—45 lb (20.4 kg)	1826P	Perform Better	2
Lifting chain—60 lb (27.2 kg)	1827P	Perform Better	2
TRX suspension trainer	2030P	Perform Better	4
Wall chin-up bar	5738P	Perform Better	4
Bravo functional trainer	8810	Cybex	2
The Trainer	6650	Perform Better	2
ECT	7701	Perform Better	2
Ultimate Sandbag (Power package: 19 in. × 9 in. outer shell with two 5-20 lb inner sand bags)	9081S	Perform Better	2
Ultimate Sandbag (Strength package: 27 in. × 10 in. outer shell with two 20-40 lb inner sand bags)	9082S	Perform Better	2
Ultimate Sandbag (Burly package: 27 in. × 13 in. outer shell with three 20-40 lb inner sand bags)	9083S	Perform Better	4
Wall-mount rack	3680S	Perform Better	3

(continued)

Table 22.2 *(continued)*

Equipment	Item number	Vendor	Number needed
Bulldog collar	50398	Power Systems	12
5 ft (1.5 m) Olympic training bar	6745	Power Systems	4
Pure Strength Olympic bar	3024-3241	Power Systems	4
Glute/ham developer	46118	Power Systems	2
9 ft (2.7 m) Big Iron half rack	19000	Cybex	2
Locking bench	19100	Cybex	2
York Bumper Grip plates—5 lb (2.3 kg)	2905-5	Power Systems	8
York Bumper Grip plates—10 lb (4.5 kg)	2905-5	Power Systems	8
York Bumper Grip plates—25 lb (11.3 kg)	2905-5	Power Systems	8
York Bumper Grip plates—35 lb (15.9 kg)	2905-5	Power Systems	8
York Bumper Grip plates (45 lb (20.4 kg)	2905-5	Power Systems	8
Smart Hurdle III	3120	Power Systems	12
Arc Trainer	750A	Cybex	2

Adapted from R- FC 4-740-02N, Facility Criteria, Navy and Marine Corps Fitness Centers, HITT Center, April 1, 2014, Appendix C, C-2.

Table 22.3 U.S. Army Physical Fitness School (USAPFS) Strength and Conditioning Equipment List

Item	Quantity	Item	Quantity	Item	Quantity
Sorinex Base Camp package		Sorinex Mighty Mitts dip/chin bar	8 each	Roller pad	16 each
Racks	8 each			Sorinex functional cable column dual handle	1 each
Sandwich hook	8 pairs	Eleiko PL competition set—435 kg (959 lb)	1 each		
24 in. (61 cm) safety bar	8 pairs			Sorinex Firebreather ring set	10 pairs
Utility pin	128 each	PLAE performance flooring	Flooring based on facility square footage	GymAware power tool kit	2 each
Indexing chin bar (45° rotating handles)	8 each			Sorinex glute ham roller	14 each
Utility seat	8 each			Sorinex Olympic Fat Bar	2 each
Roller pad	8 pairs	Bolt-on utility seat with two-bar storage	8 each	Diamond bar	4 each
4 ft (122 cm) safety and utility strap spotter pack	8 pairs	Utility seats	8 each	Troy curl bar	4 each
Landmine attachment	8 each	Sorinex 0-90 NP bench	8 each	Sandbag Advance PKG Elite	4 each
Utility pin	128 each	Intek urethane dumbbell set—5-50 lb (2-23 kg)	1 set	Box squat boxes with rubber top	4 each
Sorinex 0-90 NP bench	4 each	Intek urethane dumbbell set—55-100 lb (25-45 kg)	1 set	Farmer's walk handles	8 each
Iron Bear kettlebell piece	9 each			10 in. (25 cm) log bar	4 each
Iron Bear dumbbell piece	9 each	Intek urethane dumbbell set—105-125 lb (48-57 kg)	1 set	Sorinex speed sled	4 each
Iron Bear medicine ball piece	9 each	Sorinex 38 ft (12 m) custom monkey rig	1 each	Sorinex Bosco Elite bumper plate—45 lb (20 kg)	64 each
Iron Bear side	12 each				
XL Series competition bench	1 each	Base Camp rope machine with Hogline rope system	2 each	Sorinex Bosco Elite bumper plate—25 lb (11 kg)	64 each
Tactical plate storage rack	1 each	XL Series Diablo dip bar	4 each	Sorinex Bosco Elite bumper plate—10 lb (5 kg)	40 each
Exercise band set	8 each	Sorinex seated calf-tib machine	1 each		
Sorinex 1/2 in. (13 mm) and 5/8 in. (16 mm) chains	10 pairs	Sorinex bar and trigger rollers	8 each	Sorinex Bosco Elite bumper plate—5 lb (2 kg)	56 each
Sorinex spider low row	1 each	Selectorized low row	1 each	Sorinex Bosco Elite bumper plate—2.5 lb (1 kg)	56 each
Sorinex 45° leg press	1 each	Selectorized lat machine	1 each		
Sorinex XL Series wall ball gong	8 each				

U.S. Army Physical Fitness School Sorinex Equipment Quote No. 4985, Customer No. C01047, November 21, 2014, pages 1-4.

Table 22.4 U.S. Navy Functional Equipment List

Item	Quantity	Item	Quantity	Item	Quantity
Double power station (rack, bench, platform)	1	Triple-tier dumbbell rack (15 pairs): bottom two levels for dumbbells, top level for kettlebells	1	Olympic curl bar—26 lb (12 kg), 5 ft (1.5 m) (black)	1
Glute/ham bench (split pad, linear)	1	Band attachment	1	Olympic spring lock collar	3
Step-up box with plywood, no logo	1	Vertical medicine ball rack	1	Medicine balls 4 lb (2 kg) 6 lb (3 kg) 8 lb (4 kg) 10 lb (5 kg) 12 lb (5.5 kg) 15 lb (7 kg) 18 lb (8 kg) 20 lb (9 kg) 25 lb (11 kg) 30 lb (14 kg)	1 each
Olympic lifting bar—20 kg (44 lb), 1 1/8 in. (3 cm) shaft, 1800# test zinc	2	Kettlebells 5 lb (2 kg) 15 lb (7 kg) 20 lb (9 kg) 25 lb (11 kg) 30 lb (14 kg) 35 lb (16 kg) 40 lb (18 kg) 45 lb (20 kg) 50 lb (23 kg) 55 lb (25 kg) 60 lb (27 kg) 70 lb (32 kg) 75 lb (43 kg) 80 lb (36 kg) 85 lb (39 kg) 90 lb (41 kg) 95 lb (43 kg) 100 lb (45 kg)	4 each		
45 lb (20 kg) bumper plate	8				
35 lb (16 kg) bumper plate	4				
25 lb (11 kg) bumper plate	4				
10 lb (5 kg) bumper plate	4			TRX strap	2
Olympic plates—rubber grip 10 lb (5 kg) 5 lb (2 kg) 2.5 lb (1 kg)	4 each			Power sled (plate loaded), including harness and belt	1
Deluxe dumbbells 5 lb (2 kg) 10 lb (5 kg) 15 lb (7 kg) 20 lb (9 kg) 25 lb (11kg) 30 lb (14 kg) 35 lb (16 kg) 40 lb (18 kg) 45 lb (20 kg) 50 lb (23 kg) 55 lb (25 kg) 60 lb (27 kg)	10 pairs total			Double ladder	1
				Battling rope—50 ft (15 m)	1
				Weightlifting band	1

Adapted from R- FC 4-740-02N, Facility Criteria, Navy and Marine Corps Fitness Centers, April 1, 2014, Table 4-27, Functional Fitness.

Table 22.5 U.S. Air Force Fitness Facility Equipment and Supply List

Item	Item	Item
Cardiorespiratory	Computer	**Football**
Upright stationary bicycle	Guest chairs	Football equipment cart
Recumbent stationary bicycle	File cabinet	Goalpost and pads (2 posts and pads per field)
Stair-climber	Shelves	Markers (5 per field)
Treadmill	**Individual workstations**	Down box, pole, and chain set
Elliptical	Desk and workspace	Extra point tees
Total body machine	Chair	Kicking tees
Selectorized resistance training	Computer	Jerseys with reversible numbers (minimum of 4 sets of 25 jerseys)
Leg press	File cabinet	Footballs (minimum of 2)
Leg curl	Shelves	Flags (minimum of 22 sets)
Leg extension	**Common work area**	Scorecards
Standing/seated leg abduction	Fax machine	Pylons (8 per field)
Standing/seated leg adduction	Copier	**Basketball**
Bench press	File cabinet	Jerseys with reversible numbers (8 sets of 15 jerseys)
Overhead press	Shelves	One basketball
Cable lat pulldown	Meeting table	Nylon nets
Compound row	Chairs	Scorebooks
Pec deck fly	**Break area**	Court cleaner
Arm curl	Refrigerator	Scoreboards
Triceps press	Microwave	Shot clocks (if not on scoreboard)
Crunch	Coffeemaker	**Tennis**
Back extension	Table	Balls
Weighted assisted dip	Chairs	Rackets
Cable crossover	**Lobby**	Windscreens
High/low pull	Sofa and chairs	Court repair kit
Miscellaneous items	TV screen	Tennis net
Outdoor bleachers	**Free weight resistance training**	Replacement post
All-purpose mower	Power rack	Sponge roller
Four wheeler	Smith machine	**Softball**
Athletic field marker for paint	Combination pull-up/dip	Bats and softballs (2 minimum per game)
Athletic field marker for chalk	Olympic bench	Scorebooks
Exercise room equipment	Olympic incline	Base set and plugs
Step platforms	Olympic decline	Catcher helmet and chest protector
Trampolines	Adjustable incline	Field drag mats
BOSU balls	Incline leg press	Fence crown
Abdominal benches	Preacher curl	Storage shed
Neo hex dumbbells	Set—5-50 lb (2-23 kg) rubber- or vinyl-coated dumbbells	Batter's box template
Yoga mats	Beauty Bell dumbbells with rack	Field rake and tamp
Jump ropes	Twin-tiered dumbbell racks	Grass and sod roller
Stretch bands	E-Z curl bar	Infield lip broom
Medicine ball, stability ball	5 ft (152 cm) Olympic bar	Field-marking dust
HR monitors	7 ft (213 cm) Olympic bar	Clay-drying agent
Plyo boxes	Weight plates—up to 45 lb (20 kg)	Foul pole (2 per field)
Core ball	Weight tree	Dry-line chalker
Exercise mats	**Racquetball and squash**	String winder
Furnishings and office equipment	Racquetball rackets with wrist straps	Pitching mound
Offices	Impact-resistant eye protection	Scorer's table
Desk and workspace	Racquetballs	Windscreen
Chair		

Table adapted from FC 4-740-02F, September 26, 2006; and Air Force Fitness and Sports Services Activity Standards.

Table 22.6 SOF Weight Training Equipment for a Small Facility

Item	Quantity	Item	Quantity
9 ft (2.7 m) power rack	8	Uesaka 45 lb (20 kg) bumper plate	36
Power rack band attachment	8	Diamond rubber 10 lb (5 kg) bumper plate	12
6 by 8 ft (1.8 by 2.4 m) Olympic platform	4	Ader 9 lb (4 kg) kettlebell	2
Reverse rhino hook bar catch	8	Ader 13 lb (6 kg) kettlebell	2
Belt squat	2	Ader 18 lb (8 kg) kettlebell	2
VMO (vastus medialis oblique) developer	2	Ader 26 lb (12 kg) kettlebell	4
Full-body squat apparatus	2	Ader 35 lb (16 kg) kettlebell	4
Reverse back extension apparatus	2	Ader 44 lb (20 kg) kettlebell	4
Hamstring/glute bench	2	Ader 53 lb (24 kg) kettlebell	4
Three-tier medicine ball rack	1	Ader 62 lb (28 kg) kettlebell	2
Band and chain storage rack	1	Ader 70 lb (32 kg) kettlebell	2
Lever-action bench	8	Ader 80 lb (36 kg) kettlebell	2
Multiangle dumbbell bench	4	Ader 88 lb (40 kg) kettlebell	1
Decline dumbbell bench	2	Ader 97 lb (44 kg) kettlebell	1
Bumper plate rack (small)	2	5-50 lb (2-23 kg) urethane dumbbells	3 sets
Bumper plate rack (large)	3	55-100 lb (25-45 kg) urethane dumbbells	3 sets
Three-tier dumbbell rack	5	105-150 lb (48-68 kg) urethane dumbbells	3 sets
Freestanding chalk bowl	4	20-110 lb (9-50 kg) urethane barbells	2 sets
Rack dip attachment	8	Barbell rack	2
Rack dip attachment storage unit	2	2.5 lb (1 kg) urethane plate	16
Nine-bar vertical storage unit	2	5 lb (2 kg) urethane plate	16
Mastiff bar—2 in. (5 cm) thick	1	10 lb (5 kg) urethane plate	24
Mastiff bar—2 3/8 in. (6 cm) thick	1	35 lb (16 kg) urethane plate	24
Mastiff bar—3 in. (8 cm) thick	1	45 lb (20 kg) urethane plate	72
Uesaka 20 kg (44 lb) training bar	12	Speedboard	2
Uesaka 25 lb (11 kg) bumper plate	12	Rower	4
Uesaka 35 lb (16 kg) bumper plate	12		

Adapted from T.K. Kelly et al., 2013, *Technical report: An assessment of the Army's tactical human optimization, rapid rehabilitation and reconditioning program* (Santa Monica, CA: Rand Corporation), 1-3, 23-27, 41-43.

Table 22.7 SOF Cardio Equipment for a Small Facility

Item	Quantity
Woodway Desmo Pro treadmill	4
Speedboard	2
VersaClimber (multistation configuration)	1
Elliptical	2
Jacob's ladder	2

Adapted from T.K. Kelly et al., 2013, *Technical report: An assessment of the Army's tactical human optimization, rapid rehabilitation and reconditioning program* (Santa Monica, CA: Rand Corporation), 1-3, 23-27, 41-43.

Table 22.8 SOF Miscellaneous Training Equipment for a Small Facility

Item	Quantity	Item	Quantity
Foam roller—3 ft (91 cm) long, 6 in. (15 cm) round	15	84 lb (38.1 kg) weighted vest	4
Foam roller—1 ft (30 cm) long, 6 in. (15 cm) round	30	Slastix All-Purpose Pro resistance band (medium)	6
Stretch strap	10	Slastix All-Purpose Pro resistance band (heavy)	6
First Place 4 lb (1.8 kg) medicine ball	4	Slastix All-Purpose Pro resistance band (extra heavy)	6
First Place 6 lb (2.7 kg) medicine ball	4	Slastix All-Purpose Pro resistance band (super heavy)	6
First Place 8 lb (3.6 kg) medicine ball	4	Mobility arch	12
First Place 10 lb (4.5 kg) medicine ball	6	King crab sled (blue)	3
First Place 12 lb (5.4 kg) medicine ball	6	Crab sled (blue)	3
First Place 15 lb (6.8 kg) medicine ball	6	Belt harness	6
First Place 18 lb (8.2 kg) medicine ball	6	Shoulder harness	6
First Place 20 lb (9.1 kg) medicine ball	6	Just Jump/Vertec vertical jump test apparatus	2
First Place 25 lb (11.3 kg) medicine ball	6	Functional trainer	4
First Place 30 lb (3.6 kg) medicine ball	6	Stand for trainer	4
Dynamax Stout 12 lb (5.4 kg) medicine ball	4	Infinity 6-pack frame	1
Dynamax Stout 14 lb (6.4 kg) medicine ball	4	Infinity 6-pack attachments	6
Dynamax Hefty 16 lb (7.3 kg) medicine ball	4	Air compressor	1
Dynamax Hefty 18 lb (8.2 kg) medicine ball	4	Accessory pack	6
Dynamax Burly 20 lb (9.1 kg) medicine ball	4	6 in. (15 cm) Banana Step	12
ABC speed/agility ladder	4	12 in. (30 cm) Banana Step	24
12 in. (30 cm) cone	24	18 in. (46 cm) Banana Step	12
12 in. (30 cm) saucer cones	3	24 in. (61 cm) Banana Step	12
20 lb (9.1 kg) weighted vest	4	40 lb (18.1 kg) weighted vest	4

Adapted from T.K. Kelly et al., 2013, *Technical report: An assessment of the Army's tactical human optimization, rapid rehabilitation and reconditioning program* (Santa Monica, CA: Rand Corporation), 1-3, 23-27, 41-43.

Table 22.9 SOF Testing and Evaluation Equipment for a Small Facility

Item	Quantity
Woodway Desmo treadmill	1
Cosmed Fitmate Pro cardiopulmonary testing apparatus	1
NeuroCom Balance Manager SMART EquiTest System	1
Static 18 in. by 60 in. (46 cm by 152 cm) force plate	1
InVision Design Package	1
BOD POD Gold Standard Body Composition Tracking System	1
Fusion Chart Software	1

Adapted from T.K. Kelly et al., 2013, *Technical report: An assessment of the Army's tactical human optimization, rapid rehabilitation and reconditioning program* (Santa Monica, CA: Rand Corporation), 1-3, 23-27, 41-43.

Table 22.10 SOF Sports Medicine Equipment for a Small Facility

Item	Quantity
Treatment table	4
Hydroculator	1
E-Stim and Ultrasound Combo unit	4
Hi-lo mat table	1
Treatment table wedge/tumble form	Gross
Hand dynamometer	1
Shortwave diathermy unit	1
Iontophoresis unit	2
Shuttle leg press	1
Biodex isokinetic dynamometer	1
Functional trainer	1
Pneumatic compression unit	4
Dumbbells (assorted)—1-20 lb (0.5-9 kg)	Gross
Stool	4
Slant board	1
Balance pads (assorted)	Gross
Mechanical traction table	2
Ice machine	1
Game Ready cryotherapy unit	6
HydroWorx 2000 pool with treadmill	1
HydroWorx PolarPlunge pool	1
HydroWorx ThermalPlunge pool	1
Physical measurement tools (e.g., goniometer)	Gross
Paraffin bath	1
AlterG Anti-Gravity Treadmill	1
Bike	1
Biodex balance system	1
Cuff weights (assorted)	Gross
Medicine balls (assorted)—1-25 lb (0.5-9 kg)	Gross
Freezer	1
Stackable steps	Gross
Slide board	Gross

Adapted from T.K. Kelly et al., 2013, *Technical report: An assessment of the Army's tactical human optimization, rapid rehabilitation and reconditioning program* (Santa Monica, CA: Rand Corporation), 1-3, 23-27, 41-43.

Table 22.11 SOF Mental Skills Training Equipment for a Small Facility

Item	Quantity
Nike Sensory Station (also known as SPARQ Sensory Station)	1
Interactive metronome	2
Laptop (large screen, fully equipped for handling all software)	10
Nike Strobe sensory training glasses	30
CogniSens NeuroTracker	1
Dynavision iSpan	1
ProComp Infiniti biofeedback system (software, hardware, headset/visor sensor)	10
emWave2 coherence software	10
Weapon laser simulator (visual acuity skill transfer)	1

Adapted from T.K. Kelly et al., 2013, *Technical report: An assessment of the Army's tactical human optimization, rapid rehabilitation and reconditioning program* (Santa Monica, CA: Rand Corporation), 1-3, 23-27, 41-43.

Table 22.12 Law Enforcement and Public Safety Center Equipment List

	Facility size		
	Large	**Medium**	**Small**
Cardiorespiratory			
Treadmill	4	2	1
Elliptical machine	4	2	1
Cycle ergometer	4	2	1
Rower	4	2	1
Stair-climber	2	1	1
Prehabilitation/rehabilitation			
Foam roller	10	6	2
Exercise ball	10	6	2
Free weight			
Power rack	10	5	3
Adjustable bench	10	5	4
Olympic weight plates up to 45 lb (20 kg)	10 sets	5 sets	3 sets
5-100 lb (2-45 kg) rubber- or vinyl-coated dumbbells	4 sets	3 sets	2 sets
Dumbbell rack	4	3	2
Olympic barbell (revolving sleeve with solid end piece)	10	5	4
5-20 kg (11-44 lb) bumper plates	10	5	4
Hexagon barbell	6	4	3
Nonbouncing medicine ball	20	10	5
Medicine ball	20	10	5
Suspension trainer	10	6	4
4-40 kg (9-88 lb) kettlebells	4 sets	3 sets	2 sets
Bands and tubing			
Mini band	4 each	3 each	2 each
0.5-2 in. (13-51 mm) Superbands	4 each	3 each	2 each
Testing and measuring			
Physician scale	2	1	1
Circumference tape	2	1	1
Sit-and-reach box	4	2	1
Body-fat caliper	4	2	1
Hand dynamometer	4	2	1
HR monitor	2	1	1

Table 22.13 Fire and Rescue and Emergency Personnel Center Equipment List

Size	1 engine (2-5 people)	1 engine, 1 medic (4-8 people)	1 engine, 1 apparatus, 1 medic (6-15 people)
Cardiorespiratory			
Treadmill	1	1	2
Elliptical machine		1	1
Cycle ergometer		1	1
Rower	1	1	1
Stair-climber			1
Rehabilitation/prehabilitation			
Foam roller	1	2	3
Exercise ball	1	1	2
Free weight			
Power rack	1	1	2
Adjustable bench	1	2	2
Olympic weight plates up to 45 lb (20 kg)	1 set	1 set	2 sets
5-100 lb (2-45 kg) rubber- or vinyl-coated dumbbells	1 set	1 set	2 sets
Dumbbell rack	1	1	2
Olympic barbell (revolving sleeve with solid end piece)	1	1	2
5-20 kg (11-44 lb) bumper plates	1 set	1 set	2 sets
Hexagon barbell	1	1	1
Nonbouncing medicine ball	1	1	2
Medicine ball	1	1	2
Suspension trainer	1	1	2
4-40 kg (9-88 lb) kettlebells	1 set	1 set	2 sets
Bands and tubing			
Mini band	1	1	1
0.5-2 in. (13-51 mm) Superbands	1 each	1 each	2 each
Testing and measuring			
Physician scale	2 each	1 each	1 each
Circumference tape	1 each	2 each	2 each
Sit-and-reach box	1 each	2 each	2 each
Body-fat caliper	1 each	2 each	2 each
Hand dynamometer	1 each	2 each	2 each
HR monitor	1 each	2 each	2 each

Table 22.14 Calculating Equipment Space Requirements

Area	Examples	Formula
Prone and supine exercises	Bench press Lying triceps extension	**Formula:** Actual weight bench length (6-8 ft [1.8-2.4 m]) + safety space cushion of 3 ft (0.9 m) *multiplied by* a suggested user space for a weight bench width of 7 ft (2.1 m) + a safety space cushion of 3 ft (0.9 m) **Example 1:** If using a 6 ft weight bench for the bench press exercise, (6 ft + 3 ft) × (7 ft + 3 ft) = 90 ft² **Example 2 (metric approximations):** If using a 2 m weight bench for the bench press exercise, (2 m [bench] + 1 m [safety space]) × (2 m [user space] + 1 m [safety space]) = 9 m²
Standing exercises	Biceps curl Upright row	**Formula:** Actual bar length (4-7 ft [1.2-2.1 m]) + a double-wide safety space cushion of 6 ft (1.8 m) *multiplied by* a suggested user space for a standing exercise width of 4 ft (1.2 m) **Example 1:** If using a 4 ft curl bar for the biceps curl exercise, (4 ft + 6 ft) × 4 ft = 40 ft² **Example 2 (metric approximations):** If using a 1 m curl bar for the biceps curl exercise, (1 m [bar] + 2 m [safety space]) × 1 m (user space) = 3 m²
Standing exercises in a rack	Back squat Shoulder press	**Formula:** Actual bar length (5-7 ft [1.5-2.1 m]) + a double-wide safety space cushion of 6 ft (1.8 m) *multiplied by* a suggested user space for a standing exercise (from a rack) width of 8 to 10 ft (2.4-3 m) **Example 1:** If using a 7 ft Olympic bar for the back squat exercise, (7 ft + 6 ft) × 10 ft = 130 ft² **Example 2 (metric approximations):** If using a 2 m Olympic bar for the back squat exercise, (2 m [bar] + 2 m [safety space]) × 3 m (safety space) = 12 m²
Olympic lifting area	Power clean	**Formula:** Lifting platform height (typically 8 ft [2.4 m]) + perimeter walkway safety space cushion of 4 ft (1.2 m) *multiplied by* a lifting platform width (typically 8 ft [2.4 m]) + perimeter walkway safety space cushion of 4 ft (1.2 m) **Example 1:** (8 ft + 4 ft) × (8 ft + 4 ft) = 144 ft² **Example 2 (metric approximations):** (2.5 m [platform] + 1 m [safety space]) × (2.5 m [platform] + 1 m [safety space]) = 12.25 m²

Reprinted from NSCA, 2016, *Essentials of strength training and conditioning*, 4th ed., edited by G.G. Haff and N.T. Triplett (Champaign, IL: Human Kinetics), 631.

Answers to Study Questions

Chapter 1
1. c, 2. b, 3. c, 4. d

Chapter 2
1. a, 2. d, 3. c, 4. c, 5. b, 6. b

Chapter 3
1. b, 2. c, 3. b, 4. b

Chapter 4
1. d, 2. c, 3. b, 4. a

Chapter 5
1. b, 2. a, 3. c, 4. b

Chapter 6
1. d, 2. b, 3. b, 4. b

Chapter 7
1. a, 2. c, 3. d, 4. d

Chapter 8
1. a, 2. a, 3. d, 4. c

Chapter 9
1. c, 2. c, 3. b, 4. d

Chapter 10
1. d, 2. b, 3. a, 4. d

Chapter 11
1. a, 2. b, 3. b, 4. d

Chapter 12
1. b, 2. a, 3. c, 4. d

Chapter 13
1. a, 2. c, 3. d, 4. b

Chapter 14
1. a, 2. d, 3. a, 4. b

Chapter 15
1. a, 2. a, 3. c, 4. b

Chapter 16
1. b, 2. b, 3. c, 4. b

Chapter 17
1. d, 2. a, 3. a, 4. d

Chapter 18
1. a, 2. d, 3. a, 4. c

Chapter 19
1. b, 2. b, 3. a, 4. b, 5. c

Chapter 20
1. a, 2. b, 3. c, 4. a, 5. a

Chapter 21
1. c, 2. a, 3. a, 4. a

Chapter 22
1. b, 2. b, 3. a, 4. a, 5. b

References

Chapter 1

1. Baur, DM, Christophi, CA, Tsismenakis, AJ, Cook, EF, and Kales, SN. Cardiorespiratory fitness predicts cardiovascular risk profiles in career firefighters. *J Occup Environ Med* 53:1155-1160, 2011.

2. Butler, RJ, Contreras, M, Burton, LC, Plisky, PJ, Goode, A, and Kiesel, K. Modifiable risk factors predict injuries in firefighters during training academies. *Work* 46:11-17, 2013.

3. Cook, G, Burton, L, Hoogenboom, BJ, and Voight, M. Functional movement screening: The use of fundamental movements as an assessment of function—part 2. *Int J Sports Phys Ther* 9:549-563, 2014.

4. Cook, G, Burton, L, Hoogenboom, BJ, and Voight, M. Functional movement screening: The use of fundamental movements as an assessment of function—part 1. *Int J Sports Phys Ther* 9:396-409, 2014.

5. Dennison, KJ, Mullineaux, DR, Yates, JW, and Abel, MG. The effect of fatigue and training status on firefighter performance. *J Strength Cond Res* 26:1101-1109, 2012.

6. Fahy, R, Leblanc, P, and Molis, J. *Firefighter fatalities in the United States, 2013*. Quincy, MA: National Fire Protection Association, 2014.

7. Farioli, A, Yang, J, Teehan, D, Baur, DM, Smith, DL, and Kales, SN. Duty-related risk of sudden cardiac death among young US firefighters. *Occup Med* 64:428-435, 2014.

8. Lehance, C, Binet, J, Bury, T, and Croisier, JL. Muscular strength, functional performances and injury risk in professional and junior elite soccer players. *Scand J Med Sci Sports* 19:243-251, 2009.

9. Lisman, P, O'Connor, FG, Deuster, PA, and Knapik, JJ. Functional movement screen and aerobic fitness predict injuries in military training. *Med Sci Sports Exerc* 45:636-643, 2013.

10. McMaster, DT, Gill, N, Cronin, J, and McGuigan, M. A brief review of strength and ballistic assessment methodologies in sport. *Sports Med* 44:603-623, 2014.

11. Myer, GD, Kushner, AM, Brent, JL, Schoenfeld, BJ, Hugentobler, J, Lloyd, RS, Vermeil, A, Chu, DA, Harbin, J, and McGill, SM. The back squat: A proposed assessment of functional deficits and technical factors that limit performance. *Strength Cond J* 36:4-27, 2014.

12. National Strength and Conditioning Association. Strength & conditioning professional standards and guidelines. July 8, 2009. www.nsca.com/uploaded Files/NSCA/Resources/PDF/Education/Tools_and_Resources/NSCA_strength_and_conditioning_pro fessional_standards_and_guidelines.pdf. Accessed August 22, 2016.

13. National Strength and Conditioning Association. TSAC professionals. www.nsca.com/tsac-professionals. Accessed August 22, 2016.

14. Smith DL. Firefighter fitness: improving performance and preventing injuries and fatalities. *Curr Sports Med Rep* 10: 167-172, 2011.

15. Varvarigou, V, Farioli, A, Korre, M, Sato, S, Dahabreh, IJ, and Kales, SN. Law enforcement duties and sudden cardiac death among police officers in United States: Case distribution study. *BMJ* 349:g6534, 2014.

Chapter 2

1. American College of Sports Medicine (ACSM). *ACSM's Guidelines for Exercise Testing and Prescription*. 9th ed. Philadelphia: Lippincott Williams & Wilkins, 456, 2014.

2. Ashor, AW, Lara, J, Siervo, M, Celis-Morales, C, Oggioni, C, Jakovljevic, DG, and Mathers, JC. Exercise modalities and endothelial function: a systematic review and dose-response meta-analysis of randomized controlled trials. *Sports Med* 45(2):279-296, 2015.

3. Åstrand, P-O, Rodahl, K, Dahl, HA, and Strømme, SB. *Textbook of Work Physiology: Physiological Bases of Exercise*. 4th ed. Champaign, IL: Human Kinetics, 649, 2003.

4. Bunt, JC. Hormonal alterations due to exercise. *Sports Med* 3(5):331-345, 1986.

5. Convertino, VA, Brock, PJ, Keil, LC, Bernauer, EM, and Greenleaf, JE. Exercise training-induced hypervolemia: role of plasma albumin, renin, and vasopressin. *J Appl Physiol* 48(4):665-669, 1980.

6. Davies, CTM. Limitations to the prediction of maximum oxygen intake from cardiac frequency measurements. *J Appl Physiol* 24(5):700-706, 1968.

7. Effron, MB. Effects of resistance training on left ventricular function. *Med Sci Sports Exerc* 21:694-697, 1989.

8. Fleck, SJ, and Kraemer, WJ. *Designing Resistance Training Programs*. 4th ed. Champaign, IL: Human Kinetics, 507, 2014.

9. Galbo, H. *Hormonal and Metabolic Adaptation to Exercise*. New York: Thieme-Stratton, 116, 1983.

10. Gledhill, N, Cox, D, and Jamnik, R. Endurance athletes' stroke volume does not plateau: major advantage is diastolic function. *Med Sci Sports Exerc* 26(9):1116-1121, 1994.

11. Green, DJ, Maiorana, A, O'Driscoll, G, and Taylor, R. Effect of exercise training on endothelium-derived nitric oxide function in humans. *J Physiol* 561(Pt 1):1-25, 2004.

12. Huston, TP, Puffer, JC, and MacMillan, W. The athletic heart syndrome. *N Engl J Med* 313(1):24-32, 1985.

13. Jasperse, JL, and Laughlin, MH. Endothelial function and exercise training: evidence from studies using animal models. *Med Sci Sports Exerc* 48:445-454, 2006.

14. Keul, J, Dickhuth, HH, Simon, G, and Lehmann, M. Effect of static and dynamic exercise on heart volume, contractility, and left ventricular dimensions. *Circ Res* 48(6 Pt 2):I162-I170, 1981.

15. Kjaer, M, and Lange, K. Adrenergic regulation of energy metabolism. In *Sports Endocrinology*. Warren, MP, and Constantini, NW, eds. Totowa, NJ: Humana Press, 181-188, 2000.

16. MacDougall, JD, Tuxen, D, Sale, DG, Moroz, JR, and Sutton, JR. Arterial blood pressure response to heavy resistance exercise. *J Appl Physiol* 58(3):785-790, 1985.

17. Mahler, DA, Shuhart, CR, Brew, E, and Stukel, TA. Ventilatory responses and entrainment of breathing during rowing. *Med Sci Sports Exerc* 23(2):186-192, 1991.

18. Maiorana, A, Thijssen, DHJ, and Green, DJ. Resistance exercise and adaptation in vascular structure and function. In *Effects of Exercise on Hypertension From Cells to Physiological Systems*. Pescatello, LS, ed. Totowa, NJ: Human Press, 137-156, 2015.

19. McCartney, N. Acute responses to resistance training and safety. *Med Sci Sports Exerc* 31(1):31-37, 1999.

20. Morganroth, J, Maron, BJ, Henry, WL, and Epstein, SE. Comparative left ventricular dimensions in trained athletes. *Ann Intern Med* 82:521, 1975.

21. Naylor, LH, O'Driscoll, G, Fitzsimmons, M, Arnolda, LF, and Green, DJ. Effects of training resumption on conduit arterial diameter of elite rowers. *Med Sci Sports Exerc* 38(1):86-92, 2006.

22. Ogawa, T, Spina, RJ, Martin III, WH, Kohrt, WM, Schechtman, KB, Holloszy, JO, and Ehsani, AA. Effects of aging, sex, and physical training on cardiovascular responses to exercise. *Circulation* 86(2):494-503, 1992.

23. Plowman, SA, and Smith, DL. *Exercise Physiology for Health, Fitness, and Performance*. Philadelphia: Lippincott Williams & Wilkins, 2014.

24. Poliner, LR, Dehmer, GJ, Lewis, SE, Parkey, RW, Blomqvist, CG, and Willerson, JT. Left ventricular performance in normal subjects: a comparison of the response to exercise in the upright and supine positions. *Circulation* 62(3):528-534, 1980.

25. Prior, BM, Lloyd, PG, Yang, HT, and Terjung, RL. Exercise-induced vascular remodeling. *Exerc Sport Sci Rev* 31:26-33, 2003.

26. Richardson, RS, Noyszewski, EA, Kendrick, KF, Leigh, JS, and Wagner, PD. Myoglobin O_2 desaturation during exercise. Evidence of limited O_2 transport. *J Clin Invest* 96(4):1916-1992, 1995.

27. Rønnestad, BR, Nygaard, H, and Raastad, T. Physiological elevation of endogenous hormones results in superior strength training adaptation. *Eur J Appl Physiol* 111(9):2249-2259, 2011.

28. Rowland, T. Endurance athletes' stroke volume response to progressive exercise: a critical review. *Sports Med* 39(8):687-695, 2009.

29. Spence, AL, Naylor, LH, Carter, HH, Buck, CL, Dembo, L, Murray, CP, Watson, P, Oxborough, D, George, KP, and Green, DJ. A prospective randomised longitudinal MRI study of left ventricular adaptation to endurance and resistance exercise training in humans. *J Physiol* 589(22):5443-5452, 2011.

30. Spence, AL, Carter, HH, Naylor, LH, and Green, DJ. A prospective randomized longitudinal study involving 6 months of endurance or resistance exercise: conduit artery adaptations in humans. *J Physiol* 591(5):1265-1275, 2013.

31. Stone, MH, Fleck, SJ, Triplett, NT, and Kraemer, WJ. Health- and performance-related potential of resistance training. *Sports Med* 11(4):210-234, 1991.

32. Walther, C, Gielen, S, and Hambrecht, R. The effect of exercise training on endothelial function in cardiovascular disease in humans. *Exerc Sport Sci Rev* 32(4):129-134, 2004.

33. Wilmore, JH, Royce, J, Girandola, RN, Katch, FI, and Katch, VL. Physiological alterations resulting from a 10-week program of jogging. *Med Sci Sports* 2(1):7-14, 1970.

Chapter 3

1. Brenner, HR, and Falls, DL. Neuromuscular junction: neuronal regulation of gene transcription at the vertebrate. In *Developmental Neurobiology*. Lemke, G, ed. Burlington, MA: Pearson, 544-552, 2009.

2. Deschenes, MR, and Leathrum, CM. Gender-specific neuromuscular adaptations to unloading in isolated rat soleus muscles. *Muscle Nerve* (in press), 2016.

3. Duchateau, J, Semmler, JG, and Enoka, RM. Training adaptations in the behavior of human motor units. *J Appl Physiol* 101:1766-1775, 2006.

4. Franzini-Armstrong, C, and Jorgensen, AO. Structure and development of E–C coupling units in skeletal muscle. *Ann Rev Physiol* 56:509-534, 1994.

5. Guadalupe-Grau, A, Fuentes, T, Guerra, B, and Calbet, JA. Exercise and bone mass in adults. *Sports Med* 39:439-468, 2009.

6. Hamill, J, and Knutzen, KM. *Biomechanical Basis of Human Movement*. 2nd ed. Baltimore: Lippincott Williams & Wilkins, 3-103, 2009.

7. Harwood, B, Choi, I, and Rice, CL. Reduced motor unit discharge rates of maximal velocity dynamic contractions in response to a submaximal dynamic fatigue protocol. *J Appl Physiol* 113:1821-1830, 2012.

8. Henneman, E. The size principle: a deterministic output emerges from a set of probabilistic connections. *J Exp Biol* 115:105-112, 1985.

9. Kraemer, WJ, Fleck, SJ, and Deschenes, MR. *Exercise Physiology: Integrating Theory and Application*. Baltimore: Lippincott Williams & Wilkins, 69-102, 2012.

10. Marieb, EN, and Mallatt, J. *Human Anatomy*. 2nd ed. Menlo Park, CA: Benjamin/Cummings, 118-135, 1997.

11. Pascoe, MA, Holmes, MR, Stuart, DG, and Enoka, RM. Discharge characteristics of motor units during long-duration contractions. *Exp Physiol* 99:1387-1398, 2014.

12. Peltonen, H, Hakkinen, K, and Avela, J. Neuromuscular responses to different resistance loading protocols using pneumatic and weight stack devices. *J Electromyogr Kinesiol* 23:118-124, 2013.

13. Pette, D, and Staron, RS. Myosin isoforms, muscle fiber types, and transitions. *Microsc Res Techniq* 50:500-509, 2000.

14. Ranieri, F, and Di Lazzaro, V. The role of motor neuron drive in muscle fatigue. *Neuromuscular Disord* 22:S157-S161, 2012.

15. Schiaffino, S, Gorza, L, Sartore, S, Saggin, L, Ausoni, S, Vianello, M, Gundersen, K, and Lomo, T. Three myosin heavy chain isoforms in type 2 skeletal muscle fibres. *J Muscle Res Cell Motil* 10:197-205, 1989.

16. Schiaffino, S, and Reggiani, C. Fiber types in mammalian skeletal muscles. *Physiological Reviews* 91:1447-1531, 2011.

17. Sherwood, L. *Human Physiology: From Cells to Systems*. Belmont, CA: Brooks/Cole, Cengage Learning, 258-303, 2010.

18. Smerdu, V, and Soukup, T. Demonstration of myosin heavy chain isoforms in rat and humans: the specificity of available monoclonal antibodies used in immuno-histochemical and immunoblotting methods. *Eur J Histochem* 52:179-190, 2008.

19. Stanfield, CL. *Principles of Human Physiology*. 5th ed. Boston: Pearson, 322-358, 2013.

20. Walker, S, Davis, L, Avela, J, and Hakkinen, K. Neuromuscular fatigue during dynamic maximal strength and hypertrophic resistance loadings. *J Electromyogr Kinesiol* 22:356-362, 2012.

21. Widmaier, EP, Raff, H, and Strang, KT. *Vander's Human Physiology: The Mechanisms of Body Function*. 13th ed. New York: McGraw-Hill, 250-279, 2011.

Chapter 4

1. Haff, GG, and Triplett, NT.. *Essentials of Strength Training and Conditioning* 4th ed. Champaign, IL: Human Kinetics, 2016.

2. Barnard, RJ, Edgerton, VR, Furukawa, T, and Peter, JB. Histochemical, biochemical, and contractile properties of red, white, and intermediate fibers. *Am J Physiol* 220(2):410-414, 1971.

3. Cerretelli, P, Ambrosoli, G, and Fumagalli, M. Anaerobic recovery in man. *Eur J Appl Physiol* 34(3):141-148, 1975.

4. Farrell, PA, Wilmore, JH, Coyle, EF, Billing, JE, and Costill, DL. Plasma lactate accumulation and distance running performance. 1979. *Med Sci Sports Exerc* 25(10):1091-1097, 1993.

5. Gastin, PB. Energy system interaction and relative contribution during maximal exercise. *Sports Med* 31(10):725-741, 2001.

6. Gavin, TP, Robinson, CB, Yeager, RC, England, JA, Nifong, LW, and Hickner, RC. Angiogenic growth factor response to acute systemic exercise in human skeletal muscle. *J Appl Physiol* 96(1):19-24, 2004.

7. Gollnick, PD, Bayly, WM, and Hodgson, DR. Exercise intensity, training, diet, and lactate concentration in muscle and blood. *Med Sci Sports Exerc* 18(3):334-340, 1986.

8. Hettinger, T. *Isometrsiche Muskeltraining*. Stuttgart, Germany: Fischer Verlag, 1966.

9. Hickson, RC, Foster, C, Pollock, ML, Galassi, TM, and Rich, S. Reduced training intensities and loss of aerobic power, endurance, and cardiac growth. *J Appl Physiol* 58(2):492-499, 1985.

10. Hickson, RC , Bomze, HA, and Hollozy, JO. Linear increase in aerobic power induced by a strenuous program of endurance exercise. *J Appl Physiol* 42(3):372-376, 1977.

11. Hickson, RC, and Rosenkoetter, MA. Reduced training frequencies and maintenance of increased aerobic power. *Med Sci Sports Exerc* 13(1):13-16, 1981.

12. Hill, AV. Muscular exercise, lactic acid and the supply and utilization of oxygen. *Proceedings of the Royal Society of London. Series B, Containing Papers of a Biological Character* 97(681):84-138, 1924.

13. Hortobagyi, T, Houmard, JA, Stevenson, JR, Fraser, DD, Johns, RA, and Israel, RG. The effects of detraining on power athletes. *Med Sci Sports Exer* 25(8):929-935, 1993.

14. Knuttgen, H, and Kraemer, WJ. Terminology and measurement in exercise performance. *J Appl Sport Sci Res* 1(1):1-10, 1987.

15. Mazzeo, RS, Brooks, GA, Schoeller, DA, and Budinger, TF. Disposal of blood [1-13C]lactate in humans during rest and exercise. *J Appl Physiol* 60(1):232-241, 1986.

16. McArdle, WD, Katch, FI, and Katch, VL. *Exercise Physiology: Nutrition, Energy and Human Performance*. Baltimore: Lippincott Williams & Wilkins, 1-533, 2010.

17. Opie, LH, and Newsholme, EA. The activities of fructose 1,6-diphosphatase, phosphofructokinase and phosphoenolpyruvate carboxykinase in white muscle and red muscle. *Biochem J* 103(2):391-399, 1967.

18. Ronnestad, BR, Nymark, BS, and Raastad, T. Effects of in-season strength maintenance training frequency in professional soccer players. *J Strength Cond Res* 25(10):2653-2660, 2011.

19. Rowell, L. *Human Cardiovascular Control*. New York: Oxford, 327-367, 1993.

20. Rozenek, R, Rosenau, L, Rosenau, P, and Stone, MH. The effect of intensity on heart rate and blood lactate response to resistance exercise. *J Strength Cond Res* 7(1):51-54, 1993.

21. Sjodin, B, and Jacobs, I. Onset of blood lactate accumulation and marathon running performance. *Int J Sports Med* 2(1):23-26, 1981.

22. Tanaka, K, Matsuura, Y, Kumagai, S, Matsuzaka, A, Hirakoba, K, and Asano, K. Relationships of anaerobic threshold and onset of blood lactate accumulation with endurance performance. *Eur J Appl Physiol* 52(1):51-56, 1983.

23. York, JW, Oscai, LB, and Penney, DG. Alterations in skeletal muscle lactate dehydrogenase isozymes following exercise training. *Biochem Biophys Res Commun* 61(4):1387-1393, 1974.

24. Zatsirosky, V, and Kraemer, W. *The Science and Practice of Strength Training*. Champaign, IL: Human Kinetics, 1-167, 2006.

Chapter 5

1. Academy of Nutrition and Dietetics, Dietitians of Canada, and American College of Sports Medicine. Position of the Academy of Nutrition and Dietetics, Dietitians of Canada, and American College of Sports Medicine: nutrition and athletic performance. *J Acad Nutr Diet* 116:501-528, 2016.

2. Adibi, SA, and Morse, EL. Intestinal transport of dipeptides in man: relative importance of hydrolysis and intact absorption. *J Clin Invest* 50:2266-2275, 1971.

3. American College of Sports Medicine. Position stand: exercise and fluid replacement. *Med Sci Sports Exerc* 39:377-390, 2007.

4. American College of Sports Medicine. Position stand: the female athlete triad. *Med Sci Sports Exerc* 39:1867-1882, 2007.

5. American Diabetes Association/Academy of Nutrition and Dietetics (formerly American Dietetic Association). Choose your foods: exchange lists for diabetes (pamphlet). 2008. www.diabetes.org or www.eatright.org.

6. American Dietetic Association. Position of the American Dietetic Association: vegetarian diets. *J Am Diet Assoc* 109:1266-1282, 2009.

7. American Dietetic Association, Dietitians of Canada, and American College of Sports Medicine. Position of the American Dietetic Association, Dietitians of Canada, and American College of Sports Medicine: nutrition and athletic performance. *J Am Diet Assoc* 109:509-527, 2009.

8. Andersen, NE, Karl, JP, Cable, SJ, Williams, KW, Rood, JC, Young, AJ, Lieberman, HR, and McClung, JP. Vitamin D status in female military personnel during combat training. *J Int Soc Sports Nutr* 7:38, 2010.

9. Anderson, JW, Baird, P, Davis, RH, Ferreri, S, Knudtson, M, Koraym, A, Waters, V, and Williams, CL. Health benefits of dietary fiber. *Nutr Rev* 67:188-205, 2009.

10. Anderson, JJB. Minerals. In *Krause's Food, Nutrition, and Diet Therapy*. 11th ed. Mahan, LK, and Escott-Stump, S, eds. Philadelphia: Saunders, 141, 2004.

11. Armstrong, LE, Pumerantz, AC, Roti, MW, Judelson, DA, Watson, G, Dias, JC, Sökmen, B, Casa, DJ, Maresh, CM, Lieberman, H, and Kellogg, M. Fluid, electrolyte, and renal indices of hydration during 11 days of controlled caffeine consumption. *Int J Sport Nutr Exerc Metab* 15:252-265, 2005.

12. Astrup, A, Dyerberg, J, Elwood, P, Hermansen, K, Hu, FB, Jakobsen, MU, Kok, FJ, Krauss, RM, Lecerf, JM, LeGrand, P, Nestel, P, Risérus, U, Sanders, T, Sinclair, A, Stender, S, Tholstrup, T, and Willett, WC. The role of reducing intakes of saturated fat in the prevention of cardiovascular disease: where does the evidence stand in 2010? *Am J Clin Nutr* 93:684-688, 2011.

13. Atkinson, FS, Foster-Powell, K, and Brand-Miller, JC. International tables of glycemic index and glycemic load values: 2008. *Diabetes Care* 31:2281-2283, 2008.

14. Bingham, SA, Day, NE, Luben, R, Ferrari, P, Slimani, N, Norat, T, Clavel-Chapelon, F, Kesse, E, Nieters, A, Boeing, H, Tjønneland, A, Overvad, K, Martinez, C, Dorronsoro, M, Gonzalez, CA, Key, TJ, Trichopoulou, A, Naska, A, Vineis, P, Tumino, R, Krogh, V, Bueno-de-Mesquita, HB, Peeters, PHM, Berglund, G, Hallmans, G, Lund, E, Skeie, G, Kaaks, R, and Riboli, E. Dietary fibre in food and protection against colorectal cancer in the European Prospective Investigation into Cancer and Nutrition (EPIC): an observational study. *Lancet* 361:1496-1501, 2003.

15. Boirie, Y, Dangin, M, Gachon, P, Vasson, M-P, Maubois, J-L, and Beaufrére, B. Slow and fast dietary proteins differently modulate postprandial protein accretion. *Proc Natl Acad Sci* 94:14930-14935, 1997.

16. Bonci, L. *Sports Nutrition for Coaches*. Champaign, IL: Human Kinetics, 36-42, 106, 115-123, 2009.

17. Brand-Miller, J, Wolever, TMS, Foster-Powell, K, and Colagiuri, S. *The New Glucose Revolution: The Authoritative Guide to the Glycemic Index*. New York: Marlowe, 32, 33, 38-40, 2003.

18. Breen, L, and Churchward-Venne, TA. Leucine: a nutrient 'trigger' for muscle anabolism, but what more? *J Physiol* 590(Pt 9): 2065-2066, 2012.

19. Buell, JL, Franks, R, Ransone, J, Powers, ME, Laquale, KM, Carlson-Phillips, A. National Athletic Trainers' Association position statement: evaluation of dietary supplements for performance nutrition. *J Athl Training* 48(1):124, 2013.

20. Buford, TW, Kreider, RB, Stout, JR, Greenwood, M, Campbell, B, Spano, M, Ziegenfuss, T, Lopez H, Landis, J, and Antonio, J. International Society of Sports Nutrition position stand: creatine supplementation and exercise. *J Int Soc Sports Nutr* 4:6, 2007.

21. Burk, A, Timpmann, S, Medijainen, L, Vahi, M, and Oopik, V. Time-divided ingestion pattern of casein-based protein supplement stimulates an increase in fat-free body mass during resistance training in young, untrained men. *Nutr Res* 29:405-413, 2009.

22. Burke, LM, Collier, GR, and Hargreaves, M. Muscle glycogen storage after prolonged exercise: effect of the glycemic index of carbohydrate feedings. *J Appl Physiol* 75:1019-1023, 1993.

23. Burke, LM, Claassen, A, Hawley, JA, and Noakes, TD. Carbohydrate intake during prolonged cycling minimizes effect of glycemic index of preexercise meal. *J Appl Physiol* 85:2220-2226, 1998.

24. Burke, LM, Collier, GR, Broad, EM, Davis, PG, Martin, DT, Sanigorski, AJ, and Hargreaves, M. Effect of alcohol intake on muscle glycogen storage after prolonged exercise. *J Appl Physiol* 95:983-990, 2003.

25. Burke, LM, Hawley, JA, Wong, SHS, and Jeukendrup, AE. Carbohydrates for training and competition. *J Sports Sci*, 2011. doi: 10.1080/02640414.2011.585473.

26. Campbell, B, Kreider, RB, Ziegenfuss, T, La Bounty, P, Roberts, M, Burke, D, Landis, J, Lopez, H, and Antonio, J. International Society of Sports Nutrition position stand: protein and exercise. *J Int Soc Sports Nutr* 4:8, 2007.

27. Cannell, JJ, Hollis, BW, Sorenson, MB, Taft, TN, and Anderson, JJB. Athletic performance and vitamin D. *Med Sci Sports Exerc* 41:1102-1110, 2009.

28. Carlson, A. Consultation and development of athlete plans. In *NSCA's Guide to Sport and Exercise Nutrition.* Campbell, B, and Spano, M, eds. Champaign, IL: Human Kinetics, 223-247, 2011.

29. Chatard, J-C, Mujika, I, Guy, C, and Lacour, J-R. Anemia and iron deficiency in athletes. *Sports Med* 27:229-240, 1999.

30. Clark, N. *Nancy Clark's Sports Nutrition Guidebook.* 4th ed. Champaign, IL: Human Kinetics, 111, 112, 123, 167-181, 2008.

31. Clarkson, PM. Tired blood: iron deficiency in athletes and effects of iron supplementation. Gatorade Sports Science Institute. *Sports Sci Exch* 3:1-5, 1990.

32. Coombes, JS, and McNaughton, LR. Effects of branched-chain amino acid supplementation on serum creatine kinase and lactate dehydrogenase after prolonged exercise. *J Sports Med Phys Fitness* 40:240-246, 2000.

33. Cribb, PJ, and Hayes, A. Effects of supplement timing and resistance exercise on skeletal muscle hypertrophy. *Med Sci Sports Exerc* 38:1918-1925, 2006.

34. Dangin, M, Boirie, Y, Guillet, C, and Beaufrère, B. Influence of the protein digestion rate on protein turnover in young and elderly subjects. *J Nutr* 132:3228S-3233S, 2002.

35. Dangin, M, Guillet, C, Garcia-Rodenas, C, Gachon, P, Bouteloup-Demange, C, Reiffers-Magnani, K, Fauquant, J, Ballévre, O, and Beaufrére, B. The rate of protein digestion affects protein gain differently during aging in humans. *J Physiol* 549(Pt 2):635-644, 2003.

36. Dattilo, M, Antunes, HKM, Medeiros, A, Neto, MN, Souza, HS, Tufik, S, and de Mello, MT. Sleep and muscle recovery: endocrinological and molecular basis for a new and promising hypothesis. *Med Hypotheses* 77:220-222, 2011.

37. Del Coso, J, Estevez, E, and Mora-Rodriguez, R. Caffeine during exercise in the heat: thermoregulation and fluid-electrolyte balance. *Med Sci Sports Exerc* 41:164-173, 2009.

38. DeMarco, HM, Sucher, KP, Cisar, CJ, and Butterfield, GE. Pre-exercise carbohydrate meals: application of glycemic index. *Med Sci Sports Exerc* 31:164-170, 1999.

39. Departments of the Army, Navy, and Air Force. Nutrition standards and education. Army Regulation 40-25, BUMEDINST 10110.6, AFI 44-141. June 15, 2001. http://armypubs.army.mil/epubs/pdf/R40_25.pdf. Accessed May 31, 2015.

40. Donnelly, JE, Smith, B, Jacobsen, DJ, Kirk, E, DuBose, K, Hyder, M, and Bailey, B. The role of exercise for weight loss and maintenance. *Best Pract Res Clin Gastroenterol* 18:1009-1029, 2004.

41. Elsner, KL, and Kolkhorst, FW. Metabolic demands of simulated firefighting tasks. *Ergonomics* 51:1418-1425, 2008.

42. Evans, WJ. Exercise and protein metabolism. *World Rev Nutr Diet* 71:21-33, 1993.

43. FAO/WHO. *FAO Food and Nutrition Paper 51. Protein quality evaluation: report of a joint FAO/WHO expert consultation.* FAO/WHO, 1991.

44. Febbraio, MA, Keenan, J, Angus, DJ, Campbell, SE, and Garnham, AP. Preexercise carbohydrate ingestion, glucose kinetics, and muscle glycogen use: effect of the glycemic index. *J Appl Physiol* 89:1845-1851, 2000.

45. Febbraio, MA, and Stewart, KL. CHO feeding before prolonged exercise: effect of glycemic index on muscle glycogenolysis and exercise performance. *J Appl Physiol* 81:1115-1120, 1996.

46. Fernandes, G, Velangi, A, and Wolever, TM. Glycemic index of potatoes commonly consumed in North America. *J Am Diet Assoc* 105:557-562, 2005.

47. Food and Agricultural Organization of the United Nations (FAO). Carbohydrates in human nutrition. Chapter 1—the role of carbohydrates in nutrition. 1998. www.fao.org/docrep/w8079e/w8079e07.htm. Accessed March 17, 2016.

48. Forrest KY, and Stuhldreher WL. Prevalence and correlates of vitamin D deficiency in US adults. *Nutr Res* 31(1):48-54, 2011.

49. Fuchs, CS, Giovanucci, EL, Colditz, GA, Hunter, DJ, Stampfer, MJ, Rosner, B, Speizer, FE, and Willet, WC. Dietary fiber and the risk of colorectal cancer and adenoma in women. *N Engl J Med* 340:169-176, 1999.

50. Gleeson, M. Can nutrition limit exercise-induced immunodepression? *Nutr Rev* 64:119-131, 2006.

51. Godfrey, RJ, Madgwick, Z, and Whyte, GP. The exercise-induced growth hormone response in athletes. *Sports Med* 33:599-613, 2003.

52. Grandjean, AC, Reimers, KJ, Bannick, KE, and Haven, MC. The effect of caffeinated, non-caffeinated, caloric, and non-caloric beverages on hydration. *J Am Coll Nutr* 19:591-600, 2000.

53. Greenleaf, JE. Problem: thirst, drinking behavior, and involuntary dehydration. *Med Sci Sports Exerc* 24:645-656, 1992.

54. Greer, BK, Woodard, JL, White, JP, Arguello, EM, and Haymes, EM. Branched-chain amino acid supplementation and indicators of muscle damage after endurance exercise. *Int J Sport Nutr Exerc Metab* 17:595-607, 2007.

55. Guezennec, CY, Satabin, P, Duforez, F, Koziet, J, and Antoine, JM. The role of type and structure of complex carbohydrates response to physical exercise. *Int J Sports Med* 14:224-231, 1993.

56. Haller, CA, and Benowitz, NL. Adverse cardiovascular and central nervous system events associated with dietary supplements containing ephedra alkaloids. *N Engl J Med* 343:1833-1838, 2000.

57. Hannan, MT, Tucker, KL, Dawson-Hughes, B, Cupples, LA, Felson, DT, and Kiel, DP. Effect of dietary protein on bone loss in elderly men and women: the Framingham Osteoporosis Study. *J Bone Miner Res* 15:2504-2512, 2000.

58. Hargreaves, M, Costill, DL, Fink, WJ, King, DS, and Fielding, RA. Effect of pre-exercise carbohydrate feedings on endurance cycling performance. *Med Sci Sports Exerc* 19:33-36, 1987.

59. Hargreaves, M, Hawley, JA, and Jeukendrup, A. Pre-exercise carbohydrate and fat ingestion: effects on metabolism and performance. *J Sports Sci* 22:31-38, 2004.

60. Harvard Health Publications, Harvard Medical School. Time for more vitamin D. www.health.harvard.edu/newsweek/time-for-more-vitamin-d.htm. November 25, 2011.

61. Heacock, PM, Hertzler, SR, and Wolf, BW. Fructose pre-feeding reduces the glycemic response to a high-glycemic index starchy food in humans. *J Nutr* 132:2601-2604, 2002.

62. Heaney, RP, and Layman, DK. Amount and type of protein influences bone health. *Am J Clin Nutr* 87(Suppl):1567S-1570S, 2008.

63. Hertzler, S. Expert opinion: probiotics, prebiotics, and human health. In *Perspectives in Nutrition*. 6th ed. Wardlaw, GM, Hampl, JS, and DiSilvestro, RA, eds. New York: McGraw-Hill Higher Education, 98-99, 2004.

64. Hoffman, JR, and Falvo, MJ. Protein—which is best? *J Sports Sci Med* 3:118-130, 2004.

65. Holick, MF. Vitamin D deficiency. *N Engl J Med* 357:266-281, 2007.

66. Hughes, GJ, Ryan, DJ, Mukherjea, R, and Schasteen, CS. Protein digestibility-corrected amino acid scores for soy protein isolates and concentrate: criteria for evaluation. *J Agric Food Chem* 59:12707-12712, 2011.

67. Hulmi, JJ, Lockwood, CM, and Stout, JR. Effect of protein/essential amino acids and resistance training on skeletal muscle hypertrophy: a case for whey protein. *Nutr Metab* 7:51, 2010.

68. Human Performance Resource Center. Protein requirements table. http://hprc-online.org/nutrition/files/ProteinRequirementsTable_120914.jpg/view. Accessed March 29, 2016.

69. Hunter, JE, Zhang, J, and Kris-Etherton, PM. Cardiovascular disease risk of dietary stearic acid compared with other saturated, and unsaturated fatty acids: a systematic review. *Am J Clin Nutr* 91:46-63, 2010.

70. Institute of Medicine. *Dietary Reference Intakes for calcium and vitamin D*. Washington, DC: National Academies Press, 7, 2011. www.nap.edu/catalog/13050/dietary-reference-intakes-for-calcium-and-vitamin-d. Accessed May 31, 2015.

71. Institute of Medicine. *Dietary Reference Intakes for energy, carbohydrate, fiber, fat, fatty acids, cholesterol, protein, and amino acids*. Washington, DC: National Academies Press, 340, 349-361, 389, 391, 423, 464-471, 494-505, 645, 689, 2005.

72. Institute of Medicine. *Dietary Reference Intakes: the essential guide to nutrient requirements*. Washington, DC: National Academies Press, 8, 82-84, 147, 156, 159-161, 328, 330, 537, 2006.

73. Institute of Medicine. *Dietary Reference Intakes for vitamin a, vitamin k, arsenic, boron, chromium, copper, iodine, iron, manganese, molybdenum, nickel, silicon, vanadium, and zinc*. Washington, DC: National Academies Press, 292-313, 2001.

74. Institute of Medicine. *Dietary Reference Intakes for water, potassium, sodium, chloride, and sulfate*. Washington, DC: National Academies Press, 75, 80, 81, 105-115, 133-134, 156, 158, 537, 2005.

75. Ivy, JL. Dietary strategies to promote glycogen synthesis after exercise. *Can J Appl Physiol* 26(Suppl):S236-S245, 2001.

76. Ivy, JL. Regulation of muscle glycogen repletion, muscle protein synthesis and repair following exercise. *J Sports Sci Med* 3:131-138, 2004.

77. Ivy, JL, Goforth HW, Damon BM, McCauley TR, Parsons EC, and Price TB. Early postexercise muscle glycogen recovery is enhanced with a carbohydrate-protein supplement. *J Appl Physiol* 93:1337-1344, 2002.

78. Ivy, JL, Katz, AL, Cutler, CL, Sherman, M, and Coyle, EF. Muscle glycogen synthesis after exercise: effect of time of carbohydrate ingestion. *J Appl Physiol* 64:1480-1485, 1988.

79. Jackman, SR, Witard, OC, Jeukendrup, AE, and Tipton, KD. Branched-chain amino acid ingestion can ameliorate soreness from eccentric exercise. *Med Sci Sports Exerc* 42:962-970, 2010.

80. Jeukendrup, AE. Carbohydrate intake during exercise performance. *Nutrition* 20:669-677, 2004.

81. Karp, JR, Johnston, JD, Tecklenburg, S, Mickleborough, TD, Fly, AD, and Stager, JM. Chocolate milk as a post-exercise recovery aid. *Int J Sport Nutr Exerc Metab* 16:78-91, 2006.

82. Kirwan, JP, Cyr-Campbell, D, Campbell, WW, Scheiber, J, and Evans, WJ. Effects of moderate and high glycemic index meals on metabolism and exercise performance. *Metabolism* 50:849-855, 2001.

83. Kirwan, JP, O'Gorman, D, and Evans, WJ. A moderate glycemic meal before endurance exercise can enhance performance. *J Appl Physiol* 84:53-59, 1998.

84. Koba, T, Hamada, K, Sakurai, M, Matsumoto, K, Hayase, H, Imaizumi, K, Tsujimoto, H, and Mitsuzono, R. Branched-chain amino acids supplementation attenuates the accumulation of blood lactate dehydrogenase during distance running. *J Sports Med Phys Fitness* 47:316-322, 2007.

85. La Bounty, PM, Campbell, BI, Wilson, J, Galvan, E, Berardi, J, Kleiner, SM, Kreider, RB, Stout, JR, Ziegenfuss, T, Spano, M, Smith, A, and Antonio, J. International Society of Sports Nutrition position stand: meal frequency. *J Int Soc Sports Nutr* 8:4, 2011.

86. LaCroix, M, Bos, C, Léonil, J, Airinei, G, Luengo, C, Daré, S, Benamouzig, R, Fouillet, H, Fauquant, J, Tomé, D, and Gaudichon, C. Compared with casein or total milk protein, digestion of milk soluble proteins is too rapid to sustain the anabolic postprandial amino acid requirement. *Am J Clin Nutr* 84:1070-1079, 2006.

87. Lattimer, JM, and Haub, MD. Effects of dietary fiber and its components on metabolic health. *Nutrients* 2:1266-1289, 2010.

88. Lemon, PWR. Is increased dietary protein necessary or beneficial for individuals with a physically active lifestyle? *Nutr Rev* 54:S169-S175, 1996.

89. Lemon, PWR, Tarnopolsky, MA, MacDougall, JD, and Atkinson, SA. Protein requirements and muscle mass/strength changes during intensive training in novice bodybuilders. *J Appl Physiol* 73:767-775, 1992.

90. Levenhagen, DK, Carr, C, Carlson, MG, Maron, DJ, Borel, MJ, and Flakoll, PJ. Postexercise protein intake enhances whole-body and leg protein accretion in humans. *Med Sci Sports Exerc* 34:828-837, 2002.

91. Levenhagen, DK, Greshem, JD, Carlson, MG, Maron, DJ, Borel, MJ, and Flakoll, PJ. Postexercise nutrient timing in humans is critical to recovery of leg glucose and protein homeostasis. *Am J Physiol Endocrinol Metab* 280:E982-E993, 2001.

92. Lewis, S, Burmeister, S, and Brazier, J. Effect of the prebiotic oligofructose on relapse of *Clostridum difficile*-associated diarrhea: a randomized controlled study. *Clin Gastroenterol Hepatol* 3:442-448, 2005.

93. Li, Z, Treyzon, L, Chen, S, Yan, E, Thames, G, and Carpenter, CL. Protein-enriched meal replacements do not adversely affect liver, kidney, or bone density: an outpatient randomized controlled trial. *Nutr J* 9:72, 2010.

94. Lichtenstein, AH, Appel, LJ, Brands, M, Carnethon, M, Daniels, S, Franch, HA, Franklin, B, Kris-Etherton, P, Harris, WS, Howard, B, Karanja, N, Lefevre, M, Rudel, L, Sacks, F, Van Horn, L, Winston, M, and Wylie-Rosett, J. Diet and lifestyle recommendations revision 2006 (AHA scientific statement). *Circulation* 114:82-96, 2006.

95. Macfarlane, S, Macfarlane, GT, and Cummings, JH. Review article: prebiotics in the gastrointestinal tract. *Aliment Pharmacol Ther* 24:701-714, 2006.

96. Manore, M, and Thompson, J. *Sport Nutrition for Health and Performance*. Champaign, IL: Human Kinetics, 69, 2000.

97. Matsumoto, K, Koba, T, Hamada, K, Sakurai, M, Higuchi, T, and Miyata, H. Branched-chain amino acid supplementation attenuates muscle soreness, muscle damage, and inflammation during an intensive training program. *J Sports Med Phys Fitness* 49:424-431, 2009.

98. Maughan, R. Fluid and carbohydrate intake during exercise. In *Clinical Sports Nutrition*. 3rd ed. Burke, LM, and Deakin, V, eds. Sydney, Australia: McGraw-Hill Australia, 395, 2006.

99. McClung, JP, Karl, JP, Cable, SJ, Williams, KW, Young, AJ, and Lieberman, HR. Longitudinal decrements in iron status during military training in female soldiers. *Br J Nutr* 102:605-609, 2009.

100. McGinley, C, Shafat, A, and Donnelly, AE. Does antioxidant vitamin supplementation protect against muscle damage? *Sports Med* 39:1011-1032, 2009.

101. McNaughton, L, and Preece, D. Alcohol and its effects on sprint and middle distance running. *Br J Sports Med* 20:56-59, 1986.

102. Mettler, S, Mitchell, N, and Tipton, KD. Increased protein intake reduces lean body mass loss during weight loss in athletes. *Med Sci Sports Exerc* 42(2):326-337, 2010.

103. Mondazzi, L, and Arcelli, E. Glycemic index in sport nutrition. *J Am Coll Nutr* 28:455S-463S, 2009.

104. Moore, DR, Robinson, MJ, Fry, JL, Tang, JE, Glover, EI, Wilkinson, SB, Prior, T, Tarnopolsky, MA, and Phillips, SM. Ingested protein dose response of muscle and albumin protein synthesis after resistance exercise in young men. *Am J Clin Nutr* 89:161-168, 2009.

105. Morris, CJ, Aeschbach, D, and Scheer, FAJL. Circadian system, sleep, and endocrinology. *Mol Cell Endocrinol* 5:91-104, 2012.

106. Nieman, DC, Henson, DA, McAnulty, SR, McAnulty, LS, Morrow, JD, Ahmed, A, and Heward, CH. Vitamin E and immunity after the Kona Triathlon World Championship. *Med Sci Sports Exerc* 36:1328-1335, 2004.

107. Noakes, TD, Goodwin, N, Rayner, BL, Branken, T, and Taylor, RKN. Water intoxication: a possible complication during endurance exercise. *Med Sci Sports Exerc* 17:370-375, 1985.

108. Ogan, D, and Pritchett, K. Vitamin D and the athlete: risks, recommendations, and benefits. *Nutrients* 5:1856-1868, 2013. www.ncbi.nlm.nih.gov/pmc/articles/PMC3725481.

109. Pagana, KD, and Pagana, TJ. *Mosby's Manual of Diagnostic and Laboratory Tests*. St. Louis: Mosby, 210-212, 1998.

110. Pasiakos, SM, Montain, SJ, and Young, AJ. Protein supplementation in U.S. military personnel. *J Nutr* 143(11):1815S-1819S, 2013. doi: 10.3945/jn.113.175968. [e-pub ahead of print].

111. Paul, GL. The rationale for consuming protein blends in sports nutrition. *J Am Coll Nutr* 28:464S-472S, 2009.

112. Peeling, P, Dawson, B, Goodman, C, Landers, G, and Trinder, D. Athletic induced iron deficiency: new insights into the role of inflammation, cytokines, and hormones. *Eur J Appl Physiol* 103:381-391, 2008.

113. Pennings, B, Boirie, Y, Senden, JMG, Gijsen, AP, Kuipers, H, and van Loon, LJC. Whey protein stimulates postprandial muscle protein accretion more effectively than do casein and casein hydrolysate in older men. *Am J Clin Nutr* 93:997-1005, 2011.

114. Pennington, JAT. *Bowes & Church's Food Values of Portions Commonly Used.* 17th ed. Philadelphia: Lippincott Williams & Wilkins, 299, 1998.

115. Powers, S, Nelson, WB, and Larson-Meyer, E. Antioxidant and vitamin D supplements for athletes: sense or nonsense? *J Sports Sci*, 2011. doi: 10.1080/02640414.2011.602098.

116. Reidy, PT, Walker, DK, Dickinson, JM, Gundermann, DM, Drummond, MJ, Timmerman, KL, Cope, MB, Mukherjea, R, Jennings, K, Volpi, E, and Rasmussen, BB. Soy-dairy protein blend and whey protein ingestion after resistance exercise increases amino acid transport and transporter expression in human skeletal muscle. *J Appl Physiol* 116:1353-1364, 2014.

117. Reidy, PT, Walker, DK, Dickinson, JM, Gundermann, DM, Drummond, MJ, Timmerman, KL, Fry, CS, Borack, MS, Cope, MB, Mukherjea, R, Jennings, K, Volpi, E, and Rasmussen, BB. Protein blend ingestion following resistance exercise promotes human muscle protein synthesis. *J Nutr* 143:410-416, 2013.

118. Reitelseder, S, Agergaard, J, Doessing, S, Helmark, IC, Lund, P, Kristensen, NB, Frystyk, J, Flyvbjerg, A, Schjerling, P, van Hall, G, Kjaer, M, and Holm, L. Whey and casein labeled with L-[1-13C]leucine and muscle protein synthesis: effect of resistance exercise and protein ingestion. *Am J Physiol Endocrinol Metab* 300:E231-E242, 2011.

119. Res, PT, Groen, B, Pennings, B, Beelen, M, Wallis, GA, Gijsen, AP, Senden, JMG, and Van Loon, LJC. Protein ingestion before sleep improves postexercise overnight recovery. *Med Sci Sports Exerc* 44:1560-1569, 2012.

120. Rivière A, Selak M, Lantin D, Leroy F, and De Vuyst L. Bifidobacteria and butyrate-producing colon bacteria: importance and strategies for their stimulation in the human gut. *Front Microbiol* 7:979, 2016.

121. Romijn, JA, Coyle, EF, Sidossis, LS, Gastaldelli, A, Horowitz, JF, Endert, E, and Wolfe, RR. Regulation of endogenous fat and carbohydrate metabolism in relation to exercise intensity and duration. *Am J Physiol Endocrinol Metab* 28:E380-E391, 1993.

122. Ruxton, CH, and Hart, VA. Black tea is not significantly different from water in the maintenance of normal hydration in human subjects: results from a randomized controlled trial. *Br J Nutr* 106:588-595, 2011.

123. Ryan, M. *Sports Nutrition for Endurance Athletes.* 2nd ed. Boulder, CO: Velo Press, 115-123, 2007.

124. Schaafsma, G. The protein digestibility-corrected amino acid score. *J Nutr* 130:1865S-1867S, 2000.

125. Sharp, CPM, and Pearson, DR. Amino acid supplements and recovery from high-intensity training. *J Strength Cond Res* 24:1125-1130, 2010.

126. Shimomura, Y, Inaguma, A, Watanabe, S, Yamamoto, Y, Muramatsu, Y, Bajotto, G, Sato, J, Shimomura, N, Kobayahsi, H, and Mawatari, K. Branched-chain amino acid supplementation before squat exercise and delayed-onset muscle soreness. *Int J Sport Nutr Exerc Metab* 20:236-244, 2010.

127. Shirreffs, SM, and Maughan, RJ. Restoration of fluid balance after exercise-induced dehydration: effects of alcohol consumption. *J Appl Physiol* 83:1152-1158, 1997.

128. Spano, M. Basic nutrition factors in health. In *Essentials of Strength Training and Conditioning.* 4th ed. Haff, GG, and Triplett, NT, eds. Champaign, IL: Human Kinetics, 175-200, 2016.

129. Sparks, MJ, Selig, SS, and Febbraio, MA. Pre-exercise carbohydrate ingestion: effect of the glycemic index on endurance exercise performance. *Med Sci Sports Exerc* 30:844-849, 1998.

130. Stannard, SR, Thompson, MW, and Brand-Miller, JC. The effect of glycemic index on plasma glucose and lactate levels during incremental exercise. *Int J Sport Nutr Exerc Metab* 10:51-61, 2000.

131. Stellingwerf, T, Maughan, RJ, and Burke, LM. Nutrition for power sports: middle-distance running, track cycling, rowing, canoeing/kayaking, and swimming. *J Sports Sci*, 2011. doi: 10.1080./02640414.2011.589469.

132. Stevenson, E, Williams, C, and Biscoe, H. The metabolic response to high carbohydrate meals with different glycemic indices consumed during recovery from prolonged strenuous exercise. *Int J Sport Nutr Exerc Metab* 15:291-307, 2005.

133. Stevenson, EJ, Williams, C, Mash, LE, Phillips, B, and Nute, ML. Influence of high-carbohydrate mixed meals with different glycemic indexes on substrate utilization during subsequent exercise in women. *Am J Clin Nutr* 84:354-360, 2006.

134. Tang, JE, Moore, DR, Kujbida, GW, Tarnopolsky, MA, and Phillips, SM. Ingestion of whey hydrolysate, casein, or soy protein isolate: effects on mixed muscle protein synthesis at rest and following resistance exercise in young men. *J Appl Physiol* 107:987-992, 2009.

135. Tharion, WJ, Lieberman, HR, Montain, SJ, Young, AJ, Baker-Fulco, CJ, DeLany, JP, and Hoyt, RW. Energy requirements of military personnel. *Appetite* 44:47-65, 2005.

136. Tholstrup, T, Hjerpsted, J, and Raff, M. Palm olein increases plasma cholesterol moderately compared with olive oil in healthy individuals. *Am J Clin Nutr* 94:1426-1432, 2011.

137. Thomas, DE, Brotherhood, JR, and Brand, JC. Carbohydrate feeding before exercise: effect of glycemic index. *Int J Sports Med* 12:180-186, 1991.

138. Thomas, DE, Brotherhood, JR, and Miller, JB. Plasma glucose levels after prolonged strenuous exercise correlate inversely with glycemic response to food consumed before exercise. *Int J Sport Nutr* 4:361-373, 1994.

139. Tipton, KD. Nutrition for acute exercise-induced injuries. *Ann Nutr Metab* 57(Suppl 2):43-53, 2010.

140. Tipton, KD, Elliott, TA, Cree, MG, Wolf, SE, Sanford, AP, and Wolfe, RR. Ingestion of casein and whey proteins result in muscle anabolism after resistance exercise. *Med Sci Sports Exerc* 36:2073-2081, 2004.

141. Tokunaga, T. Novel physiological function of fructooligosaccharides. *Biofactors* 21:89-94, 2004.

142. Tomomatsu, H. Health effects of oligosaccharides. *Food Techn* 48:61-65, 1994.

143. U.S. Army. 2011. Soldier life: Meals, Ready-to-Eat. www.goarmy.com/soldier-life/fitness-and-nutrition/components-of-nutrition.html. Accessed November 21, 2011.

144. U.S. Department of Agriculture, Agricultural Research Service. USDA National Nutrient Database for Standard Reference Release 27. www.nal.usda.gov/fnic/foodcomp/search. Accessed May 31, 2015.

145. U.S. Department of Agriculture, Agricultural Research Service, Beltsville Human Nutrition Research Center, and Food Surveys Research Group (Beltsville, MD). Continuing Survey of Food Intakes by Individuals 1994-96, 1998 and Diet and Health Knowledge Survey 1994-96: Documentation (csfii9498_documentation updated.pdf) or Data Files (csfii9498_data.exe). www.ars.usda.gov. Accessed November 27, 2011.

146. U.S. Department of Agriculture and U.S. Department of Health and Human Services. *Scientific report of the 2015 Dietary Guidelines Advisory Committee.* February 2015. https://health.gov/dietaryguidelines/2015-scientific-report/PDFs/Scientific-Report-of-the-2015-Dietary-Guidelines-Advisory-Committee.pdf.

147. Van Hall, G, Shirreffs, SU, and Calbet, JAL. Muscle glycogen resynthesis during recovery from cycle exercise: no effect of additional protein ingestion. *J Appl Physiol* 88:1631-1636, 2000.

148. Volek, JS, Volk, BM, Gomez, AL, Kunces, LJ, Kupchak, BR, Freidenreich, DJ, Aristizabal, JC, Saenz, C, Dunn-Lewis, C, Ballard, KD, Quann, EE, Kawiecki, DL, Flanagan, SD, Comstock, BA, Fragala, MS, Earp, JE, Fernandez, ML, Bruno, RS, Ptolemy, AS, Kellogg, MD, Maresh, CM, and Kraemer, WJ. Whey protein supplementation during resistance training augments lean body mass. *J Am Coll Nutr* 32:122-135, 2013.

149. Wardlaw, GM, Hampl, JS, and DiSilvestro, RA. *Perspectives in Nutrition.* 6th ed. New York: McGraw-Hill, 303, 311, 313, 358-359, 403, 420, 441, 477, 2004.

150. Wee, S-L, Williams, C, Gray, S, and Horabin, J. Influence of high and low glycemic index meals on endurance running capacity. *Med Sci Sports Exerc* 31:393-399, 1999.

151. West, DWD, Burd, NA, Coffey, VG, Baker, SK, Burke, LM, Hawley, JA, Moore, DR, Stellingwerf, T, and Phillips, SM. Rapid aminoacidemia enhances myofibrillar protein synthesis and anabolic intramuscular signaling responses after resistance exercise. *Am J Clin Nutr* 94:795-803, 2011.

152. Williams, MH. *Nutrition for Health, Fitness and Sport.* 6th ed. New York: McGraw-Hill, 84, 142, 2002.

153. Wish, JB. Assessing iron status: beyond serum ferritin and transferrin saturation. *Clin J Am Soc Nephrol* 1:S4-S8, 2006.

154. Wolever, TMS, and Miller, JB. Sugars and blood glucose control. *Am J Clin Nutr* 62(Suppl):212S-227S, 1995.

155. Wood, SM, Kennedy, JS, Arsenault, JE, Thomas, JE, Buch, RH, Shippee, RL, DeMichele, SJ, Winship, TR, Schaller, JP, Montain, S, and Cordle, CT. Novel nutritional immune formula maintains host defense mechanisms. *Mil Med* 11:975-985, 2005.

156. Wu, C-L, Nicholas, C, Williams, C, Took, A, and Hardy, L. The influence of high-carbohydrate meals with different glycaemic indices on substrate utilization during subsequent exercise. *Br J Nutr* 90:1049-1056, 2003.

157. Wu, C-L, and Williams, C. A low glycemic index meal before exercise improves endurance running capacity in men. *Int J Sport Nutr Exerc Metab* 16:510-527, 2006.

Chapter 6

1. Army Regulation 40-25: nutrition standards and education. Washington, DC: Department of the Army, 2001.

2. *2015-2020 Dietary Guidelines for Americans.* Washington, DC: U.S. Department of Health and Human Services and U.S. Department of Agriculture, 2015.

3. Alaunyte, I, Stojceska, V, and Plunkett, A. Iron and the female athlete: a review of dietary treatment methods for improving iron status and exercise performance. *J Int Soc Sports Nutr* 12:38, 2015.

4. Askew, E, Munro, I, Sharp, M, Siegel, S, Popper, R, Rose, M, Hoyt, R, Martin, J, Reynolds, K, and Lieberman, H. Nutritional status and physical and mental performance of special operations soldiers consuming the ration, lightweight, or the meal, ready-to-eat military field ration during a 30-day field training exercise. DTIC Document, 1987.

5. Askew, EW. Nutrition and performance at environmental extremes. DTIC Document, 1994.

6. Askew, EW. Environmental and physical stress and nutrient requirements. *Am J Clin Nutr* 61:631S-637S, 1995.

7. Bailey, DM, and Davies, B. Acute mountain sickness; prophylactic benefits of antioxidant vitamin supplementation at high altitude. *High Alt Med Biol* 2:21-29, 2001.

8. Baker-Fulco, CJ, Bathalon, GP, Bovill, ME, and Lieberman, HR. Military Dietary Reference Intakes: rationale for tabled values. DTIC Document, 2001.

9. Barclay, C, and Loiselle, D. Dependence of muscle fatigue on stimulation protocol: effect of hypocaloric diet. *J Appl Physiol* 72:2278-2284, 1992.

10. Barlas, FM, Higgins, WB, Pflieger, JC, and Diecker, K. 2011 Health related behaviors survey of active duty military personnel. DTIC Document, 2013.

11. Baughman, P, Fekedulegn, D, Andrew, ME, Joseph, PN, Dorn, JM, Violanti, JM, and Burchfiel, CM. Central adiposity and subclinical cardiovascular disease in police officers. *ISRN Obesity*, 2013.

12. Bonci, CM, Bonci, LJ, Granger, LR, Johnson, CL, Malina, RM, Milne, LW, Ryan, RR, and Vanderbunt, EM. National Athletic Trainers' Association position statement: preventing, detecting, and managing disordered eating in athletes. *J Athl Training* 43:80-108, 2008.

13. Bouchama, A, and Knochel, JP. Heat stroke. *N Engl J Med* 346:1978-1988, 2002.

14. Carbone, JW, McClung, JP, and Pasiakos, SM. Skeletal muscle responses to negative energy balance: effects of dietary protein. *Adv Nutr* 3:119-126, 2012.

15. Chao, W-H, Askew, EW, Roberts, DE, Wood, SM, and Perkins, JB. Oxidative stress in humans during work at moderate altitude. *J Nutr* 129:2009-2012, 1999.

16. Chiuve, SE, Sampson, L, and Willett, WC. The association between a nutritional quality index and risk of chronic disease. *Am J Prev Med* 40:505-513, 2011.

17. Costello, RB, Lentino, CV, Boyd, CC, O'Connell, ML, Crawford, CC, Sprengel, ML, and Deuster, PA. The effectiveness of melatonin for promoting healthy sleep: a rapid evidence assessment of the literature. *Nutr J* 13:1, 2014.

18. Costill, DL, Sherman, WM, Fink, WJ, Maresh, C, Witten, M, and Miller, JM. The role of dietary carbohydrates in muscle glycogen resynthesis after strenuous running. *Am J Clin Nutr* 34:1831-1836, 1981.

19. Cuddy, JS, Sol, JA, Hailes, WS, and Ruby, BC. Work patterns dictate energy demands and thermal strain during wildland firefighting. *Wilderness Environ Med* 26:221-226, 2015.

20. de Oliveira, EP, and Burini, RC. Carbohydrate-dependent, exercise-induced gastrointestinal distress. *Nutrients* 6:4191-4199, 2014.

21. Deuster, P. Nutritional armor for the warfighter: can omega-3 fatty acids enhance stress resilience, wellness, and military performance? *Mil Med* 179:185-191, 2014.

22. Flakoll, PJ, Judy, T, Flinn, K, Carr, C, and Flinn, S. Postexercise protein supplementation improves health and muscle soreness during basic military training in Marine recruits. *J Appl Physiol* 96:951-956, 2004.

23. Funderburk, LK, Daigle, K, and Arsenault, JE. Vitamin D status among overweight and obese soldiers. *Mil Med* 180:237-240, 2015.

24. Ganio, MS, Armstrong, LE, Casa, DJ, McDermott, BP, Lee, EC, Yamamoto, LM, Marzano, S, Lopez, RM, Jimenez, L, and Le Bellego, L. Mild dehydration impairs cognitive performance and mood of men. *Br J Nutr* 106:1535-1543, 2011.

25. Gilsanz, V, Kremer, A, Mo, AO, Wren, TA, and Kremer, R. Vitamin D status and its relation to muscle mass and muscle fat in young women. *J Clin Endocr Metab* 95:1595-1601, 2010.

26. Grimaldi, AS, Parker, BA, Capizzi, JA, Clarkson, PM, Pescatello, LS, White, CM, and Thompson, PD. 25(OH) vitamin D is associated with greater muscle strength in healthy men and women. *Med Sci Sports Exerc* 45:157, 2013.

27. Hall, WL. Dietary saturated and unsaturated fats as determinants of blood pressure and vascular function. *Nutr Res Rev* 22:18-38, 2009.

28. Halson, SL. Sleep in elite athletes and nutritional interventions to enhance sleep. *Sports Med* 44:13-23, 2014.

29. Henning, PC, Park, B-S, and Kim, J-S. Physiological decrements during sustained military operational stress. *Mil Med* 176:991-997, 2011.

30. Hill, NE, Stacey, MJ, and Woods, DR. Energy at high altitude. *J R Army Med Corps* 157:43-48, 2011.

31. Holick, MF. Sunlight and vitamin D for bone health and prevention of autoimmune diseases, cancers, and cardiovascular disease. *Am J Clin Nutr* 80:1678S-1688S, 2004.

32. Holick, MF, Binkley, NC, Bischoff-Ferrari, HA, Gordon, CM, Hanley, DA, Heaney, RP, Murad, MH, and Weaver, CM. Evaluation, treatment, and prevention of vitamin D deficiency: an Endocrine Society clinical practice guideline. *J Clin Endocr Metab* 96:1911-1930, 2011.

33. Holick, MF, Binkley, NC, Bischoff-Ferrari, HA, Gordon, CM, Hanley, DA, Heaney, RP, Murad, MH, and Weaver, CM. Guidelines for preventing and treating vitamin D deficiency and insufficiency revisited. *J Clin Endocrinol Metab* 97:1153-1158, 2012.

34. Hoyt, RW, and Honig, A. Body fluid and energy metabolism at high altitude. *Compr Physiol Suppl* 14:1277-1289, 1996.

35. Jeukendrup, A, and Gleeson, M. *Sport Nutrition: An Introduction to Energy Production and Performance.* Champaign, IL: Human Kinetics, 2010.

36. Jitnarin, N, Poston, WS, Haddock, CK, Jahnke, SA, and Day, RS. Accuracy of body mass index-defined obesity status in US firefighters. *Saf Health Work* 5:161-164, 2014.

37. Johnson, NJ, and Luks, AM. High-altitude medicine. *Med Clin North Am* 100:357-369, 2016.

38. Kales, SN, Soteriades, ES, Christophi, CA, and Christiani, DC. Emergency duties and deaths from heart disease among firefighters in the United States. *N Engl J Med* 356:1207-1215, 2007.

39. Kenefick, RW, Hazzard, MP, Mahood, NV, and Castellani, JW. Thirst sensations and AVP responses at rest and during exercise-cold exposure. *Med Sci Sports Exerc* 36:1528-1534, 2004.

40. Larsen, B, Snow, R, and Aisbett, B. Effect of heat on firefighters' work performance and physiology. *J Therm Biol* 53:1-8, 2015.

41. Lieberman, HR, Niro, P, Tharion, WJ, Nindl, BC, Castellani, JW, and Montain, SJ. Cognition during sustained operations: comparison of a laboratory simulation to field studies. *Aviat Space Envir MD* 77:929-935, 2006.

42. Lowden, A, Moreno, C, Holmbäck, U, Lennernäs, M, and Tucker, P. Eating and shift work—effects on habits, metabolism, and performance. *Scand J Work Environ Health* 36:150-162, 2010.

43. Margolis, LM, Crombie, AP, McClung, HL, McGraw, SM, Rood, JC, Montain, SJ, and Young, AJ. Energy requirements of US Army Special Operation Forces during military training. *Nutrients* 6:1945-1955, 2014.

44. Margolis, LM, Murphy, NE, Martini, S, Spitz, MG, Thrane, I, McGraw, SM, Blatny, J-M, Castellani, JW, Rood, JC, and Young, AJ. Effects of winter military training on energy balance, whole-body protein balance, muscle damage, soreness, and physical performance. *Appl Physiol Nutr ME* 39:1395-1401, 2014.

45. Margolis, LM, Rood, J, Champagne, C, Young, AJ, and Castellani, JW. Energy balance and body composition during US Army special forces training. *Appl Physiol Nutr ME* 38:396-400, 2013.

46. McClung, JP, Karl, JP, Cable, SJ, Williams, KW, Nindl, BC, Young, AJ, and Lieberman, HR. Randomized, double-blind, placebo-controlled trial of iron supplementation in female soldiers during military training: effects on iron status, physical performance, and mood. *Am J Clin Nutr* 90:124-131, 2009.

47. McClung, JP, Karl, JP, Cable, SJ, Williams, KW, Young, AJ, and Lieberman, HR. Longitudinal decrements in iron status during military training in female soldiers. *Br J Nutr* 102:605-609, 2009.

48. Milledge, J. Respiratory water loss at altitude. *Newsletter ISMM* 2:5-7, 1992.

49. Mitchell, KS, Mazzeo, SE, Schlesinger, MR, Brewerton, TD, and Smith, BN. Comorbidity of partial and subthreshold PTSD among men and women with eating disorders in the national comorbidity survey—replication study. *Int J Eat Disord* 45:307-315, 2012.

50. Montain, S, and Jonas, WB. Nutritional armor: omega-3 for the warfighter. *Mil Med* 179:1-1, 2014.

51. Montain, SJ. Hydration recommendations for sport 2008. *Curr Sports Med Rep* 7:187-192, 2008.

52. Moore, DR, Robinson, MJ, Fry, JL, Tang, JE, Glover, EI, Wilkinson, SB, Prior, T, Tarnopolsky, MA, and Phillips, SM. Ingested protein dose response of muscle and albumin protein synthesis after resistance exercise in young men. *Am J Clin Nutr* 89:161-168, 2009.

53. Nindl, BC, Barnes, BR, Alemany, JA, Frykman, PN, Shippee, RL, and Friedl, KE. Physiological consequences of US Army Ranger training. *Med Sci Sports Exerc* 39:1380, 2007.

54. Nolte, HW, Noakes, TD, and Nolte, K. Ad libitum vs. restricted fluid replacement on hydration and performance of military tasks. *Aviat Space Environ Med* 84:97-103, 2013.

55. Oliver, SJ, Golja, P, and Macdonald, JH. Carbohydrate supplementation and exercise performance at high altitude: a randomized controlled trial. *High Alt Med Biol* 13:22-31, 2012.

56. Panel NOEIE. Clinical guidelines on the identification, evaluation, and treatment of overweight and obesity in adults. Betheseda, MD: National Heart, Lung, and Blood Institute (NHLBI), 1998.

57. Pasiakos, SM, Austin, KG, Lieberman, HR, and Askew, EW. Efficacy and safety of protein supplements for US Armed Forces personnel: consensus statement. *J Nutr* 143:1811S-1814S, 2013.

58. Pasiakos, SM, Cao, JJ, Margolis, LM, Sauter, ER, Whigham, LD, McClung, JP, Rood, JC, Carbone, JW, Combs, GF, and Young, AJ. Effects of high-protein diets on fat-free mass and muscle protein synthesis following weight loss: a randomized controlled trial. *FASEB J* 27:3837-3847, 2013.

59. Pasiakos, SM, Margolis, LM, and Orr, JS. Optimized dietary strategies to protect skeletal muscle mass during periods of unavoidable energy deficit. *FASEB J* 29:1136-1142, 2015.

60. Poos, MI, Costello, R, and Carlson-Newberry, SJ; Institute of Medicine (US) Committee on Military Nutrition Research. *Nutritional needs in cold and in high-altitude environments*. Washington, DC: National Academies Press, 1999.

61. Raines, J, Snow, R, Nichols, D, and Aisbett, B. Fluid intake, hydration, work physiology of wildfire fighters working in the heat over consecutive days. *Ann Occup Hyg* 59:554-565, 2015.

62. Reynold, RD. Effects of cold and altitude on vitamin and mineral requirements. In *Nutritional Needs in Cold and in High-Altitude Environments: Applications for Military Personnel in Field Operations*. Marriott, BM, and Carlson, SJ, eds. Washington, DC: National Academies Press, Institute of Medicine Committee on Military Nutrition Research, 215-244, 1996.

63. Riddle, JR, Smith, TC, Smith, B, Corbeil, TE, Engel, CC, Wells, TS, Hoge, CW, Adkins, J, Zamorski, M, and Blazer, D. Millennium Cohort: the 2001–2003 baseline prevalence of mental disorders in the US military. *J Clin Epidemiol* 60:192-201, 2007.

64. Rodriguez, NR, DiMarco, NM, and Langley, S. Position of the American Dietetic Association, Dietitians of Canada, and the American College of Sports Medicine: nutrition and athletic performance. *J Am Diet Assoc* 109:509-527, 2009.

65. Rosen, CJ, Abrams, SA, Aloia, JF, Brannon, PM, Clinton, SK, Durazo-Arvizu, RA, Gallagher, JC, Gallo, RL, Jones, G, Kovacs, CS, Manson, JE, Mayne, ST, Ross, AC, Shapses, SA, and Taylor, CL. IOM committee members respond to Endocrine Society vitamin D guideline. *J Clin Endocrinol Metab* 97:1146-1152, 2012.

66. Rosenbloom, C, and Coleman, E. *Sports Nutrition: A Practice Manual for Professionals*. Chicago: Academy of Nutrition and Dietetics, 2012.

67. Sawka, MN, Burke, LM, Eichner, ER, Maughan, RJ, Montain, SJ, and Stachenfeld, NS. American College of Sports Medicine position stand. Exercise and fluid replacement. *Med Sci Sports Exerc* 39:377-390, 2007.

68. Scofield, DE, and Kardouni, JR. The tactical athlete: a product of 21st century strength and conditioning. *Strength Condit J* 37:2-7, 2015.

69. Sharp, MA, Knapik, JJ, Walker, LA, Burrell, L, Frykman, PN, Darakjy, SS, Lester, ME, and Marin, RE. Physical fitness and body composition after a 9-month deployment to Afghanistan. DTIC Document, 2008.

70. Sharp, RL. Role of sodium in fluid homeostasis with exercise. *J Am Coll Nutr* 25:231S-239S, 2006.

71. Smith, DL, Fehling, PC, Frisch, A, Haller, JM, Winke, M, and Dailey, MW. The prevalence of cardiovascular disease risk factors and obesity in firefighters. *J Obes* 908267, 2012.

72. Smith, TJ, White, A, Hadden, L, and Marriott, BP. Associations between mental health disorders and body mass index among military personnel. *Am J Health Behav* 38:529-540, 2014.

73. Stocks, JM, Taylor, NA, Tipton, MJ, and Greenleaf, JE. Human physiological responses to cold exposure. *Aviat Space Environ Med* 75:444-457, 2004.

74. Teucher, B, Olivares, M, and Cori, H. Enhancers of iron absorption: ascorbic acid and other organic acids. *Int J Vitam Nutr Res* 74:403-419, 2004.

75. Tharion, WJ, Lieberman, HR, Montain, SJ, Young, AJ, Baker-Fulco, CJ, Delany, JP, and Hoyt, RW. Energy requirements of military personnel. *Appetite* 44:47-65, 2005.

76. Tharion, WJ, Szlyk, PC, and Rauch, TM. Fluid loss and body rehydration effects on marksmanship performance. DTIC Document, 1989.

77. Umhau, JC, George, DT, Heaney, RP, Lewis, MD, Ursano, RJ, Heilig, M, Hibbeln, JR, and Schwandt, ML. Low vitamin D status and suicide: a case-control study of active duty military service members. *PLoS One* 8:e51543, 2013.

78. U.S. Department of Health and Human Services, Office of Dietary Supplements (ODS). Iron: dietary supplement fact sheet. Washington, DC: National Institutes of Health, 2016.

79. Verde, T, Shephard, RJ, Corey, P, and Moore, R. Sweat composition in exercise and in heat. *J Appl Physiol Respir Environ Exerc Physiol* 53:1540-1545, 1982.

80. Wehr, E, Pilz, S, Boehm, BO, März, W, and Obermayer, PB. Association of vitamin D status with serum androgen levels in men. *Clin Endocrinol (Oxf)* 73:243-248, 2010.

81. Wentz, L, Berry-Cabán, C, Eldred, J, and Wu, Q. Vitamin D correlation with testosterone concentration in us army special operations personnel. *FASEB J* 29:733-735, 2015.

82. Wentz, L, Eldred, J, Henry, M, and Berry-Caban, C. Clinical relevance of optimizing vitamin d status in soldiers to enhance physical and cognitive performance. *J Spec Oper Med* 14:58-66, 2013.

83. Westerterp, KR, and Saris, WH. Limits of energy turnover in relation to physical performance, achievement of energy balance on a daily basis. *J Sports Sci* 9:1-15, 1991.

84. Yanovich, R, Karl, J, Yanovich, E, Lutz, L, Williams, K, Cable, S, Young, A, Pasiakos, S, and McClung, J. Effects of basic combat training on iron status in male and female soldiers: a comparative study. *US Army Med Dep J* Apr-Jun:67-73, 2015.

Chapter 7

1. Albertson, TE, Chenoweth, JA, Colby, DK, and Sutter, ME. The changing drug culture: use and misuse of appearance- and performance-enhancing drugs. *FP Essentials* 441:30-43, 2016.

2. Angell, P, Chester, N, Green, D, Somauroo, J, Whyte, G, and George, K. Anabolic steroids and cardiovascular risk. *Sports Med* 42:119-134, 2012.

3. Baguet, A, Reyngoudt, H, Pottier, A, Everaert, I, Callens, S, Achten, E, and Derave, W. Carnosine loading and washout in human skeletal muscles. *J Appl Physiol* 106:837-842, 2009.

4. Bailey, SJ, Vanhatalo, A, Winyard, PG, and Jones, AM. The nitrate-nitrite-nitric oxide pathway: its role in human exercise physiology. *Eur J Sport Sci* 12:309-320, 2011.

5. Bassini-Cameron, A, Monteiro, A, Gomes, A, Werneck-de-Castro, JP, and Cameron, L. Glutamine protects against increases in blood ammonia in football players in an exercise intensity-dependent way. *Br J Sports Med* 42:260-266, 2008.

6. Bays, HE. Safety considerations with omega-3 fatty acid therapy. *Am J Cardiol* 99:35C-43C, 2007.

7. Bescos, R, Sureda, A, Tur, JA, and Pons, A. The effect of nitric-oxide-related supplements on human performance. *Sports Med* 42:99-117, 2012.

8. Bhasin, S, Cunningham, GR, Hayes, FJ, Matsumoto, AM, Snyder, PJ, Swerdloff, RS, and Montori, VM. Testosterone therapy in adult men with androgen deficiency syndromes: an endocrine society clinical practice guideline. *J Clin Endocrinol Metab* 91:1995-2010, 2006.

9. Bird, SR, Goebel, C, Burke, LM, and Greaves, RF. Doping in sport and exercise: anabolic, ergogenic, health and clinical issues. *Ann Clin Biochem* 53:196-221, 2016.

10. Blomstrand, E. A role for branched-chain amino acids in reducing central fatigue. *J Nutr* 136:544S-547S, 2006.

11. Blomstrand, E, Eliasson, J, Karlsson, HK, and Kohnke, R. Branched-chain amino acids activate key enzymes in protein synthesis after physical exercise. *J Nutr* 136:269S-273S, 2006.

12. Branch, JD. Effect of creatine supplementation on body composition and performance: a meta-analysis. *Int J Sport Nutr Exerc Metab* 13:198-226, 2003.

13. Brown, GA, Vukovich, M, and King, DS. Testosterone prohormone supplements. *Med Sci Sports Exerc* 38:1451-1461, 2006.

14. Brown, GA, Vukovich, MD, Sharp, RL, Reifenrath, TA, Parsons, KA, and King, DS. Effect of oral DHEA on serum testosterone and adaptations to resistance training in young men. *J Appl Physiol* 87:2274-2283, 1999.

15. Buchman, AL. Glutamine: commercially essential or conditionally essential? A critical appraisal of the human data. *Am J Clin Nutr* 74:25-32, 2001.

16. Buford, TW, Kreider, RB, Stout, JR, Greenwood, M, Campbell, B, Spano, M, Ziegenfuss, T, Lopez, H, Landis, J, and Antonio, J. International Society of Sports Nutrition position stand: creatine supplementation and exercise. *J Int Soc Sports Nutr* 4:6, 2007.

17. Candow, DG, and Chilibeck, PD. Potential of creatine supplementation for improving aging bone health. *J Nutr Health Aging* 14:149-153, 2010.

18. Carvalho-Peixoto, J, Alves, RC, and Cameron, LC. Glutamine and carbohydrate supplements reduce ammonemia increase during endurance field exercise. *Appl Physiol Nutr Metab* 32:1186-1190, 2007.

19. Cohen, PA, Bloszies, C, Yee, C, and Gerona, R. An amphetamine isomer whose efficacy and safety in humans has never been studied, beta-methylphenylethylamine (BMPEA), is found in multiple dietary supplements. *Drug Test Anal* 8(3-4):328-333, 2015.

20. Cohen, PA, Maller, G, DeSouza, R, and Neal-Kababick, J. Presence of banned drugs in dietary supplements following FDA recalls. *JAMA* 312:1691-1693, 2014.

21. Cohen, PA, Travis, JC, and Venhuis, BJ. A methamphetamine analog (N,alpha-diethyl-phenylethylamine) identified in a mainstream dietary supplement. *Drug Test Anal* 6:805-807, 2014.

22. Cohen, PA, Travis, JC, and Venhuis, BJ. A synthetic stimulant never tested in humans, 1,3-dimethylbutylamine (DMBA), is identified in multiple dietary supplements. *Drug Test Anal* 7:83-87, 2015.

23. Cury-Boaventura, MF, Levada-Pires, AC, Folador, A, Gorjao, R, Alba-Loureiro, TC, Hirabara, SM, Peres, FP, Silva, PR, Curi, R, and Pithon-Curi, TC. Effects of exercise on leukocyte death: prevention by hydrolyzed whey protein enriched with glutamine dipeptide. *Eur J Appl Physiol* 103(3):289-294, 2008.

24. Demant, TW, and Rhodes, EC. Effects of creatine supplementation on exercise performance. *Sports Med* 28:49-60, 1999.

25. Deuster, PA, Faraday, MM, Chrousos, GP, and Poth, MA. Effects of dehydroepiandrosterone and alprazolam on hypothalamic-pituitary responses to exercise. *J Clin Endocrinol Metab* 90: 4777-4783, 2005.

26. Devries, MC, and Phillips, SM. Supplemental protein in support of muscle mass and health: advantage whey. *J Food Sci* 80(Suppl 1):A8-A15, 2015.

27. Doherty, M, and Smith, PM. Effects of caffeine ingestion on rating of perceived exertion during and after exercise: a meta-analysis. *Scand J Med Sci Sports* 15:69-78, 2005.

28. Evans-Brown, M, Kimergard, A, McVeigh, J, Chandler, M, and Brandt, SD. Is the breast cancer drug tamoxifen being sold as a bodybuilding dietary supplement? *BMJ* 348:g1476, 2014.

29. Ferrando, AA, Sheffield-Moore, M, Yeckel, CW, Gilkison, C, Jiang, J, Achacosa, A, Lieberman, SA, Tipton, K, Wolfe, RR, and Urban, RJ. Testosterone administration to older men improves muscle function: molecular and physiological mechanisms. *Am J Physiol Endocrinol Metab* 282:E601-E607, 2002.

30. Food and Drug Administration. Safety. July 2013. www.fda.gov/Safety.

31. Garcia-de-Lorenzo, A, Zarazaga, A, Garcia-Luna, PP, Gonzalez-Huix, F, Lopez-Martinez, J, Mijan, A, Quecedo, L, Casimiro, C, Usan, L, and del Llano, J. Clinical evidence for enteral nutritional support with glutamine: a systematic review. *Nutrition* 19:805-811, 2003.

32. Givens, ML, and Deuster, P. Androgens and androgen derivatives: science, myths, and theories: explored from a special operations perspective. *J Spec Oper Med* 15:98-104, 2015.

33. Gonzalez, AM, Walsh, AL, Ratamess, NA, Kang, J, and Hoffman, JR. Effect of a pre-workout energy supplement on acute multi-joint resistance exercise. *J Sports Sci Med* 10:261-266, 2011.

34. Green, GA. Drug testing in sport: hGH (human growth hormone). *Virtual Mentor* 16:547-551, 2014.

35. Greenhaff, PL, Bodin, K, Soderlund, K, and Hultman, E. Effect of oral creatine supplementation on skeletal muscle phosphocreatine resynthesis. *Am J Physiol* 266:E725-E730, 1994.

36. Hamazaki, T, Colleran, H, Hamazaki, K, Matsuoka, Y, Itomura, M, and Hibbeln, J. The safety of fish oils for those whose risk of injury is high. *Mil Med* 179:134-137, 2014.

37. Handelsman, DJ. Indirect androgen doping by oestrogen blockade in sports. *Br J Pharmacol* 154:598-605, 2008.

38. Harris, RC, Sale, C, and Delves, SK. Modification of the ergogenic effects of creatine loading by caffeine. *Med Sci Sports Exerc* 37:S348-S349, 2005.

39. Harris, RC, Tallon, MJ, Dunnett, M, Boobis, L, Coakley, J, Kim, HJ, Fallowfield, JL, Hill, CA, Sale, C, and Wise, JA. The absorption of orally supplied beta-alanine and its effect on muscle carnosine synthesis in human vastus lateralis. *Amino Acids* 30:279-289, 2006.

40. Hartgens, F, and Kuipers, H. Effects of androgenic-anabolic steroids in athletes. *Sports Med* 34:513-554, 2004.

41. Haussinger, D, Roth, E, Lang, F, and Gerok, W. Cellular hydration state: an important determinant of protein catabolism in health and disease. *Lancet* 341:1330-1332, 1993.

42. Havenetidis, K. The use of creatine supplements in the military. *J R Army Med Corps*, 2015. [e-pub ahead of print].

43. Healy, ML, Gibney, J, Russell-Jones, DL, Pentecost, C, Croos, P, Sonksen, PH, and Umpleby, AM. High dose growth hormone exerts an anabolic effect at rest and during exercise in endurance-trained athletes. *J Clin Endocrinol Metab* 88:5221-5226, 2003.

44. Hoffman, JR, Landau, G, Stout, JR, Hoffman, MW, Shavit, N, Rosen, P, Moran, DS, Fukuda, DH, Shelef, I, Carmom, E, and Ostfeld, I. Beta-alanine ingestion increases muscle carnosine content and combat specific performance in soldiers. *Amino Acids* 47:627-636, 2015.

45. Hulmi, JJ, Lockwood, CM, and Stout, JR. Effect of protein/essential amino acids and resistance training on skeletal muscle hypertrophy: a case for whey protein. *Nutr Metab* 7:51, 2010.

46. Institute of Medicine. *Nutrient Composition of Rations for Short-Term, High-Intensity Combat Operations.* Washington, DC: National Academies Press, 2005.

47. Jager, R, Purpura, M, Shao, A, Inoue, T, and Kreider, RB. Analysis of the efficacy, safety, and regulatory status of novel forms of creatine. *Amino Acids* 40:1369-1383, 2011.

48. Jones, G. Caffeine and other sympathomimetic stimulants: modes of action and effects on sports performance. *Essays Biochem* 44:109-123, 2008.

49. Joy, JM, Lowery, RP, Wilson, JM, Purpura, M, De Souza, EO, Wilson, SM, Kalman, DS, Dudeck, JE, and Jager, R. The effects of 8 weeks of whey or rice protein supplementation on body composition and exercise performance. *Nutr J* 12:86, 2013.

50. Kadi, F, Eriksson, A, Holmner, S, Butler-Browne, GS, and Thornell, LE. Cellular adaptation of the trapezius muscle in strength-trained athletes. *Histochem Cell Biol* 111:189-195, 1999.

51. Kamimori, GH, McLellan, TM, Tate, CM, Voss, DM, Niro, P, and Lieberman, HR. Caffeine improves reaction time, vigilance and logical reasoning during extended periods with restricted opportunities for sleep. *Psychopharmacology* 232:2031-2042, 2015.

52. Keisler, BD, and Armsey, TD, 2nd. Caffeine as an ergogenic aid. *Curr Sports Med Rep* 5:215-219, 2006.

53. Kendall, KL, Moon, JR, Fairman, CM, Spradley, BD, Tai, CY, Falcone, PH, Carson, LR, Mosman, MM, Joy, JM, Kim, MP, Serrano, ER, and Esposito, EN. Ingesting a preworkout supplement containing caffeine, creatine, beta-alanine, amino acids, and B vitamins for 28 days is both safe and efficacious in recreationally active men. *Nutr Res* 34:442-449, 2014.

54. Knapik, JJ, Steelman, RA, Hoedebecke, SS, Farina, EK, Austin, KG, and Lieberman, HR. A systematic review and meta-analysis on the prevalence of dietary supplement use by military personnel. *BMC Complem Altern M* 14:143, 2014.

55. Ko, R, Low Dog, T, Gorecki, DK, Cantilena, LR, Costello, RB, Evans, WJ, Hardy, ML, Jordan, SA, Maughan, RJ, Rankin, JW, Smith-Ryan, AE, Valerio, LG, Jr, Jones, D, Deuster, P, Giancaspro, GI, and Sarma, ND. Evidence-based evaluation of potential benefits and safety of beta-alanine supplementation for military personnel. *Nutr Rev* 72:217-225, 2014.

56. Kraemer, RR, Durand, RJ, Acevedo, EO, Johnson, LG, Kraemer, GR, Hebert, EP, and Castracane, VD. Rigorous running increases growth hormone and insulin-like growth factor-I without altering ghrelin. *Exp Biol Med* 229:240-246, 2004.

57. Kraemer, WJ, Marchitelli, L, Gordon, SE, Harman, E, Dziados, JE, Mello, R, Frykman, P, McCurry, D, and Fleck, SJ. Hormonal and growth factor responses to heavy resistance exercise protocols. *J Appl Physiol* 69:1442-1450, 1990.

58. Kreider, RB, Ferreira, M, Wilson, M, and Almada, AL. Effects of calcium beta-hydroxy-beta-methylbutyrate (HMB) supplementation during resistance-training on markers of catabolism, body composition and strength. *Int J Sports Med* 20:503-509, 1999.

59. Lansley, KE, Winyard, PG, Bailey, SJ, Vanhatalo, A, Wilkerson, DP, Blackwell, JR, Gilchrist, M, Benjamin, N, and Jones, AM. Acute dietary nitrate supplementation improves cycling time trial performance. *Med Sci Sports Exerc* 43:1125-1131, 2011.

60. Leder, BZ, Rohrer, JL, Rubin, SD, Gallo, J, and Longcope, C. Effects of aromatase inhibition in elderly men with low or borderline-low serum testosterone levels. *J Clin Endocrinol Metab* 89:1174-1180, 2004.

61. Legault, Z, Bagnall, N, and Kimmerly, DS. The influence of oral L-glutamine supplementation on muscle strength recovery and soreness following unilateral knee extension eccentric exercise. *Int J Sport Nutr Exerc Metab* 25:417-426, 2015.

62. Levenhagen, DK, Gresham, JD, Carlson, MG, Maron, DJ, Borel, MJ, and Flakoll, PJ. Postexercise nutrient intake timing in humans is critical to recovery of leg glucose and protein homeostasis. *Am J Physiol Endocrinol Metab* 280:E982-E993, 2001.

63. Lewis, MD, and Bailes, J. Neuroprotection for the warrior: dietary supplementation with omega-3 fatty acids. *Mil Med* 176:1120-1127, 2011.

64. Lieberman, HR, Tharion, WJ, Shukitt-Hale, B, Speckman, KL, and Tulley, R. Effects of caffeine, sleep loss, and stress on cognitive performance and mood during U.S. Navy SEAL training. Sea-Air-Land. *Psychopharmacology* 164:250-261, 2002.

65. Lind, DS. Arginine and cancer. *J Nutr* 134:2837S-2841S, 2853S, 2004.

66. Lindqvist, AS, Moberg, T, Eriksson, BO, Ehrnborg, C, Rosen, T, and Fahlke, C. A retrospective 30-year follow-up study of former Swedish-elite male athletes in power sports with a past anabolic androgenic steroids use: a focus on mental health. *Br J Sports Med* 47:965-969, 2013.

67. Matsumoto, K, Mizuno, M, Mizuno, T, Dilling-Hansen, B, Lahoz, A, Bertelsen, V, Munster, H, Jordening, H, Hamada, K, and Doi, T. Branched-chain amino acids and arginine supplementation attenuates skeletal muscle proteolysis induced by moderate exercise in young individuals. *Int J Sports Med* 28:531-538, 2007.

68. McLellan, TM. Protein supplementation for military personnel: a review of the mechanisms and performance outcomes. *J Nutr* 143:1820S-1833S, 2013.

69. Miller, SL, Tipton, KD, Chinkes, DL, Wolf, SE, and Wolfe, RR. Independent and combined effects of amino acids and glucose after resistance exercise. *Med Sci Sports Exerc* 35:449-455, 2003.

70. Molfino, A, Gioia, G, Rossi Fanelli, F, and Muscaritoli, M. Beta-hydroxy-beta-methylbutyrate supplementation in health and disease: a systematic review of randomized trials. *Amino Acids* 45:1273-1292, 2013.

71. Naclerio, F, Larumbe-Zabala, E, Cooper, R, Allgrove, J, and Earnest, CP. A multi-ingredient containing carbohydrate, proteins L-glutamine and L-carnitine attenuates fatigue perception with no effect on performance, muscle damage or immunity in soccer players. *PloS one* 10:e0125188, 2015.

72. Neff, LM, Culiner, J, Cunningham-Rundles, S, Seidman, C, Meehan, D, Maturi, J, Wittkowski, KM, Levine, B, and Breslow, JL. Algal docosahexaenoic acid affects plasma lipoprotein particle size distribution in overweight and obese adults. *J Nutr* 141:207-213, 2011.

73. Nissen, SL, and Sharp, RL. Effect of dietary supplements on lean mass and strength gains with resistance exercise: a meta-analysis. *J Appl Physiol* 94:651-659, 2003.

74. Ormsbee, MJ, Mandler, WK, Thomas, DD, Ward, EG, Kinsey, AW, Simonavice, E, Panton, LB, and Kim, JS. The effects of six weeks of supplementation with multi-ingredient performance supplements and resistance training on anabolic hormones, body composition, strength, and power in resistance-trained men. *J Int Soc Sports Nutr* 9:49, 2012.

75. Ormsbee, MJ, Thomas, DD, Mandler, WK, Ward, EG, Kinsey, AW, Panton, LB, Scheett, TP, Hooshmand, S, Simonavice, E, and Kim, JS. The effects of pre- and post-exercise consumption of multi-ingredient performance supplements on cardiovascular health and body fat in trained men after six weeks of resistance training: a stratified, randomized, double-blind study. *Nutr Metab* 10:39, 2013.

76. Panton, LB, Rathmacher, JA, Baier, S, and Nissen, S. Nutritional supplementation of the leucine metabolite beta-hydroxy-beta-methylbutyrate (HMB) during resistance training. *Nutrition* 16:734-739, 2000.

77. Park, BS, Henning, PC, Grant, SC, Lee, WJ, Lee, SR, Arjmandi, BH, and Kim, JS. HMB attenuates muscle loss during sustained energy deficit induced by calorie restriction and endurance exercise. *Metabolism* 62:1718-1729, 2013.

78. Plumb, JO, Otto, JM, and Grocott, MP. "Blood doping" from Armstrong to prehabilitation: manipulation of blood to improve performance in athletes and physiological reserve in patients. *Extrem Physiol Med* 5:5, 2016.

79. Potteiger, JA, Carper, MJ, Randall, JC, Magee, LJ, Jacobsen, DJ, and Hulver, MW. Changes in lower leg anterior compartment pressure before, during, and after creatine supplementation. *J Athl Train* 37:157-163, 2002.

80. Rae, C, Digney, AL, McEwan, SR, and Bates, TC. Oral creatine monohydrate supplementation improves brain performance: a double-blind, placebo-controlled, cross-over trial. *Proc Biol Sci* 270:2147-2150, 2003.

81. Rahnema, CD, Crosnoe, LE, and Kim, ED. Designer steroids—over-the-counter supplements and their androgenic component: review of an increasing problem. *Andrology* 3:150-155, 2015.

82. Rennie, MJ, Bohe, J, Smith, K, Wackerhage, H, and Greenhaff, P. Branched-chain amino acids as fuels and anabolic signals in human muscle. *J Nutr* 136:264S-268S, 2006.

83. Rohle, D, Wilborn, C, Taylor, L, Mulligan, C, Kreider, R, and Willoughby, D. Effects of eight weeks of an alleged aromatase inhibiting nutritional supplement 6-OXO (androst-4-ene-3,6,17-trione) on serum hormone profiles and clinical safety markers in resistance-trained, eugonadal males. *J Int Soc Sports Nutr* 4:13, 2007.

84. Roy, BD. Milk: the new sports drink? A Review. *J Int Soc Sports Nutr* 5:15, 2008.

85. Shei, RJ, Lindley, MR, and Mickleborough, TD. Omega-3 polyunsaturated fatty acids in the optimization of physical performance. *Mil Med* 179:144-156, 2014.

86. Shimazaki, M, and Martin, JL. Do herbal agents have a place in the treatment of sleep problems in long-term care? *J Am Med Dir Assoc* 8:248-252, 2007.

87. Shimomura, Y, Yamamoto, Y, Bajotto, G, Sato, J, Murakami, T, Shimomura, N, Kobayashi, H, and Mawatari, K. Nutraceutical effects of branched-chain amino acids on skeletal muscle. *J Nutr* 136:529S-532S, 2006.

88. Sinha-Hikim, I, Roth, SM, Lee, MI, and Bhasin, S. Testosterone-induced muscle hypertrophy is associated with an increase in satellite cell number in healthy, young men. *Am J Physiol Endocrinol Metab* 285:E197-E205, 2003.

89. Smith, AE, Fukuda DH, Kendall KL, and Stout JR. The effects of a pre-workout supplement containing caffeine, creatine, and amino acids during three weeks of high-intensity exercise on aerobic and anaerobic performance. *J Int Soc Sports Nutr* 7:10, 2010.

90. Smith AE, Stout, JR, Kendall, KL, Fukuda, DH, and Cramer, JT. Exercise-induced oxidative stress: the effects of beta-alanine supplementation in women. *Amino Acids* 43:77-90, 2012.

91. Smith, AE, Walter, AA, Graef, JL, Kendall, KL, Moon, JR, Lockwood, CM, Fukuda, DH, Beck, TW, Cramer, JT, and Stout, JR. Effects of beta-alanine supplementation and high-intensity interval training on endurance performance and body composition in men: a double-blind trial. *J Int Soc Sports Nutr* 6:5, 2009.

92. Smith-Ryan, AE, Fukuda, DH, Stout, JR, and Kendall, KL. High-velocity intermittent running: effects of beta-alanine supplementation. *J Strength Cond Res* 26:2798-2805, 2012.

93. Smith-Ryan, AE, Fukuda, DH, Stout, JR, and Kendall, KL. The influence of beta-alanine supplementation on markers of exercise-induced oxidative stress. *Appl Physiol Nutr Metab* 39:38-46, 2014.

94. Smith-Ryan, AE, Ryan, ED, Fukuda, DH, Costa, PB, Cramer, JT, and Stout, JR. The effect of creatine loading on neuromuscular fatigue in women. *Med Sci Sports Exerc* 46:990-997, 2014.

95. Sobolewski, EJ, Thompson, BJ, Smith, AE, and Ryan, ED. The physiological effects of creatine supplementation on hydration: a review. *Am J Lifestyle Med* 5:320-327, 2011.

96. Spillane, M, Schwarz, N, Leddy, S, Correa, T, Minter, M, Longoria, V, and Willoughby, DS. Effects of 28 days of resistance exercise while consuming commercially available pre- and post-workout supplements, NO-Shotgun® and NO-Synthesize® on body composition, muscle strength and mass, markers of protein synthesis, and clinical safety markers in males. *Nutr Metab* 8:78, 2011.

97. Spradley, BD, Crowley, KR, Tai, CY, Kendall, KL, Fukuda, DH, Esposito, EN, Moon, SE, and Moon, JR. Ingesting a pre-workout supplement containing caffeine, B-vitamins, amino acids, creatine, and beta-alanine before exercise delays fatigue while improving reaction time and muscular endurance. *Nutr Metab* 9:28, 2012.

98. Stokes, K. Growth hormone responses to sub-maximal and sprint exercise. *Growth Horm IGF Res* 13:225-238, 2003.

99. Sullivan, PG, Geiger, JD, Mattson, MP, and Scheff, SW. Dietary supplement creatine protects against traumatic brain injury. *Ann Neurol* 48:723-729, 2000.

100. Sureda, A, and Pons, A. Arginine and citrulline supplementation in sports and exercise: ergogenic nutrients? *Med Sport Sci* 59:18-28, 2012.

101. Syrotuik, DG, and Bell, GJ. Acute creatine monohydrate supplementation: a descriptive physiological profile of responders vs. nonresponders. *J Strength Cond Res* 18:610-617, 2004.

102. Tharion, WJ, Shukitt-Hale, B, and Lieberman, HR. Caffeine effects on marksmanship during high-stress military training with 72 hour sleep deprivation. *Aviat Space Environ Med* 74:309-314, 2003.

103. Tipton, KD, Borsheim, E, Wolf, SE, Sanford, AP, and Wolfe, RR. Acute response of net muscle protein balance reflects 24-h balance after exercise and amino acid ingestion. *Am J Physiol Endocrinol Metab* 284:E76-E89, 2003.

104. Trexler, ET, Smith-Ryan, AE, Melvin, MN, Roelofs, EJ, and Wingfield, HL. Effects of pomegranate extract on blood flow and running time to exhaustion. *Appl Physiol Nutr Metab* 39:1038-1042, 2014.

105. Trexler, ET, Smith-Ryan, AE, Stout, JR, Hoffman, JR, Wilborn, CD, Sale, C, Kreider, RB, Jager, R, Earnest, CP, Bannock, L, Campbell, B, Kalman, D, Ziegenfuss, TN, and Antonio, J. International society of sports nutrition position stand: beta-alanine. *J Int Soc Sports Nutr* 12:30, 2015.

106. Twycross-Lewis, R, Kilduff, LP, Wang, G, and Pitsiladis, YP. The effects of creatine supplementation on thermoregulation and physical (cognitive) performance: a review and future prospects. *Amino Acids* 48:1843-1855, 2016.

107. U.S. Anti-Doping Agency. High risk dietary supplement list. Accessed July 2, 2015. www.supplement411.org/hrl/.

108. Van Gammeren, D, Falk, D, and Antonio, J. Effects of norandrostenedione and norandrostenediol in resistance-trained men. *Nutrition* 18:734-737, 2002.

109. Van Marken Lichtenbelt, WD, Hartgens, F, Vollaard, NB, Ebbing, S, and Kuipers, H. Bodybuilders' body composition: effect of nandrolone decanoate. *Med Sci Sports Exerc* 36:484-489, 2004.

110. Wallace, MB, Lim, J, Cutler, A, and Bucci, L. Effects of dehydroepiandrosterone vs androstenedione supplementation in men. *Med Sci Sports Exerc* 31:1788-1792, 1999.

111. Walsh, AL, Gonzalez, AM, Ratamess, NA, Kang, J, and Hoffman, JR. Improved time to exhaustion following ingestion of the energy drink Amino Impact. *J Int Soc Sports Nutr* 7:14, 2010.

112. Wilmore, D. Enteral and parenteral arginine supplementation to improve medical outcomes in hospitalized patients. *J Nutr* 134:2863S-2867S, 2895S, 2004.

113. World Anti-Doping Agency. The 2015 Prohibited List. September 20, 2014. http://list.wada-ama.org/. Accessed July 1, 2015.

114. Yarasheski, KE, Campbell, JA, Smith, K, Rennie, MJ, Holloszy, JO, and Bier, DM. Effect of growth hormone and resistance exercise on muscle growth in young men. *Am J Physiol* 262:E261-E267, 1992.

Chapter 8

1. Enrolled Acts and Resolutions of Congress, 1789-1996. An Act to Regulate and Improve the Civil Service of the United States, January 16, 1883. https://catalog.archives.gov/id/5730369. Accessed July 1, 2015.

2. International Association of Fire Chiefs (IAFC). Candidate Physical Ability Test (CPAT). www.iafc.org/Operations/content.cfm?ItemNumber=1174. Accessed Feb 18, 2015.

3. War Department Field Manual FM 21-20. *Physical Training*. Washington, DC: United States Government Printing Office, 1946.

4. Department of the Army Field Manual FM 21-20. *Physical Training*. Washington, DC: Headquarters, Department of the Army, 1957.

5. Department of the Army Field Manual 21-20. *Physical Readiness Training*. Washington, DC: Headquarters, Department of the Army, 1973.

6. Fitness and Amateur Sport and Canadian Association of Sports Sciences. *Canadian Standardized Test of Fitness (CSTF): Operations Manual (for 15 to 69 Years of Age)*. Government of Canada: Fitness and Amateur Sport, 1986.

7. *2nd Blue Ribbon Panel on Military Physical Readiness: Military Physical Performance Testing*. Norfolk, VA: NSCA, 2013.

8. Defence Technology Agency (DTA). Case study: Land Combat Test (LCFT) for the New Zealand Army. www.dta.mil.nz/?page_id=1193. Accessed May 18, 2016.

9. Tat, OH. New IPPT motivates SAF servicemen and women to do well and keep fit. www.mindef.gov.sg/imindef/resourcelibrary/cyberpioneer/topics/articles/news/2015/mar/09mar15_news.html. Accessed May 18, 2016.

10. HIPAA for Professionals. www.hhs.gov/hipaa/for-professionals/index.html. Accessed May 5, 2016.

11. Amiri-Khorasani, M, Sahebozamani, M, Tabrizi, KG, and Yusof, AB. Acute effect of different stretching methods on Illinois agility test in soccer players. *J Strength Cond Res* 24:2698-2704, 2010.

12. Bilzon, JL, Scarpello, EG, Bilzon, E, and Allsopp, AJ. Generic task-related occupational requirements for Royal Naval personnel. *Occup Med* 52:503-510, 2002.

13. Bonneau, J, and Brown, J. Physical ability, fitness and police work. *J Clin Forensic Med* 2:157-164, 1995.

14. Crowder, TA, Ferrara, AL, and Levinbook, MD. Creation of a criterion-referenced Military Optimal Performance Challenge. *Mil Med* 178:1085-1101, 2013.

15. Deci, EL, and Ryan, RM. Conceptualizations of intrinsic motivation and self-determination. In *Intrinsic Motivation and Self-Determination in Human Behavior.* Deci, EL, and Ryan, RM, eds. New York: Plenum, 3-40, 1985. http://link.springer.com/book/10.1007%2F978-1-4899-2271-7.

16. Doyle, T, Billing, D, Drain, J, Linnane, D, Carr, A, Hann, D, Hunt, A, Fogarty, A, Carstairs, G, Silk, A, Best, S, Tofari, P, Savage, R, and Lewis, M. *Physical Employment Standards (PES) for Australian Defence Force Employment Categories Currently Restricted to Women, Part B: Physical Employment Assessments and Standards.* Victoria, Australia: Human Protection and Performance Division, Australian Department of Defence, 2015.

17. Gillet, N, Berjot, S, and Gobancé, L. A motivational model of performance in the sport domain. *Eur J Sport Sci* 9:151-158, 2009.

18. Gledhill, N, and Jamnik, VK. Characterization of the physical demands of firefighting. *Can J Sport Sci* 17:207-213, 1992.

19. Gomez-Merino, D, Drogou, C, Chennaoui, M, Tiollier, E, Mathieu, J, and Guezennec, CY. Effects of combined stress during intense training on cellular immunity, hormones and respiratory infections. *Neuroimmunomodulation* 12:164-172, 2005.

20. Gould, D. Goal setting for peak performance. In *Applied Sport Psychology.* 2nd ed. Williams, JM, ed. Mountain View, CA: Mayfield, 158, 1993.

21. Greenberg, GJ, and Berger, RA. A model to assess one's ability to apprehend and restrain a resisting suspect in police work. *J Occup Med* 25:809-813, 1983.

22. Gumieniak, RJ, Jamnik, VK, and Gledhill, N. Physical fitness bona fide occupational requirements for safety-related physically demanding occupations; test development considerations. *Health and Fitness Journal of Canada* 4:47-52, 2004.

23. Gumieniak, RJ, Jamnik, VK, and Gledhill, N. Catalog of Canadian fitness screening protocols for public safety occupations that qualify as a bona fide occupational requirement. *J Strength Cond Res* 27:1168-1173, 2013.

24. Gunther, CM, Burger, A, Rickert, M, Crispin, A, and Schulz, CU. Grip strength in healthy Caucasian adults: reference values. *J Hand Surg Am* 33:558-565, 2008.

25. Gutman, A, Koppes, LL, and Vodanovich, SJ. *EEO Law and Personnel Practices.* Florence, KY: Psychology Press, 443, 70-71, 2011.

26. Hauschild, V, DeGroot, D, Hall, S, Deaver, K, Hauret, K, Grier, T, and Jones, B. *Correlations Between Physical Fitness Tests and Performance of Military Tasks: A Systematic Review and Meta-Analyses.* Aberdeen Proving Ground, MD: Army Public Health Command, 2014.

27. National Fire Protection Association (NFPA). *NFPA 1583: Standard on Health-Related Fitness Programs for Fire Department Members.* Quincy, MA: National Fire Protection Association, 2015.

28. Heyward, VH, Gibson, AL, eds. Principles of assessment, prescription, and exercise program adherence. In *Advanced Fitness Assessment and Exercise Prescription.* 6th ed. Champaign, IL: Human Kinetics, 40-43, 2014.

29. Jaenen, S. Identification of common military tasks: optimizing operational physical fitness. In *RTO-TR-HFM-080—Optimizing Operational Physical Fitness.* NSaT Organization, ed. NATO Science and Technology Organization, 342, 2009. www.cso.nato.int/pubs/rdp.asp?RDP=RTO-TR-HFM-080.

30. Köhler, O. Kraftleistungen bei Einzel-und Gruppenabeit [Physical performance in individual and group situations]. *Industrielle Psychotechnik* 3:274-282, 1926.

31. Köhler, O. Über den Gruppenwirkungsgrad der menschlichen Körperarbeit und die Bedingung optimaler Kollektivkraftreaktion [Group efficiency in physical work and the condition of optimal collective strength reaction]. *Industrielle Psychotechnik* 4:209-226, 1927.

32. Locke, EA, and Latham, GP. Building a practically useful theory of goal setting and task motivation: a 35-year odyssey. *Am Psychol* 57:705-717, 2002.

33. Mazzetti, SA, Kraemer, WJ, Volek, JS, Duncan, ND, Ratamess, NA, Gomez, AL, Newton, RU, Hakkinen, K, and Fleck, SJ. The influence of direct supervision of resistance training on strength performance. *Med Sci Sports Exerc* 32:1175-1184, 2000.

34. McGuigan, M. Administration, scoring, and interpretation of selected tests. In *Essentials of Strength Training and Conditioning.* 4th ed. Haff, GG, and Triplett, NT, eds. Champaign, IL: Human Kinetics, 252-253, 261, 350-390, 2016.

35. Michaelides, MA, Parpa, KM, Henry, LJ, Thompson, GB, and Brown, BS. Assessment of physical fitness aspects and their relationship to firefighters' job abilities. *J Strength Cond Res* 25: 956-965, 2011.

36. National Fire Protection Association (NFPA) and Technical Committee on Fire Fighter Professional Q. *NFPA 1001: Fire Fighter Professional Qualifications.* Quincy, MA: National Fire Protection Association, 1974.

37. Palmer, B, Carroll, JW, and Mirza, AT. *A Review of Firefighter Physical Fitness/Wellness Programs: Options for the Military.* Brooks Air Force Base, TX: Do Defense, 1998.

38. Payne, W, and Harvey, J. A framework for the design and development of physical employment tests and standards. *Ergonomics* 53:858-871, 2010.

39. Raycroft, JE. *Mass Physical Training.* Washington, DC: U.S. Infantry Association, 6-9, 1920.

40. Rayson, MP. *Gender and Bio-Medical Aspects of Performance in the Infantry and Royal Armoured Corps.* AHS (Army), ed. Farnham, UK: Optimal Performance Limited, 76, 2000.

41. Reilly, T. Canada's Physical Fitness Standard for the Land Force: a global comparison. *Canadian Army J* 13(2):12, 2010.

42. Reynolds, K, Cosio-Lima, L, Bovill, M, Tharion, W, Williams, J, and Hodges T. A comparison of injuries, limited-duty days, and injury risk factors in infantry, artillery, construction engineers, and special forces soldiers. *Mil Med* 174:702-708, 2009.

43. Rhea, MR, Alvar, BA, and Gray, R. Physical fitness and job performance of firefighters. *J Strength Cond Res* 18:348-352, 2004.

44. Ricciardi, R, Deuster, PA, and Talbot, LA. Effects of gender and body adiposity on physiological responses to physical work while wearing body armor. *Mil Med* 172:743-748, 2007.

45. Rodiguez, A, Sanchez, J, Rodriguez-Marroyo, JA, and Villa, JG. Effects of seven weeks of static hamstring stretching on flexibility and sprint performance in young soccer players according to their playing position. *J Sports Med Phys Fitness*, 2015. [e-pub ahead of print].

46. Scofield, DE, and Kardouni, JR. The tactical athlete: a product of 21st century strength and conditioning. *Strength Cond J* 37:2-7, 2015.

47. Shephard, RJ, and Bonneau, J. Assuring gender equity in recruitment standards for police officers. *Can J Appl Physiol* 27:263-295, 2002.

48. Sothmann, MS, Gebhardt, DL, Baker, TA, Kastello, GM, and Sheppard, VA. Performance requirements of physically strenuous occupations: validating minimum standards for muscular strength and endurance. *Ergonomics* 47:864-875, 2004.

49. Spiering, BA, Walker, LA, Hendrickson, NR, Simpson, K, Harman, EA, Allison, SC, and Sharp, MA. Reliability of military-relevant tests designed to assess soldier readiness for occupational and combat-related duties. *Mil Med* 177:663-668, 2012.

50. Spivoc, M. Elements of clarification on the Canadian Armed Forces' proposed FORCE Incentive Program: a response to Major Draho's "An Alternate View of Incentivized Fitness in the Canadian Armed Forces." *Canadian Military J* 15:55-58, 2015.

51. Sporis, G, Jukic, I, Bok, D, Vuleta, D, Jr, and Harasin, D. Impact of body composition on performance in fitness tests among personnel of the Croatian navy. *Coll Antropol* 35:335-339, 2011.

52. Szivak, TK, and Kraemer, WJ. Physiological readiness and resilience: pillars of military preparedness. *J Strength Cond Res* 29(Suppl 11):S34-S39, 2015.

53. Warr, BJ, Alvar, BA, Dodd, DJ, Heumann, KJ, Mitros, MR, Keating, CJ, and Swan, PD. How do they compare? An assessment of predeployment fitness in the Arizona National Guard. *J Strength Cond Res* 25:2955-2962, 2011.

54. Weinberg, R, and Butt, J. Goal-setting and sport performance: research findings and practical applications. In *Routledge Companion to Sport and Exercise Psychology: Global Perspectives and Fundamental Concepts.* Papaioannou, AG, and Hackfort, D, eds. New York: Routledge, 343-355, 2014.

55. Williams, AG, Rayson, MP, and Jones, DA. Training diagnosis for a load carriage task. *J Strength Cond Res* 18:30-34, 2004.

56. Zeno, SA, Purvis, D, Crawford, C, Lee, C, Lisman, P, and Deuster, PA. Warm-ups for military fitness testing: rapid evidence assessment of the literature. *Med Sci Sports Exerc* 45:1369-1376, 2013.

Chapter 9

1. Abel, MG, Mortara, AJ, and Pettitt, RW. Evaluation of circuit-training intensity for firefighters. *J Strength Cond Res* 25:2895-2901, 2011.

2. Abel, MG, Sell, K, and Dennison, K. Design and implementation of fitness programs for firefighters. *Strength Cond J* 33:31-42, 2011.

3. Ahtiainen, JP, Pakarinen, A, Alen, M, Kraemer, WJ, and Häkkinen, K. Short vs. long rest period between the sets in hypertrophic resistance training: influence on muscle strength, size, and hormonal adaptations in trained men. *J Strength Cond Res* 19:572-582, 2005.

4. Anderson, KG, and Behm, DG. Maintenance of EMG activity and loss of force output with instability. *J Strength Cond Res* 18:637-640, 2004.

5. Augustsson, J, Thomee, R, Hornstedt, P, Lindblom, J, Karlsson, J, and Grimby, G. Effect of pre-exhaustion exercise on lower-extremity muscle activation during a leg press exercise. *J Strength Cond Res* 17:411-416, 2003.

6. Baker, D, and Newton, RU. Acute effect on power output of alternating an agonist and antagonist muscle exercise during complex training. *J Strength Cond Res* 19:202-205, 2005.

7. Barnard, RJ, and Duncan, HW. Heart rate and ECG responses of firefighters. *J Occup Med* 17:247-250, 1975.

8. Behm, DG, and Anderson, KG. The role of instability with resistance training. *J Strength Cond Res* 20:716-722, 2006.

9. Behm, DG, and Sale, DG. Intended rather than actual movement velocity determines the velocity-specific training response. *J Appl Physiol* 74:359-368, 1993.

10. Blackburn, JR, and Morrissey, MC. The relationship between open and closed kinetic chain strength of the lower limb and jumping performance. *J Orthop Sports Phys Ther* 27:430-435, 1998.

11. Boyer, BT. A comparison of the effects of three strength training programs on women. *J Appl Sports Sci Res* 4:88-94, 1990.

12. Brandl, SG, and Stroshine, MS. The physical hazards of police work revisited. *Police Q* 15:262-282, 2012.

13. Clark, JG, Jackson, MS, Schaeffer, PM, and Sharpe, EG. Training SWAT teams: implications for improving tactical units. *J Crim Just* 28:407-413, 2000.

14. Cormie, P, McCaulley, GO, and McBride, JM. Power versus strength-power jump squat training: influence on the load-power relationship. *Med Sci Sports Exerc* 39:996-1003, 2007.

15. Cressey, E, Hartman, B, and Robertson, M. *Assess and Correct: Breaking Barriers to Unlock Performance*. Indianapolis: Assess and Correct, 61-137, 2009.

16. Cuddy, JS, Slivka, DR, Hailes, WS, and Ruby, BC. Factors of trainability and predictability associated with military physical fitness test success. *J Strength Cond Res* 25:3486-3494, 2011.

17. DeLorme, TW, and Watkins, AL. Techniques of progressive resistance exercise. *Arch Phys Med Rehabil* 29:263-273, 1948.

18. Gledhill, N, and Jamnik, VK. Characterization of the physical demands of firefighting. *Can J Sport Sci* 17:207-213, 1992.

19. Haff, GG, Berninger, D, and Caulfield, S. Exercise technique for alternative modes and nontraditional implement training. In *Essentials of Strength Training and Conditioning*. 4th ed. Haff, GG, and Triplett, NT, eds. Champaign, IL: Human Kinetics, 409-438, 2016.

20. Harman, EA, Gutekunst, DJ, Frykman, PN, Nindl, BC, Alemany, JA, Mello, RP, and Sharp, MA. Effects of two different eight-week training programs on military physical performance. *J Strength Cond Res* 22:524-534, 2008.

21. Harris, NK, Woulfe, CJ, Wood, MR, Dulson, DK, Gluchowski, AK, and Keogh, JB. Acute physiological responses to strongman training compared to traditional strength training. *J Strength Cond Res* 30:1397-1408, 2016.

22. Hatfield, DL, Kraemer, WJ, Spiering, BA, Hakkinen, K, Volek, JS, Shimano, T, Spreuwenberg, LP, Silvestre, R, Vingren, JL, Fragala, MS, Gomez, AL, Fleck, SJ, Newton, RU, and Maresh, CM. The impact of velocity of movement on performance factors in resistance exercise. *J Strength Cond Res* 20:760-766, 2006.

23. Henning, PC, Khamoui, AV, and Brown, LE. Preparatory strength and endurance training for U.S. Army basic combat training. *Strength Cond J* 33:48-57, 2011.

24. Hoffman, JR, Kraemer, WJ, Fry, AC, Deschenes, M, and Kemp, DM. The effect of self-selection for frequency of training in a winter conditioning program for football. *J Appl Sport Sci Res* 3:76-82, 1990.

25. Issurin, VB. New horizons for the methodology and physiology of training periodization. *Sports Med* 40:189-206, 2010.

26. Jamnik, VK, Thomas, SG, Shaw, JA, and Gledhill, N. Identification and characterization of the critical physically demanding tasks encountered by correctional officers. *Appl Physiol Nutr Metab* 35:45-48, 2010.

27. Jones, EJ, Bishop, PA, Woods, AK, and Green, JM. Cross-sectional area and muscular strength: a brief review. *Sports Med* 38:987-994, 2008.

28. Jones, K, Hunter, G, Fleisig, G, Escamilla, R, and Lemak, L. The effects of compensatory acceleration on upperbody strength and power in collegiate football players. *J Strength Cond Res* 13:99-105, 1999.

29. Kawamori, N, Crum, AJ, Blumert, PA, Kulik, JR, Childers, JT, Wood, JA, Stone, MH, and Haff, GG. Influence of different relative intensities on power output during the hang power clean: identification of the optimal load. *J Strength Cond Res* 19:698-708, 2005.

30. Kawamori, N, and Haff, GG. The optimal training load for the development of muscular power. *J Strength Cond Res* 18:675-684, 2004.

31. Knapik, JJ. The influence of physical fitness training on the manual material handling capability of women. *Appl Ergon* 28:339-345, 1997.

32. Knapik, JJ, Reynolds, KL, and Harman, E. Soldier load carriage: historical, physiological, biomechanical, and medical aspects. *Mil Med* 169:45-56, 2004.

33. Kraemer, WJ, Mazzetti, SA, Nindl, BC, Gotshalk, LA, Volek, JS, Bush, JA, Marx, JO, Dohi, K, Gomez, AL, Miles, M, Fleck, SJ, Newton, RU, and Häkkinen, K. Effect of resistance training on women's strength/power and occupational performances. *Med Sci Sports Exerc* 33:1011-1025, 2001.

34. Kraemer, WJ, Patton, JF, Gordon, SE, Harman, EA, Deschenes, MR, Reynolds, K, Newton, RU, Triplett, NT, and Dziados, JE. Compatibility of high-intensity strength and endurance training on hormonal and skeletal muscle adaptations. *J Appl Physiol* 78:976-989, 1995.

35. Kraemer, WJ, and Ratamess, NA. Fundamentals of resistance training: progression and exercise prescription. *Med Sci Sport Exerc* 36:674-678, 2004.

36. Kraemer, WJ, and Szivak, TK. Strength training for the warfighter. *J Strength Cond Res* 26:S107-S118, 2012.

37. Kraemer, WJ, Vescovi, JD, Volek, JS, Nindl, BC, Newton, RU, Patton, JF, Dziados, JE, French, DN, and Häkkinen, K. Effects of concurrent resistance and aerobic training on load-bearing performance and the Army Physical Fitness Test. *Mil Med* 169:994-1000, 2004.

38. Krieger, JW. Single versus multiple sets of resistance exercise: a meta-regression. *J Strength Cond Res* 23:1890-1901, 2009.

39. Kuruganti, U, Parker, P, Rickards, J, Tingley, M, and Sexsmith, J. Bilateral isokinetic training reduces the bilateral leg strength deficit for both old and young adults. *Eur J Appl Physiol* 94:175-179, 2005.

40. Lemon, PWR, and Hermiston, RT. The human energy cost of firefighting. *J Occup Med* 19:558-562, 1977.

41. Lloyd, RS, and Faigenbaum, AD. Age- and sex-related differences and their implications for resistance exercise. In *Essentials of Strength Training and Conditioning*. 4th ed. Haff, GG, and Triplett, NT, eds. Champaign, IL: Human Kinetics, 136-154, 2016.

42. Maddigan, ME, Button, DC, and Behm, DG. Lower-limb and trunk muscle activation with back squats and weighted sled apparatus. *J Strength Cond Res* 28:3346-3353, 2014.

43. Mangine, GT, Ratamess, NA, Hoffman, JR, Faigenbaum, AD, Kang, J, and Chilakos, A. The effects of combined ballistic and heavy resistance training on maximal lower- and upper-body strength in recreationally-trained men. *J Strength Cond Res* 22:132-139, 2008.

44. Manning, JE, and Griggs, TR. Heart rates in firefighters using light and heavy breathing equipment: similar near-maximal exertion in response to multiple work load conditions. *J Occup Med* 25:215-218, 1983.

45. Marcinik, EJ, Hodgdon, JA, Mittleman, K, and O'Brien, JJ. Aerobic/callisthenic and aerobic/circuit weight training programs for Navy men: a comparative study. *Med Sci Sports Exerc* 17:482-487, 1985.

46. Marcinik, EJ, Hodgdon, JA, O'Brien, JJ, and Mittleman, K. Fitness changes of Naval women following aerobic-based programs featuring callisthenic or circuit weight training exercises. *Eur J Appl Physiol Occup Physiol* 54:244-249, 1985.

47. McBride, JM, Cormie, P, and Deane, R. Isometric squat force output and muscle activity in stable and unstable conditions. *J Strength Cond Res* 20:915-918, 2006.

48. Munn, J, Herbert, RD, and Gandevia, SC. Contralateral effects of unilateral resistance training: a meta-analysis. *J Appl Physiol* 96:1861-1866, 2004.

49. Munn, J, Herbert, RD, Hancock, MJ, and Gandevia, SC. Resistance training for strength: effect of number of sets and contraction speed. *Med Sci Sports Exerc* 37:1622-1626, 2005.

50. Nindl, BC, Alvar, BA, Dudley, JR, Favre, MW, Martin, GJ, Sharp, MA, Warr, BJ, Stephenson, MD, and Kraemer, WJ. Executive summary from the National Strength and Conditioning Association's Second Blue Ribbon Panel on military physical readiness: military physical performance testing. *J Strength Cond Res* 29:S216-S220, 2015.

51. Nindl, BC, Barnes, BR, Alemany, JA, Frykman, PN, Shippee, RL, and Friedl, KE. Physiological consequences of U.S. Army Ranger training. *Med Sci Sports Exerc* 39:1380-1387, 2007.

52. Page, P, Frank, CC, and Lardner, R. *Assessment and Treatment of Muscle Imbalance: The Janda Approach*. Champaign, IL: Human Kinetics, 5-245, 2010.

53. Pawlak, R, Clasey, JL, Palmer, T, Symons, TB, and Abel, MG. The effect of a novel tactical training program on physical fitness and occupational performance in firefighters. *J Strength Cond Res* 29:578-588, 2015.

54. Peterson, MD, Dodd, DJ, Alvar, BA, Rhea, MR, and Favre, M. Undulating training for development of hierarchical fitness and improved firefighter job performance. *J Strength Cond Res* 22:1683-1695, 2008.

55. Peterson, MD, Pistilli, E, Haff, GG, Hoffman, EP, and Gordon, PM. Progression of volume load and muscular adaptation during resistance exercise. *Eur J Appl Physiol* 111:1063-1071, 2011.

56. Peterson, MD, Rhea, MR, and Alvar, BA. Maximizing strength development in athletes: a meta-analysis to determine the dose–response relationship. *J Strength Cond Res* 18:377-382, 2004.

57. Pincivero, DM, Lephart, SM, and Karunakara, RG. Effects of rest interval on isokinetic strength and functional performance after short-term high intensity training. *Br J Sports Med* 31:229-234, 1997.

58. Pryor, RR, Colburn, D, Crill, MT, Hostler, DP, and Suyama, J. Fitness characteristics of a suburban special weapons and tactics team. *J Strength Cond Res* 26:752-757, 2012.

59. Ratamess, NA. *ACSM's Foundations of Strength Training and Conditioning*. Philadelphia: Wolters Kluwer Lippincott Williams & Wilkins, 192-330, 2012.

60. Ratamess, NA, Chiarello, CM, Sacco, AJ, Hoffman, JR, Faigenbaum, AD, Ross, R, and Kang, J. The effects of rest interval length on acute bench press performance: the influence of gender and muscle strength. *J Strength Cond Res* 26:1817-1826, 2012.

61. Ratamess, NA, Chiarello, CM, Sacco, AJ, Hoffman, JR, Faigenbaum, AD, Ross, R, and Kang, J. The effects of rest interval length manipulation of the first upper-body resistance exercise in sequence on acute performance of subsequent exercises in men and women. *J Strength Cond Res* 26:2929-2938, 2012.

62. Ratamess, NA, Falvo, MJ, Mangine, GT, Hoffman, JR, Faigenbaum, AD, and Kang, J. The effect of rest interval length on metabolic responses to the bench press exercise. *Eur J Appl Physiol* 100:1-17, 2007.

63. Ratamess, NA, Rosenberg, JG, Kang, J, Sundberg, S, Izer, KA, Levowsky, J, Rzeszutko, C, Ross, RE, and Faigenbaum, AD. Acute oxygen uptake and resistance exercise performance using different rest interval lengths: the influence of maximal aerobic capacity and exercise sequence. *J Strength Cond Res* 28:1875-1888, 2014.

64. Ratamess, NA, Rosenberg, JG, Klei, S, Dougherty, BM, Kang, J, Smith, C, Ross, RE, and Faigenbaum, AD. Comparison of the acute metabolic responses to traditional resistance, body-weight, and battling rope exercises. *J Strength Cond Res* 29:47-57, 2015.

65. Rhea, MR, and Alderman, BL. A meta-analysis of periodized versus nonperiodized strength and power training programs. *Res Q Exerc Sport* 75:413-422, 2004.

66. Rhea, MR, Alvar, BA, Burkett, LN, and Ball, SD. A meta-analysis to determine the dose response for strength development. *Med Sci Sports Exerc* 35:456-464, 2003.

67. Rhea, MR, Ball, SD, Phillips, WT, and Burkett, LN. A comparison of linear and daily undulating periodized programs with equated volume and intensity for strength. *J Strength Cond Res* 16:250-255, 2002.

68. Rhea, MR, Phillips, WT, Burkett, LN, Stone, WJ, Ball, SD, Alvar, BA, and Thomas, AB. A comparison of linear and daily undulating periodized programs with equated volume and intensity for local muscular endurance. *J Strength Cond Res* 17:82-87, 2003.

69. Roberts, MA, O'Dea, J, Boyce, A, and Mannix, ET. Fitness levels of firefighter recruits before and after a supervised exercise training program. *J Strength Cond Res* 16:271-277, 2002.

70. Robinson, JM, Stone, MH, Johnson, RL, Penland, CM, Warren, BJ, and Lewis, RD. Effects of different weight training exercise/rest intervals on strength, power, and high intensity exercise endurance. *J Strength Cond Res* 9:216-221, 1995.

71. Santtila, M, Häkkinen, K, Karavirta, L, and Kyrolainen, H. Changes in cardiovascular performance during an 8-week military basic training period combined with added endurance or strength training. *Mil Med* 173:1173-1179, 2008.

72. Santtila, M, Häkkinen, K, Kraemer, WJ, and Kyrolainen, H. Effects of basic training on acute physiological responses to a combat loaded run test. *Mil Med* 175:273-279, 2010.

73. Santtila, M, Kyrolainen, H, and Häkkinen, K. Changes in maximal and explosive strength, electromyography, and muscle thickness of lower and upper extremities induced by combined strength and endurance training in soldiers. *J Strength Cond Res* 23:1300-1308, 2009.

74. Schiotz, MK, Potteiger, JA, Huntsinger, PG, and Denmark, DC. The short-term effects of periodized and constant-intensity training on body composition, strength, and performance. *J Strength Cond Res* 12:173-178, 1998.

75. Schoenfeld, BJ. The mechanisms of muscle hypertrophy and their application to resistance training. J Strength Cond Res. 24: 2857-2872, 2010.

76. Schoenfeld, BJ, Peterson, MD, Ogborn, D, Contreras, B, and Sonmez, GT. Effects of low- vs. high-load resistance training on muscle strength and hypertrophy in well-trained men. *J Strength Cond Res* 29:2954-2963, 2015.

77. Schoenfeld, BJ, Pope, ZK, Benik, FM, Hester, GM, Sellers J, Nooner, JL, Schnaiter, JA, Bond-Williams, KE, Carter, AS, Ross, CL, Just, BL, Henselmans, M, and Krieger, JW. Longer inter-set rest periods enhance muscle strength and hypertrophy in resistance-trained men. *J Strength Cond Res*. [e-pub ahead of print].

78. Schoenfeld, BJ, Ratamess, NA, Peterson, MD, Contreras, B, Tiryaki-Sonmez, G, and Alvar, BA. Effects of different volume-equated resistance training loading strategies on muscular adaptations in well-trained men. *J Strength Cond Res* 28:2909-2918, 2014.

79. Sell, TC, Abt, JP, Crawford, K, Lovalekar, M, Nagai, T, Deluzio, JB, Smalley, BW, McGrail, MA, Rowe, RS, Cardin, S, and Lephart, SM. Warrior model for human performance and injury prevention: Eagle tactical athlete program (ETAP) part 1. *J Spec Oper Med* 10:2-21, 2010.

80. Senna, G, Willardson, JM, de Salles, BF, Scudese, E, Carneiro, F, Palma, A, and Simao, R. The effect of rest interval length on multi- and single-joint exercise performance and perceived exertion. *J Strength Cond Res* 25:3157-3162, 2011.

81. Sheppard, JM, and Triplett, NT. Program design for resistance training. In *Essentials of Strength Training and Conditioning*. 4th ed. Haff, GG, and Triplett, NT, eds. Champaign, IL: Human Kinetics, 439-469, 2016.

82. Simao, R, Farinatti, PTV, Polito, MD, Maior, AS, and Fleck, SJ. Influence of exercise order on the number of repetitions performed and perceived exertion during resistive exercises. *J Strength Cond Res* 19:152-156, 2005.

83. Smith, S. *Tactical Fitness*. Hobart, NY: Hatherleigh Press, 21-171, 2014.

84. Souza-Junior, TP, Willardson, JM, Bloomer, R, Leite, RD, Fleck, SJ, Oliveira, PR, and Simao, R. Strength and hypertrophy responses to constant and decreasing rest intervals in trained men using creatine supplementation. *J Int Soc Sports Nutr* 8:1-11, 2011.

85. Stone, M, Plisk, S, and Collins, D. Training principles: evaluation of modes and methods of resistance training—a coaching perspective. *Sports Biomech* 1:79-103, 2002.

86. United States Army. *FM 7-22 Army Physical Readiness Training*. Washington, DC: Department of the Army, 1-1–10-20, 2012.

87. Vilaça-Alves, J, Geraldes, L, Fernandes, HM, Vaz, L, Farjalla, R, Saavedra, F, and Reis, VM. Effects of pre-exhausting the biceps brachii muscle on the performance of the front lat pull-down exercise using different handgrip positions. *J Hum Kinet* 42:157-163, 2014.

88. Willardson, JM, and Burkett, LN. A comparison of 3 different rest intervals on the exercise volume completed during a workout. *J Strength Cond Res* 19:23-26, 2005.

89. Willardson, JM, and Burkett, LN. The effect of different rest intervals between sets on volume components and strength gains. *J Strength Cond Res* 22:146-152, 2008.

90. Williams, AG, Rayson, MP, and Jones, DA. Resistance training and the enhancement of the gains in material-handling ability and physical fitness of British Army recruits during basic training. *Ergonomics* 45:267-279, 2002.

Chapter 10

1. Baker, D, Wilson, G, and Carlyon, R. Periodization: the effect on strength of manipulating volume and intensity. *J Strength Cond Res* 8:235-242, 1994.

2. Bompa, TO. Antrenamentul in perooda, pregatitoare. *Caiet Pentre Sporturi Nautice* 3:22-24, 1956.

3. Bompa, TO. Criteria pregatirii a unui plan departra ani. *Cultura Fizica si Sport* 2:11-19, 1968.

4. Bompa, TO, and Carrera, MC. *Periodization Training for Sports: Science-Based Strength and Conditioning Plans for 20 Sports.* Champaign, IL: Human Kinetics, 11-19, 2005.

5. Bompa, TO, and Haff, GG. *Periodization: Theory and Methodology of Training.* Champaign, IL: Human Kinetics, 125-556, 2009.

6. Bondarchuk, A. Periodization of sports training. *Leg-kaya Atletika* 12:8-9, 1986.

7. Bondarchuk, AP. Constructing a training system. *Track Tech* 102:254-269, 1988.

8. Bosquet, L, Montpetit, J, Arvisais, D, and Mujika, I. Effects of tapering on performance: a meta-analysis. *Med Sci Sports Exerc* 39:1358-1365, 2007.

9. Brink, MS, Visscher, C, Arends, S, Zwerver, J, Post, WJ, and Lemmink, KA. Monitoring stress and recovery: new insights for the prevention of injuries and illnesses in elite youth soccer players. *Br J Sports Med* 44:809-815, 2010.

10. Bruin, G, Kuipers, H, Keizer, HA, and Vander Vusse, GJ. Adaptation and overtraining in horses subjected to increasing training loads. *J Appl Physiol* 76:1908-1913, 1994.

11. Bullock, SH, Jones, BH, Gilchrist, J, and Marshall, SW. Prevention of physical training-related injuries recommendations for the military and other active populations based on expedited systematic reviews. *Am J Prev Med* 38:S156-S181, 2010.

12. Chiu, LZF, and Barnes, JL. The fitness-fatigue model revisited: implications for planning short- and long-term training. *NSCA J* 25:42-51, 2003.

13. Counsilman, JE, and Counsilman, BE. *The New Science of Swimming.* Englewood Cliffs, NJ: Prentice Hall, 229-244, 1994.

14. Cristea, A, Korhonen, MT, Hakkinen, K, Mero, A, Alen, M, Sipila, S, Viitasalo, JT, Koljonen, MJ, Suominen, H, and Larsson, L. Effects of combined strength and sprint training on regulation of muscle contraction at the whole-muscle and single-fibre levels in elite master sprinters. *Acta Physiol (Oxf)* 193:275-289, 2008.

15. Dick, FW. *Sports Training Principles.* London: A and C Black, 217-254, 2002.

16. Dolney, TJ, and Sheridan, SC. The relationship between extreme heat and ambulance response calls for the city of Toronto, Ontario, Canada. *Environmental Research* 101:94-103, 2006.

17. Fleck, S, and Kraemer, WJ. *Designing Resistance Training Programs.* 4th ed. Champaign, IL: Human Kinetics, 16-61, 2014.

18. Foster, C. Monitoring training in athletes with reference to overtraining syndrome. *Med Sci Sports Exerc* 30:1164-1168, 1998.

19. Fry, AC. The role of training intensity in resistance exercise overtraining and overreaching. In *Overtraining in Sport.* Kreider, RB, Fry, AC, and O'Toole, ML, eds. Champaign, IL: Human Kinetics, 107-127, 1998.

20. Fry, RW, Morton, AR, and Keast, D. Overtraining in athletes. An update. *Sports Med* 12:32-65, 1991.

21. Fry, RW, Morton, AR, and Keast, D. Periodisation and the prevention of overtraining. *Can J Sport Sci* 17:241-248, 1992.

22. Fry, RW, Morton, AR, and Keast, D. Periodisation of training stress—a review. *Can J Sport Sci* 17:234-240, 1992.

23. Gabbett, T, King, T, and Jenkins, D. Applied physiology of rugby league. *Sports Med* 38:119-138, 2008.

24. Garcia-Pallares, J, Sanchez-Medina, L, Carrasco, L, Diaz, A, and Izquierdo, M. Endurance and neuromuscular changes in world-class level kayakers during a periodized training cycle. *Eur J Appl Physiol* 106:629-638, 2009.

25. Garhammer, J. Periodization of strength training for athletes. *Track Tech* 73:2398-2399, 1979.

26. Haff, GG. Periodization: let the science guide our program design. In *United Kingdom Strength and Conditioning Conference.* Belfast, Ireland, 2008.

27. Haff, GG. Periodization of training. In *Conditioning for Strength and Human Performance.* Brown, LE, and Chandler, J, eds. Philadelphia: Wolters Kluwer, Lippincott, Williams & Wilkins, 326-345, 2012.

28. Haff, GG. Peaking for competition in individual sports. In *High-Performance Training for Sports.* Joyce, D, and Lewindon, D, eds. Champaign, IL: Human Kinetics, 524-540, 2014.

29. Haff, GG. Periodization strategies for youth development. In *Strength and Conditioning for Young Athletes: Science and Application.* Lloyd, RS, and Oliver, JL, eds. London: Routledge, Taylor & Francis Group, 149-168, 2014.

30. Haff, GG. The essentials of periodisation. In *Strength and Conditioning for Sports Performance.* Jeffreys, I, and Moody, J, eds. Abingdon, Oxon: Routledge, 404-448, 2016.

31. Haff, GG, and Haff, EE. Training integration and periodization. In *Strength and Conditioning Program Design.* Hoffman, J, ed. Champaign, IL: Human Kinetics, 209-254, 2012.

32. Haff, GG, Kraemer, WJ, O'Bryant, HS, Pendlay, G, Plisk, S, and Stone, MH. Roundtable discussion: periodization of training—part 1. *NSCA J* 26:50-69, 2004.

33. Harre, D. Principles of athletic training. In *Principles of Sports Training: Introduction to the Theory and Methods of Training.* Harre, D, ed. Berlin: Sportverlag, 73-94, 1982.

34. Harre, D. *Principles of Sports Training.* Berlin: Democratic Republic: Sportverlag, 73-94, 1982.

35. Harre, D. *Trainingslehre.* Berlin: Sportverlag, 73-94, 1982.

36. Harris, GR, Stone, MH, O'Bryant, HS, Proulx, CM, and Johnson, RL. Short-term performance effects of high power, high force, or combined weight-training methods. *J Strength Cond Res* 14:14-20, 2000.

37. Hooper, SL, Mackinnon, LT, and Ginn, EM. Effects of three tapering techniques on the performance, forces and psychometric measures of competitive swimmers. *Eur J Appl Physiol Occup Physiol* 78:258-263, 1998.

38. Impellizzeri, FM, Rampinini, E, and Marcora, SM. Physiological assessment of aerobic training in soccer. *J Sports Sci* 23:583-592, 2005.

39. Issurin, V. Block periodization versus traditional training theory: a review. *J Sports Med Phys Fitness* 48:65-75, 2008.

40. Issurin, V. *Block Periodization: Breakthrough in Sports Training.* Muskegon Heights, MI: Ultimate Athlete Concepts, 1-213, 2008.

41. Izquierdo, M, Ibanez, J, Gonzalez-Badillo, JJ, Ratamess, NA, Kraemer, WJ, Häkkinen, K, Bonnabau, H, Granados, C, French, DN, and Gorostiaga, EM. Detraining and tapering effects on hormonal responses and strength performance. *J Strength Cond Res* 21:768-775, 2007.

42. Jeffreys, I. Quadrennial planning for the high school athlete. *Strength and Cond J* 30:74-83, 2008.

43. Kentta, G, and Hassmen, P. Overtraining and recovery. A conceptual model. *Sports Medicine* 26:1-16, 1998.

44. Kraemer, WJ, and Fleck, SJ. *Optimizing Strength Training: Designing Nonlinear Periodization Workouts.* Champaign, IL: Human Kinetics, 1-245, 2007.

45. Kukushkin, GI. *System of Physical Education in the USSR.* Moscow: Raduga, 128-174, 1983.

46. Kurz, T. *Science of Sports Training.* Island Pond, VT: Stadion, 293-341, 2001.

47. Matveyev, L. *Periodization of Sports Training.* Moskow: Fizkultura i Sport, 1965.

48. Matveyev, L. About the construction of training. *Modern Athlete and Coach* 32:12-16, 1994.

49. Matveyev, LP. *Periodisterung Des Sportlichen Trainings.* Moscow: Fizkultura i Sport, 86-298, 1972.

50. Matveyev, LP. *Fundamentals of Sports Training.* Moscow: Fizkultua i Sport, 86-298, 1977.

51. Minetti, AE. On the mechanical power of joint extensions as affected by the change in muscle force (or cross-sectional area), ceteris paribus. *Eur J Appl Physiol* 86:363-369, 2002.

52. Mujika, I, Goya, A, Padilla, S, Grijalba, A, Gorostiaga, E, and Ibanez, J. Physiological responses to a 6-d taper in middle-distance runners: influence of training intensity and volume. *Med Sci Sports Exerc* 32:511-517, 2000.

53. Mujika, I, and Padilla, S. Scientific bases for precompetition tapering strategies. *Med Sci Sports Exerc* 35:1182-1187, 2003.

54. Nádori, L. *Training and Competition.* Budapest: Sport, 1962.

55. Nádori, L. *Theory of Training and Exercise.* Budapest: Sport, 1968.

56. Nádori, L, and Granek, I. *Theoretical and Methodological Basis of Training Planning With Special Considerations Within a Microcycle.* Lincoln, NE: NSCA, 1-63, 1989.

57. Olbrect, J. *The Science of Winning: Planning, Periodizing, and Optimizing Swim Training.* Luton, England: Swimshop, 1-200, 2000.

58. Ozolin, N. Athlete's training system for competition. In *The Role and Sequence of Using Different Training-Load Intensity.* Bondarchuk, A, ed. Escondido: Sports Training, 202-204, 1971.

59. Plisk, SS, and Stone, MH. Periodization strategies. *Strength and Cond* 25:19-37, 2003.

60. Rhea, MR, Ball, SD, Phillips, WT, and Burkett, LN. A comparison of linear and daily undulating periodized programs with equated volume and intensity for strength. *J Strength Cond Res* 16:250-255, 2002.

61. Rhea, MR, Phillips, WT, Burkett, LN, Stone, WJ, Ball, SD, Alvar, BA, and Thomas, AB. A comparison of linear and daily undulating periodized programs with equated volume and intensity for local muscular endurance. *J Strength Cond Res* 17:82-87, 2003.

62. Rowbottom, DG. Periodization of training. In *Exercise and Sport Science.* Garrett, WE, and Kirkendall, DT, eds. Philadelphia: Lippicott Williams & Wilkins, 499-512, 2000.

63. Sell, TC, Abt, JP, Crawford, K, Lovalekar, M, Nagai, T, Deluzio, JB, Smalley, BW, McGrail, MA, Rowe, RS, Cardin, S, and Lephart, SM. Warrior model for human performance and injury prevention: Eagle Tactical Athlete Program (ETAP) part I. *J Spec Oper Med* 10:2-21, 2010.

64. Sell, TC, Abt, JP, Crawford, K, Lovalekar, M, Nagai, T, Deluzio, JB, Smalley, BW, McGrail, MA, Rowe, RS, Cardin, S, and Lephart, SM. Warrior model for human performance and injury prevention: Eagle Tactical Athlete Program (ETAP) part II. *J Spec Oper Med* 10:22-33, 2010.

65. Selye, H. *The Stress of Life.* New York: McGraw-Hill, 1-324, 1956.

66. Siff, MC. *Supertraining.* Denver: Supertraining Institute, 319-336, 2003.

67. Siff, MC, and Verkhoshansky, YU. *Supertraining.* Denver: Supertraining International, 319-336, 1999.

68. Smith, DJ. A framework for understanding the training process leading to elite performance. *Sports Med* 33:1103-1126, 2003.

69. Stone, MH, Keith, R, Kearney, JT, Wilson, GD, and Fleck, SJ. Overtraining: a review of the signs and symptoms of overtraining. *Journal of Applied Sport Science Research* 5:35-50, 1991.

70. Stone, MH, and O'Bryant, HO. *Weight Training: A Scientific Approach.* Edina, MN: Burgess, 1987.

71. Stone, MH, Stone, ME, and Sands, WA. *Principles and Practice of Resistance Training.* Champaign, IL: Human Kinetics, 241-295, 2007.

72. Verkhoshansky, YU. Perspectives in the development of speed-strength preparation in the development of jumpers. *Track and Field* 9:11-12, 1966.

73. Verkhoshansky, YU. *Osnovi Spetsialnoi Silovoi Podgotovki i Sporte (Fundamentals of Special Strength Training in Sport).* Moscow: Fizkultura i Sport, 117-144, 1977.

74. Verkhoshansky, YU. *Programming and Organization of Training.* Moscow: Fizkultura i Sport, 1-136, 1985.

75. Verkhoshansky, YU. *Fundamentals of Special Strength Training in Sport.* Livonia, MI: Sportivny Press, 117-144, 1986.

76. Verkhoshansky, YU. *Special Strength Training: A Practical Manual for Coaches.* Muskegon Heights, MI: Ultimate Athlete Concepts, 117-144, 2006.

77. Verkhoshansky, YU. Theory and methodology of sport preparation: block training system for top-level athletes. *Teoria i Practica Physicheskoj Culturi* 4:2-14, 2007.

78. Viru, A. Some facts about microcycles. *Mod Athlete Coach* 28:29-32, 1990.

79. Viru, A. *Adaptations in Sports Training.* Boca Raton, FL: CRC Press LLC, 241-295, 1995.

80. Wong, HT, and Lai, PC. Weather inference and daily demand for emergency ambulance services. *Emerg Med J* 29:60-64, 2012.

81. Zamparo, P, Antonutto, G, Capelli, C, Girardis, M, Sepulcri, L, and di Prampero, PE. Effects of elastic recoil on maximal explosive power of the lower limbs. *Eur J Appl Physiol* 75:289-297, 1997.

82. Zatsiorsky, VM. Basic concepts of training theory. In *Science and Practice of Strength Training.* Champaign, IL: Human Kinetics, 3-19, 1995.

83. Zatsiorsky, VM, and Kraemer, WJ. *Science and Practice of Strength Training.* Champaign, IL: Human Kinetics, 108-135, 2006.

Chapter 11

1. Haff, GG, Triplett, NT., eds. *Essentials of Strength Training and Conditioning.* 4th ed. Champaign, IL: Human Kinetics, 353-357, 2016.

2. Herbert, L, and Miller, G. Newer heavy load lifting methods help firms reduce back injuries. *Occup Health Saf* 56:57-60, 1987.

3. Kushner, AM, Brent, JL, Schoenfeld, BJ, Hugentobler, J, Lloyd, RS, Vermeil, A, Chu, DA, Harbin, J, McGill, SM, and Myer, GD. The back squat: targeted training techniques to correct functional deficits and technical factors that limit performance. *Strength and Conditioning Journal* 37(2):13-60, 2015.

4. Shellock, FG, and Prentice, WE. Warming up and stretching for improved physical performance and prevention of sports-related injuries. *Sports Med* 2(4):267-278, 1985.

Chapter 12

1. Abrahams, M. Mechanical behavior of tendon in vitro. *Med Biol Eng Comput* 5(5):433-443, 1967.

2. Alter, MJ. *Sport Stretch.* 2nd ed. Champaign, IL: Human Kinetics, 1998.

3. Arazi, H, Nia, FR, Hakimi, M, and Mohamadi, MA. The effect of PNF stretching combined with resistance training on strength, muscle volume and flexibility in non-athlete male students. *Sport Sci* 5(1):85-90, 2012.

4. Arroyo-Morales, M, Olea, N, Martinez, M, Moreno-Lorenzo, C, Díaz-Rodríguez, L, and Hidalgo-Lozano, A. Effects of myofascial release after high-intensity exercise: a randomized clinical trial. *J. Manip Physiol Therap* 31(3):217-223. 2008.

5. Baechle, T, and Earle, R. *Essentials of Strength and Conditioning.* 2nd ed. Champaign, IL: Human Kinetics, 322-329, 2000.

6. Barnes, MF. The basic science of myofascial release: morphologic change in connective tissue. *J Bodyw Mov Ther* 1(4):231-238, 1997.

7. Bradley, PS, Olsen, PD, and Portas, MD. The effect of static, ballistic, and proprioceptive neuromuscular facilitation stretching on vertical jump performance. *J Strength Cond Res* 21(1):223-226, 2007.

8. Cherry, DB. Review of physical therapy alternatives for reducing muscle contracture. *Phys Ther* 60(7):877-881, 1980.

9. Cipriani, D, Abel, B, and Pirrwitz, D. A comparison of two stretching protocols on hip range of motion: implications for total daily stretch duration. *J Strength Cond Res* 17(2):274-278, 2003.

10. Condon, SM, and Hutton, RS. Soleus muscle electromyographic activity and ankle dorsiflexion range of motion during four stretching procedures. *Phys Ther* 67(1):24-30, 1987.

11. Cornelius, WL. Flexibility: the effective way. *Strength Cond J* 7(3):62-64, 1985.

12. Costa, PB, Graves, BS, Whitehurst, M, and Jacobs, PL. The acute effects of different durations of static stretching on dynamic balance performance. *J Strength Cond Res* 23(1):141-147, 2009.

13. Curran, PF, Fiore, RD, and Crisco, JJ. A comparison of the pressure exerted on soft tissue by 2 myofascial rollers. *J Sport Rehabil* 17(4):432, 2008

14. Da Costa, BR, and Vieira, ER. Stretching to reduce work-related musculoskeletal disorders: a systematic review. *J Rehabil Med* 40(5):321-328, 2008.

15. Dalleck, LC, Atwood, JP, Prins, RL, Buchanan, CA, and Curry, MA. Developing a comprehensive exercise prescription: the optimal order for cardiorespiratory, resistance, flexibility, and neuromotor. *J Fit Res* 3(2):13-25, 2014.

16. Davis, DS, Ashby, PE, McCale, KL, McQuain, JA, and Wine, JM. The effectiveness of 3 stretching techniques on hamstring flexibility using consistent stretching parameters. *J Strength Cond Res* 19(1):27-32, 2005.

17. Eston, RG, Rowlands, AV, Coulton, D, McKinnery, J, and Gleeson, NP. Effect of flexibility training on symptoms of exercise-induced muscle damage: a preliminary study. *J Exerc Sci Fit* 5(1):33-39, 2007.

18. Etnyre, BR, and Abraham, LD. Gains in range of ankle dorsiflexion using three popular stretching techniques. *Am J Phys Med Rehab* 65(4):189-196, 1986.

19. Ettinger, WH, Burns, R, Messier, SP, Applegate, W, Rejeski, WJ, Morgan, T, Shumaker, S, Berry, MJ, O'Toole, M, Monu, J, and Craven, T. A randomized trial comparing aerobic exercise and resistance exercise with a health education program in older adults with knee osteoarthritis: the Fitness Arthritis and Seniors Trial. *J Am Med Assoc* 277(1):25-31, 1997.

20. Fleck, S, and Kraemer, W. *Designing Resistance Training Programs.* 3rd ed. Champaign, IL: Human Kinetics, 141-147, 2004.

21. Foran, B. *High-Performance Sports Conditioning.* Champaign, IL: Human Kinetics, 49-61, 2001.

22. Galloway, SD, and Watt, JM. Massage provision by physiotherapists at major athletics events between 1987 and 1998. *Brit J Sport Med* 38(2):235-237, 2004.

23. Gaudreault, N, Fuentes, A, Mezghani, N, Gauthier, VO, and Turcot, K. Relationship between knee walking kinematics and muscle flexibility in runners. *J Sport Rehabil* 22(4):279-287, 2013.

24. Goodwin, JE, Glaister, M, Howatson, G, Lockey, RA, and McInnes, G. Effect of preperformance lower-limb massage on thirty-meter sprint running. *J Strength Cond Res* 21(4):1028-1031, 2007.

25. Haff, GG, and Triplett, T. *Essentials of Strength Training and Conditioning.* 4th ed. Champaign, IL: Human Kinetics, 320-328, 2016.

26. Handrakis, JP, Southard, VN, Abreu, JM, Aloisa, M, Doyen, MR, Echevarria, LM, Hwang, H, Samuels, C, Venegas, SA, and Douris, PC. Static stretching does not impair performance in active middle-aged adults. *J Strength Cond Res* 24(3):825-830, 2010.

27. Healey, KC, Hatfield, DL, Blanpied, P, Dorfman, LR, and Riebe, D. The effects of myofascial release with foam rolling on performance. *J Strength Cond Res* 28(1):61-68, 2014.

28. Herda, TJ, Cramer, JT, Ryan, ED, McHugh, MP, and Stout, JR. Acute effects of static versus dynamic stretching on isometric peak torque, electromyography, and mechanomyography of the biceps femoris muscle. *J Strength Cond Res* 22(3):809-817, 2008.

29. Heyward, VH, and Gibson, A. *Advanced Fitness Assessment and Exercise Prescription.* 7th ed. Champaign, IL: Human Kinetics, 305-308, 2014.

30. Holt, LE, Travis, TM, and Okita, T. Comparative study of three stretching techniques. *Percept Motor Skill* 31(2):611-616, 1970.

31. Hough, PA, Ross, EZ, and Howatson, G. Effects of dynamic and static stretching on vertical jump performance and electromyographic activity. *J Strength Cond Res* 23(2):507-512, 2009.

32. Hrysomallis, C. Hip adductors' strength, flexibility, and injury risk. *J Strength Cond Res* 23(5):1514-1517, 2009.

33. Johns, RJ, and Wright, V. Relative importance of various tissues in joint stiffness. *J Appl Physiol* 17(5):824-828, 1962.

34. Johnston, AP, De Lisio, M, and Parise, G. Resistance training, sarcopenia, and the mitochondrial theory of aging. *Appl Physiol Nutr Me* 33(1):191-199, 2007.

35. Kendall, FP, McCreary, EK, Provance, PG, Rodgers, MM, and Romani, WA. *Muscles: Testing and Function with Posture and Pain.* 5th ed. Baltimore: Lippincott Williams & Wilkins, 31-37, 2005.

36. MacDonald, GZ, Penney, MD, Mullaley, ME, Cuconato, AL, Drake, CD, Behm, DG, and Button, DC. An acute bout of self-myofascial release increases range of motion without a subsequent decrease in muscle activation or force. *J Strength Cond Res* 27(3):812-821, 2013.

37. Magnusson, SP, Simonsen, EB, Aagaard, P, Gleim, GW, McHugh, MP, and Kjaer, M. Viscoelastic response to repeated static stretching in the human hamstring muscle. *Scand J Med Sci Sports* 5(6):342-347, 1995.

38. Magnusson, SP, Simonsen, EB, Dyhre-Poulsen, P, Aagaard, P, Mohr, T, and Kjaer, M. Viscoelastic stress relaxation during static stretch in human skeletal muscle in the absence of EMG activity. *Scand J Med Sci Sports* 6(6):323-328, 1996.

39. Mattacola, CG, Perrin, DH, Gansneder, BM, Allen, JD, and Mickey, CA. A comparison of visual analog and graphic rating scales for assessing pain following delayed onset muscle soreness. *J Sport Rehab* 6:38-46, 1997.

40. McHugh, MP, and Cosgrave, CH. To stretch or not to stretch: the role of stretching in injury prevention and performance. *Scand J Med Sci Sports* 20:169-181, 2010.

41. McHugh, MP, and Nesse, M. Effect of stretching on strength loss and pain after eccentric exercise. *Med Sci Sports Exer* 40(3):566, 2008.

42. Moore, MA, and Hutton, RS. Electromyographic investigation of muscle stretching techniques. *Med Sci Sports Exer* 12(5):322-329, 1979.

43. Mori, H, Ohsawa, H, Tanaka, TH, Taniwaki, E, Leisman, G, and Nishijo, K. Effect of massage on blood flow and muscle fatigue following isometric lumbar exercise. *Med Sci Monitor* 10(5):CR173-CR178, 2004.

44. Nelson, RT, and Bandy, WD. Eccentric training and static stretching improve hamstring flexibility of high school males. *J Athl Training* 39(3):254, 2004.

45. Ogai, R, Yamane, M, Matsumoto, T, and Kosaka, M. Effects of petrissage massage on fatigue and exercise performance following intensive cycle pedalling. *Br J Sports Med* 42(10):834-838, 2008.

46. Perrier, ET, Pavol, MJ, and Hoffman, MA. The acute effects of a warm-up including static or dynamic stretching on counter-movement jump height, reaction time, and flexibility. *J Strength Cond Res* 25(7):1925-1931, 2011.

47. Reis, ES, Pereira, GB, Sousa, NF, Tibana, RA, Silva, MF, Araujo, M, and Prestes, J. Acute effects of proprioceptive neuromuscular facilitation and static stretching on maximal voluntary contraction and muscle electromyographical activity in indoor soccer players. *Clin Physiol Funct I* 33(6):418-422, 2013.

48. Rubini, EC, Costa, AL, and Gomes, PS. The effects of stretching on strength performance. *Sports Med* 37(3):213-224, 2007.

49. Ryan, ED, Beck, TW, Herda, TJ, Hull, HR, Hartman, MJ, Stout, JR, and Cramer, JT. Do practical durations of stretching alter muscle strength? A dose–response study. *Med Sci Sports Exer* 40(8):1529-1537, 2008.

50. Ryba, TV, and Kaltenborn, JM. The benefits of yoga for athletes: the body. *Athlet Ther Today* 11(2):32-34, 2006.

51. Sady, SP, Wortman, MV, and Blanke, D. Flexibility training: ballistic, static or proprioceptive neuromuscular facilitation? *Arch Phys Med Rehab* 63(6):261-263, 1982.

52. Sefton, J. Myofascial release for athletic trainers. Part 1: theory and session guidelines. *Athl Ther Today* 9:48-49, 2004.

53. Sexton, P, and Chambers, J. The importance of flexibility for functional range of motion. *Athl Ther Today* 11(3):13-17, 2006.

54. Small, K, McNaughton, L, and Matthews, M. A systematic review into the efficacy of static stretching as part of a warm-up for the prevention of exercise-related injury. *Res Sports Med* 16(3):213-231, 2008.

55. Smith, CA. The warm-up procedure: to stretch or not to stretch. A brief review. *J Orthop Sports Phys Ther* 19(1):12-17, 1994.

56. Swann, E, and Graner, SJ. Uses of manual-therapy techniques in pain management. *IJATT* 7(4), 2010.

57. Sauers, E, August, A, and Snyder, A. Fauls stretching routine produces acute gains in throwing shoulder mobility in collegiate baseball players. *J Sport Rehab* 16(1):28-40, 2007.

58. Tanigawa, MC. Comparison of the hold-relax procedure and passive mobilization on increasing muscle length. *Phys Ther* 52(7):725-735, 1972.

59. Thacker, SB, Gilchrist, J, Stroup, DF, and Kimsey Jr, CD. The impact of stretching on sports injury risk: a systematic review of the literature. *Med Sci Sports Exer* 36(3):371-378, 2004.

60. Tsolakis, C, and Bogdanis, GC. Acute effects of two different warm-up protocols on flexibility and lower limb explosive performance in male and female high level athletes. *J Sports Sci Med* 11(4):669-675, 2012.

61. Voss, DE, Ionta, MK, and Myers, BJ. *Proprioceptive Neuromuscular Facilitation, PNF: Patterns and Techniques.* Chicago: Rehabilitation Institute of Chicago, 1985.

62. Wang, K, McCarter, R, Wright, J, Beverly, J, and Ramirez-Mitchell, R. Regulation of skeletal muscle stiffness and elasticity by titin isoforms: a test of the segmental extension model of resting tension. *Proc Natl Acad Sci USA* 88(16):7101-7105, 1991.

63. Weerapong, P, Hume, PA, and Kolt, GS. The mechanisms of massage and effects on performance, muscle recovery and injury prevention. *Sports Med* 35(3):235-256, 2005.

64. Weinberg, R, Jackson, A, and Kolodny, K. The relationship of massage and exercise to mood enhancement. *Sport Psychol* 2:202-211, 1988.

65. Wiktorsson-Moller, M, Öberg, B, Ekstrand, J, and Gillquist, J. Effects of warming up, massage, and stretching on range of motion and muscle strength in the lower extremity. *Am J Sports Med* 11(4):249-252, 1983.

66. Winchester, JB, Nelson, AG, Landin, D, Young, MA, and Schexnayder, IC. Static stretching impairs sprint performance in collegiate track and field athletes. *J Strength Cond Res* 1533-4287/22(1):13-18, 2008.

67. Young, WB, and Behm, DG. Should static stretching be used during a warm-up for strength and power activities? *Strength and Cond J* 24(6):33-37, 2002.

Chapter 13

1. Alexander, RM. *Principles of Animal Locomotion.* Princeton, NJ: Princeton University Press, 2003.

2. Allerheiligen, B, and Rogers, R. Plyometrics program design. *Strength Cond* 17:26-31, 1995.

3. Allerheiligen, B, and Rogers, R. Plyometrics program design, part 2. *Strength Cond* 17:33-39, 1995.

4. Prentice, WE. *Arnheim's Principles of Athletic Training: A Competency Based Approach.* 15th ed. New York: McGraw-Hill Education, 613, 2013.

5. Blacker, SD, Carter, JM, Wilkinson, DM, Richmond, VL, Rayson, MP, and Peattie, M. Physiological responses of police officers during job simulations wearing chemical, biological, radiological and nuclear personal protective equipment. *Ergonomics* 56:137-147, 2013.

6. Behm, DG, Anderson, K, and Curnew, RS. Muscle force and activation under stable an unstable conditions. *J Strength Cond Res* 16:416-422, 2002.

7. Bodyen, H. Power training for sprinters. In *Sprints and Relays.* 1st ed. Jarver, J, ed. Mountain View, CA: TAFNEWS Press, 65-68, 1978.

8. Britton, C, Lynch, CF, Ramirez, M, Torner, J, Buresh, C, and Peek-Asa, C. Epidemiology of injuries to wildland firefighters. *Am J Emer Med* 31:339-345, 2013.

9. Casa, DJ, Csillan, D, Armstrong, LE, Baker, LB, Bergeron, MF, Buchanan, VM, Carroll, MJ, Cleary, MA, Eichner, ER, Ferrara, MS, and Fitzpatrick, TD. Preseason heat-acclimatization guidelines for secondary school athletics. *J Athletic Training* 44:332-333, 2009.

10. Chmielewski, TL, Myer, GD, Kauffman, D, and Tillman, SM. Plyometric exercise in the rehabilitation of athletes: physiological responses and clinical application. *J Orthop Sports Phys Ther* 36:308-320, 2006.

11. Cissik, JM, and Barnes, M. *Sports Speed and Agility.* 2nd ed. Monterey Bay, CA: Coaches Choice, 41-75, 2011.

12. Chumanov, ES, Heiderscheit, BC, and Thelen, DG. The effect of speed and influence of individual muscles on hamstring mechanisms during the swing phase of sprinting. *J Biomech* 40:3555-3562, 2007.

13. Dawes, J, and Lentz, D. Methods of improving power for acceleration for the non-track athlete. *Strength Cond J* 34:44-51. 2012.

14. Dawes, JJ, Orr, RM, Elder, CL, Krall, K, Stierli, M, and Schilling, B. Relationship between selected measures of power and strength and linear running speed amongst special weapons and tactics police officers. *J Aust Strength Cond* 23:22-26, 2015.

15. DeMaio, M, Onate, J, Swain, D, Morrison, S. Ringleb, S, and Naiak, D. Physical performance decrements in military personnel wearing personal protective equipment (PPE). In *Human Performance Enhancement for NATO Military Operations*, P2-1-P2-6, 2009.

16. DeWeese, B, and Nimphius, S. Program design and technique for speed and agility training. In *Essentials of Strength Training and Conditioning.* Haff, G, and Triplett, T, eds. Champaign, IL: Human Kinetics, 522-558, 2016.

17. DiVencenzo, HR, Morgan, AL, Laurent, CM, and Keylock, KT. Metabolic demands of law enforcement personal protective equipment during drills tasks. *Ergonomics* 57:1760-1765, 2014.

18. Dreger, RW, Jones, RL, and Petersen, SR. Effects of the self-contained breathing apparatus and fire protective clothing on maximal oxygen uptake. *Ergonomics* 49:911-920, 2006.

19. Funk, DC, Swank, AM, Mikla, BM, Fagan, TA, and Farr, BK. Impact of prior exercise on hamstring flexibility: a comparison of proprioceptive neuromuscular facilitation and static stretching. *J Strength Cond Res* 17:489-492, 2003.

20. Gagua, E. Sprint reflections. In *Sprints and Relays.* 4th ed. Jarver, J, ed. Mountain View, CA: TAFNEWS Press, 20-26, 1995.

21. Gillman, GM. 300 yard shuttle run. *Nat Strength Cond Assoc J* 5:46, 1983.

22. Harman, EA, Gutekunst, DJ, Frykman, PN, Bradley CN, Alemany, JJ, Mello, RP, and Sharp, MA. Effects of two different eight-week training programs on military physical performance. *J Strength Cond Res* 22:524-534, 2008.

23. Ham, K, and Young, BA. Deterministic model of the vertical jump: implications for training. *J Strength Cond Res* 21:967-972, 2007

24. Hauret, KG, Jones, BH, Bullock, SH, Canham-Chervak, M, and Canada, S. Musculoskeletal injuries: description of an under-recognized injury problem among military personnel. *Am J Prev Med* 38:S61-S70, 2010.

25. Henderson, NE. Injuries and injury risk factors among men and women in U.S. Army combat medic advanced individual training. *Military Med* 165:647, 2000.

26. Henry, GJ, Dawson, B, Lay, BS, and Young, WB. Relationships between reactive agility movement time and unilateral vertical, horizontal and lateral jumps. *J Strength Cond Res* 30:2514-2521, 2016.

27. Herda, TJ, and Cramer, JT. Bioenergetics of exercise and training. In *Essentials of Strength and Conditioning.* 4th ed. Haff, G, and Triplett, T, eds. Champaign, IL: Human Kinetics, 60, 2016.

28. Holcomb, WR, Kleiner, DM, and Chu, DA. Plyometrics: considerations for safe and effective training. *Strength Cond J* 20:36-39, 1998.

29. Jeffreys, I. Motor learning: applications for agility, part 1. *Strength Cond J* 28:72-76, 2006.

30. Jeffreys, I. Warm-up and flexibility training. In *Essentials of Strength Training and Conditioning.* 4th ed. Haff, G, and Triplett, T, eds. Champaign, IL: Human Kinetics, 317-350, 2016.

31. Knudson, D. Correcting the use of the term "power" in the strength and conditioning literature. *J Strength Cond Res* 23:1902-1908, 2009.

32. Little, T, and Williams, AG. Specificity of acceleration, maximum speed and agility in professional soccer players. *J Strength Cond Res* 19:76-78, 2005

33. McBride, J. Biomechanics. In *Essentials of Strength Training and Conditioning.* 4th ed. Haff, G, and Triplett, T, eds. Champaign, IL: Human Kinetics, 25-28, 2016.

34. McNeely, E. Introduction to plyometrics: converting strength to power. *NSCA's Perf Train J* 6:19-22, 2005.

35. Michaelides, MA, Parpa, KM, Henry, LJ, Thompson, GB, and Brown, BS. Assessment of physical fitness aspect and their relationship to firefighters' job abilities. *J Strength Cond Res* 25:956-965, 2011.

36. Paradisis, GP, Pappas, PT, Theodorou, AS, Zacharogiannis, EG, Skordilis, EK, and Smirniotou, AS. Effects of static and dynamic stretching on sprint and jump performance in boys and girls. *J Strength Cond Res* 28:154-160, 2014.

37. Park, K, Hur, P, Rosengren, KS, Horn, GP, and Hsiao-Wecksler, ET. Effect of load carriage on gait due to firefighting air bottle configuration. *Ergonomics* 33:882-891, 2010.

38. Park, K, Rosengren, KS, Horn, GP, Smith, DL, and Hsiao-Wecksler, ET. Assessing gait changes in firefighters due to fatigue and protective clothing. *Safety Science* 49:719-726, 2011.

39. Peterson, MD, Dodd, DJ, Alvar, BA, Rhea, MR, and Favre, M. Undulation training for development of hierarchical fitness and improved firefighter job performance. *J Strength Cond Res* 22:1683-1695, 2008.

40. Potach, DH, and Chu, DA. Program design and technique for plyometric training. In *Essentials of Strength and Conditioning.* 4th ed. Haff, G, and Triplett, T, eds. Champaign, IL: Human Kinetics, 471-520, 2016.

41. Rhea, MR, Alvar, BA, and Gray, R. Physical fitness and job performance of firefighters. *J Strength Cond Res* 18:348-352, 2004.

42. Saunders, PU, Pyne, DB, Telford, RD, and Hawley, JA. Factors affecting running economy in trained distance runners. *Sports Med* 34:465-485, 2004.

43. Schmidt, RA, and Lee, TD. *Motor Learning and Performance: From Principles to Application.* Champaign, IL: Human Kinetics, 9, 2014.

44. Schmidt, RA, and Wrisberg, CA. *Motor Learning and Performance: A Site-Based Learning Approach.* 4th ed. Champaign, IL: Human Kinetics, 2008.

45. Sell, KM. *Development of minimal physical fitness test standards for firefighters.* Doctoral dissertation, University of Utah, 2006.

46. Sheppard, JM, Young, WB, Doyle, T, Sheppard, TA, and Newton, RU. An evaluation of a new test of reactive agility and its relationship to sprint speed and change of direction speed. *J Sci Med Sport* 9:342-349, 2006.

47. Sheppard, RJ, and Bonneau, J. Assuring gender equity in recruitment standards for police officers. *Can J Applied Physiol* 27:263-295, 2002.

48. Stanish, HI, Wood, TM, and Campagna, P. Prediction of performance on the RCMP Physical Ability Requirement Evaluation. *J Occup Envir Med* 41:669-677, 1999.

49. Stone, MH, Stone, M, and Sands, W. *Principles and Practice of Resistance Training.* Champaign, IL: Human Kinetics, 203, 2007.

50. Wathen, D. Literature review explosive/plyometric drills. *Natl Strength Cond Assoc J* 15:46-48, 1993.

51. Zemke, B, and Wright, G. The use of strongman type implements and training to increase sport performance in collegiate athletes. *Strength Cond J* 33:1-7, 2011.

Chapter 14

1. Abramson, AK. Cycling Bike Fit Task Force: First consensus statement on definitions and key concepts. 2013. www.fitkitsystems.com/wp-content/uploads/2015/10/Medicine_of_Cycling_Bike_Fit_Consensus_Statement.pdf.

2. Baris, D, Garrity, TJ, Telles, JL, Heineman, EF, Olshan, A, and Zahm, SH. Cohort mortality study of Philadelphia firefighters. *Am J Ind Med* 39:463-476, 2001.

3. Beaton, R, Murphy, S, Johnson, C, Pike, K, and Corneil, W. Exposure to duty-related incident stressors in urban firefighters and paramedics. *J Trauma Stress* 11:821-828, 1998.

4. Blair, SN, Kampert, JB, Kohl, HW, Barlow, CE, Macera, CA, Paffenbarger, RS, and Gibbons, LW. Influences of cardiorespiratory fitness and other precursors on cardiovascular disease and all-cause mortality in men and women. *JAMA* 276:205-210, 1996.

5. Bolognesi, M. Ventilatory threshold and maximal oxygen uptake during cycling and running in duathletes. *Med Sport* 50:209-216, 1997.

6. Borg, GA. Psychophysical bases of perceived exertion. *Med Sci Sports Exerc* 14:377-381, 1982.

7. Carraro, A, Gobbi, E, Ferri, I, Benvenuti, P, and Zanuso, S. Enjoyment perception during exercise with aerobic machines. *Percept Mot Skills* 119:146-155, 2014.

8. Clemente Suarez, VJ, and Gonzalez-Rave, JM. Four weeks of training with different aerobic workload distributions—effect on aerobic performance. *Eur J Sport Sci* 14(Suppl 1):S1-S7, 2014.

9. Cordain, L, Tucker, A, Moon, D, and Stager, JM. Lung volumes and maximal respiratory pressures in collegiate swimmers and runners. *Res Q Exerc Sport* 61:70-74, 1990.

10. Cornelissen, VA, and Fagard, RH. Effects of endurance training on blood pressure, blood pressure-regulating mechanisms, and cardiovascular risk factors. *Hypertension* 46:667-675, 2005.

11. Daniels, J. *Daniels' Running Formula.* Champaign, IL: Human Kinetics, 47-63, 2014.

12. El-Kader, SMA. Aerobic exercise training improves cardiopulmonary fitness among firefighters. *Eur J Gen Med* 7:352-358, 2010.

13. Fontaine, M. Shoulder impingement: the keys to dealing with swimmer's shoulder. *ACA News* 10:20-21, 2014.

14. Foss, O, and Hallen, J. The most economical cadence increases with increasing workload. *Eur J Appl Physiol* 92:443-451, 2004.

15. Gellish, RL, Goslin, BR, Olson, RE, McDonald, A, Russi, GD, and Moudgil, VK. Longitudinal modeling of the relationship between age and maximal heart rate. *Med Sci Sports Exerc* 39:822-829, 2007.

16. Gettman, LR, Pollock, ML, Durstine, JL, Ward, A, Ayres, J, and Linnerud, AC. Physiological responses of men to 1, 3, and 5 day per week training programs. *Res Q* 47:638-646, 1976.

17. Gibala, MJ, Little, JP, van Essen, M, Wilkin, GP, Burgomaster, KA, Safdar, A, Raha, S, and Tarnopolsky, MA. Short-term sprint interval versus traditional endurance training: similar initial adaptations in human skeletal muscle and exercise performance. *J Physiol* 575:901-911, 2006.

18. Gist, NH, Fedewa, MV, Dishman, RK, and Cureton, KJ. Sprint interval training effects on aerobic capacity: a systematic review and meta-analysis. *Sports Med* 44:269-279, 2014.

19. Haddad, M, Padulo, J, and Chamari, K. The usefulness of session rating of perceived exertion for monitoring training load despite several influences on perceived exertion. *Int J Sports Physiol Perform* 9:882-883, 2014.

20. Haskell, WL, Lee, I-M, Pate, RR, Powell, KE, Blair, SN, Franklin, BA, Macera, CA, Heath, GW, Thompson, PD, and Bauman, A. Physical activity and public health: updated recommendation for adults from the American College of Sports Medicine and the American Heart Association. *Circulation* 116:1081, 2007.

21. Hessl, SM. Police and corrections. *Occup Med* 16:39-49, 2001.

22. Hootman, JM, Macera, CA, Ainsworth, BE, Martin, M, Addy, CL, and Blair, SN. Association among physical activity level, cardiorespiratory fitness, and risk of musculoskeletal injury. *Am J Epidemiol* 154:251-258, 2001.

23. Hue, O, Le Gallais, D, Chollet, D, Boussana, A, and Prefaut, C. The influence of prior cycling on biomechanical and cardiorespiratory response profiles during running in triathletes. *Eur J Appl Physiol Occup Physiol* 77:98-105, 1998.

24. Hydren, JR, and Cohen, BS. Current scientific evidence for a polarized cardiovascular endurance training model. *J Strength Cond Res* 29:3523-3530, 2015.

25. Jamnik, VK, Thomas, SG, Shaw, JA, and Gledhill, N. Identification and characterization of the critical physically demanding tasks encountered by correctional officers. *Appl Physiol Nutr Metab* 35:45-58, 2010.

26. Jones, BH, Cowan, DN, and Knapik, JJ. Exercise, training and injuries. *Sports Med* 18:202-214, 1994.

27. Kales, SN, Soteriades, ES, Christophi, CA, and Christiani, DC. Emergency duties and deaths from heart disease among firefighters in the United States. *N Engl J Med* 356:1207-1215, 2007.

28. Kilpatrick, MW, Martinez, N, Little, JP, Jung, ME, Jones, AM, Price, NW, and Lende, DH. Impact of high-intensity interval duration on perceived exertion. *Med Sci Sports Exerc* 47:1038-1045, 2015.

29. LaTourrette, T, Loughran, DS, and Seabury, SA. *Occupational Safety and Health for Public Safety Employees: Assessing the Evidence and the Implications for Public Policy.* Santa Monica, CA: Rand Corporation, 15-40, 2008.

30. Laursen, PB. Training for intense exercise performance: high-intensity or high-volume training? *Scand J Med Sci Sports* 20(Suppl 2):1-10, 2010.

31. Lee, SJ, and Hidler, J. Biomechanics of overground vs. treadmill walking in healthy individuals. *J Appl Physiol* 104:747-755, 2008.

32. Milanovic, Z, Sporis, G, and Weston, M. Effectiveness of high-intensity interval training (HIT) and continuous endurance training for $\dot{V}O_2$max improvements: a systematic review and meta-analysis of controlled trials. *Sports Med* 45:1469-1481, 2015.

33. Nielsen, RO, Buist, I, Parner, ET, Nohr, EA, Sorensen, H, Lind, M, and Rasmussen, S. Foot pronation is not associated with increased injury risk in novice runners wearing a neutral shoe: a 1-year prospective cohort study. *Br J Sports Med* 48:440-447, 2014.

34. Oliveira, C, Simões, M., and Bezerra, P. Exercise intensity in different exercise modes. In *Aerobic Exercise: Health Benefits, Types and Common Misconceptions.* Simmon, J, and Brown, A, eds. Hauppauge, NY: Nova Science, 155-170, 2013.

35. Perna, F, Bryner, R, Donley, D, Kolar, M, Hornsby, G, Sauers, J, Ullrich, I, and Yeater, R. Effect of diet and exercise on quality of life and fitness parameters among obese individuals. *J Exerc Physiol Online* 1, 1999.

36. Pierce, E, Weltman, A, Seip, R, and Snead, D. Effects of training specificity on the lactate threshold and $\dot{V}O_2$ peak. *Int J Sports Med* 11:267-272, 1990.

37. Potteiger, JA, and Webber, SF. Rating of perceived exertion and heart rate as indicators of exercise intensity in different environmental temperatures. *Med Sci Sports Exerc* 26:791-796, 1994.

38. Pryor, RR, Colburn, D, Crill, MT, Hostler, DP, and Suyama, J. Fitness characteristics of a suburban special weapons and tactics team. *J Strength Cond Res* 26:752-757, 2012.

39. Purvis, JW, and Cukiton, KJ. Ratings of perceived exertion at the anaerobic threshold. *Ergonomics* 24:295-300, 1981.

40. Reinking, MF, Austin, TM, and Hayes, AM. A survey of exercise-related leg pain in community runners. *Int J Sports Phys Ther* 8:269-276, 2013.

41. Reis, JF, Alves, FB, Bruno, PM, Vleck, V, and Millet, GP. Effects of aerobic fitness on oxygen uptake kinetics in heavy intensity swimming. *Eur J Appl Physiol* 112:1689-1697, 2012.

42. Reuter, BH, and Dawes, JJ. Program design and technique for aerobic endurance training. In *Essentials of Strength Training and Conditioning.* 4th ed. Haff, GG, and Triplett, NT, eds. Champaign, IL: Human Kinetics, 559-582, 2015.

43. Rhea, MR. Applications of Exercise Research to Fire Fighter Health and Fitness. Arizona State University, 2004.

44. Rhea, MR. Needs analysis and program design for police officers. *Strength Cond J* 37:30-34, 2015.

45. Ricciardi, R, Deuster, PA, and Talbot, LA. Metabolic demands of body armor on physical performance in simulated conditions. *Mil Med* 173:817-824, 2008.

46. Riley, PO, Paolini, G, Della Croce, U, Paylo, KW, and Kerrigan, DC. A kinematic and kinetic comparison of overground and treadmill walking in healthy subjects. *Gait Posture* 26:17-24, 2007.

47. Robergs, RA, and Landwehr, R. The surprising history of the "HRmax = 220 – age" equation. *J Exerc Physiol* 5:1-10, 2002.

48. Ronnestad, BR, Hansen, J, and Ellefsen, S. Block periodization of high-intensity aerobic intervals provides superior training effects in trained cyclists. *Scand J Med Sci Sports* 24:34-42, 2014.

49. Ronnestad, BR, Hansen, J, Thyli, V, Bakken, TA, and Sandbakk, O. 5-week block periodization increases aerobic power in elite cross-country skiers. *Scand J Med Sci Sports* 26:140-146, 2016.

50. Sarzynski, MA, Rankinen, T, Earnest, CP, Leon, AS, Rao, DC, Skinner, JS, and Bouchard, C. Measured maximal heart rates compared to commonly used age-based prediction equations in the Heritage Family Study. *Am J Hum Biol* 25:695-701, 2013.

51. Schneider, DA, Lacroix, KA, Atkinson, GR, Troped, PJ, and Pollack, J. Ventilatory threshold and maximal oxygen uptake during cycling and running in triathletes. *Med Sci Sports Exerc* 22:257-264, 1990.

52. Scribbans, TD, Vecsey, S, Hankinson, PB, Foster, WS, and Gurd, BJ. The effect of training intensity on V̇O₂max in young healthy adults: a meta-regression and meta-analysis. *Int J Exerc Sci* 9:230-247, 2016.

53. Sepkowitz, KA, and Eisenberg, L. Occupational deaths among healthcare workers. *Emerg Infect Dis* 11:1003-1008, 2005.

54. Simpson, RJ, Graham, SM, Florida-James, GD, Connaboy, C, Clement, R, and Jackson, AS. Perceived exertion and heart rate models for estimating metabolic workload in elite British soldiers performing a backpack load-carriage task. *Appl Physiol Nutr Metab* 35:650-656, 2010.

55. Skinner, JS, Jaskolski, A, Jaskolska, A, Krasnoff, J, Gagnon, J, Leon, AS, Rao, DC, Wilmore, JH, and Bouchard, C. Age, sex, race, initial fitness, and response to training: the HERITAGE Family Study. *J Appl Physiol (1985)* 90:1770-1776, 2001.

56. Sloth, M, Sloth, D, Overgaard, K, and Dalgas, U. Effects of sprint interval training on V̇O₂max and aerobic exercise performance: a systematic review and meta-analysis. *Scand J Med Sci Sports* 23:e341-e352, 2013.

57. Smith, DL. Firefighter fitness: improving performance and preventing injuries and fatalities. *Curr Sports Med Rep* 10:167-172, 2011.

58. Tanaka, H. Effects of cross-training. *Sports Med* 18:330-339, 1994.

59. Tovin, BJ. Prevention and treatment of swimmer's shoulder. *N Am J Sports Phys Ther* 1:166-175, 2006.

60. Treloar, AK, and Billing, DC. Effect of load carriage on performance of an explosive, anaerobic military task. *Mil Med* 176:1027-1031, 2011.

61. Wenger, HA, and Bell, GJ. The interactions of intensity, frequency and duration of exercise training in altering cardiorespiratory fitness. *Sports Med* 3:346-356, 1986.

62. Wollack and Associates. *Multijurisdictional Law Enforcement Physical Skills Survey*. Sacramento, CA: Author, 1992.

Chapter 15

1. American College of Sports Medicine (ACSM) position stand. Progression models in resistance training for healthy adults. *Med Sci Sports Exerc* 41:687-708, 2009.

2. *Army Physical Readiness Training.* U.S. Army, ed. Headquarters, Dept. of the Army, 434, 2012.

3. *FM 7-0 training units and developing leaders for full spectrum operations.* U.S. Army, ed. February 2011.

4. Abel, MG, Mortara, AJ, and Pettitt, RW. Evaluation of circuit-training intensity for firefighters. *J Strength Cond Res* 25:2895-2901, 2011.

5. Abel, MG, Sell, K, and Dennison, K. Design and implementation of fitness programs for firefighters. *Strength Cond J* 33:31-42, 2011.

6. Adams, J, Cheng, D, Lee, J, Shock, T, Kennedy, K, and Pate, S. Use of the bootstrap method to develop a physical fitness test for public safety officers who serve as both police officers and firefighters. *Proc (Bayl Univ Med Cent)* 27:199-202, 2014.

7. Adams, K, O'Shea, JP, O'Shea, KL, and Climstein, M. The effect of six weeks of squat, plyometric and squat-plyometric training on power production. *J Appl Sport Sci Res* 6:36-41, 1992.

8. Anderson, GS, Plecas, D, and Segger, T. Police officer physical ability testing: re-evaluating a selection criterion. *Policing* 24:23, 2001.

9. Arabatzi, F, Kellis, E, and Saez-Saez De Villarreal, E. Vertical jump biomechanics after plyometric, weight lifting, and combined (weight lifting + plyometric) training. *J Strength Cond Res* 24:2440-2448, 2010.

10. Babcock, L, Escano, M, D'Lugos, A, Todd, K, Murach, K, and Luden, N. Concurrent aerobic exercise interferes with the satellite cell response to acute resistance exercise. *Am J Physiol Regul Integr Comp Physiol* 302:R1458-R1465, 2012.

11. Baechle, TR, and Earle, RW. Learning how to manipulate training variables to maximize results. In *Weight Training: Steps to Success.* 4th ed. Champaign, IL: Human Kinetics, 177-188, 2011.

12. Berryman, N, Maurel, D, and Bosquet, L. Effect of plyometric vs. dynamic weight training on the energy cost of running. *J Strength Cond Res* 24:1818-1825, 2010.

13. Bonneau, J, and Brown, J. Physical ability, fitness and police work. *J Clin Forensic Med* 2:157-164, 1995.

14. Boyce, RW, Jones, GR, Schendt, KE, Lloyd, CL, and Boone, EL. Longitudinal changes in strength of police officers with gender comparisons. *J Strength Cond Res* 23:2411-2418, 2009.

15. Carlson, MJ, and Jaenen, SP. The development of a preselection physical fitness training program for Canadian Special Operations Regiment applicants. *J Strength Cond Res* 26(Suppl 2):S2-S14, 2012.

16. Chicharro, JL, Lopez-Mojares, LM, Lucia, A, Perez, M, Alvarez, J, Labanda, P, Calvo, F, and Vaquero, AF. Overtraining parameters in special military units. *Aviat Space Environ Med* 69:562-568, 1998.

17. Coutts, AJ, Murphy, AJ, and Dascombe, BJ. Effect of direct supervision of a strength coach on measures of muscular strength and power in young rugby league players. *J Strength Cond Res* 18:316-323, 2004.

18. Coutts, KD. Kinetic differences of two volleyball jumping techniques. *Med Sci Sports Exerc* 14:57-59, 1982.

19. De Villarreal, ES, Izquierdo, M, and Gonzalez-Badillo, JJ. Enhancing jump performance after combined vs. maximal power, heavy-resistance, and plyometric training alone. *J Strength Cond Res* 25:3274-3281, 2011.

20. Dean, C. *The modern warrior's combat load—dismounted operations in Afghanistan.* U.S. Army Center for Army Lessons Learned, Task Force Devil Combined Arms Assessment Team. 2003.

21. Dhahbi, W, Chaouachi, A, Padulo, J, Behm, DG, and Chamari, K. Five-meter rope-climbing: a commando-specific power test of the upper limbs. *Int J Sports Physiol Perform* 10:509-515, 2015.

22. Fatouros, IG, Jamurtas, AZ, Leontsini, D, Taxildaris, K, Aggelousis, N, Kostopoulos, N, and Buckenmeyer, P. Evaluation of plyometric exercise training, weight training, and their combination on vertical jumping performance and leg strength. *J Strength Cond Re* 14:470-476, 2000.

23. Fernandez-Fernandez, J, Sanz-Rivas, D, Kovacs, MS, and Moya, M. In-season effect of a combined repeated sprint and explosive strength training program on elite junior tennis players. *J Strength Cond Res* 29:351-357, 2015.

24. Fleck, SJ, and Kraemer, WJ. *Designing Resistance Training Programs.* Champaign, IL: Human Kinetics, 1-62, 179-296, 2014.

25. Folland, JP, and Williams, AG. The adaptations to strength training: morphological and neurological contributions to increased strength. *Sports Med* 37:145-168, 2007.

26. Gabriel, DA, Kamen, G, and Frost, G. Neural adaptations to resistive exercise: mechanisms and recommendations for training practices. *Sports Med* 36:133-149, 2006.

27. Gomez-Merino, D, Drogou, C, Chennaoui, M, Tiollier, E, Mathieu, J, and Guezennec, CY. Effects of combined stress during intense training on cellular immunity, hormones and respiratory infections. *Neuroimmunomodulation* 12:164-172, 2005.

28. Gould, D. Goal setting for peak performance. In *Applied Sport Psychology.* 2nd ed. Williams, JM, ed. Mountain View, CA: Mayfield, 158, 1993.

29. Grieco, CR, Cortes, N, Greska, EK, Lucci, S, and Onate, JA. Effects of a combined resistance-plyometric training program on muscular strength, running economy, and VO$_2$peak in division I female soccer players. *J Strength Cond Res,* 26: 2570-2576, 2012.

30. Gumieniak, RJ, Jamnik, VK, and Gledhill, N. Physical fitness bona fide occupational requirements for safety-related physically demanding occupations: test development considerations. *HFJC* 4:47-52, 2004.

31. Gumieniak, RJ, Jamnik, VK, and Gledhill, N. Catalog of Canadian fitness screening protocols for public safety occupations that qualify as a bona fide occupational requirement. *J Strength Cond Res* 27:1168-1173, 2013.

32. Hamill, BP. Relative safety of weightlifting and weight training. *J Strength Cond Res* 8:53-57, 1994.

33. Harman, EA, Gutekunst, DJ, Frykman, PN, Nindl, BC, Alemany, JA, Mello, RP, and Sharp, MA. Effects of two different eight-week training programs on military physical performance. *J Strength Cond Res* 22:524-534, 2008.

34. Hedrick, A. Training for hypertrophy. *Strength Cond J,* 17:22-29, 1995.

35. Hendrickson, NR, Sharp, MA, Alemany, JA, Walker, LA, Harman, EA, Spiering, BA, Hatfield, DL, Yamamoto, LM, Maresh, CM, Kraemer, WJ, and Nindl, BC. Combined resistance and endurance training improves physical capacity and performance on tactical occupational tasks. *Eur J Appl Physiol* 109:1197-1208, 2010.

36. Heneweer, H, Picavet, HS, Staes, F, Kiers, H, and Vanhees, L. Physical fitness, rather than self-reported physical activities, is more strongly associated with low back pain: evidence from a working population. *Eur Spine J* 21:1265-1272, 2012.

37. Hollander, IE, and Bell, NS. Physically demanding jobs and occupational injury and disability in the U.S. Army. *Mil Med* 175:705-712.

38. Hollander, IE, and Bell, NS. Physically demanding jobs and occupational injury and disability in the U.S. Army. *Mil Med* 175:705-712, 2010.

39. Israetel, MA, McBride, JM, Nuzzo, JL, Skinner, JW, and Dayne, AM. Kinetic and kinematic differences between squats performed with and without elastic bands. *J Strength Cond Res* 24:190-194, 2010.

40. Jones, TW, Howatson, G, Russell, M, and French, DN. Performance and neuromuscular adaptations following differing ratios of concurrent strength and endurance training. *J Strength Cond Res* 27:3342-3351, 2013.

41. Kennedy-Armbruster, C, Evans, EM, Sexauer, L, Peterson, J, and Wyatt, W. Association among functional-movement ability, fatigue, sedentary time, and fitness in 40 years and older active duty military personnel. *Mil Med* 178:1358-1364, 2013.

42. Knapik, JJ. Extreme conditioning programs: potential benefits and potential risks. *J Spec Oper Med* 15:108-113, 2015.

43. Knapik, JJ, Reynolds, KL, and Harman, E. Soldier load carriage: historical, physiological, biomechanical, and medical aspects. *Mil Med* 169:45-56, 2004.

44. Knapik, JJ, Rieger, W, Palkoska, F, Van Camp, S, and Darakjy, S. United States Army physical readiness training: rationale and evaluation of the physical training doctrine. *J Strength Cond Res* 23:1353-1362, 2009.

45. Knapik, JJ, Sharp, MA, Canham-Chervak, M, Hauret, K, Patton, JF, and Jones, BH. Risk factors for training-related injuries among men and women in basic combat training. *Med Sci Sports Exerc* 33:946-954, 2001.

46. Kraemer, WJ, and Koziris, LP. Muscle strength training: techniques and considerations. *Phys Ther Pract* 2:54-68, 1992.

47. Kraemer, WJ, Mazzetti, SA, Nindl, BC, Gotshalk, LA, Volek, JS, Bush, JA, Marx, JO, Dohi, K, Gomez, AL, Miles, M, Fleck, SJ, Newton, RU, and Hakkinen, K. Effect of resistance training on women's strength/power and occupational performances. *Med Sci Sports Exerc* 33:1011-1025, 2001.

48. Kraemer, WJ, Nindl, BC, Gotshalk, LA, Harman, FS, Volek, JS, Tokeshi, SA, Meth, S, Bush, JA, Etzweiler, SW, Fredman, BS, Sebastianelli, WJ, Putukian, M, Newton, RU, Hakkinen, K, and Fleck, S. Prediction of military relevant occupational tasks in women from physical performance components. In *Advances in Occupational Ergonomics and Safety*. Kumar, S, ed. Burke, VA: IOS Press, 719-722, 1998.

49. Kraemer, WJ, and Szivak, TK. Strength training for the warfighter. *J Strength Cond Res* 26(Suppl 2):S107-S118, 2012.

50. Kraemer, WJ, Vescovi, JD, Volek, JS, Nindl, BC, Newton, RU, Patton, JF, Dziados, JE, French, DN, and Hakkinen, K. Effects of concurrent resistance and aerobic training on load-bearing performance and the Army physical fitness test. *Mil Med* 169:994-999, 2004.

51. Krieger, JW. Single versus multiple sets of resistance exercise: a meta-regression. *J Strength Cond Res* 23:1890-1901, 2009.

52. Lagestad, P, and van den Tillaar, R. A comparison of training and physical performance of police students at the start and the end of three-year police education. *J Strength Cond Res* 28:1394-1400, 2014.

53. Lande, RG. Stress in service members. *Psychiatr Clin North Am* 37:547-560, 2014.

54. Larsen, B, Netto, K, and Aisbett, B. The effect of body armor on performance, thermal stress, and exertion: a critical review. *Mil Med* 176:1265-1273, 2011.

55. Lattari, E, Arias-Carrion, O, Monteiro-Junior, RS, Mello Portugal, EM, Paes, F, Menendez-Gonzalez, M, Silva, AC, Nardi, AE, and Machado, S. Implications of movement-related cortical potential for understanding neural adaptations in muscle strength tasks. *Int Arch Med* 7:9, 2014.

56. Mala, J, Szivak, TK, Flanagan, SD, Comstock, BA, Laferrier, JZ, Maresh, CM, and Kraemer, WJ. The role of strength and power during performance of high intensity military tasks under heavy load carriage. *US Army Med Dep J* Apr-Jun:3-11, 2015.

57. Mayer, JM, Quillen, WS, Verna, JL, Chen, R, Lunseth, P, and Dagenais, S. Impact of a supervised worksite exercise program on back and core muscular endurance in firefighters. *Am J Health Promot* 29:165-172, 2015.

58. Mazzetti, SA, Kraemer, WJ, Volek, JS, Duncan, ND, Ratamess, NA, Gomez, AL, Newton, RU, Hakkinen, K, and Fleck, SJ. The influence of direct supervision of resistance training on strength performance. *Med Sci Sports Exerc* 32:1175-1184, 2000.

59. McDonough, SL, Phillips, J, and Twilbeck, T. Determining best practices to reduce occupational health risks in firefighters. *J Strength Cond Res* 29(7):2041-2044, 2015.

60. McGuigan, M. Administration, scoring, and interpretation of selected tests. In *Essentials of Strength Training and Conditioning*. 4th ed. Haff, G, and Triplett, T, eds. Champaign, IL: Human Kinetics, 261, 350-390, 2016.

61. Melchiorri, G, and Rainoldi, A. Muscle fatigue induced by two different resistances: elastic tubing versus weight machines. *J Electromyogr Kinesiol* 21:954-959, 2011.

62. Michaelides, MA, Parpa, KM, Henry, LJ, Thompson, GB, and Brown, BS. Assessment of physical fitness aspects and their relationship to firefighters' job abilities. *J Strength Cond Res* 25:956-965, 2011.

63. Michaelides, MA, Parpa, KM, Thompson, J, and Brown, B. Predicting performance on a firefighter's ability test from fitness parameters. *Res Q Exerc Sport* 79:468-475, 2008.

64. Moritani, T, and deVries, HA. Neural factors versus hypertrophy in the time course of muscle strength gain. *Am J Phys Med* 58:115-130, 1979.

65. Naclerio, FJ, Colado, JC, Rhea, MR, Bunker, D, and Triplett, NT. The influence of strength and power on muscle endurance test performance. *J Strength Cond Res* 23:1482-1488, 2009.

66. Niebuhr, DW, Scott, CT, Powers, TE, Li, Y, Han, W, Millikan, AM, and Krauss, MR. Assessment of recruit motivation and strength study: preaccession physical fitness assessment predicts early attrition. *Mil Med* 173:555-562, 2008.

67. Nindl, BC, Castellani, JW, Warr, BJ, Sharp, MA, Henning, PC, Spiering, BA, and Scofield, DE. Physiological Employment Standards III: physiological challenges and consequences encountered during international military deployments. *Eur J Appl Physiol* 113:2655-2672, 2013.

68. Otto, RM, and Carpinelli, RN. A critical analysis of the single versus multiple set debate. *JEPonline* 9:32-57, 2006.

69. Paavolainen, L, Hakkinen, K, Hamalainen, I, Nummela, A, and Rusko, H. Explosive-strength training improves 5 km running time by improving running economy and muscle power. *J Appl Physiol* 86:1527-1533, 1999.

70. Pawlak, R, Clasey, J, Palmer, T, Symons, B, and Abel, MG. The effect of a novel tactical training program on physical fitness and occupational performance in firefighters. *J Strength Cond Res* 29:578-588, 2015.

71. Pawlak, R, Clasey, JL, Palmer, T, Symons, TB, and Abel, MG. The effect of a novel tactical training program on physical fitness and occupational performance in firefighters. *J Strength Cond Res* 29:578-588, 2015.

72. Payne, W, and Harvey, J. A framework for the design and development of physical employment tests and standards. *Ergonomics* 53:858-871, 2010.

73. Pelham, TW, Holt, LE, and White, H. Physical training of combat diving candidates: implications for the prevention of musculoskeletal injuries. *Work* 30:423-431, 2008.

74. Perez-Schindler, J, Hamilton, DL, Moore, DR, Baar, K, and Philp, A. Nutritional strategies to support concurrent training. *Eur J Sport Sci* 15:41-52, 2015.

75. Peterson, MD, Dodd, DJ, Alvar, BA, Rhea, MR, and Favre, M. Undulation training for development of hierarchical fitness and improved firefighter job performance. *J Strength Cond Res* 22:1683-1695, 2008.

76. Pincivero, DM, Lephart, SM, and Karunakara, RG. Effects of rest interval on isokinetic strength and functional performance after short-term high intensity training. *Br J Sports Med* 31:229-234, 1997.

77. Potach, DH, and Chu, DA. Program design and technique for plyometric training. In *Essentials of Strength Training and Conditioning*. 4th ed. Haff, G, and Triplett, NT, eds. Champaign, IL: Human Kinetics, 476-479, 2016.

78. Potach, DH, and Grindstaff, TL. Rehabilitation and reconditioning. In *Essentials of Strength Training and Conditioning*. 4th ed. Haff, G, and Triplett, NT, eds. Champaign, IL: Human Kinetics, 609-611, 2016.

79. Pryor, RR, Colburn, D, Crill, MT, Hostler, DP, and Suyama, J. Fitness characteristics of a suburban special weapons and tactics team. *J Strength Cond Res* 26:752-757, 2012.

80. Pugh, JK, Faulkner, SH, Jackson, AP, King, JA, and Nimmo, MA. Acute molecular responses to concurrent resistance and high-intensity interval exercise in untrained skeletal muscle. *Physiol Rep* 3(4), 2015.

81. Radcliffe, JN, Comfort, P, and Fawcett, T. The psychological strategies included by strength and conditioning coaches in applied strength and conditioning. *J Strength Cond Res* 29(9):2641-2654, 2015.

82. Ramirez-Campillo, R, Alvarez, C, Henriquez-Olguin, C, Baez, EB, Martinez, C, Andrade, DC, and Izquierdo, M. Effects of plyometric training on endurance and explosive strength performance in competitive middle- and long-distance runners. *J Strength Cond Res* 28:97-104, 2014.

83. Rhea, MR, Alvar, BA, and Gray, R. Physical fitness and job performance of firefighters. *J Strength Cond Res* 18:348-352, 2004.

84. Richmond, SR, and Godard, MP. The effects of varied rest periods between sets to failure using the bench press in recreationally trained men. *J Strength Cond Res* 18:846-849, 2004.

85. Robinson, JM, Stone, MH, Johnson, RL, Penland, CM, Warren, BJ, and Lewis, RD. Effects of different weight training exercise/rest intervals on strength, power, and high intensity exercise endurance. *J Strength Cond Res* 9:216-221, 1995.

86. Rohde, U, Sievert, A, Ruther, T, Witzki, A, and Leyk, D. Concept for a predeployment assessment of basic military fitness in the German Armed Forces. *J Strength Cond Res* 29(Suppl 11):S211-S215, 2015.

87. Rossomanno, CI, Herrick, JE, Kirk, SM, and Kirk, EP. A 6-month supervised employer-based minimal exercise program for police officers improves fitness. *J Strength Cond Res* 26:2338-2344, 2012.

88. Sale, DG. Neural adaptation to resistance training. *Med Sci Sports Exerc* 20:S135-S145, 1988.

89. Saunders, PU, Telford, RD, Pyne, DB, Peltola, EM, Cunningham, RB, Gore, CJ, and Hawley, JA. Short-term plyometric training improves running economy in highly trained middle and long distance runners. *J Strength Cond Res* 20:947-954, 2006.

90. Sharp, MA, Harman, EA, Boutilier, BE, Bovee, MW, and Kraemer, WJ. Progressive resistance training program for improving manual materials handling performance. *Work* 3:62-68, 1993.

91. Sheppard, JM, and Triplett, NT. Program design for resistance training. In *Essentials of Strength Training and Conditioning*. 4th ed. Haff, G, and Triplett, NT, eds. Champaign, IL: Human Kinetics, 441-442, 447-466, 2016.

92. Sporis, G, Harasin, D, Bok, D, Matika, D, and Vuleta, D. Effects of a training program for special operations battalion on soldiers' fitness characteristics. *J Strength Cond Res* 26:2872-2882, 2012.

93. Spurrs, RW, Murphy, AJ, and Watsford, ML. The effect of plyometric training on distance running performance. *Eur J Appl Physiol* 89:1-7, 2003.

94. Stevenson, MW, Warpeha, JM, Dietz, CC, Giveans, RM, and Erdman, AG. Acute effects of elastic bands during the free-weight barbell back squat exercise on velocity, power, and force production. *J Strength Cond Res* 24:2944-2954, 2010.

95. Stone, MH, and O'Bryant, HS. *Weight Training: A Scientific Approach*. Minneapolis: Burgess, 104-190, 1987.

96. Storer, TW, Dolezal, BA, Abrazado, ML, Smith, DL, Batalin, MA, Tseng, CH, and Cooper, CB. Firefighter health and fitness assessment: a call to action. *J Strength Cond Res* 28:661-671, 2014.

97. Strating, M, Bakker, RH, Dijkstra, GJ, Lemmink, KA, and Groothoff, JW. A job-related fitness test for the Dutch police. *Occup Med* 60:255-260, 2010.

98. Szivak, TK, Kraemer, WJ, Nindl, BC, Gotshalk, LA, Volek, JS, Gomez, AL, Dunn-Lewis, C, Looney, DP, Comstock, BA, Hooper, DR, Flanagan, SD, and Maresh, CM. Relationships of physical performance tests to military-relevant tasks in women. *US Army Med Dep J* Apr-Jun:20-26, 2014.

99. Tesch, PA. Training for bodybuilding. In *The Encyclopedia of Sports Medicine: Strength and Power in Sport*. Komi, PV, ed. Malden, MA: Blackwell Scientific, 370-381, 1992.

100. Tesch, PA, and Larsson, L. Muscle hypertrophy in bodybuilders. *Eur J Appl Physiol Occup Physiol* 49:301-306, 1982.

101. Thompson, BJ, Stock, MS, Shields, JE, Luera, MJ, Munayer, IK, Mota, JA, Carrillo, EC, and Olinghouse, KD. Barbell deadlift training increases the rate of torque development and vertical jump performance in novices. *J Strength Cond Res* 29:1-10, 2015.

102. Turner, AM, Owings, M, and Schwane, JA. Improvement in running economy after 6 weeks of plyometric training. *J Strength Cond Res* 17:60-67, 2003.

103. Vaara, JP, Kyrolainen, H, Niemi, J, Ohrankammen, O, Hakkinen, A, Kocay, S, and Hakkinen, K. Associations of maximal strength and muscular endurance test scores with cardiorespiratory fitness and body composition. *J Strength Cond Res* 26:2078-2086, 2012.

104. Vickers Jr, RR. *Physical abilities and military task performance: a replication and extension.* San Diego: NHR CENTER, 2009.

105. Willardson, JM, and Burkett, LN. A comparison of 3 different rest intervals on the exercise volume completed during a workout. *J Strength Cond Res* 19:23-26, 2005.

106. Willardson, JM, and Burkett, LN. The effect of different rest intervals between sets on volume components and strength gains. *J Strength Cond Res* 22:146-152, 2008.

107. Williams, AG, Rayson, MP, and Jones, DA. Resistance training and the enhancement of the gains in material-handling ability and physical fitness of British Army recruits during basic training. *Ergonomics* 45:267-279, 2002.

Chapter 16

1. American Physical Therapy Association (APTA). Guidelines: physical therapist scope of practice. March 2014. www.apta.org/uploadedFiles/APTAorg/About_Us/Policies/Practice/ScopePractice.pdf. Accessed May 27, 2015.

2. Beach, TA, Frost, DM, Clark, JM, Maly, MR, and Callaghan, JP. Unilateral ankle immobilization alters the kinematics and kinetics of lifting. *Work* 47(2):221-234, 2014.

3. Bompa, TO, and Haff, GG. *Periodization: Theory and Methodology of Training.* 5th ed. Champaign, IL: Human Kinetics, 99-103, 2009.

4. Brukner, P, and Kahn, K. *Brukner and Kahn's Clinical Sports Medicine.* 4th ed. North Ryde NSW: McGraw-Hill Australia, 6-10, 25-40, 245-246, 2012.

5. Buist, I, Bredeweg, SW, van Mechelen, W, Lemmink, KA, Pepping, GJ, and Diercks, RL. No effect of a graded training program on the number of running-related injuries in novice runners: a randomized controlled trial. *Am J Sports Med* 36(1):33-39, 2008.

6. Bullock, SH, Jones, BH, Gilchrist, J, and Marshall, SW. Prevention of physical training–related injuries: recommendations for the military and other active populations based on expedited systematic reviews. *Am J Prev Med* 38(1S):S156-S181, 2010.

7. Byrd, JWT, Jones, KS, Schmitz, LMR, and Doner, GP. Hip arthroscopy in the warrior athlete: 2 to 10 year outcomes. *J Hip Preserv Surg* 3(1):68-71, 2016.

8. Cameron, KL, and Owens, BD. The burden and management of sports-related musculoskeletal injuries and conditions within the U.S. military. *Clin Sports Med* 33:573-589, 2014.

9. Chen, MR, and Dragoo, JL. The effect of nonsteroidal anti-inflammatory drugs on tissue healing. *Knee Surg Sports Traumatol Arthrosc* 21(3):540-549, 2013.

10. Chinn, L, and Hertel, J. Rehabilitation of ankle and foot injuries in athletes. *Clin Sports Med* 29(1):157-167, 2010.

11. Durall, CJ, Manske, RC, and Davies, GJ. Avoiding shoulder injury from resistance training. *Strength Cond J* 23(5):10, 2001.

12. Escamilla, RF, Fleisig, GS, Lowry, TM, Barrentine, SW, and Andrews, JR. Effects of technique variations on knee biomechanics during the squat and leg press. *Med Sci Sports Exerc* 33(6):984-998, 2001.

13. Escamilla, RF, Fleisig, GS, Zheng, N, Lander, JE, Barrentine, SW, Andrews, JR, Bergemann, BW, and Moorman III, CT. A three-dimensional biomechanical analysis of the squat during varying stance widths. *Med Sci Sports Exerc* 33(9):1552-1566, 2001.

14. Fees, M, Decker, T, Snyder-Mackler, L, and Axe, MJ. Upper extremity weight-training modifications for the injured athlete. A clinical perspective. *Am J Sports Med* 26(5):732-742, 1998.

15. Fonseca, ST, Ocarino, JM, Silva, PL, and Aquino, CF. Integration of stress and their relationship to the KC. In *Scientific Foundations and Principles of Practice in Musculoskeletal Rehabilitation.* Magee, DJ, Zachazewski, JE, and Quillen, WS, eds. St. Louis: Saunders Elsevier, 476-486, 2007.

16. Fontana, HDB, Haupenthal, A, Ruschel, C, Hubert, M, Ridehalgh, C, and Roesler, H. Effect of gender, cadence, and water immersion on ground reaction forces during stationary running. *J Orthop Sports Phys Ther* 42(5):437-443, 2012.

17. French, D. Adaptations to anaerobic programs. In *Essentials of Strength and Conditioning.* 4th ed. Haff, GG, and Triplett, NT, eds. Champaign, IL: Human Kinetics, 87-114, 2016.

18. Frost, DM, Beach, TA, Callaghan, JP, and McGill, SM. Exercise-based performance enhancement and injury prevention for firefighters: contrasting the fitness and movement-related adaptations to two training methodologies. *J Strength Cond Res* 29(9):2441-2459, 2015.

19. Fry, AC, Smith, JC, and Schilling, BK. Effect of knee position on hip and knee torques during the barbell squat. *J Strength Cond Res* 17:629-633, 2003.

20. Fukuda, TY, Fingerhut, D, Moreira, VC, Camarini, PMF, Scodeller, NF, Duarte, A, Martinelli, M, and Bryk, FF. Open kinetic chain exercises in a restricted range of motion after anterior cruciate ligament reconstruction: a randomized controlled clinical trial. *Am J Sports Med* 41:788-794, 2013.

21. George, SZ, Childs, JD, Teyhen, DS, Wu, SS, and Wright, AC. Predictors of occurrence and severity of first time low back pain episodes: findings from a military inception cohort. *PLoS ONE* 7(2):e30597, 2012. doi:10.1371/journal.pone.0030597.

22. Granter, R. Treatments use for musculoskeletal conditions: more choices and more evidence. In *Brukner and Kahn's Clinical Sports Medicine.* 4th ed. Brukner, P, ed. North Ryde, NSW: McGraw-Hill Australia, 164-209, 2012.

23. Hale, SA, Fergus, A, Axmacher, R, and Kiser, K. Bilateral improvements in lower extremity function after unilateral balance training in individuals with chronic ankle instability. *J Athl Train* 49(2):181-191, 2014.

24. Hauret, KG, Jones, BH, Bullock, SH, Canham-Chervak, MC, Canada, S, Mitchener, TA, and Moore, S. Musculoskeletal injuries: description of an under-recognized injury problem among military personnel. *Am J Prev Med* 38(1S):S61-S70, 2010.

25. Hegedus, EJ, McDonough, SM, Bleakley, C, Baxter, D, and Cook, CE. Clinician-friendly lower extremity physical performance measures in athletes: a systematic review of measurement properties and correlation with injury, part 2. The tests for the hip, thigh, foot and ankle including the Star Excursion Balance Test. *Br J Sports Med* 49(10):649-656, 2015.

26. Hegedus, EJ, McDonough, SM, Bleakley, C, Cook, CE, and Baxter, D. Clinician-friendly lower extremity physical performance measures in athletes: a systematic review of measurement properties and correlation with injury, part 1. The tests for knee function including the hop tests. *Br J Sports Med* 49(10):642-648, 2015.

27. Hooper, DR, Szivak, TK, DiStefano, LJ, Comstock, BA, Dunn-Lewis, C, Apicella, JM, Kelly, NA, Creighton, BC, Volek, JS, Maresh, CM, and Kraemer, WJ. Effects of resistance training fatigue on joint biomechanics. *J Strength Cond Res* 27(1):146-153, 2013.

28. Jacobs, JM, Cameron, KL, and Bojescul, JA. Lower extremity stress fractures in the military. *Clin Sports Med* 33:591-613, 2014.

29. Jarvinen, TAH, Jarvinen, M, and Kalimo, H. Regeneration of injured skeletal muscle after the injury. *Muscles Ligaments Tendons J* 3(4):337-345, 2013.

30. Jeffreys, I. A multidimensional approach to enhancing recovery. *Strength Cond J* 27(15):78-85, 2005.

31. Jones, BH, Canham-Chervak, MC, Canada, S, Mitchener, TA, and Moore, S. Medical surveillance of injuries in the U.S. military descriptive epidemiology and recommendations for improvement. *Am J Prev Med* 38(1S):S42-S60, 2010.

32. Kannus, P, Parkkari, J, Jarvinen, TLN, and Jarvinen, M. Basic science and clinical studies coincide: active treatment approach is needed after a sports injury. *Scand J Med Sci Sports* 13(3):1540-1544, 2003.

33. Kisner, C, and Colby, LA. *Therapeutic Exercise: Foundation and Techniques*. Philadelphia: F.A. Davis, 315-329, 2012.

34. Knapik, JJ, Graham, B, Cobbs, A, Thompson, D, and Jones, BH. A prospective investigation of injury incidence and injury risk factors among army recruits in military police training. *BMC Musculoskelet Disord* 14:32, 2013.

35. Knapik, JJ, Hauret, KG, Arnold, S, Canham-Chervak, M, Mansfield, AJ, Hoedebecke, EL, and McMillian, D. Injury and fitness outcomes during implementation of Physical Readiness Training. *Int J Sports Med* 24:372-381, 2003.

36. Knapik, JJ, Sharp, MA, Canham-Chervak, M, Hauret, K., Patton, JF, and Jones, BH. Risk factors for training-related injuries among men and women in basic combat training. *Med Sci Sports Exerc* 33:946-954, 2001.

37. Kollock, RO, Andrews, C, Johnston, A, Elliot, T, Wilson, AE, Games, KE, and Sefton, JM. A meta-analysis to determine if lower extremity muscle strengthening should be included in military knee-overuse injury-prevention programs. *J Athl Train*, March 2016. [e-pub ahead of print].

38. Lawrence, RL, Braman, JP, Staker, JL, Laprade, RF, and Ludewig, PM. Comparison of 3-dimensional shoulder complex kinematics in individuals with and without shoulder pain, part 2: glenohumeral joint. *J Orthop Sports Phys Ther* 44(9):646-655, 2014.

39. Lehr, ME, Plisky, PJ, Butler, RJ, Fink, ML, Kiesel, KB, and Underwood, FB. Field-expedient screening and injury risk algorithm categories as predictors of noncontact lower extremity injury. *Scand J Med Sci Sports* 23:e225-e232, 2013.

40. Malanga, GA, Yan, N, and Stark, J. Mechanisms and efficacy of heat and cold therapies for musculoskeletal injury. *Postgrad Med* 127(1):57-65, 2015.

41. Malliaras, P, Barton, CJ, Reeves, ND, and Langberg, H. Achilles and patellar tendinopathy loading programmes: a systematic review comparing clinical outcomes and identifying potential mechanisms for effectiveness. *Sports Med* 43(4):267-286, 2013.

42. McGill, SM. *Low Back Disorders: Evidence-Based Prevention and Rehabilitation*. 3rd ed. Champaign, IL: Human Kinetics, 97-151, 2016.

43. McKeon, PO, Hertel, J, Bramble, D, and Davis, I. The foot core system: a new paradigm for understanding intrinsic foot muscle function. *Br J Sports Med* 49:290, 2015.

44. Meeusen, R, Duclos, M, Foster, C, Fry, A, Gleeson, M, Nieman, D, Raglin, J, Rietjens, G, Steinacker, J, and Urhausen, A. Prevention, diagnosis and treatment of the overtraining syndrome: joint consensus statement of the European College of Sport Science and the American College of Sports Medicine. *Eur J Sport Sci* 13(1):1-24, 2013.

45. Moore, JH, Goffar, SL, Teyhen, DS, Pendergrass, TL, Childs, JD, and Ficke, JR. The role of U.S. military physical therapists during recent combat campaigns. *Phys Ther* 93:1268-1275, 2013.

46. Nabeel, I, Baker, BA, McGrail Jr, MP, and Flottemesch, TJ. Correlation between physical activity, fitness, and musculoskeletal injuries in police officers. *Minn Med* 90(9):40-43, 2007.

47. Nagura, T, Dyrby, CO, Alexander, EJ, and Andriacchi, TP. Mechanical loads at the knee joint during deep flexion. *J Orthop Res* 20:881-886, 2002.

48. National Athletic Trainers' Association (NATA). Athletic training education overview. www.nata.org/athletic-training-education-overview. Accessed May 27, 2015.

49. National Strength and Conditioning Association (NSCA). Professional Standards and Guidelines Task Force. Strength and conditioning professional standards and guidelines. July 2009. www.nsca.com/uploadedFiles/NSCA/Resources/PDF/Education/Tools_and_Resources/NSCA_strength_and_conditioning_professional_standards_and_guidelines.pdf. Accessed September 26, 2015.

50. National Fire Protection Association (NFPA). Firefighter injuries in the United States. November 2014. www.nfpa.org/research/reports-and-statistics/the-fire-service/fatalities-and-injuries/firefighter-injuries-in-the-united-states. Accessed May 29, 2015.

51. Nindl, BC, Jones, BH, Van Arsdale, SJ, Kelly, K, and Kraemer, WJ. Operational physical performance and fitness in military women: physiological, musculoskeletal injury, and optimized physical training considerations for successfully integrating women into combat-centric military occupations. *Mil Med* 181(1 Suppl):50-62, 2016. doi:10.7205/MILMED-D-15-00382.

52. Noehren, B, Pohl, MB, Sanchez, Z, Cunningham, T, and Lattermann, C. Proximal and distal kinematics in female runners with patellofemoral pain. *Clin Biomech* 27:366-371, 2012.

53. Orr, R, Pope, R, Johnston, V, and Coyle, J. Load carriage and its force impact. *ADFJ* 185:52-63, 2011.

54. Owens, BD. The incidence and characteristics of shoulder instability at the United States Military Academy. *Am J Sports Med* 35(7):1168-1173, 2007.

55. Pagnani, MJ, and Warren, RF. Stabilizers of the glenohumeral joint. *J Shoulder Elbow Surg* 3(3):173-190, 1994.

56. Pollock, ML, Gettman, LR, Milesis, CA, Bah, MD, Durstine, L, and Johnson, RB. Effects of frequency and duration of training on attrition and incidence of injury. *Med Sci Sports* 9(1):31-36, 1977.

57. Purdam, CR, Jonsson, P, Alfredson, H, Lorentzon, R, Cook, JL, and Khan, KM. A pilot study of the eccentric decline squat in the management of painful chronic patellar tendinopathy. *BJSM* 38:395-397, 2004.

58. Quigley, EJ, and Richards, JG. The effects of cycling on running mechanics. *J App Biomech* 12:470-479, 1996.

59. Rauh, MJ, Macera, CA, Trone, DW, Shaffer, RA, and Brodine, SK. Epidemiology of stress fracture and lower-extremity overuse injuries in female recruits. *Med Sci Sports Exerc* 38:1571-1577, 2006.

60. Schoenfeld, BJ. The use of nonsteroidal anti-inflammatory drugs for exercise-induced muscle damage: implications for skeletal muscle development. *Sports Med* 42(12):1017-1028, 2012.

61. Schoenfeld, BJ. Squatting kinematics and kinetics and their application to exercise performance. *J Strength Cond Res* 24(12):3497-3506, 2010.

62. Seabury SA, and McLaren CF. The frequency, severity, and economic consequences of musculoskeletal injuries to firefighters in California. Santa Monica, CA: RAND Corporation, 12, 2010.

63. Sharma, P, and Maffulli, N. Tendon injury and tendinopathy: healing and repair. *J Bone Joint Surg Am* 87:187-202, 2005.

64. Silbernagel, KG, and Crossley, KM. A proposed return-to-sport program for patients with midportion Achilles tendinopathy: rationale and implementation. *J Orthop Sports Phys Ther* 44(11):876-886, 2015.

65. Slivka, DR, Hailes, WS, Cuddy, JS, and Ruby, BC. Effects of 21 days of intensified training on markers of overtraining. *J Strength Cond Res* 24(10):2604-2612, 2010.

66. Swinton, PA, Stewart, A, Agouris, I, Keogh, JWL, and Lloyd, R. A biomechanical analysis of straight and hexagonal barbell deadlifts using submaximal loads. *J Strength Cond Res* 25(7):2000-2009, 2011.

67. Reichard, AA, and Jackson, LL. Occupational injuries among emergency responders. *Am J Ind Med* 53:1-11, 2010

68. Teyhen, DS, Shaffer, SW, Butler, RJ, Goffar, SL, Kiesel, KB, Rhon, DI, Williamson, JN, and Plisky, PJ. What risk factors are associated with musculoskeletal injury in U.S. Army Rangers? A prospective prognostic study. *Clin Orthop Relat Res*, May 27, 2015. [e-pub ahead of print].

69. USACHPPM REPORT NO. 21-KK-08QR-08. Recommendations for prevention of physical training (PT)-related injuries: results of a systematic evidence-based review by the Joint Services Physical Training Injury Prevention Work Group (JSPTIPWG) U.S. Army Center for Health Promotion and Preventive Medicine. July 2008. www.dtic.mil/dtic/tr/fulltext/u2/a484873.pdf. Accessed May 29, 2015.

70. Van den Bekerom, M, Struiis, P, Blankevoort, L, Welling, L, and Kerkhoffs, G. What is the evidence for rest, ice, compression, and elevation therapy in the treatment of ankle sprains in adults? *J Athl Train* 47(4):435-443, 2012.

71. Wall, BT, Dirks, ML, Snidjers, T, Senden, JMG, Dolmans, J, and van Loon, LJC. Substantial skeletal muscle loss occurs during only 5 days of disuse. *Acta Physiol* 210:600-611, 2014.

72. Wall, PD, Fernandez, M, Griffin, DR, and Foster, NE. Nonoperative treatment for femoroacetabular impingement: a systematic review of the literature. *PM&R* 5(5):418-426, 2013.

73. Warden, SJ, Davis, IS, and Fredericson, M. Management and prevention of bone stress injuries in long-distance runners. *J Orthop Sports Phys Ther* 44(10):749-765, 2014.

74. Wilkinson, DM, Blacker, SD, Richmond, VL, Horner, FE, Rayson, MP, Spiess, A, and Knapik, JJ. Injuries and injury risk factors among British army infantry soldiers during predeployment training. *Inj Prev* 17(6):381-387, 2011.

75. Witvrouw, E, Callaghan, MJ, Stefanik, JJ, Noehren, B, Bazett-Jones, DM, Earl-Boehm, JE, Davis, IS, Powers, CM, McConnell, J, Crossley, KM. Patellofemoral pain: consensus statement from the 3rd International Patellofemoral Pain Research Retreat. *Br J Sports Med* 48:411-414, 2014.

Chapter 17

1. Abel, MG, Mortara, AJ, and Pettitt, RW. Evaluation of circuit-training intensity for firefighters. *J Strength Cond Res* 25:2895-2901, 2011.

2. Abel, MG, Palmer, TG, and Trubee, N. Exercise program design for structural firefighters. *Strength Cond J* 37:11, 2015.

3. Abel, MG, Sell, K, and Dennison, K. Design and implementation of fitness programs for firefighters. *Strength Cond J* 33:31-42, 2011.

4. Abel, MG, Triplett, NT, Dawes, J, Pettitt, RW, Pawlak, R, and Havener, K. Effect of a single bout of heavy resistance training on subsequent fireground performance. In *Proceedings of the National Strength and Conditioning Association Conference, Orlando, FL, 8-11 July, 2015. J Strength Cond Res*, in press.

5. American College of Sports Medicine (ACSM). *ACSM's Guidelines for Exercise Testing and Prescription*. 9th ed. Philadelphia: Lippincott Williams & Wilkins, 40-59, 88-93, 2014.

6. Assadi, SN, Esmaily, H, and Mostaan, L. (2013). Comparison of sensory–neural hearing between firefighters and office workers. *Int J Prev Med* 4:115, 2013.

7. Astrand, P-O, Rodahl, K, Dahl, HA, and Stromme, SB. *Work Physiology: Physiological Basis of Exercise*. 4th ed. Champaign, IL: Human Kinetics, 2003.

8. Barr, D, Gregson, W, and Reilly, T. The thermal ergonomics of firefighting reviewed. *Appl Ergonomics* 41:161-172, 2010.

9. Barr, D, Reilly, T, and Gregson, W. The impact of different cooling modalities on the physiological responses in firefighters during strenuous work performed in high environmental temperatures. *Eur J of Appl Physiol* 111:959-967, 2011.

10. Barregard, L, Sällsten, G, Gustafson, P, Andersson, L, Johansson, L, Basu, S, and Stigendal, L. Experimental exposure to wood-smoke particulates in healthy humans: effects on markers of inflammation, coagulation, and lipid peroxidation. *Inhal Toxicol* 18:845-853, 2006.

11. Bartsch, P, and Gibbs, SR. Effect of altitude on the heart and lungs. *Circulation* 116:2191-2202, 2007.

12. Baur, DM, Christophi, CA, and Kales, SN. Metabolic syndrome is inversely related to cardiorespiratory fitness in male career firefighters. *J Strength Cond Res* 26:2331-2337, 2012.

13. Baur, DM, Christophi, CA, Tsismenakis, AJ, Cook, EF, and Kales, SN. Cardiorespiratory fitness predicts cardiovascular risk profiles in career firefighters. *J Occup Environ Med* 53:1155-1160, 2011.

14. Behm, DG, Drinkwater, EJ, Willardson, JM, and Cowley, PM. The use of instability to train the core musculature. *Appl Physiol Nutr Metab* 35:91-108, 2010.

15. Bilzon, JL, Scarpello, EG, Smith, CV, Ravenhill, NA, and Rayson, MP. Characterization of the metabolic demands of simulated shipboard Royal Navy fire-fighting tasks. *Ergonomics* 44:766-780, 2001.

16. Binkley, HM, Beckett, J, Casa, DJ, Kleiner, DM, and Plummer, PE. National Athletic Trainers' Association position statement: exertional heat illnesses. *J Athl Training* 37:329-343, 2002.

17. Britton, C, Lynch, CF, Ramirez, M, Torner, J, Buresh, C, and Peek-Asa, C. Epidemiology of injuries to wildland firefighters. *Am Journal Emer Med* 31:339-345, 2013.

18. Britton, C, Lynch, CF, Torner, J, and Peek-Asa, C. Fire characteristics associated with firefighter injury on large federal wildland fires. *Ann Epidemiol* 23:37-42, 2013.

19. Brooks, GA, Fahey, TD, and Baldwin, KM. *Exercise Physiology: Human Bioenergetics and its Application*. 4th ed. Columbus, OH: McGraw-Hill, 543-565, 2005.

20. Broome, RE, Lyman, Z, and Told, J. Mind-body integrative training: firefighter personal protective equipment (PPE). *IFSJLM* 8:59-65, 2014.

21. Carey, MG, Al-Zaiti, SS, Dean, GE, Sessanna, L, and Finnell, DS. Sleep problems, depression, substance use, social bonding, and quality of life in professional firefighters. *J Occup Environ Med* 53:928-933, 2011.

22. Castellani, JW, Young, AJ, Ducharme, MB, Giesbrecht, GG, Glickman, E, and Sallis, RE. American College of Sports Medicine position stand: prevention of cold injuries during exercise. *Med Sci Sports Exerc* 38:2012-2029, 2006.

23. Cheung, SS. *Advanced Environmental Exercise Physiology*. Champaign, IL: Human Kinetics, 2010.

24. Chiou, SS, Turner, N, Zwiener, J, Weaver, DL, and Haskell, WE. Effect of boot weight and sole flexibility on gait and physiological responses of firefighters in stepping over obstacles. *Hum Factors* 54:373-386, 2012.

25. Craig, FN, and Moffitt, JT. Efficiency of evaporative cooling from wet clothing. *J Appl Physiol* 36:313-316, 1974.

26. Davis, PO, Dotson, CO, and Laine, D. Relationship between simulated firefighting tasks and physical performance measures. *Med Sci Sports Exer* 14:65-71, 1982.

27. Dennison, KJ, Mullineaux, DR, Yates, JW, and Abel, MG. The effect of fatigue and training status on firefighter performance. *J Strength Cond Res* 26:1101-1109, 2012.

28. Domitrovich, JW. *Wildland Firefighter Health and Safety Report #14*. United States Forest Service: MTDC, 2011.

29. Domitrovich, JW. *Wildland firefighter health and safety*. Doctoral dissertation, University of Montana, 2011.

30. Domitrovich, JW, and Sharkey, BJ. *Heat illness education for wildland firefighters. 1051-2316P-MTDC*. United States Forest Service: MTDC, 2010.

31. Dorman, LE, and Havenith, G. The effects of protective clothing on energy consumption during different activities. *Eur J Appl Physiol* 105:463-470, 2009.

32. Dreger, RW, Jones, RL, and Petersen, SR. Effects of the self-contained breathing apparatus and fire protective clothing on maximal oxygen uptake. *Ergonomics* 49:911-920, 2006.

33. Dreger, RW, and Paradis, S. Clinical study and technical report by NAIT University. March 7, 2013. www.training mask.com/clinicals/clinical-study-and-technical-report-by-nait-university.

34. Eves, ND, Petersen, SR, and Jones, RL. Hyperoxia improves maximal exercise with the self-contained breathing apparatus (SCBA). *Ergonomics* 45:829-839, 2002.

35. Fahy, RF. U.S. firefighter fatalities due to sudden cardiac death, 1995-2004. *NFPA J* 99:44-47, 2005.

36. Fahy, RF. *U.S. Firefighter Deaths Related to Training, 1996-2005.* Quincy, MA: National Fire Protection Association, 2006.

37. Fahy, RF. *Wildland Firefighter Fatalities, 1999-2008.* Quincy, MA: National Fire Protection Association, 2009.

38. Fahy, RF. *Firefighter Fatalities due to Heat Stroke in the United States, 1999 to 2011.* Quincy, MA: National Fire Protection Association, 2011.

39. Fahy, RF. *U.S. Firefighter Deaths Related to Training, 2001-2010.* Quincy, MA: National Fire Protection Association, 2012.

40. Fahy, RF, LeBlanc, PR, and Molis, JL. *Firefighter Fatalities in the United States, 2010.* Quincy, MA: National Fire Protection Association, 2011.

41. Fahy, RF, LeBlanc, PR, and Molis, JL. *Firefighter Fatalities in the United States, 2013.* Quincy, MA: National Fire Protection Association, 2014.

42. Feairheller, DL. Blood pressure and heart rate responses in volunteer firefighters while wearing personal protective equipment. *Blood Press Monit* 20:194-198, 2015.

43. Fent, KW, and Evans, DE. Assessing the risk to firefighters from chemical vapors and gases during vehicle fire suppression. *J Environ Monit* 13:536-543, 2011.

44. Fire Service Institute (FSI). *Firefighter Fatalities and Injuries: The Role of Heat Stress and PPE.* University of Illinois Fire Service Institute: Firefighter Life Safety Research Center, 2008.

45. Fogarity, AL, Armstrong, KA, Gordon, CJ, Groeller, H, Woods, BF, Stocks, JM, and Taylor, NAS. Cardiovascular and thermal consequences of protective clothing: a comparison of clothed and unclothed states. *Ergonomics* 47:1073-1086, 2004.

46. Foster, JA, and Roberts, GV. *Measurements of Firefighting Environment. Central Fire Brigades Advisory Council, Joint Committee on Fire Research Report 61/1994.* Wetherby, UK: ODPM, 1994.

47. Frost, DM, Beach, TAC, Callaghan, JP, and McGill, SM. Exercise-based performance enhancement and injury prevention for firefighters: contrasting the fitness- and movement-related adaptations to two training methodologies. *J Strength Cond* 29:2441-2459, 2015.

48. Garcia-Pallares, J, and Izquierdo, M. Strategies to optimize concurrent training of strength and aerobic fitness for rowing and canoeing. *Sports Med* 41:329-343, 2011.

49. Gasser, GA, and Brooks, GA. Metabolic bases of excess post-exercise oxygen consumption: a review. *Med Sci Sport Exer* 16:29-43, 1984.

50. Gavin, TP. Clothing and thermoregulation during exercise. *Sports Med* 33:941-947, 2003.

51. Gledhill, N, and Jamnik, VK. Characterization of the physical demands of firefighting. *Can J Sports Sci* 17:207-213, 1992.

52. Gleeson, M. Immune function and exercise. *Eur J Sport Sci* 4:52-66, 2004.

53. Haff, GG, and Triplett, NT. *Essentials of Strength and Conditioning.* 4th ed. Champaign, IL: Human Kinetics, 2016.

54. Hartman, J. Bearing the cold: tips for cold weather exercise. *TSAC Report* 40:4-7, 2016.

55. Haynes, HJG, and Stein, GP. *US Fire Department Profile 2014.* Quincy, MA: National Fire Protection Association, 3, 2016.

56. Heil, DP. Estimating energy expenditure in wildland fire fighters using a physical activity monitor. *Appl Ergonomics* 33:405-413, 2002.

57. Hilton, AD. *Occupationally acquired hearing loss among civilian and active fire-fighters.* Thesis, University of Texas, 2002.

58. Holmer, I, and Gavhed, D. Classification of metabolic and respiratory demands in fire fighting activity with extreme workloads. *Appl Ergonomics* 38:45-52, 2007.

59. Horn, GP, Blevins, S, Fernhall, B, and Smith, DL. Core temperature and heart rate response to repeated bouts of firefighting activities. *Ergonomics* 56:1465-1473, 2013.

60. Hur, P, Rosengren, KS, Horn, GP, Smith, DL, and Hsiao-Wecksler, ET. Effect of protective clothing and fatigue on functional balance of firefighters. *J Ergonomics* S2:004, 2013.

61. Issurin, V. Block periodization versus traditional training theory: a review. *J Sports Med Phys Fitness* 48:65-75, 2008.

62. International Association of Fire Fighters (IAFF). *Fire service joint labor management wellness-fitness task force: candidate physical ability test program summary.* www.iaff.org/hs/cpat/cpat_index.html. Accessed May 12, 2015.

63. International Association of Fire Fighters (IAFF) and International Association of Fire Chiefs (IAFC). *IAFF/IAFC Fire Service Joint Labor Management Wellness Fitness Initiative.* 3rd ed. Washington, DC: IAFF, 7, 2008.

64. International Association of Fire Fighters (IAFF), International Association of Fire Chiefs (IAFC), and American Council on Exercise (ACE). *The IAFF/IAFC/ACE Peer Fitness Trainer Resource Manual.* Monterey, CA: Healthy Learning, 2003.

65. Jahnke, SA, Poston, WSC, Haddock, CK, and Jitnarin, N. Obesity and incident injury among career firefighters in the central United States. *Obesity* 21:1505-1508, 2013.

66. Karter, MJ. *Patterns of firefighter fireground injuries. Report.* Quincy, MA: National Fire Protection Association, 2009.

67. Karter, MJ, and Molis, JL. U.S. firefighter injuries, 2010. *NFPA J* Nov/Dec, 2011.

68. Karter, MJ, and Molis, JL. U.S. firefighters injuries, 2013. *NFPA J* Nov/Dec, 2014.

69. Kuehl, KS, Kisbu-Sakarya, Y, Elliot, DL, Moe, EL, Defrancesco, CA, Mackinnon, DP, Lockhart, G, Goldberg, L, and Kuehl, HE. Body mass index as a predictor of firefighter injury and workers' compensation claims. *J Occup Environ Med* 54:579-582, 2012.

70. Kizakevich, PN, McCartney, ML, Hazucha, MJ, Sleet, LH, Jochem, WJ, Hackney, AC, and Bolick, K. Noninvasive ambulatory assessment of cardiac function in healthy men exposed to carbon monoxide during upper and lower body exercise. *Eur J Appl Physiol Occup Physiol* 83:7-16, 2000.

71. Leetun, DT, Ireland, ML, Wilson, JD, Ballantyne, BT, and Davis, IM. Core stability measures as risk factors for lower extremity injuries in athletes. *Med Sci Sports Exer* 36:926-934, 2004.

72. Leveritt, M, Abernethy, PJ, Barry, BK, and Logan, PA. Concurrent strength and endurance training: a review. *Sports Med* 28:413-427, 1999.

73. Lord, C, Netto, K, Petersen, A, Nichols, D, Drain, J, Phillips, M, and Aisbett, B. Validating "fit for duty" tests for Australian volunteer firefighters suppressing bushfires. *Appl Ergonomics* 43:191-197, 2012.

74. Mangan, RJ. Injuries, illnesses, and fatalities among wildland firefighters. *Fire Manag Today* 62:36-40, 2002.

75. Martin, D, and Windsor, J. From mountain to bedside: understanding the clinical relevance of human acclimatisation to high-altitude hypoxia. *J Postgrad Med* 84:622-627, 2008.

76. Merry, TL, Ainslie, PN, and Cotter, JD. Effects of aerobic fitness on hypohydration-induced physiological strain and exercise impairment. *Acta Physiol* 198:179-190, 2010.

77. Michaelides, MA, Parpa, KM, Henry, LJ, Thompson, GB, and Brown, BS. Assessment of physical fitness aspects and their relationship to firefighters' job abilities. *J Strength Cond Res* 25:956-965, 2011.

78. Miranda, AI, Martins, V, Cascão, P, Amorim, JH, Valente, J, Borrego, C, Ferreira, AJ, Cordeiro, CR, Viegas, DX, and Ottmar, R. Wildland smoke exposure values and exhaled breath indicators in firefighters. *J Toxicol Env Health, Part A* 75:831-843, 2012.

79. National Fire Protection Association (NFPA). *NFPA 1977: Standard on Protective Clothing and Equipment for Wildland Firefighting.* Quincy, MA: NFPA, 9, 2011.

80. National Fire Protection Association (NFPA). *NFPA 1051: Standard for Wildland Firefighter Professional Qualifications.* Quincy, MA: NFPA, 2012.

81. National Fire Protection Association (NFPA). *NFPA 1582: Standard on Comprehensive Occupational Medical Program for Fire Departments.* Quincy, MA: NFPA, 18, 2013.

82. National Fire Protection Association (NFPA). *NFPA 1500: Standard on Fire Department Occupational Safety and Health Program.* Quincy, MA: NFPA, 6, 9, 2013.

83. National Fire Protection Association (NFPA). *NFPA 1971: Standard on Protective Ensembles for Structural Firefighting and Proximity Firefighting.* Quincy, MA: NFPA, 16, 2013.

84. National Fire Protection Association (NFPA). *NFPA 1583: Standard on Health-Related Fitness Programs for Firefighters.* Quincy, MA: NFPA, 1583-1586, 2015.

85. National Institute for Occupational Safety and Health (NIOSH). *Criteria for a recommended standard: occupational exposure to hot environments.* Cincinnati: U.S. Department of Health and Human Services, Public Health Service, Centers for Disease Control and Prevention, National Institute for Occupational Safety and Health, DHHS (NIOSH) Publication No. 86-113, 1986.

86. National Institute for Occupational Safety and Health (NIOSH). *Wildland firefighter dies from hyperthermia and exertional heatstroke while conducting mop-up operations—Texas. A summary of a NIOSH firefighter fatality investigation.* Report #2011-17, 2012.

87. National Institute for Occupational Safety and Health (NIOSH). *Health hazard evaluation report: evaluation of chemical exposures during firefighter training exercises involving smoke simulant.* Cincinnati: U.S. Department of Health and Human Services, Centers for Disease Control and Prevention, National Institute for Occupational Safety and Health, NIOSH HETA Report No. 2012-0028-3190, 2013.

88. National Volunteer Fire Council (NVFC) and United States Fire Administration (USFA). *Retention and Recruitment for the Volunteer Emergency Services: Challenges and Solutions.* NVFC-USFA (FA-310), 6-10, 2007.

89. National Wildfire Coordinating Group (NWCG). *Wildland Fire Incident Management Field Guide PMS 210 (Formerly Fireline Handbook PMS 410).* Boise: NWCG, 3-18, 2014.

90. Nunneley, SA. Heat stress in protective clothing: interactions among physical and physiological factors. *Scand J Work Env Health* 15:52-57, 1989.

91. O'Connell, ER, Thomas, PC, Cady, LD, and Karwasky, RJ. Energy costs of simulated stair climbing as a job-related task in firefighting. *J Occup Med* 28:282-284, 1986.

92. Park, H, Kim, S, Morris, K, Moukperian, M, Moon, Y, and Stull, J. Effect of firefighters' personal protective equipment on gait. *Appl Ergonomics* 48:42-48, 2015.

93. Pawlak, R, Clasey, J, Palmer, T, Symons, B, and Abel, MG. The effect of a novel tactical training program on physical fitness and occupational performance in firefighters. *J Strength Cond Res* 29:578-588, 2014.

94. Perroni, F, Tessitore, A, Cortis, C, Lupo, C, D'Artibale, E, Cignitti, L, and Capranica, L. Energy cost and energy sources during simulated firefighting activity. *J Strength Cond Res* 24:3457-3463, 2010.

95. Phillips, M, Payne, W, Lord, C, Netto, K, Nichols, D, and Aisbett, B. Identification of physically demanding tasks performed during bushfire suppression by Australian rural firefighters. *Appl Ergonomics* 43:435-441, 2012.

96. Poplin, GS, Harris, RB, Pollack, KM, Peate, WF, and Burgess, JL. Beyond the fireground: injuries in the fire service. *Injury Prev* 18:228-233, 2012.

97. Poplin, GS, Roe, DJ, Peate, W, Harris, RB, and Burgess, JL. The association of aerobic fitness with injuries in the fire service. *Am J Epidemiol* 179:149-155, 2014.

98. Poston, WS, Haddock, CK, Jahnke, SA, Jitnarin, N, Tuley, BC, and Kales, SN. The prevalence of overweight, obesity, and substandard fitness in a population-based firefighter cohort. *J Occup Env Med* 53:266-273, 2011.

99. Poston, WS, Jitnarin, N, Haddock, CK, Jahnke, SA, and Tuley, BC. Obesity and injury-related absenteeism in a population-based firefighter cohort. *Obesity* 19:2076-2081, 2013.

100. Reinhardt, TE, and Ottmar, RD. Baseline measurements of smoke exposure among wildland firefighters. *J Occup Environ Hyg* 1:593-606, 2004.

101. Rhea, MR, Alvar, BA, and Gray, R. Physical fitness and job performance of firefighters. *J Strength Cond Res* 18:348-352, 2004.

102. Romet, T, and Frim, J. Physiological responses of firefighting activities. *Eur J Appl Physiol* 56:633-638, 1987.

103. Rosengren, KS, Hsiao-Wecksler, ET, and Horn, G. Fighting fires without falling: effects of equipment design and fatigue on firefighter's balance and gait. *Ecol Psychol* 26:167-175, 2014.

104. Ruby, BC, Leadbetter III, GW, Armstrong, DW, and Gaskill, SE. Wildland firefighter load carriage: effects on transit time and physiological responses during simulated escape to safety zone. *Int J Wildland Fire* 12:111-116, 2003.

105. Rutstein, DD, Mullan, RJ, Frazier, TM, Halperin, WE, Melius, JM, and Sestito, JP. Sentinel health events (occupational): a basis for physician recognition and public health surveillance. *Am J Public Health* 73:1054-1062, 1983.

106. Schlader, ZJ, Simmons, SE, Stannard, SR, and Mündel, T. Skin temperature as a thermal controller of exercise intensity. *Eur J Appl Physiol* 111:1631-1639, 2011.

107. Seabury, SA, and McLaren, CF. *The frequency, severity, and economic consequences of musculoskeletal injuries to firefighters in California.* Santa Monica, CA: RAND Corporation, 13-14, 2010.

108. Selkirk, GA, and McLellan, TM. Physical work limits for Toronto firefighters in warm environments. *J Occup Environ Hyg* 1:199-212, 2004.

109. Sell, KM, and Livingston, B. Mid-season physical fitness profile of interagency hotshot firefighters. *Int J Wildland Fire* 21:773-777, 2012.

110. Sharkey, BJ, and Gaskill, SE. *Fitness and Work Capacity.* 3rd ed. PMS 304-2. Boise: National Wildfire Coordinating Group NFES, 1596, 2009.

111. Sharkey, BJ, and Davis, PO. Job-related tests. In *Hard Work: Defining Physical Work Performance Requirements.* Champaign, IL: Human Kinetics, 46-47, 2008.

112. Sharman, JE, Cockcroft, JR, and Coombes, JS. Cardiovascular implications of exposure to traffic air pollution during exercise. *QJM* 97:637-643, 2004.

113. Sheaff, AK, Bennett, A, Hanson, ED, Kim, Y-S, Hsu, J, Shim, JK, Edwards, ST, and Hurley, BF. Physiological determinants of the candidate physical ability test in firefighters. *J Strength Cond Res* 24:3112-3122, 2010.

114. Smith, DL. Firefighter fitness: improving and performance and preventing injuries and fatalities. *Curr Sports Med Reports* 10:167-172, 2011.

115. Smith, DL, Fehling, PC, Hultquist, EM, Lefferts, WK, Barr, DA, Storer, TW, and Cooper, CB. Firefighter's personal protective equipment and the chronotropic index. *Ergonomics* 55:1243-1251, 2012.

116. Smith, DL, Manning, TS, and Petruzzello, SJ. Effect of strenuous live-fire drills on cardiovascular and psychological responses of recruit firefighters. *Ergonomics* 44:244-254, 2001.

117. Smith, DL, Petruzzello, SJ, Kramer, JM, and Misner, JE. Physiological, psychophysical, and psychological responses of firefighters to firefighting training drills. *Aviat Space Envir Med* 67:1063-1068, 1996.

118. Smith, DL, Petruzzello, SJ, Kramer, JM, and Misner, JE. The effects of different thermal environments on the physiological and psychological responses of firefighters to a training drill. *Ergonomics* 40:500-510, 1997.

119. Son, SY, Lee, JY, and Tochihara, Y. Occupational stress and strain in relation to personal protective equipment of Japanese firefighters assessed by a questionnaire. *Ind Health* 51:214-222, 2013.

120. Soteriades, ES, Smith, DL, Tsismenakis, AJ, Baur, DM, and Kales, SN. Cardiovascular disease in US firefighters: a systematic review. *Cardiol Rev* 19:202-215, 2011.

121. Soteriades, ES, Targino, MC, Talias, MA, Hauser, R, Kawachi, I, Christiani, DC, and Kales, SN. Obesity and risk of LVH and ECG abnormalities in US firefighters. *J Occup Environ Med* 53:867-871, 2011.

122. Sothmann, MS, Saupe, K, Jasenof, D, and Blaney, J. Heart rate response of firefighters to actual emergencies: implications for cardiorespiratory fitness. *J Occup Med* 34:797-800, 1992.

123. Strickland, M, and Petersen, S. *Analysis of predictive tests of aerobic fitness for wildland firefighters.* Paper presented at annual meeting of the Canadian Society for Exercise Physiology, Canmore, CA, 1999.

124. Throne, LC, Bartholomew, JB, Craig, J, and Farrar, RP. Stress reactivity in firefighters: an exercise intervention. *Int J Stress Management* 7:235-246, 2000.

125. Tubbs, RL. Noise and hearing loss in firefighting. *Occup Med* 10:843-856, 1995.

126. U.S. Bureau of Labor Statistics (BLS). Firefighters. 2011. www.bls.gov. Accessed May 10, 2015.

127. U.S. Fire Administration (USFA). *Fire and Emergency Medical Services Ergonomics: A Guide for Understanding and Implementing an Ergonomics Program in Your Department.* Emmitsburg, MD: USFA, 1996.

128. U.S. Fire Administration (USFA). *Health and Wellness Guide for the Volunteer Fire and Emergency Services.* FA-321/February, 2, 2009.

129. Von Heimburg, ED, Rasmussen, AK, and Medbo, JI. Physiological responses of firefighters and performance predictors during a simulated rescue of hospital patients. *Ergonomics* 49:111-126, 2006.

130. Wendt, D, Van Loon, LJ, and Lichtenbelt, WDM. Thermoregulation during exercise in the heat. *Sports Med* 37:669-682, 2007.

131. Westerlind, KC. Physical activity and cancer prevention: mechanisms. *Med Sci Sport Exer* 35:1834-1840, 2003.

132. Williams-Bell, FM, Villar, R, Sharratt, MT, and Hughson, RL. Physiological demands of the firefighter candidate physical ability test. *Med Sci Sports Exer* 41:653-662, 2009.

133. Windsor, JS, and Rodway, GW. Heights and haematology: the story of haemoglobin at altitude. *J Postgrad Med* 83:148-151, 2007.

134. Wong, KC. Physiology and pharmacology of hypothermia. *Western J Med* 138:227-232, 1983.

135. Yang, J, Teehan, D, Farioli, A, Baur, DM, Smith, D, and Kales, SN. Sudden cardiac death among firefighters ≤45 years of age in the United States. *Am J Cardiol* 112:1962-1967, 2013.

Chapter 18

1. ACSM (American College of Sports Medicine). Position stand—exercise and fluid replacement. *Med Sci Sport Exer* 39:377-390, 2007.

2. Åkerstedt, T. Shift work and disturbed sleep/wakefulness. *Occup Med* 53:89-94, 2003.

3. Alpert, GP, and Dunham, RG. *An analysis of police use-of-force data.* Washington, DC: National Institute of Justice, 1998.

4. Anderson, G, Zutz, A, and Plecas, D. Police officer back health. *J Crim Justice Res* 2:2, 2011.

5. Anderson, GS, Plecas, D, and Segger, T. Police officer physical ability testing—re-validating a selection criterion. *Policing* 24:8-31, 2001.

6. Arizona Peace Officer Standards and Training Board. Arizona Administrative Code. Revised statutes. 2007. http://apps.azsos.gov/public_services/Title_13/13-04.pdf.

7. Arvey, RD, Landon, TE, Nutting, SM, and Maxwell, SE. Development of physical ability tests for police officers: a construct validation approach. *J Appl Psychol* 77:996, 1992.

8. Attwells, R, Birrell, SA, Hooper, RH, and Mansfield, NJ. Influence of carrying heavy loads on soldier's posture, movements and gait. *Ergonomics* 49:1527-1537, 2006.

9. Exercise and Sports Science Australia (ESSA). Adult Pre-Exercise Screening System. 2011. www.essa.org.au/wp-content/uploads/2011/09/Screen-tool-version-v1.1.pdf.

10. Australian Associated Press. Police officer who shot man dead at Westfield Parramatta deserves bravery award. *Sydney Morning Herald.* New South Wales, Australia, 2014. www.smh.com.au/nsw/police-officer-who-shot-man-dead-at-westfield-parramatta-deserves-bravery-award-20140120-313zz.html.

11. Australian Centre for Posttraumatic Mental Health. *Australian Guidelines for the Treatment of Acute Stress Disorder and Posttraumatic Stress Disorder.* Melbourne, Victoria: ACPMH, 2013.

12. Barba, J. *Law Order* Jun:60, 2005. www.hendonpub.com/resources/article_archive/results/details?id=4076.

13. Battié, MC, Videman, T, Gibbons, LE, Manninen, H, Gill, K, Pope, M, and Kaprio, J. Occupational driving and lumbar disc degeneration: a case control study. *Lancet* 360:1369-1374, 2002.

14. Binkley, HM, Beckett, J, Casa, DJ, Kleiner, DM, and Plummer, PE. National Athletic Trainers' Association (NATA) position statement: exertional heat illnesses. *J Athl Training* 37:329, 2002.

15. Birrell, SA, Hooper, RH, and Haslam, RA. The effect of military load carriage on ground reaction forces. *Gait Posture* 26:611-614, 2007.

16. Birzer, ML, and Craig, DE. Gender differences in police physical ability test performance. *Am J Police* 15:93-108, 1996.

17. Bissett, D, Bissett, J, and Snell, C. Physical agility tests and fitness standards: perceptions of law enforcement officers. *Police Prac Res* 13:208-223, 2012.

18. Black Dog Institute. Expert guidelines: Diagnosis and treatment of post-traumatic stress disorder in emergency service workers. www.blackdoginstitute.org.au/docs/PTSD_Guidelines_final.pdf. Accessed September 13, 2016.

19. Blacker, SD, Carter, JM, Wilkinson, DM, Richmond, VL, Rayson, MP, and Peattie, M. Physiological responses of police officers during job simulations wearing chemical, biological, radiological and nuclear personal protective equipment. *Ergonomics* 56:137-147, 2013.

20. Bock, C, and Orr, R. Use of the Functional Movement Screen in a tactical population: a review. *J Mil Veterans Health* 23:31-40, 2015.

21. Bonneau, J, and Brown, J. Physical ability, fitness and police work. *J Clin Forensic Med* 2:157-164, 1995.

22. Boyce, RW, Jones, GR, Schendt, KE, Lloyd, CL, and Boone, EL. Longitudinal changes in strength of police officers with gender comparisons. *J Strength Cond Res* 23:2411-2418, 2009.

23. Buchheit, M. 30-15 Intermittent Fitness Test et répétition de sprints. *Sci Sport* 23:26-28, 2008.

24. Buchheit, M. The 30-15 Intermittent Fitness Test: accuracy for individualizing interval training of young intermittent sport players. *J Strength Cond Res* 22:365-374, 2008.

25. Buchheit, M, Laursen, PB, Millet, GP, Pactat, F, and Ahmaidi, S. Predicting intermittent running performance: critical velocity versus endurance index. *Int J Sports Med*, 2007. [e-pub ahead of print].

26. Carbone, PD, Carlton, SD, Stierli, M, and Orr, RM. The impact of load carriage on the marksmanship of the tactical police officer: a pilot study. *J Aust Strength Cond* 22:50-57, 2014.

27. Carlier IV, Lamberts RD, and Gersons BP. Risk factors for posttraumatic stress symptomatology in police officers: a prospective analysis. *J Nerv Ment Dis* 185:498-506, 1997.

28. Carlton, A, and Orr, RM. The effects of fluid loss on physical performance: a critical review. *JSHS* 4:357-363, 2015.

29. Carlton, SD, Orr, R, Stierli, M, and Carbone, PD. The impact of load carriage on mobility and marksmanship of the tactical response officer. *J Aust Strength Cond* 22:23-27, 2013.

30. Chao, W-H, Askew, EW, Roberts, DE, Wood, SM, and Perkins, JB. Oxidative stress in humans during work at moderate altitude. *J Nutr* 129:2009-2012, 1999.

31. Cheuvront, SN, Goodman, DA, Kenefick, RW, Montain, SJ, and Sawka, MN. Impact of a protective vest and spacer garment on exercise-heat strain. *Eur J Appl Physiol* 102:577-583, 2008.

32. Collingwood, TR. Physical fitness standards: measuring job relatedness. *Police Chief* 2:31-37, 1995.

33. Cook, JM, Sakr, CJ, Redlich, CA, and DeLoreto, AL. Elevated blood lead levels related to the use of firearms. *J Occup Env Med* 57:e136-e138, 2015.

34. Copay, AG, and Charles, MT. Police academy fitness training at the Police Training Institute, University of Illinois. *Policing* 21:416-431, 1998.

35. Dawes, J. Basic training concepts. *Tactical Strength Cond* January:4.1-4.2, 2008.

36. Decker, A, Orr, R, and Hinton, B. Physiological demands of law enforcement occupational tasks in Australian police officers. *JSCR* (submitted for publication).

37. Dempsey, PC, Handcock, PJ, and Rehrer, NJ. Impact of police body armour and equipment on mobility. *Appl Ergon* 44:957-961, 2013.

38. Deuster, PA, and Silverman, MN. Physical fitness: a pathway to health and resilience. *US Army Med Dep J* Oct-Dec:24-35, 2013.

39. Docherty, D, and Hodgson, M. Complex training revisited: a review of its current status as a viable training approach. *Strength Cond J* 26:52-57, 2004.

40. Fleck, SJ, and Kraemer, WJ. *Designing Resistance Training Programs*. 3rd ed. Champaign, IL: Human Kinetics, 278-286, 2004.

41. Ford, P, De Ste Croix, M, Lloyd, R, Meyers, R, Moosavi, M, Oliver, J, Till, K, and Williams, C. The Long-Term Athlete Development model: physiological evidence and application. *J Sports Sci* 29:389-402, 2011.

42. Freitas de Salles, B, Simao, R, Miranda, F, de Silva Novaes, J, Lemos, A, and Willardson, J. Rest interval between sets in strength training. *Sports Med* 39:765-777, 2009.

43. Gächter, M, Savage, DA, and Torgler, B. Retaining the thin blue line: what shapes workers' willingness not to quit the current. CREMA Working Paper Series 2009-28, Center for Research in Economics, Management and the Arts (CREMA).

44. Gambetta, V. *Athletic Development: The Art & Science of Functional Sports Conditioning*. Champaign, IL: Human Kinetics, 177-209, 2007.

45. Garbarino, S, De Carli, F, Nobili, L, Mascialino, B, Squarcia, S, Penco, MA, Beelke, M, and Ferrilla, F. Sleepiness and sleep disorders in shift workers: a study on a group of Italian police officers. *Sleep* 25:648-653, 2002.

46. Gerber, M, Kellmann, M, Elliot, C, Hartmann, T, Brand, S, Holsboer-Trachsler, E, and Pühse, U. Perceived fitness protects against stress-based mental health impairments among police officers who report good sleep. *J Occup Health* 55:376-384, 2013.

47. Gyi, D, and Porter, J. Musculoskeletal problems and driving in police officers. *Occup Med* 48:153-160, 1998.

48. Haff, GG, and Travis Triplett, N. *Essentials of Strength Training and Conditioning*. 4th ed. Champaign, IL: Human Kinetics, 177-209, 439-468, 2016.

49. Hamada, T, Sale, DG, and MacDougall, DJ. Postactivation potentiation in endurance-trained male athletes. *Med Sci Sports Exerc* 32(2):403-411, 2000.

50. Härmä, M. Ageing, physical fitness and shiftwork tolerance. *Appl Ergon* 27:25-29, 1996.

51. Hecker, A, and Wheeler, K. Impact of hydration and energy intake on performance. *J NATA* 19:4-9, 1994.

52. Holmes, M, McKinnon, C, Dickerson, CR, and Callaghan, J. The effects of police duty belt and seat design changes on lumbar spine posture, driver contact pressure and discomfort. *Ergonomics* 56:126-136, 2013.

53. Kang, J-H, and Chen, S-C. Effects of an irregular bedtime schedule on sleep quality, daytime sleepiness, and fatigue among university students in Taiwan. *BMC Public Health* 9:1-6, 2009.

54. Karp, JR. Interval training for the fitness professionals. *Strength Cond J* 22(24):64-69, 2000.

55. Kinoshita, H. Effects of different loads and carrying systems on selected biomechanical parameters describing walking gait. *Ergonomics* 28:1347-1362, 1985.

56. Knapik, JJ, Reynolds, KL, and Harman, E. Soldier load carriage: historical, physiological, biomechanical, and medical aspects. *Mil Med* 169:45-56, 2004.

57. Kraemer, WJ, and Ratamess, NA. Fundamentals of resistance training: progression and exercise prescription. *Med Sci Sports Exerc* 36(4):674-688, 2004.

58. Laursen, PB, Shing, CM, Peake, JM, Coombes, JS, and Jenkins, DG. The scientific basis for high intensity training: optimizing training programmes and maximising performance in highly trained endurance athletes. *Med Sci Sports Exerc* 34:1801-1807, 2002.

59. Lloyd, R, and Cooke, CB. Kinetic changes associated with load carriage using two rucksack designs. *Ergonomics* 43:1331-1341, 2000.

60. Loefstedt, H, Selden, A, Storeus, L, and Bodin, L. Blood lead in Swedish police officers. *Am J Ind Med* 35:519-522, 1999.

61. Lorentz, J, Hill, L, and Samimi, B. Occupational needlestick injuries in a metropolitan police force. *Am J Prev Med* 18:146-150.

62. Lyne, A. Man arrested in Gatton after dramatic car chase. *Gatton Star Newspaper*. Brisbane, 2014. www.sunshinecoastdaily.com.au/news/man-arrested-gatton-after-dramatic-car-chase/2244373.

63. Marmolejo, AP. *Stress management with routine physical fitness amongst law enforcement officers*. Texas State University at San Marcos, 2010.

64. McArdle, WD, Katch, FI, and Katch, VL. *Essentials of Exercise Physiology*. New York: Wolters Kluwer Health, 623, 2010.

65. McEntire, SJ, Suyama, J, and Hostler, D. Mitigation and prevention of exertional heat stress in firefighters: a review of cooling strategies for structural firefighting and hazardous materials responders. *Prehosp Emerg Care* 17:241-260, 2013.

66. McGill, S, Frost, D, Lam, T, Finlay, T, Darby, K, and Andersen, J. Fitness and movement quality of emergency task force police officers: an age-grouped database with comparison to populations of emergency services personnel, athletes and the general public. *Int J Ind Ergonom* 43:146-153, 2013.

67. McKinnon, C, Callaghan, J, and Dickerson, C. Evaluation of the influence of mobile data terminal location on physical exposures during simulated police patrol activities. *Appl Ergon* 43:859-867, 2012.

68. McKinnon, CD, Callaghan, JP, and Dickerson, CR. Field quantification of physical exposures of police officers in vehicle operation. *Int J Occup Saf Ergo* 17:61-68, 2011.

69. McLellan, TM, Sleno, NJ, Bossi, LL, Pope, JI, Adam, JJ, Thompson, JJ, and Narlis, C. *Heat stress of tactical assault, fragmentation and load-bearing vests worn over combat clothing*. Toronto: Defence R&D Canada, 2003.

70. Meakin, JR, Smith, FW, Gilbert, FJ, and Aspden, RM. The effect of axial load on the sagittal plane curvature of the upright human spine in vivo. *J Biomech* 41:2850-2854, 2008.

71. Meir, R, Diesel, W, and Archer, E. Developing a prehabilitation program in a collision sport: a model developed within English Premiership rugby union football. *Strength Cond J* 29:50-62, 2007.

72. Minick, KI, Kiesel, KB, Burton, L, Taylor, A, Plisky, P, and Butler, RJ. Interrater reliability of the functional movement screen. *J Strength Cond Res* 24:479-486, 2010.

73. Monk, TH, and Folkard, S. *Making Shiftwork Tolerable*. Boca Raton, FL: CRC Press, 1992, 14.

74. Occupational Safety and Health Administration (OSHA). About work/rest schedules. United States Department of Labor. www.osha.gov/SLTC/heatillness/heat_index/work_rest_schedules.html.

75. Orloff, HA, and Rapp, CM. The effects of load carriage on spinal curvature and posture. *Spine* 29:1325-1329, 2004.

76. Orr, R, Johnston, V, Coyle, J, and Pope, R. Reported load carriage injuries of the Australian Army soldier. *J Occup Rehab* 25:316-322, 2014.

77. Orr, R, Pope, R, Stierli, M, and Hinton, B. A functional movement screen profile of police recruits and attested officers. *J Athl Training* 17:296, 2016.

78. Orr, R, and Stierli, M. Injuries common to tactical personnel (a multidisciplinary review). Presented at 2013 Australian Strength and Conditioning Association International Conference on Applied Strength and Conditioning, Melbourne, 2013.

79. Orr, R, Stierli, M, Amabile, ML, and Wilkes, B. The impact of a structured reconditioning program on the physical attributes and attitudes of injured police officers: a pilot study. *J Aust Strength Cond* 21:42, 2013.

80. Orr, RM, Ford, KR, and Stierli, MJ. Implementation of an ability-based training program in police force recruits. *J Strength Cond Res*, 2015. [e-pub ahead of print].

81. Orr, RM, Pope, R, Stierli, M, and Hinton, B. A Functional Movement Screen profile of an Australian state police force: a retrospective cohort study. *BMC Musculoskelet Disord* 17:296, 2016.

82. Peterson, MD, Rhea, MR, and Alvar, BA. Applications of the dose–response for muscular strength development: a review of meta-analytic efficacy and reliability for designing training prescription. *J Strength Cond Res* 19:950-958, 2005.

83. Peto, J, Matthews, FE, Hodgson, JT, and Jones, JR. Continuing increase in mesothelioma mortality in Britain. *Lancet* 345:535-539, 1995.

84. Polcyn, AF, Bensel, CK, Harman, E, and Obusek, JP. The effects of load weight: a summary analysis of maximal performance, physiological and biomechanical results from four studies of load carriage systems. In *RTO Meeting Proceedings 56: Soldier Mobility: Innovations in Load Carriage System Design and Evaluation*. Kingston, Canada: Research and Technology Organisation/North Atlantic Treaty Organization, 2000.

85. Rajaratnam, SW, Barger, LK, Lockley, SW, Shea, SA, Wang, W, Landrigan, CP, O'Brien, CS, Qadri, S, Sullivan, JP, Cade, BE, Epstein, LJ, White, DP, and Dzeisler, CA. Sleep disorders, health, and safety in police officers. *J Am Med Assoc* 306:2567-2578, 2011.

86. Ramey, SL, Perkhounkova, Y, Moon, M, Tseng, H-C, Wilson, A, Hein, M, Hood, K, and Franke, WD. Physical activity in police beyond self-report. *J Occup Env Med* 56:338-343, 2014.

87. Rhea, MR. Needs analysis and program design for police officers. *Strength Cond J* 37:30-34, 2015.

88. Rhea, MR. Needs analysis and program design for police officers. *Strength Cond J* 37:30-34, 2015.

89. Sale, DG. Postactivation potentiation: role in human performance. *Exercise Sport Sci R* 30(3):138-143, 2002.

90. Smith, CA, Chimera, NJ, Wright, NJ, and Warren, M. Interrater and intrarater reliability of the functional movement screen. *J Strength Cond Res* 27:982-987, 2013.

91. Smolander, J, Louhevaara, V, and Oja, P. Policemen's physical fitness in relation to the frequency of leisure-time physical exercise. *Int Arch Occup Environ Health* 20(6):295-305, 1984.

92. Snook, SH, and Ciriello, VM. The effects of heat stress on manual handling tasks. *Am Ind Hyg Assoc* 35:681-685, 1974.

93. Snyder, S. Introduction to tactical strength and conditioning. *Tactical Strength Cond Rep* 2:2.1-2.2, 2007.

94. Soroka, A, and Sawicki, B. Physical activity levels as a quantifier in police officers and cadets. *Int J Occup Med Environ Health* 27:498-505, 2014.

95. Takahashi, R. Power training for judo: plyometric training with medicine balls. *Strength Cond J* 14:66-71, 1992.

96. The Audit Office of New South Wales. Managing injured police: NSW Police Force (performance audit). 2008. www.audit.nsw.gov.au.

97. Vila, B, Morrison, GB, and Kenney, DJ. Improving shift schedule and work-hour policies and practices to increase police officer performance, health, and safety. *Police Quart* 5:4-24, 2002.

98. Violanti, JM, Fekedulegn, D, Andrew, ME, Charles, LE, Hartley, TA, Vila, B, and Burchfiel, CM. Shift work and the incidence of injury among police officers. *Am J Ind Med* 55:217-227, 2012.

99. Williams, JJ, and Westall, D. SWAT and non-SWAT police officers and the use of force. *J Crim Just* 31:469-474, 2003.

100. Wilmore, JH, Costill, DL, and Kenney, L. *Physiology of Sport and Exercise.* Champaign, IL: Human Kinetics, 2012, 286.

101. Wilson, A, Hinton, B, and Orr, R. Profiling the daily tasks of an Australian state police force. *J Health Saf Environ* (submitted).

102. Yessis, M. A strength and power training program for football lineman. *NSCA J* 5:30-36, 1983.

Chapter 19

1. Abt, JP, Sell, TC, Lovalekar, MT, Keenan, KA, Bozich, AJ, Morgan, JS, Kane, SF, Benson, PJ, and Lephart, SM. Injury epidemiology of U.S. Army special operations forces. *Mil Med* 179:1106-1112, 2014.

2. Armstrong, LE, Casa, DJ, Millard-Stafford, M, Moran, DS, Pyne, SW, and Roberts, WO. American College of Sports Medicine position stand:. Exertional heat illness during training and competition. *Med Sci Sports Exerc* 39:556-572, 2007.

3. Anderson, MK, Grier, T, Canham-Chervak, M, Bushman, TT, and Jones, BH. Occupation and other risk factors for injury among enlisted U.S. Army soldiers. *Public Health* 129:531-538, 2015.

4. Armstrong, LE. Heat acclimatization. In *Encyclopedia of Sports Medicine and Science.* Fahey, TD, ed. Internet Society for Sport Science, 1998.

5. Bompa, TO, and Haff, GG. *Periodization: theory and methodology of training.* Champaign, IL: Human Kinetics, 123-256, 2009.

6. Brawley, S, Fairbanks, K, Nguyen, W, Blivin, S, and Frantz, E. Sports medicine training room clinic model for the military. *Mil Med* 177:135-138, 2012.

7. Carow, S, Haniuk, E, Cameron, K, Padua, D, Marshall, S, DiStefano, L, de la Motte, S, Beutler, A, and Gerber, J. Risk of lower extremity injury in a military cadet population after a supervised injury-prevention program. *J Athl Training*, 2014. [e-pub ahead of print].

8. Casa, DJ, Csillan, D, Armstrong, LE, Baker, LB, Bergeron, MF, Buchanan, VM, Carroll, MJ, Cleary, MA, Eichner, ER, Ferrara, MS, Fitzpatrick, TD, Hoffman, JR, Kenefick, RW, Klossner, DA, Knight, JC, Lennon, SA, Lopez, RM, Matava, MJ, O'Connor, FG, Peterson, BC, Rice, SG, Robinson, BK, Shriner, RJ, West, MS, and Yeargin, SW. Preseason heat-acclimatization guidelines for secondary school athletics. *J Athl Training* 44:332-333, 2009.

9. Casa, DJ, DeMartini, JK, Bergeron, MF, Csillan, D, Eichner, ER, Lopez, RM, Ferrara, MS, Miller, KC, O'Connor, F, Sawka, MN, and Yeargin, SW. National Athletic Trainers' Association position statement: exertional heat illnesses. *J Athl Training* 50:986-1000, 2015.

10. Cheuvront, SN, Kenefick, RW, and Zambraski, EJ. Spot urine concentrations should not be used for hydration assessment: a methodology review. *Int J Sport Nutr Exerc Metab* 25:293-297, 2015.

11. Christen, J, Foster, C, Porcari, JP, and Mikat, RP. Temporal robustness of the session RPE. *Int J Sports Physiol Perform*, 2016. [e-pub ahead of print]

12. Cosio-Lima, L, Brown, K, Reynolds, KL, Gregg, R, and Perry, RA, Jr. Injury and illness incidence in a Sergeants Major Academy class. *Mil Med* 178:735-741, 2013.

13. Dean, C. *The Modern Warrior's Combat Load: Dismounted Operations in Afghanistan, April-May 2003.* Fort Leavenworth, KS: U.S. Army Center for Army Lessons Learned (CALL), 2004.

14. Evans, RK, Scoville, CR, Ito, MA, and Mello, RP. Upper body fatiguing exercise and shooting performance. *Mil Med* 168:451-456, 2003.

15. Fleck, SJ, and Kraemer, W. *Designing Resistance Training Programs.* 4th ed. Champaign, IL: Human Kinetics, 2014.

16. Friedl, KE, Knapik, JJ, Hakkinen, K, Baumgartner, N, Groeller, H, Taylor, NA, Duarte, AF, Kyrolainen, H, Jones, BH, Kraemer, WJ, and Nindl, BC. Perspectives on aerobic and strength influences on military physical readiness: report of an international military

physiology roundtable. *J Strength Cond Res* 29(Suppl 11):S10-S23, 2015.

17. Ganio, MS, Brown, CM, Casa, DJ, Becker, SM, Yeargin, SW, McDermott, BP, Boots, LM, Boyd, PW, Armstrong, LE, and Maresh, CM. Validity and reliability of devices that assess body temperature during indoor exercise in the heat. *J Athl Training* 44:124-135, 2009.

18. Garrison, M, Dembowski, S, and Shepard, N. Sports and exercise-related injuries in the military. In *Musculoskeletal Injuries in the Military*. Owens, B, and Cameron, KL, eds. New York: Springer Verlag, 317, 2015.

19. Hackett, PH, and Roach, RC. High-altitude cerebral edema. *High Alt Med Biol* 5:136-146, 2004.

20. Hauschild, VD, Schuh, A, Taylor, BJ, Canham-Chervak, M, and Jones, BH. Identification of specific activities associated with fall-related injuries, active component, U.S. Army, 2011. *MSMR* 23:2-9, 2016.

21. Henderson, NE, Knapik, JJ, Shaffer, SW, McKenzie, TH, and Schneider, GM. Injuries and injury risk factors among men and women in U.S. Army Combat Medic advanced individual training. *Mil Med* 165:647-652, 2000.

22. Hew-Butler, T, Rosner, MH, Fowkes-Godek, S, Dugas, JP, Hoffman, MD, Lewis, DP, Maughan, RJ, Miller, KC, Montain, SJ, Rehrer, NJ, Roberts, WO, Rogers, IR, Siegel, AJ, Stuempfle, KJ, Winger, JM, and Verbalis, JG. Statement of the 3rd International Exercise-Associated Hyponatremia Consensus Development Conference, Carlsbad, California, 2015. *Br J Sports Med* 49:1432-1446, 2015.

23. Hollingsworth, DJ. The prevalence and impact of musculoskeletal injuries during a pre-deployment workup cycle: survey of a Marine Corps special operations company. *J Spec Oper Med* 9:11-15, 2009.

24. Jaenen, S. Identification of common military tasks. In *Optimizing Operational Physical Fitness*. Technical Report TRHFM-080. Paris, France, 2009.

25. Johnson, NJ, and Luks, AM. High-altitude medicine. *Med Clin North Am* 100:357-369, 2016.

26. Joint Chiefs of Staff. Joint Publication 3-11. Operations in chemical, biological, radiological, and nuclear environments. October 2013. www.dtic.mil/doctrine/new_pubs/jp3_11.pdf. Accessed August 18, 2015.

27. Knapik, JJ. Injuries and injury prevention during foot marching. *J Spec Oper Med* 14:131-135, 2014.

28. Knapik, JJ. The importance of physical fitness for injury prevention: part 1. *J Spec Oper Med* 15:123-127, 2015.

29. Knapik, JJ. The importance of physical fitness for injury prevention: part 2. *J Spec Oper Med* 15:112-115, 2015.

30. Knapik, JJ, and East, WB. History of United States Army physical fitness and physical readiness training. *US Army Med Dep J* Apr-Jun:5-19, 2014.

31. Knapik, JJ, Reynolds, KL, and Harman, E. Soldier load carriage: historical, physiological, biomechanical, and medical aspects. *Mil Med* 169:45-56, 2004.

32. Kraemer, WJ, Fleck, SJ, and Deschenes, MR. *Exercise Physiology: Integrating Theory and Application*. Philadelphia: Lippincott Williams & Wilkins, 281-310, 2012.

33. Kraemer, WJ, Fleck, SJ, and Deschenes, MR. *Exercise Physiology: Integrating Theory and Application*. 2nd ed. Philadelphia: Lippincott Williams & Wilkins, 321-330, 2016.

34. Kraemer, WJ, Mazzetti, SA, Nindl, BC, Gotshalk, LA, Volek, JS, Bush, JA, Marx, JO, Dohi, K, Gomez, AL, Miles, M, Fleck, SJ, Newton, RU, and Hakkinen, K. Effect of resistance training on women's strength/power and occupational performances. *Med Sci Sports Exerc* 33:1011-1025, 2001.

35. Kraemer, WJ, and Szivak, TK. Strength training for the warfighter. *J Strength Cond Res* 26(Suppl 2):S107-S118, 2012.

36. Kraemer, WJ, Vescovi, JD, Volek, JS, Nindl, BC, Newton, RU, Patton, JF, Dziados, JE, French, DN, and Hakkinen, K. Effects of concurrent resistance and aerobic training on load-bearing performance and the Army physical fitness test. *Mil Med* 169:994-999, 2004.

37. Kraemer, W, and Fleck, S. *Optimizing Strength Training: Designing Nonlinear Periodization Workouts*. Champaign, IL: Human Kinetics, 1-73, 2007.

38. Mala, J. Improving performance of heavy load carriage during high-intensity combat-related tasks. *Strength Cond J* 37:43-52, 2015.

39. Mala, J, Szivak, TK, Flanagan, SD, Comstock, BA, Laferrier, JZ, Maresh, CM, and Kraemer, WJ. The role of strength and power during performance of high intensity military tasks under heavy load carriage. *US Army Med Dep J* Apr-Jun:3-11, 2015.

40. Mann, JB, Thyfault, JP, Ivey, PA, and Sayers, SP. The effect of autoregulatory progressive resistance exercise vs. linear periodization on strength improvement in college athletes. *J Strength Cond Res* 24:1718-1723, 2010.

41. McNamara, JM, and Stearne, DJ. Flexible nonlinear periodization in a beginner college weight training class. *J Strength Cond Res* 24:17-22, 2010.

42. Miller, JC. Shiftwork. October 2010. https://primis.phmsa.dot.gov/crm/docs/Miller2010_Shift_and_Night_Work_unpub.pdf. Accessed August 18, 2016.

43. Montain, SJ, Latzka, WA, and Sawka, MN. Fluid replacement recommendations for training in hot weather. *Mil Med* 164:502-508, 1999.

44. Morton, RL. High-altitude cardiopulmonary diseases. 2016. http://emedicine.medscape.com/article/1006029-overview. Accessed August 17, 2016.

45. Nindl, BC, Alvar, BA, Dudley JR, Favre, MW, Martin, GJ, Sharp, MA, Warr, BJ, Stephenson, MD, and Kraemer, WJ. Executive summary from the National Strength and Conditioning Association's Second Blue Ribbon Panel on Military Physical Readiness: military physical performance testing. *J Strength Cond Res* 29(Suppl 11):S216-S220, 2015.

46. Nindl, BC, Castellani, JW, Warr, BJ, Sharp, MA, Henning, PC, Spiering, BA, and Scofield, DE. Physiological Employment Standards III: physiological challenges and consequences encountered during international military deployments. *Eur J Appl Physiol* 113:2655-2672, 2013.

47. O'Connor, FG, Deuster, PA, Davis, J, Pappas, CG, and Knapik, JJ. Functional movement screening: predicting injuries in officer candidates. *Med Sci Sports Exerc* 43:2224-2230, 2011.

48. Orr, R, Knapik, JJ, and Pope, R. Avoiding program-induced cumulative overload (PICO). *J Spec Oper Med* 16:91-95, 2016.

49. Orr, RM, Pope, R, Johnston, V, and Coyle, J. Soldier occupational load carriage: a narrative review of associated injuries. *Int J Inj Contr Saf Promot* 21:388-396, 2014.

50. Pandorf, C, Harman, EA, Frykman, PN, Patton, JF, Mello, RP, and Nindl, BC. Correlates of load carriage performance among women. In *RTO Meeting Proceedings 56 Soldier Mobility: Innovations in Load Carriage System Design and Evaluation, RTO-MP-056 AC/323(HFM-043) TP/28*, Kingston.

51. Plisk, SS, and Stone, MH. Periodization strategies. *Strength Cond J* 25:19-32, 2003.

52. Raleigh, JP, Giles, MD, Scribbans, TD, Edgett, BA, Sawula, LJ, Bonafiglia, JT, Graham, RB, and Gurd, BJ. The impact of work-matched interval training on $\dot{V}O_2$peak and $\dot{V}O_2$ kinetics: diminishing returns with increasing intensity. *Appl Physiol Nutr Metab* 41:706-713, 2016.

53. Reiman, MP, and Lorenz, DS. Integration of strength and conditioning principles into a rehabilitation program. *Int J Sports Phys Ther* 6:241-253, 2011.

54. Reuter, B. *Developing Endurance*. Champaign, IL: Human Kinetics, 45-220, 2012.

55. Reynolds, K, Cosio-Lima, L, Bovill, M, Tharion, W, Williams, J, and Hodges, T. A comparison of injuries, limited-duty days, and injury risk factors in infantry, artillery, construction engineers, and special forces soldiers. *Mil Med* 174:702-708, 2009.

56. Rodriguez-Soto, AE, Jaworski, R, Jensen, A, Niederberger, B, Hargens, AR, Frank, LR, Kelly, KR, and Ward, SR. Effect of load carriage on lumbar spine kinematics. *Spine (Phila Pa 1976)* 38:E783-E791, 2013.

57. Roy, TC, Knapik, JJ, Ritland, BM, Murphy, N, and Sharp, MA. Risk factors for musculoskeletal injuries for soldiers deployed to Afghanistan. *Aviat Space Environ Med* 83:1060-1066, 2012.

58. Roy, TC, and Lopez, HP. A comparison of deployed occupational tasks performed by different types of military battalions and resulting low back pain. *Mil Med* 178:e937-e943, 2013.

59. Roy, TC, Ritland, BM, Knapik, JJ, and Sharp, MA. Lifting tasks are associated with injuries during the early portion of a deployment to Afghanistan. *Mil Med* 177:716-722, 2012.

60. Sell, TC, Pederson, JJ, Abt, JP, Nagai, T, Deluzio, J, Wirt, MD, McCord, LJ, and Lephart, SM. The addition of body armor diminishes dynamic postural stability in military soldiers. *Mil Med* 178:76-81, 2013.

61. Sih, BL, and Negus, CH. Physical training outcome predictions with biomechanics, part I: Army Physical Fitness Test modeling. *Mil Med* 181:77-84, 2016.

62. Spiering, BA, Kraemer, WJ, Anderson, JM, Armstrong, LE, Nindl, BC, Volek, JS, and Maresh, CM. Resistance exercise biology: manipulation of resistance exercise programme variables determines the responses of cellular and molecular signalling pathways. *Sports Med* 38:527-540, 2008.

63. Teyhen, DS, Shaffer, SW, Butler, RJ, Goffar, SL, Kiesel, KB, Rhon, DI, Williamson, JN, and Plisky, PJ. What risk factors are associated with musculoskeletal injury in US Army Rangers? A prospective prognostic study. *Clin Orthop Relat Res* 473:2948-2958, 2015.

64. Uhorchak, JM, Scoville, CR, Williams, GN, Arciero, RA, St Pierre, P, and Taylor, DC. Risk factors associated with noncontact injury of the anterior cruciate ligament: a prospective four-year evaluation of 859 West Point cadets. *Am J Sports Med* 31:831-842, 2003.

65. U.S. Department of the Army. Field Manual 7-22. Army physical readiness training. Washington, DC: Army Headquarters, 2012.

66. U.S. Department of the Army. Soldier's manual of common tasks, warrior skills level 1 (STP21-1-SMCT). Washington, DC: Army Headquarters, 2012.

67. U.S. Department of the Army. U.S. Army 350-29 TR. Prevention of heat and cold casualties. Washington, DC: Army Headquarters, 18 July 2016.

68. U.S. Department of the Army. Soldier's manual of common tasks, warrior leader skills levels 2, 3, and 4 (STP 21-24-SMCT). Washington, DC: Army Headquarters, 2009.

69. U.S. Department of the Army, Maneuver Center of Excellence. Master Fitness Training Course. www.benning.army.mil/tenant/wtc/mft.html.70.

70. U.S. Department of the Army, Research Institute of Environmental Medicine. Altitude acclimatization guide. 2004. www.usariem.army.mil/assets/docs/partnering/altitudeacclimatizationguide.pdf. Accessed August 18, 2016.

71. U.S. Department of the Army, Training and Doctrine Command. Army physical readiness training circular (TC 3-22.20). Washington, DC: Army Headquarters, 2010.

72. U.S. Department of Homeland Security. COMDTINST M3710.4C. Coast Guard helicopter rescue swimmer manual. Washington, DC: U.S. Department of Homeland Security, 2011.

73. U.S. Department of the Navy. Naval Military Personnel Manual (MILPERSMAN) 1220-410. SEAL/EOD/SWCC/DIVER/AIRR physical screening testing standards and procedures. Washington, DC: Navy Headquarters, 2013.

74. U.S. Department of Veterans Affairs. Military Hazardous Exposures. www.benefits.va.gov/COMPENSATION/claims-postservice-exposures-index.asp.

75. U.S. Marine Corps. All-Marine message 032/08. Quantico, VA: U.S. Marine Headquarters, 2008.

Chapter 20

1. *Army Physical Readiness Training.* US Army, ed. Headquarters, Dept. of the Army, 434, 2012.

2. Abel, MG, Sell, K, and Dennison, K. Design and implementation of fitness programs for firefighters. *Strength Cond J* 33:31-42, 2011.

3. Agency, U. *Report on the ADEA soldier's load initiative.* Fort Lewis, WA, 1987.

4. Anderson, GS, Plecas, D, and Segger, T. Police officer physical ability testing: re-evaluating a selection criterion. *Policing* 24:23, 2001.

5. Bailey, TL, McDermott, WM. *Review of research on load carrying, tentage and equipage.* Tentage and Equipage Series, Report 9. Natick, MA: U.S. Army Quartermaster Research and Development Center, 2-13, 1952.

6. Bastien, GJ, Willems, PA, Schepens, B, and Heglund, NC. Effect of load and speed on the energetic cost of human walking. *Eur J Appl Physiol* 94:76-83, 2005.

7. Beekley, MD, Alt, J, Buckley, CM, Duffey, M, and Crowder, TA. Effects of heavy load carriage during constant-speed, simulated, road marching. *Mil Med* 172:592-595, 2007.

8. Bessen, RJ, Belcher, VW, and Franklin, RJ. Rucksack paralysis with and without rucksack frames. *Military Medicine* 152:372-375, 1987.

9. Bilzon, JL, Allsopp, AJ, and Tipton, MJ. Assessment of physical fitness for occupations encompassing load-carriage tasks. *Occup Med* 51:357-361, 2001.

10. Birrell, SA, and Haslam, RA. Subjective skeletal discomfort measured using a comfort questionnaire following a load carriage exercise. *Mil Med* 174:177-182, 2009.

11. Birrell, SA, and Hooper, RH. Initial subjective load carriage injury data collected with interviews and questionnaires. *Mil Med* 172:306-311, 2007.

12. Brudvig, TJ, Gudger, TD, and Obermeyer, L. Stress fractures in 295 trainees: a one-year study of incidence as related to age, sex, and race. *Mil Med* 148:666-667, 1983.

13. Carlton, SD, and Orr, RM. The impact of occupational load carriage on carrier mobility: a critical review of the literature. *JOSE* 20:33-41, 2014.

14. Cathcart, EP, Richardson, DT, and Campbell, W. Army Hygiene Advisory Committee report 3 on the maximal load to be carried by the soldier. *Army Med Corps* 41:12-24, 1923.

15. Dalen, A, Nilsson, J, and Thorstensson, A. Factors influencing a prolonged foot march. In *FOA Report C50601-H6.* Stockholm: Karolinska Institute, 9-12, 1978.

16. Dean, C. *The modern warrior's combat load. Dismounted operations in Afghanistan, April-May 2003.* Ft. Leavenworth, KS: Army Center for Lessons Learned, 2004.

17. Dempsey, PC, Handcock, PJ, and Rehrer, NJ. Impact of police body armour and equipment on mobility. *Appl Ergon* 44:957-961, 2013.

18. DiVencenzo, HR, Morgan, AL, Laurent, CM, and Keylock, KT. Metabolic demands of law enforcement personal protective equipment during exercise tasks. *Ergonomics* 57:1760-1765, 2014.

19. Donald, JG, and Fitts Jr, WT. March fractures: a study with special reference to etiological factors. *J Bone Joint Surg Am* 29:297-300, 1947.

20. Dubik, JM, and Fullerton, TD. Soldier overloading in Grenada. *Military Rev* 67:38-47, 1987.

21. Fleck, S, and Kraemer W. *Designing Resistance Training Programs.* 4th ed. Champaign, IL: Human Kinetics, 1-62, 179-296, 2014.

22. Friedl, KE. Body composition and military performance: origins of the army standards. In *Body Composition and Physical Performance: Applications for the Military Services.* Grumstrup-Scott, J, and Marriott, BM, eds. Washington DC: National Academies Press, 31-55, 1990.

23. Fulco, CS, Lewis, SF, Frykman, PN, Boushel, R, Smith, S, Harman, EA, Cymerman, A, and Pandolf, KB. Quantitation of progressive muscle fatigue during dynamic leg exercise in humans. *J Appl Physiol* 79:2154-2162, 1995.

24. Gerber, K. *Influence of physical fitness training on the manual material handling capability and road marching performance of female soldiers.* Aberdeen Proving Ground, MD: Human Research and Engineering Directorate, U.S. Army Research Laboratory, 1996.

25. Giladi, M, Milgrom, C, Danon, Y, and Aharonson, Z. The correlation between cumulative march training and stress fractures in soldiers. *Mil Med* 150:600-601, 1985.

26. Grenier, JG, Peyrot, N, Castells, J, Oullion, R, Messonnier, L, and Morin, JB. Energy cost and mechanical work of walking during load carriage in soldiers. *Med Sci Sports Exerc* 44:1131-1140, 2012.

27. Hadid, A, Epstein, Y, Shabshin, N, and Gefen, A. Modeling mechanical strains and stresses in soft tissues of the shoulder during load carriage based on load-bearing open MRI. *J Appl Physiol* 112:597-606, 2012.

28. Haisman, MF. Determinants of load carrying ability. *Appl Ergon* 19:111-121, 1988.

29. Harman, EA, Frykman, P, Palmer, C, Lammi, E, Reynolds, K, and Backus, V. *Effects of a specifically designed physical conditioning program on the load carriage and lifting performance of female soldiers.* Natick, MA: U.S. Army Research Institute of Environmental Medicine, 1997.

30. Harman, EA, Gutekunst, DJ, Frykman, PN, Nindl, BC, Alemany, JA, Mello, RP, and Sharp, MA. Effects of two different eight-week training programs on military physical performance. *J Strength Cond Res* 22:524-534, 2008.

31. Hendrickson, NR, Sharp, MA, Alemany, JA, Walker, LA, Harman, EA, Spiering, BA, Hatfield, DL, Yamamoto, LM, Maresh, CM, Kraemer, WJ, and Nindl, BC. Combined resistance and endurance training improves physical capacity and performance on tactical occupational tasks. *Eur J Appl Physiol* 109:1197-1208, 2010.

32. Hollander, IE, and Bell, NS. Physically demanding jobs and occupational injury and disability in the U.S. Army. *Mil Med* 175:705-712, 2010.

33. Huang, TW, and Kuo, AD. Mechanics and energetics of load carriage during human walking. *J Exp Biol* 217:605-613, 2014.

34. Jaenen, S. Identification of common military tasks. Optimizing operational physical fitness. In *RTO-TR-HFM-080—Optimizing Operational Physical Fitness*. NSaT Organization, ed. Neuilly-sur-Seine, France: NATO Science and Technology Organization, 342, 2009.

35. James, CR, Atkins, LT, Dufek, JS, and Bates, BT. An exploration of load accommodation strategies during walking with extremity-carried weights. *Hum Mov Sci* 35:17-29, 2014.

36. Jaworski, RL, Jensen, A, Niederberger, B, Congalton, R, and Kelly, KR. Changes in combat task performance under increasing loads in active duty marines. *Mil Med* 180:179-186, 2015.

37. Jones, BH, Harris, JM, Vinh, TN, and Rubin, C. Exercise-induced stress fractures and stress reactions of bone: epidemiology, etiology, and classification. In *Exercise and Sport Sciences Reviews*. Pandolf, K, ed. Baltimore: Williams & Wilkins, 382, 1989.

38. Knapik, J, Bahrke, M, Staab, J, Reynolds, K, Vogel, J, and O'Connor, J. *Frequency of loaded road march training and performance on a loaded road march*. Natick, MA: U.S. Army Research Institute of Environmental Medicine, 1990.

39. Knapik, J, Daniels, W, Murphy, M, Fitzgerald, P, Drews, F, and Vogel, J. Physiological factors in infantry operations. *Eur J Appl Physiol Occup Physiol* 60:233-238, 1990.

40. Knapik, J, Harman, E, and Reynolds, K. Load carriage using packs: a review of physiological, biomechanical and medical aspects. *Appl Ergon* 27:207-216, 1996.

41. Knapik, J, Reynolds, K, Staab, J, Vogel, JA, and Jones, B. Injuries associated with strenuous road marching. *Mil Med* 157:64-67, 1992.

42. Knapik, JJ, Harman, EA, Steelman, RA, and Graham, BS. A systematic review of the effects of physical training on load carriage performance. *J Strength Cond Res* 26:585-597, 2012.

43. Knapik, J, Johnson, R, Ang, P, Meiselman, H, Bensel, C, Johnson, W, Flynn, B, Hanlon, W, Kirk, J, Harman, E, Frykman, P, and Jones B. *Road march performance of special operations soldiers carrying various loads and load distributions*. Natick, MA: Military Performance Division, U.S. Army Research Institute of Environmental Medicine, 1993.

44. Knapik, JJ, Reynolds, KL, Duplantis, KL, and Jones, BH. Friction blisters. Pathophysiology, prevention and treatment. *Sports Med* 20:136-147, 1995.

45. Knapik, JJ, Reynolds, KL, and Harman, E. Soldier load carriage: historical, physiological, biomechanical, and medical aspects. *Mil Med* 169:45-56, 2004.

46. Kraemer, WJ, Mazzetti, SA, Nindl, BC, Gotshalk, LA, Volek, JS, Bush, JA, Marx, JO, Dohi, K, Gomez, AL, Miles, M, Fleck, SJ, Newton, RU, and Hakkinen, K. Effect of resistance training on women's strength/power and occupational performances. *Med Sci Sports Exerc* 33:1011-1025, 2001.

47. Kraemer, WJ, Nindl, BC, Gotshalk, LA, Harman, FS, Volek, JS, Tokeshi, SA, Meth, S, Bush, JA, Etzweiler, SW, Fredman, BS, Sebastianelli, WJ, Putukian, M, Newton, RU, Hakkinen, K, and Fleck, S. Prediction of military relevant occupational tasks in women from physical performance components. In *Advances in Occupational Ergonomics and Safety*. Kumar, S, ed. Amsterdam: IOS Press, 719-722, 1998.

48. Kraemer, WJ, Vescovi, JD, Volek, JS, Nindl, BC, Newton, RU, Patton, JF, Dziados, JE, French, DN, and Hakkinen, K. Effects of concurrent resistance and aerobic training on load-bearing performance and the Army physical fitness test. *Mil Med* 169:994-999, 2004.

49. Kraemer, WJ, Vogel, JA, Patton, JF, Dziados, JE, and Reynolds, KL. *The effects of various physical training programs on short duration, high intensity load bearing performance and the Army Physical Fitness Test*. Natick, MA: U.S. Army Research Institute of Environmental Medicine, 1987.

50. Lothian, NV. The load carried by the soldier. *Army Med Corps* 37:342-351, 1921.

51. Lothian, NV. The load carried by the soldier. *Army Med Corps* 38:9-24, 1922.

52. Lyons, J, Allsopp, A, and Bilzon, J. Influences of body composition upon the relative metabolic and cardiovascular demands of load-carriage. *Occup Med* 55:380-384, 2005.

53. Marshall, SLA. *The Soldier's Load and the Mobility of a Nation*. Quantico, VA: Marine Corps Association, 33-47, 1980.

54. Michaelides, MA, Parpa, KM, Henry, LJ, Thompson, GB, and Brown, BS. Assessment of physical fitness aspects and their relationship to firefighters' job abilities. *J Strength Cond Res* 25:956-965, 2011.

55. Mullins, AK, Annett, LE, Drain, JR, Kemp, JG, Clark, RA, and Whyte, DG. Lower limb kinematics and physiological responses to prolonged load carriage in untrained individuals. *Ergonomics* 58:770-780, 2015.

56. Nindl, BC, and Sharp, MA. Physical training for improved occupational performance. *American College of Sports Medicine Current Comment*. 2002. www.acsm.org/AM/Template.cfm?Section= current_comments1&Template=/CM/ContentDisplay .cfm&ContentID=8651.

57. McGuigan, M. Administration, scoring, and interpretation of selected tests. In *Essentials of Strength Training and Conditioning*. 4th ed. Haff, GG, and Triplett, NT, eds. Champaign, IL: Human Kinetics, 252-253, 261, 350-390, 2016.

58. Orr, RM, Pope, R, Johnston, V, and Coyle, J. Load carriage: minimising soldier injuries through physical conditioning—a narrative review. *J Mil Veterans Health* 18:31-38, 2010.

59. Orr, RM, Pope, R, Johnston, V, and Coyle, J. Soldier occupational load carriage: a narrative review of associated injuries. *Int J Inj Contr Saf Promot* 21:388-396, 2014.

60. Pal, MS, Majumdar, D, Bhattacharyya, M, Kumar, R, and Majumdar, D. Optimum load for carriage by soldiers at two walking speeds on level ground. *Int J Ind Ergonom* 39:68-72, 2009.

61. Pandorf, CE, Harman, EA, Frykman, PN, Patton, JF, Mello, RP, and Nindl, BC. Correlates of load carriage and obstacle course performance among women. *Work* 18:179-189, 2002.

62. Park, H, Kim, S, Morris, K, Moukperian, M, Moon, Y, and Stull, J. Effect of firefighters' personal protective equipment on gait. *Appl Ergon* 48:42-48, 2015.

63. Park, K, Hur, P, Rosengren, KS, Horn, GP, and Hsiao-Wecksler, ET. Effect of load carriage on gait due to firefighting air bottle configuration. *Ergonomics* 53:882-891, 2010.

64. Patterson, MJ, Roberts, W, Lau, W, and Prigg, SK. *Gender and physical training effects on soldier physical competencies and physiological strain*. Canberra: Defence Science and Technology Organisation, 2005.

65. Peterson, MD, Dodd, DJ, Alvar, BA, Rhea, MR, and Favre, M. Undulation training for development of hierarchical fitness and improved firefighter job performance. *J Strength Cond Res* 22:1683-1695, 2008.

66. Porter, SC. The soldier's load. *Infantry* May-June:19-22, 1992.

67. Pryor, RR, Colburn, D, Crill, MT, Hostler, DP, and Suyama, J. Fitness characteristics of a suburban special weapons and tactics team. *J Strength Cond Res* 26:752-757, 2012.

68. Quesada, PM, Mengelkoch, LJ, Hale, RC, and Simon, SR. Biomechanical and metabolic effects of varying backpack loading on simulated marching. *Ergonomics* 43:293-309, 2000.

69. Reilly, T, Morris, T, and Whyte, G. The specificity of training prescription and physiological assessment: a review. *J Sports Sci* 27:575-589, 2009.

70. Renbourn, ET. The knapsack and pack: an historical and physiological survey with particular reference to the British soldier. *Army Med Corps* 100:193-200, 1954.

71. Reynolds, K, Cosio-Lima, L, Creedon, J, Gregg, R, and Zigmont, T. Injury occurrence and risk factors in construction engineers and combat artillery soldiers. *Mil Med* 167:971-977, 2002.

72. Reynolds, KL, Kaszuba, J, Mello, RP, and Patton, JF. Prolonged treadmill load carriage: acute injuries and changes in foot anthropometry. In *Technical Report T1/9*. Natick, MA: U.S. Army Research Institute of Environmental Medicine, 19, 1990.

73. Reynolds, KL, White, JS, Knapik, JJ, Witt, CE, and Amoroso, PJ. Injuries and risk factors in a 100-mile (161 km) infantry road march. *Prev Med* 28:167-173, 1999.

74. Ricciardi, R, Deuster, PA, and Talbot, LA. Metabolic demands of body armor on physical performance in simulated conditions. *Mil Med* 173:817-824, 2008.

75. Rudzki, SJ. Weight-load marching as a method of conditioning Australian Army recruits. *Mil Med* 154:201-205, 1989.

76. Sampson, JB, Leitch, D, Kirk, J, and Raisanen, G. *Front-end analysis of load bearing equipment for the U.S. Army and U.S. Marine Corps*. Natick, MA: Army Soldier Systems Command, 1995.

77. Sanders, JW, Putnam, S, Frankart, C, Frenck, RW, Monteville, MR, Riddle, MS, Rockabrand, DM, Sharp, TW, and Tribble, DR. Impact of illness and non-combat injury during Operations Iraqi Freedom and Enduring Freedom (Afghanistan). *Am J Trop Med Hyg* 73:713-719, 2005.

78. Schiotz, MK, Potteiger, J, Huntsinger, PG, and Denmark, DC. The short-term effects of periodized and constant-intensity training on body composition, strength, and performance. *J Strength Cond Res* 12:173-178, 1998.

79. Sell, TC, Pederson, JJ, Abt, JP, Nagai, T, Deluzio, J, Wirt, MD, McCord, LJ, and Lephart, SM. The addition of body armor diminishes dynamic postural stability in military soldiers. *Mil Med* 178:76-81, 2013.

80. Sharp, MA, Patton, JF, and Vogel, JA. *A database of physically demanding tasks performed by U.S. Army soldiers. Technical report no. T98-12*. Natick, MA: U.S. Army Research Institute of Environmental Medicine, 1998.

81. Vanderburgh, PM, and Flanagan, S. The backpack run test: a model for a fair and occupationally relevant military fitness test. *Mil Med* 165:418-421, 2000.

82. Visser, T, van Dijk, MJ, Collee, T, and van der Loo, H. Is intensity of duration the key factor in march training? In *International Congress on Soldiers' Performance*. Finland, 2005.

83. Von Heimburg, ED, Rasmussen, AK, and Medbo, JI. Physiological responses of firefighters and performance predictors during a simulated rescue of hospital patients. *Ergonomics* 49:111-126, 2006.

84. Williams, AG, and Rayson, MP. Can simple anthropometric and physical performance tests track training-induced changes in load-carriage ability? *Mil Med* 171:742-748, 2006.

85. Williams, AG, Rayson, MP, and Jones, DA. Effects of basic training on material handling ability and physical fitness of British Army recruits. *Ergonomics* 42:1114-1124, 1999.

86. Williams, AG, Rayson, MP, and Jones, DA. Resistance training and the enhancement of the gains in material-handling ability and physical fitness of British Army recruits during basic training. *Ergonomics* 45:267-279, 2002.

87. Williams, AG, Rayson, MP, and Jones, DA. Training diagnosis for a load carriage task. *J Strength Cond Res* 18:30-34, 2004.

Chapter 21

1. Alano, R, McEligot, A, Johnson, S, McMahan, S, Mullapudi, L, and Sassarini, F. The associations between sleep quality and eating patterns in young adults. *FASEB J* 24:lb361, 2010.

2. Alasagheirin, MH, Clark, MK, Ramey, SL, and Grueskin, EF. Body mass index misclassification of obesity among community police officers. *AAOHN J* 59:469-475, 2011.

3. Anderson, GS, Plecas, D, and Segger, T. Police officer physical ability testing—re-validating a selection criterion. *Policing* 24:8-31, 2001.

4. Australian Competition and Consumer Commission. Smokeless tobacco products. 2010. www.productsafety.gov.au/bans/smokeless-tobacco-products.

5. Bastien, M, Poirier, P, Lemieux, I, and Després, J-P. Overview of epidemiology and contribution of obesity to cardiovascular disease. *Prog Cardiovasc Dis* 56:369-381, 2014.

6. Baur, DM, Christophi, CA, and Kales, SN. Metabolic syndrome is inversely related to cardiorespiratory fitness in male career firefighters. *J Strength Cond Res* 26:2331-2337, 2012.

7. Bedno, S, Hauret, K, Loringer, K, Kao, T-C, Mallon, T, and Jones, B. Effects of personal and occupational stress on injuries in a young, physically active population: a survey of military personnel. *Mil Med* 179:1311-1318, 2014.

8. Belloc, NB, and Breslow, L. Relationship of physical health status and health practices. *Prev Med* 1:409-421, 1972.

9. Berry, L, Mirabito, AM, and Baun, WB. What's the hard return on employee wellness programs? *Harvard Bus Rev* December:1-8, 2010.

10. Blehm, C, Vishnu, S, Khattak, A, Mitra, S, and Yee, RW. Computer vision syndrome: a review. *Surv Ophthalmol* 50:253-262, 2005.

11. Bolstad-Johnson, DM, Burgess, JL, Crutchfield, CD, Storment, S, Gerkin, R, and Wilson, JR. Characterization of firefighter exposures during fire overhaul. *Am Ind Hyg Assoc* 61:636-641, 2000.

12. Bowles, SV, Picano, J, Epperly, T, and Myer, S. The LIFE program: a wellness approach to weight loss. *Mil Med* 171:1089-1094, 2006.

13. Bray, RM, Pemberton, MR, Hourani, LL, Witt, M, Olmsted, KL, Brown, JM, Weimer, B, Lance, ME, Marsden, ME, and Scheffler, S. *Department of Defense survey of health-related behaviors among active duty military personnel.* DTIC Document, 2009.

14. Busbin, JW, and Campbell, DP. Employee wellness programs: a strategy for increasing participation. *Market Health Serv* 10:22, 1990.

15. Can, SH, and Hendy, HM. Behavioral variables associated with obesity in police officers. *Ind Health* 52:240-247, 2014.

16. Carey, MG, Al-Zaiti, SS, Dean, GE, Sessanna, L, and Finnell, DS. Sleep problems, depression, substance use, social bonding, and quality of life in professional firefighters. *J Occup Environ Med* 53:928, 2011.

17. Carey, MG, Al-Zaiti, SS, Liao, L, Martin, HN, and Butler, RA. A low-glycemic nutritional fitness program to reverse metabolic syndrome in professional firefighters: results of a pilot study. *J Cardiovasc Nurs* 26:298, 2011.

18. Caux, C, O'Brien, C, and Viau, C. Determination of firefighter exposure to polycyclic aromatic hydrocarbons and benzene during firefighting using measurement of biological indicators. *Appl Occup Env Hyg* 17:379-386, 2002.

19. Cho, S, Dietrich, M, Brown, CJ, Clark, CA, and Block, G. The effect of breakfast type on total daily energy intake and body mass index: results from the Third National Health and Nutrition Examination Survey (NHANES III). *J Am Coll Nutr* 22:296-302, 2003.

20. Christeson, W, Taggart, AD, and Messner-Zidell, S. *Too fat to fight: retired military leaders want junk food out of America's schools. A report by Mission: Readiness.* Washington, DC: Mission: Readiness, Military Leaders for Kids, 2010.

21. D'Este, C, Attia, JR, Brown, AM, Gibson, R, Gibberd, R, Tavener, M, Guest, M, Horsley, K, Harrex, W, and Ross, J. Cancer incidence and mortality in aircraft maintenance workers. *Am J Ind Med* 51:16-23, 2008.

22. Da Silva, FC, Hernandez, SS, Goncalves, E, Arancibia, BA, Da Silva Castro, TL, and Da Silva, R. Anthropometric indicators of obesity in policemen: a systematic review of observational studies. *Int J Occup Med Environ Health* 27:891-901, 2014.

23. Dall, TM, Zhang, Y, Chen, YJ, Askarinam Wagner, RC, Hogan, PF, Fagan, NK, Olaiya, ST, and Tornberg, DN. Cost associated with being overweight and with obesity, high alcohol consumption, and tobacco use within the military health system's TRICARE prime-enrolled population. *Am J Health Promot* 22:120-139, 2007.

24. Daniels, RD, Kubale, TL, Yiin, JH, Dahm, MM, Hales, TR, Baris, D, Zahm, SH, Beaumont, JJ, Waters, KM, and Pinkerton, LE. Mortality and cancer incidence in a pooled cohort of US firefighters from San Francisco, Chicago and Philadelphia (1950–2009). *Occup Environ Med* 71:388-397, 2014.

25. Dawes, J, Elder, C, Hough, L, Melrose, D, and Stierli, M. Description of selected physical performance measures and anthropometric characteristics of part- and full-time special weapons and tactics teams. *J Aust Strength Cond* 21:51-57, 2013.

26. Dawes, J, Orr, R, Brandt, B, Conroy, R, and Pope, R. The effect of age on push-up performance amongst male law enforcement officers. *J Aust Strength Cond*, in press.

27. Dawson, D, and Reid, K. Fatigue, alcohol and performance impairment. *Nature* 388:235-235, 1997.

28. De Bacquer, D, Van Risseghem, M, Clays, E, Kittel, F, De Backer, G, and Braeckman, L. Rotating shift work and the metabolic syndrome: a prospective study. *Int J Epidemiol* 38:848-854, 2009.

29. Defense Health Board. *Implications of trends in obesity and overweight for the Department of Defense. "Fit to fight, fit for life."* Washington, DC: U.S. Department of Defense, 2013.

30. Department of the Army. *Army health promotion: Army regulation 600-63.* Washington, DC: Headquarters, Department of Army, 2015.

31. Dobson, M, Choi, B, Schnall, PL, Wigger, E, Garcia-Rivas, J, Israel, L, and Baker, DB. Exploring occupational and health behavioral causes of firefighter obesity: a qualitative study. *Am J Ind Med* 56:776-790, 2013.

32. Doheny, M, Linden, P, and Sedlak, C. Reducing orthopaedic hazards of the computer work environment. *Orthop Nurs* 14:7-15, 1995.

33. Ehrman, JK, Gordon, P, Visich, PS, and Keteyian, SJ. *Clinical Exercise Physiology.* Champaign, IL: Human Kinetics, 2008.

34. Ekstedt, M, Söderström, M, Åkerstedt, T, Nilsson, J, Søndergaard, H-P, and Aleksander, P. Disturbed sleep and fatigue in occupational burnout. *Scand J Work Env Hea* 32:121-131, 2006.

35. Elliot, DL, Goldberg, L, Kuehl, KS, Moe, EL, Breger, RK, and Pickering, MA. The PHLAME (Promoting Healthy Lifestyles: Alternative Models' Effects) firefighter study: outcomes of two models of behavior change. *J Occup Environ Med* 49:204-213, 2007.

36. Feyer, A. Fatigue: time to recognize and deal with an old problem. *Brit Med J* 322:808-810, 2001.

37. Franke, WD, Ramey, SL, and Shelley, MC. Relationship between cardiovascular disease morbidity, risk factors, and stress in a law enforcement cohort. *J Occup Environ Med* 44:1182-1189, 2002.

38. Fry, MJ, Magazine, MJ, and Rao, US. Firefighter staffing including temporary absences and wastage. *Oper Res* 54:353-365, 2006.

39. Gahm, GA, Swanson, RD, Lucenko, BA, and Reger, MA. History and implementation of the Fort Lewis Soldier Wellness Assessment Program (SWAP). *Mil Med* 174:721-727, 2009.

40. Gershon, RR, Lin, S, and Li, X. Work stress in aging police officers. *J Occup Environ Med* 44:160-167, 2002.

41. Giam, G. Effects of sleep deprivation with reference to military operations. *Ann Acad Med Singap* 26:88, 1997.

42. Gizlice, Z. Health conditions and behaviors among North Carolina and United States military veterans compared to non-veterans. *N C Pub Health: Special Report Series: Study Number* 133:1-7, 2002.

43. Groeger, JA, Zijlstra, F, and Dijk, DJ. Sleep quantity, sleep difficulties and their perceived consequences in a representative sample of some 2000 British adults. *J Sleep Res* 13:359-371, 2004.

44. Gu, MJK, Charles, LE, Burchfiel, CM, Fekedulegn, D, Sarkisian, MK, Andrew, ME, Ma, MC, and Violanti, JM. Long work hours and adiposity among police officers in a US Northeast City. *J Occup Environ Med* 54:1374, 2012.

45. Haddock, CK, Jitnarin, N, Poston, WS, Tuley, B, and Jahnke, SA. Tobacco use among firefighters in the central United States. *Am J Ind Med* 54:697-706, 2011.

46. Hales, T, Jackson, S, and Baldwin, T. *NIOSH alert: preventing fire fighter fatalities due to heart attacks and other sudden cardiovascular events.* Washington, DC: Department of Health and Human Services, Public Health Service, Centers for Disease Control and Prevention, and National Institute for Occupational Safety and Health, 2007-2133, 2007.

47. Härmä, M. Ageing, physical fitness and shiftwork tolerance. *Appl Ergon* 27:25-29, 1996.

48. Harrell, J, Johnston, LF, Griggs, TR, Schaefer, P, Carr Jr, EG, and Raines, BN. An occupation-based physical activity intervention program: improving fitness and decreasing obesity. *Workplace Health Saf* 44:377-384, 1996.

49. Haskell, WL, Lee, I-M, Russell, R, Powell, KE, Blair, SN, Franklin, BA, Macera, CA, Health, GW, Thompson, PD, and Bauman, A. Physical activity and public health: updated recommendation for adults from the American College of Sports Medicine and the American Heart Association. *Med Sci Sports Exerc* 39:1423-1434, 2007.

50. Hayes, JR, Sheedy, JE, Stelmack, JA, and Heaney, CA. Computer use, symptoms, and quality of life. *Optometry Vision Sci* 84:E738-E755, 2007.

51. Joseph, AM, Muggli, M, Pearson, KC, and Lando, H. The cigarette manufacturers' efforts to promote tobacco to the US military. *Mil Med* 170:874-880, 2005.

52. Kales, SN, Soteriades, ES, Christophi, CA, and Christiani, DC. Emergency duties and deaths from heart disease among firefighters in the United States. *New Engl J Med* 356:1207-1215, 2007.

53. Knutsson, A, and Nilsson, T. Tobacco use and exposure to environmental tobacco smoke in relation to certain work characteristics. *Scand J Public Healt* 26:183-189, 1998.

54. Kuehl, H, Mabry, L, Elliot, DL, Kuehl, KS, and Favorite, KC. Factors in adoption of a fire department wellness program: champ and chief model. *J Occup Environ Med* 55:424-429, 2013.

55. Kuehl, K, Elliot, D, Goldberg, L, Moe, E, Perrier, E, and Smith, J. Economic benefit of the PHLAME wellness programme on firefighter injury. *Occup Med* 63:203-209, 2013.

56. Kuehl, KS, Elliot, DL, Goldberg, L, MacKinnon, DP, Vila, BJ, Smith, J, Miocevic, M, O'Rourke, HP, Valente, MJ, and DeFrancesco, C. The safety and health improvement: enhancing law enforcement departments study: feasibility and findings. *Front Pub Health* 2:1-7, 2014.

57. Kuehl, KS, Elliot, DL, MacKinnon, DP, O'Rourke, HP, DeFrancesco, C, Miocevic, M, Valente, M, Sleigh, A, Garg, B, and McGinnis, W. The SHIELD (Safety & Health Improvement: Enhancing Law Enforcement Departments) study: mixed methods longitudinal findings. *J Occup Environ Med* 58:492-498, 2016.

58. Kuhns, JB, Maguire, ER, and Leach, NR. *Health, Safety, and Wellness Program case studies in law enforcement.* Washington, DC: Office of Community Oriented Policing Services, 2015.

59. Kyröläinen, H, Häkkinen, K, Kautiainen, H, Santtila, M, Pihlainen, K, and Häkkinen, A. Physical fitness, BMI and sickness absence in male military personnel. *Occup Med* 58:251-256, 2008.

60. Lindsey, D. Police fatigue: an accident waiting to happen. *FBI Law Enforce Bull* 76:1-6, 2007.

61. Loefstedt, H, Selden, A, Storeus, L, and Bodin, L. Blood lead in Swedish police officers. *Am J Ind Med* 35:519-522, 1999.

62. Lusa, S, Häkkänen, M, Luukkonen, R, and Viikari-Juntura, E. Perceived physical work capacity, stress, sleep disturbance and occupational accidents among firefighters working during a strike. *Work Stress* 16:264-274, 2002.

63. Ma, Y, Bertone, ER, Stanek, EJ, Reed, GW, Hebert, JR, Cohen, NL, Merriam, PA, and Ockene, IS. Association between eating patterns and obesity in a free-living US adult population. *Am J Epidemiol* 158:85-92, 2003.

64. MacDonald, D, Pope, R, and Orr, R. Differences in physical characteristics and performance measures of part-time and fulltime tactical personnel: a critical narrative review. *J Mil Vet Health* 24:45-55, 2016.

65. Marriott, BM. *Not Eating Enough: Overcoming Underconsumption of Military Operational Rations.* Washington, DC: National Academies Press, 1995.

66. McLaughlin, R, and Wittert, G. The obesity epidemic: implications for recruitment and retention of defence force personnel. *Obes Rev* 10:693-699, 2009.

67. Mensah, CE. *Impact of shift work on diet and cardiovascular health of fire-fighters in selected fire stations in the Accra metropolitan area.* University of Ghana, 2013.

68. Montain, SJ, Carvey, CE, and Stephens, MB. Nutritional fitness. *Mil Med* 175:65-72, 2010.

69. Morgan, KJ, Zabik, ME, and Stampley, GL. The role of breakfast in diet adequacy of the US adult population. *J Am Coll Nutr* 5:551-563, 1986.

70. Morimoto, K. Health and lifestyle. *Koshu Eisei* 51:135-143, 1987.

71. Murphy, PJ. *Fatigue Management During Operations: A Commander's Guide.* Puckapunyal, Australia: Doctrine Wing, Land Warfare Development Centre, 2002.

72. National Institute for Occupational Safety and Health (NIOSH). *Fire fighter collapses and dies while assisting with fire suppression efforts at a residential fire.* Ohio: U.S. Department of Health and Human Services, 2005.

73. Obst, PL, Davey, JD, and Sheehan, MC. Does joining the police service drive you to drink? A longitudinal study of the drinking habits of police recruits. *Drugs* 8:347-357, 2001.

74. Orr, R. *The Royal Military College of Duntroon. Physical conditioning optimisation review—project report.* Canberra, Australia: Department of Defence, 2010.

75. Orr, R. *The Royal Military College of Duntroon. Physical conditioning optimisation review—staff health and wellbeing report.* Canberra, Australia: Department of Defence, 2010.

76. Orr, R. The Royal Military College Physical Conditioning Optimisation review: a four-year project to improve physical health and fitness while reducing injuries. Presented at Safety in Action Conference, Melbourne, Australia, 17-19 April, 2012.

77. Orr, R, and Moorby, GM. *The physical conditioning optimisation project—a physical conditioning continuum review of the Army Recruit Training Course.* Canberra, Australia: Department of Defence, 2006.

78. Orr, R, Stierli, M, Amabile, ML, and Wilkes, B. The impact of a structured reconditioning program on the physical attributes and attitudes of injured police officers: a pilot study. *J Aust Strength Cond* 21:42-47, 2013.

79. Palmer, B, Carroll, JW, and Mirza, AT. *A review of firefighter physical fitness/wellness programs: options for the military.* DTIC Document No. CSERIAC-RA-98-003, 1998.

80. Parks, KM, and Steelman, LA. Organizational wellness programs: a meta-analysis. *J Occup Health Psych* 13:58-68, 2008.

81. Peto, J, Matthews, FE, Hodgson, JT, and Jones, JR. Continuing increase in mesothelioma mortality in Britain. *Lancet* 345:535-539, 1995.

82. Plat, M, Frings-Dresen, M, and Sluiter, J. A systematic review of job-specific workers' health surveillance activities for fire-fighting, ambulance, police and military personnel. *Int Arch Occ Env Hea* 84:839-857, 2011.

83. Poirier, P, and Eckel, RH. Obesity and cardiovascular disease. *Curr Atheroscler Rep* 4:448-453, 2002.

84. Polich, JM. Epidemiology of alcohol abuse in military and civilian populations. *Am J Public Health* 71:1125-1132, 1981.

85. Poston, WS, Haddock, C, Jitnarin, N, and Janhke, SA. A national qualitative study of tobacco use among career firefighters and department health personnel. *Nicotine Tob Res* 14:734-741, 2011.

86. Poston, WS, Haddock, CK, Jahnke, SA, Jitnarin, N, Tuley, BC, and Kales, SN. The prevalence of overweight, obesity, and substandard fitness in a population-based firefighter cohort. *J Occup Environ Med* 53:266-273, 2011.

87. Poston, WS, Jitnarin, N, Haddock, CK, Jahnke, SA, and Tuley, BC. Obesity and injury-related absenteeism in a population-based firefighter cohort. *Obesity* 19:2076-2081, 2011.

88. Poston, WS, Jitnarin, N, Haddock, CK, Jahnke, SA, and Tuley, BC. The impact of surveillance on weight change and predictors of change in a population-based firefighter cohort. *J Occup Environ Med* 54:961-968, 2012.

89. Pukkala, E, Martinsen, JI, Weiderpass, E, Kjaerheim, K, Lynge, E, Tryggvadottir, L, Sparén, P, and Demers, PA. Cancer incidence among firefighters: 45 years of follow-up in five Nordic countries. *Occup Environ Med* 43:204-211, 2014.

90. Purvis, DL, Lentino, CV, Jackson, TK, Murphy, KJ, and Deuster, PA. Nutrition as a component of the performance triad: how healthy eating behaviors contribute to soldier performance and military readiness. *US Army Med Dep J* Oct-Dec:66-78, 2013.

91. Rachele, JN, Heesch, KC, and Washington, TL. Wellness programs at firefighter and police workplaces: a systematic review. *Health Behav Policy Rev* 1:302-313, 2014.

92. Rallings, M, Martin, P, and Davey, J. A prospective study of alcohol consumption rates of first-year Australian police officers. *Policing* 28:206-220, 2005.

93. Ramey, SL, Downing, NR, and Franke, WD. Milwaukee police department retirees cardiovascular disease risk and morbidity among aging law enforcement officers. *Workplace Health Saf* 57:448-453, 2009.

94. Ramey, SL, Downing, NR, and Knoblauch, A. Developing strategic interventions to reduce cardiovascular disease risk among law enforcement officers: the art and science of data triangulation. *Workplace Health Saf* 56:54-62, 2008.

95. Ramey, SL, Perkhounkova, Y, Moon, M, Tseng, H-C, Wilson, A, Hein, M, Hood, K, and Franke, WD. Physical activity in police beyond self-report. *J Occup Environ Med* 56:338-343, 2014.

96. Rosekind, MR, Gander, PH, Gregory, KB, Smith, RM, Miller, DL, Oyung, R, Webbon, LL, and Johnson, JM. Managing fatigue in operational settings 1: physiological considerations and countermeasures. *Behav Med* 21:157-165, 1996.

97. Ruscio, B, Smith, J, Amoroso, P, Anslinger, J, Bullock, S, Burnham, B, Campbell, J, Chervak, M, Garbow, K, and Garver, R. *DoD Military Injury Prevention Priorities Working Group: leading injuries, causes and mitigation recommendations*. DTIC Document, 2006.

98. Ruxton, C, and Kirk, T. Breakfast: a review of associations with measures of dietary intake, physiology and biochemistry. *Brit J Nutr* 78:199-213, 1997.

99. Santulli, G. Epidemiology of cardiovascular disease in the 21st century: updated numbers and updated facts. *J Cardiovascular Dis* 1:1-2, 2013.

100. Smith, AP. Breakfast and mental health. *Int J Food Sci Nutr* 49:397-402, 1998.

101. Smith, B, Ryan, MA, Wingard, DL, Patterson, TL, Slymen, DJ, Macera, CA, and Team, MCS. Cigarette smoking and military deployment: a prospective evaluation. *Am J Prev Med* 35:539-546, 2008.

102. Smith, EA, Poston, WS, Haddock, CK, and Malone, RE. Installation tobacco control programs in the US military. *Mil Med* 181:596-601, 2016.

103. Smith, TJ, Marriott, BP, Dotson, L, Bathalon, GP, Funderburk, L, White, A, Hadden, L, and Young, AJ. Overweight and obesity in military personnel: sociodemographic predictors. *Obesity* 20:1534-1538, 2012.

104. Sörensen, L, Smolander, J, Louhevaara, V, Korhonen, O, and Oja, P. Physical activity, fitness and body composition of Finnish police officers: a 15-year follow-up study. *Occup Med* 50:3-10, 2000.

105. Soteriades, ES, Hauser, R, Kawachi, I, Liarokapis, D, Christiani, DC, and Kales, SN. Obesity and cardiovascular disease risk factors in firefighters: a prospective cohort study. *Obesity Res* 13:1756-1763, 2005.

106. Soteriades, ES, Smith, DL, Tsismenakis, AJ, Baur, DM, and Kales, SN. Cardiovascular disease in US firefighters: a systematic review. *Cardiol Rev* 19:202-215, 2011.

107. Steinhardt, M, Greenhow, L, and Stewart, J. The relationship of physical activity and cardiovascular fitness to absenteeism and medical care claims among law enforcement officers. *Am J Health Promot* 5:455-460, 1991.

108. Thayyil, J, Jayakrishnan, TT, Raja, M, and Cherumanalil, JM. Metabolic syndrome and other cardiovascular risk factors among police officers. *North Am J Med Sci* 4:630-635, 2012.

109. Thomas, DQ, Lumpp, SA, Schreiber, JA, and Keith, JA. Physical fitness profile of Army ROTC cadets. *J Strength Cond Res* 18:904-907, 2004.

110. Tsismenakis, AJ, Christophi, CA, Burress, JW, Kinney, AM, Kim, M, and Kales, SN. The obesity epidemic and future emergency responders. *Obesity* 17:1648-1650, 2009.

111. Van Dongen, HP, Maislin, G, Mullington, JM, and Dinges, DF. The cumulative cost of additional wakefulness: dose–response effects on neurobehavioral functions and sleep physiology from chronic sleep restriction and total sleep deprivation. *Sleep* 26:117-129, 2003.

112. Violanti, JM, Burchfiel, CM, Miller, DB, Andrew, ME, Dorn, J, Wactawski-Wende, J, Beighley, CM, Pierino, K, Joseph, PN, and Vena, JE. The Buffalo Cardio-Metabolic Occupational Police Stress (BCOPS) pilot study: methods and participant characteristics. *Ann Epidemiol* 16:148-156, 2006.

113. Violanti, JM, Hartley, TA, Gu, JK, Fekedulegn, D, Andrew, ME, and Burchfiel, CM. Life expectancy in police officers: a comparison with the US general population. *Int J Emerg Mental Hlth* 15:217, 2013.

114. Wada, T, Fukumoto, T, Ito, K, Hasegawa, Y, and Osaki, T. Relationship between the three kinds of healthy habits and the metabolic syndrome. *Obes Res Clin Pract* 3:123-132, 2009.

115. Whiteman, JA, Snyder, DA, and Ragland, JJ. The value of leadership in implementing and maintaining a successful health promotion program in the Naval Surface Force, US Pacific Fleet. *Am J Health Promot* 15:437-440, 2001.

116. World Health Organization (WHO). *Fact sheet N°311: obesity and overweight.* Geneva: WHO, 2015.

117. Zhu, K, Devesa, SS, Wu, H, Zahm, SH, Jatoi, I, Anderson, WF, Peoples, GE, Maxwell, LG, Granger, E, and Potter, JF. Cancer incidence in the US military population: comparison with rates from the SEER program. *Cancer Epidem Biomar* 18:1740-1745, 2009.

Chapter 22

1. Americans with Disabilities Act of 1990, Pub L No. 101-336, 104 Stat 328, 1990.

2. Balady, GJ, Chaitman, B, Driscoll, D, Foster, C, Froelicher, E, Gordon, N, Pate, R, Rippe, J, and Bazzarre, T. AHA/ACSM joint position statement: recommendations for cardiovascular screening, staffing, and emergency policies at health/fitness facilities. *Med Sci Sports Exerc* 30:1009-1018, 1998.

3. Baley, J, and Matthews, D. *Law and Liability in Athletics, Physical Education and Recreation.* Boston: Allyn and Bacon, 1984.

4. Department of the U.S. Air Force. Air Force Handbook 32-1084, facility requirements. https://wbdg.org/ccb/AF/AFH/ARCHIVES/32_1084.pdf, 228. Accessed April 12, 2015.

5. Department of the U.S. Army. Revised Army standard for Physical Fitness Facilities (PFF). https://mrsi.usace.army.mil/fdt/Army%20Standards/Physical%20Fitness%20Facility.pdf. Accessed April 23, 2015.

6. Eickhoff-Shemek, J. Standards of practice. In *Law for Recreation and Sport Managers.* 2nd ed. Cotton, D, Wilde, J, and Wlohan, J, eds. Dubuque, IA: Kendall/Hunt, 293-294, 2001.

7. Hurdy, A. Facility design, layout, and organization. In *Essentials of Strength Training and Conditioning.* 4th ed. Haff, G, and Triplett, T, eds. Champaign, IL: Human Kinetics, 623-640, 2016.

8. International Association of Chiefs of Police (IACP). Police facility planning guideline: a desk reference for law enforcement executives. Alexandria, VA, 2012.

9. Kelly, TK, Masi, R, Walker, B, Knapp, S, and Leuschner, KJ. *Technical report—an assessment of the Army's tactical human optimization, rapid rehabilitation and reconditioning program.* Santa Monica, CA: Rand Corporation, 1-3, 23-27, 41-43, 63-64, 2013.

10. Kroll, B. Structural and functional considerations in designing the facility, part 1. *NSCA J* 13(1):51-58. 1991.

11. National Fire Protection Agency (NFPA). *NFPA 1500: Standard on Fire Department Occupational Safety and Health Program.* Quincy, MA, 2013.

12. National Fire Protection Agency (NFPA). *NFPA 1581: Standard on Fire Department Infection Control Program.* Quincy, MA, 2013.

13. National Fire Protection Agency (NFPA). *NFPA 1582: Standard on Comprehensive Occupational Medical Program for Fire Departments.* Quincy, MA, 2013.

14. National Fire Protection Agency (NFPA). *NFPA 1583: Standard on Health-Related Programs for Fire Department Members.* Quincy, MA, 2013.

15. NetMBA Business Knowledge Center. Strategic management—SWOT analysis. www.netmba.com. Accessed May 14, 2015.

16. Takahashi, S. Facility and equipment layout and maintenance. In *NSCA's Essentials of Personal Training.* 2nd ed. Champaign, IL: Human Kinetics, 603-622, 2012.

17. Tharrett, SJ, McInnis, KJ, and Peterson, JA. *ACSM's Health/Fitness Facility Standards and Guidelines.* 3rd ed. Champaign, IL: Human Kinetics, 142-143, 2007.

18. Training Program Services Bureau. Guidelines for student safety in certified courses. Sacramento, CA, 2007.

19. Triplett, T, Williams, C, and McHenry, P. National Strength and Conditioning Association's position paper. Strength and conditioning professional standards and guidelines. 2009. www.nsca.com/uploadedFiles/NSCA/Resources/PDF/Education/Tools_and_Resources/NSCA_strength_and_conditioning_professional_standards_and_guidelines.pdf. Accessed July 25, 2015.

20. United States Access Board. Chapter 9: exercise equipment, bowling lanes, and shooting facilities. www.access-board.gov/guidelines-and-standards/recreation-facilities/backgroundregulatory-assessment/chapter-9-exercise-equipment,-bowling-lanes,-and-shooting-facilities. Accessed June 2, 2015.

21. U.S. Air Force. Air Force services facility design guide—design: fitness centers. 2005. https://wbdg.org/ccb/AF/AFDG/ARCHIVES/fitguide.pdf. Accessed June 2, 2015.

22. U.S. Department of Defense (DoD). Air Force fitness centers. FC 4-740-02F w/Change 1. www.wbdg.org/ccb/DOD/UFC/fc_4_740_02f.pdf. Accessed April 12, 2015.

23. U.S. Department of Defense (DoD). Department of Defense Instruction 1015.10—Military Morale, Welfare, and Recreation (MWR) programs. 2006. www.dtic.mil/whs/directives/corres/pdf/101510p.pdf. Accessed March 19, 2015.

24. U.S. Department of Defense (DoD). Department of Defense Morale, Welfare, and Recreation physical fitness center standards. 2005. http://download.militaryonesource.mil/12038/MOS/MWR/DoD-MWR-Physical-Fitness-Center-Standards.pdf. Accessed April 12, 2015.

25. U.S. Department of Defense (DoD). Navy and Marine Corp fitness centers. FC 4-740-02N. www.wbdg.org/ccb/DOD/UFC/fc_4_740_02n.pdf. 2014. Accessed April 23, 2015.

26. U.S. Department of Defense (DoD). Department of Defense standard practice—standard practice for Unified Facilities Criteria and unified facilities guide specifications. 2006. www.wbdg.org/ccb/FEDMIL/std3007f.pdf. Accessed April 23, 2015.

Index

About the Editors

Brent A. Alvar, PhD, CSCS,*D, RSCC*D, FNSCA, is the vice president of university research and the concentration track director for Human & Sport Performance at Rocky Mountain University of Health Professions. He is a certified strength and conditioning specialist with distinction, registered

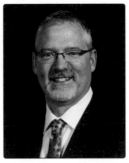

Photo courtesy of NSCA

strength and conditioning coach with distinction, and a fellow of the NSCA. Alvar was named the NSCA's Educator of the Year in 2016 and is a past member of the NSCA Board of Directors.

At Rocky Mountain University, Alvar served as the director and associate dean of university research and the codirector of the graduate program in health promotion and wellness. Alvar also served as the sport performance director and faculty member at Chandler Gilbert Community College while simultaneously having an appointment as an assistant research professor in the department of exercise and wellness at Arizona State University, where he earned his bachelor's, master's, and doctoral degrees.

Katie Sell, PhD, CSCS,*D, TSAC-F, is an associate professor and coordinator of the undergraduate exercise science program in the department of health professions at Hofstra University. Her NSCA certifications include being a certified strength and conditioning specialist with distinction and a tactical

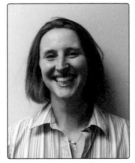

© Katie Sell

strength and conditioning facilitator. She is also an exercise physiologist certified with the American College of Sports Medicine (ACSM).

Sell has been a volunteer assistant coach for the Hofstra women's tennis program, a member of the NSCA Tactical Strength and Conditioning Special Interest Group Executive Council, and a consultant to FireFit, which is an interagency wildland firefighter fitness task group. She serves as a physical fitness standards and programming consultant with various professional firefighting departments in the Salt Lake City, Utah, region.

Sell's primary research interests are in the areas of physical activity promotion among college students and firefighter health, physical fitness, and exercise programming. She received her doctoral degree from the University of Utah, her master's degree from Southern Illinois University, and her bachelor's degree from the University of Tennessee at Martin.

Patricia A. Deuster, PhD, MPH, CNS, is a professor in the department of military and emergency medicine at the Uniformed Services University of the Health Sciences (USU) and director of the Consortium for Health and Military Performance (CHAMP), the Defense Center of Excellence in the area of human

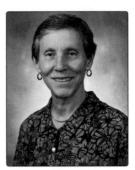

Photo courtesy of NSCA

performance optimization. A certified nutrition specialist and fellow of the American College of Sports Medicine (ACSM), Deuster is a coauthor of *The Navy SEAL Nutrition Guide* and *The Special Operations Forces Nutrition Guide* and the editor of *The Navy SEAL Physical Fitness Guide.*

Deuster received the Special Operations Medical Researcher Award in 2014 by the Special Operations Medical Association. She is a member of the Order of Military Medical Merit and has served the Department of Defense on its Dietary Supplement Subcommittee, Food and Nutrition Subcommittee, Human Performance Optimization Committee, Population Health Working Group, and Operational Supplement Safety Initiative.

Deuster received her bachelor's and master's degrees from the College of William and Mary, her PhD from the University of Maryland, and her MPH from USU. Among her athletic achievements, she has been a tennis professional, nationally ranked marathoner, and qualifier for the first women's marathon Olympic Trials in 1984.

Contributors

Mark Abel, PhD, CSCS,*D, TSAC-F,*D
University of Kentucky, Lexington

Brent A. Alvar, PhD, CSCS,*D, RSCC*D, FNSCA
Rocky Mountain University of Health
Professions, Provo, UT

Mike Barnes, MEd, CSCS, NSCA-CPT
Infinity Personal Training and Fitness, Colorado
Springs, CO

Maj. Nicholas D. Barringer, RD, CSCS,*D, CSSD
Baylor University Graduate Program in Nutrition,
U.S. Army Medical Department Center & School,
Fort Sam Houston, TX

John R. Bennett, MS, CSCS, EMT-P
Florida Firefighter Fitness Collaborative,
Seminole County Fire Department, Orlando, FL

Amanda Carlson-Phillips, MS, RD, CSSD
EXOS, Phoenix, AZ

Maj. Aaron P. Crombie, PhD, RD
Baylor University Graduate Program in Nutrition,
U.S. Army Medical Department Center and
School, Fort Sam Houston, TX

Jay Dawes, PhD, CSCS,*D, NSCA-CPT,*D, FNSCA
University of Colorado, Colorado Springs

Michael R. Deschenes, PhD
College of William & Mary, Williamsburg, VA

Patricia A. Deuster, PhD, MPH, CNS
Consortium for Health and Military Performance
(CHAMP), Uniformed Services University of the
Health Sciences, Bethesda, MD

Daniel J. Dodd, PhD, CSCS
Rocky Mountain University of Health
Professions, Provo, UT

Joseph Domitrovich, PhD
Forest Service National Technology and
Development Program, Missoula, Montana

Jason Dudley, MS, CSCS,*D, TSAC-F*D
Central Washington University, Ellensburg, WA

LTC. David Feltwell, PT, OCS, TSAC-F
Center for Initial Military Training, Fort Eustis,
VA

Patrick Gagnon, MS
Canadian Forces Morale and Welfare Services,
Ottawa, Ontario, Canada

G. Gregory Haff, PhD, CSCS,*D, FNSCA
Edith Cowan University, Western Australia

Paul C. Henning, PhD, CSCS
U.S. Army Research Institute of Environmental
Medicine (USARIEM), Natick, MA

Steve Hertzler, PhD, RD, LD
EAS Sports Nutrition/Abbott Nutrition,
Columbus, OH

Ben Hinton, MSc, CSCS
Health and Fitness Unit, NSW Police Force,
Sydney, Australia

John Hofman, Jr., MS, CSCS
911 Tactical Performance, Folsom, CA

Suzanne Jaenen, MS
National Defence Headquarters, Ottawa, Ontario,
Canada

William Kraemer, PhD, CSCS,*D, FNSCA
The Ohio State University, Columbus, OH

Raymond W. McCoy, PhD
College of William & Mary, Williamsburg, VA

Danny McMillian, PT, DSc, OCS, CSCS, TSAC-F
University of Puget Sound, Tacoma, WA

Todd Miller, PhD, CSCS,*D, TSAC-F, FNSCA
George Washington University, Milken Institute
School of Public Health, Washington, DC

Bradley C. Nindl, PhD
University of Pittsburgh, Pittsburgh, PA

Robin Orr, PhD, MPhty, BFET, TSAC-F
Bond University, Queensland, Australia

Frank A. Palkoska, MS, CSCS
U.S. Army Physical Fitness School (USAPFS),
Fort Jackson, SC

Nicholas A. Ratamess, PhD, CSCS,*D, FNSCA
The College of New Jersey, Ewing, NJ

Matthew R. Rhea, PhD, CSCS,*D
A.T. Still University, Kirksville, MO

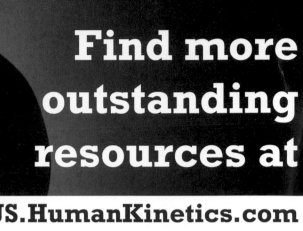
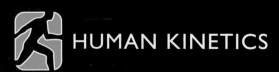

Sarah E. Sauers, MS, CSCS
U.S. Army Research Institute of Environmental
Medicine (USARIEM), Natick, MA

Brad Schoenfeld, PhD, CSCS, NSCA-CPT, FNSCA
Lehman College, Bronx, NY

Dennis E. Scofield, MEd, CSCS,*D
U.S. Army Research Institute of Environmental
Medicine (USARIEM), Natick, MA

Katie Sell, PhD, CSCS,*D, TSAC-F
Hofstra University, Hempstead, NY

Marilyn A. Sharp, MS
U.S. Army Research Institute of Environmental
Medicine (USARIEM), Natick, MA

Denise Smith, PhD
First Responder Health and Safety Laboratory,
Skidmore College, Saratoga Springs, NY

Abbie E. Smith-Ryan, PhD, CSCS,*D, FNSCA, FISSN
University of North Carolina, Chapel Hill

Barry A. Spiering, PhD, CSCS
Nike Sport Research Lab, Beaverton, OR

Mark Stephenson, MS, ATC, CSCS,*D, TSAC-F
Human Performance Program, Department of
Defense

Sgt. Mick Stierli, BPhysEd, MExSc, CSCS,*D, TSAC-F,*D
New South Wales Police Force, Sydney, Australia

Tunde Szivak, PhD, CSCS
The Ohio State University, Columbus, OH

Eric T. Trexler, MA, CSCS, CISSN
University of North Carolina, Chapel Hill

Maj. Bradley J. Warr, PhD, MPAS, CSCS
U.S. Army Research Institute of Environmental
Medicine (USARIEM), Natick, MA

Colin D. Wilborn, PhD, CSCS, ATC
University of Mary Hardin–Baylor, Belton, TX